PHARMACOLOGY ESSENTIALS

PHARMACOLOGY ESSENTIALS

Jody A. Lambright Eckler, RN, BSN

Co-Director
Phoenix Health and Education Services
Castalia, Ohio

Public Health Nurse, Tuberculosis
  Coordinator, School Nurse
Huron County Health Department
Norwalk, Ohio

Formerly, Instructor
Sandusky School of Practical Nursing
Sandusky, Ohio

Judy M. Stimmel Fair, RN, MEd

Co-Director
Phoenix Health and Education Services
Port Clinton, Ohio

Public Health Nurse,
Erie County General Health District
  Service Coordinator
Erie County Early Intervention
  Collaborative
Sandusky, Ohio

Formerly, Instructor
Sandusky School of Practical Nursing
Sandusky, Ohio

W.B. SAUNDERS COMPANY

A Harcourt Health Sciences Company

Philadelphia   London   New York   St. Louis   Montreal   Sydney   Toronto

W.B. SAUNDERS COMPANY
A Harcourt Health Sciences Company

The Curtis Center
Independence Square West
Philadelphia, Pennsylvania 19106

Library of Congress Cataloging-in-Publication Data

Eckler, Jody A. Lambright.
   Pharmacology essentials / Jody A. Lambright Eckler, Judy M.
Stimmel Fair.

      p.   cm.
   Includes bibliographical references.

   ISBN 0–7216–6486–5

   1. Pharmacology.   2. Drugs—Administration.   3. Nursing.
I. Fair, Judy M. Stimmel.   II. Title.
   [DNLM: 1. Drug Therapy—nurses' instruction.   2. Pharmacology—
nurses' instruction.   3. Drugs—nurses' instruction.   QV 55 E19p
1996]

RM300.E345   1996   615'.1—dc20

DNLM/DLC   95-19853

Pharmacology Essentials, 1st edition   ISBN 0–7216–6486–5

Printed in the United States of America

Last digit is the print number: 9   8   7   6   5

To my mother, Ruth M. Lambright, who believed in me and encouraged me to write. I wish you could have seen this, mom.

To my father, D. Garth Lambright, who taught me that girls can do anything that boys can do. Thanks, dad.

To my son, Phillip J. Eckler, who put up with hours that mom spent in front of the computer instead of with him.

But most of all to my husband, my hero, Gary A. Eckler, who made sure that everything ran like clockwork around the house while I wrote.

Thank you, thank you, thank God for you, the winds beneath my wings.

—JODY

To Roger, for providing me with physical and emotional sustenance while keeping me "chained" to the computer.

To Susan and Julianne, for your understanding and assistance through your graduation and weddings.

To mom (and dad), for never letting me say "I can't."

To Jody, for remaining my friend and partner.

To all of my nursing colleagues and all of my former students, because you each have had something to teach me.

—JUDY

ACKNOWLEDGMENTS

The authors wish to express special thanks to Ilze S. Rader, who saw the value of our book and enabled us to share our approach to the teaching of pharmacology with a whole new audience of nursing students. Special thanks to Lee Henderson for his expert guidance in the development of the entire manuscript. Thanks, also, to Roger W. Fair for helping with photography; Phillip J. Eckler and Ruth M. Lambright for agreeing to be models; Marie Thomas for fielding our numerous questions and for her careful organization; Denise Black Gold for helping with the final development of the text and illustrations; David Harvey and RoseMarie Klimowicz for their meticulous copy editing; Michael Carcel for smoothly managing the production of the book so that it ran on schedule from beginning to end; Gene Harris for his innovation and flexibility in creating and refining the book's graphic design; Karen M. Giacomucci for coordinating the drawing of the book's illustrations; Theodore G. Huff and Wieslawa B. Langenfeld for creating such instructive illustrations from our rough sketches; Lisa Lambert for sizing the illustrations and preparing them for the printer; and Maura Connor for her innovative ideas for marketing the finished book.

REVIEWERS

Nancy K. Brown, BSN, RN
Practical Nursing Department
Heart of the Ozarks Community Technical College
Springfield, Missouri

Donna Cartwright, MS, RN, NP
School of Practical Nursing
College of Eastern Utah
Price, Utah

Eileen J. Colon, BSN, RN
School of Practical Nursing
Isothermal Community College
Spindale, North Carolina

Michelle L. Dumpe, MSN, RN
School of Practical Nursing
Venango County Area Vocational-Technical School
Oil City, Pennsylvania

Margaret A. Frandina, BSN, MEd, RN
School of Practical Nursing
Buffalo Vocational-Technical Center
Buffalo, New York

Theresa M. Giudici, RN
Choffin School of Practical Nursing
Youngstown, Ohio

Joyce Harris, RN, MA
Butler County Program of Practical Nurse
Education
Hamilton, Ohio

Patricia M. Jacobson, MSN, RN
School of Practical Nursing
Bullard Havens Regional Vocational-Technical
School
Bridgeport, Connecticut

Kathleen Jesiolowski, BSN, RN
School of Practical Nursing
Lebanon County Area Vocational-Technical School
Lebanon, Pennsylvania

Yvonne B. Meinket, RN, BS, MEd
Health Occupations Program
Charlotte Vocational-Technical Center
Port Charlotte, Florida

Margaret B. Ogle, BSN, RN
School of Practical Nursing
Greenville Technical College
Greenville, South Carolina

Sally J. O'Neil, BSN, MSEd, RN
School of Practical Nursing
W.F. Kaynor Regional Vocational-Technical School
Waterbury, Connecticut

Judith M. Pelletier, RN, BSN
School of Practical Nursing
Massachusetts Bay Community College
Framingham, Massachusetts

Mary A. Sweeney, MSN, RN, C
Vocational Nursing Program
Amarillo College
Amarillo, Texas

T. Jan Woods, RN, MSN, CEN
Practical Nursing Program
Medical College of Georgia
Augusta, Georgia

TO THE STUDENT

Welcome to the study of pharmacology! *Pharmacology Essentials* is a unique textbook written specifically for nursing students and others preparing for careers in the health professions. We wrote it specifically for those of you who find pharmacology confusing or frustrating and for those of you who just plain hate it! In this text, we focus on presenting the essentials of pharmacology clearly and concisely to help you understand and remember this important content. We hope that *Pharmacology Essentials* will help make your course of study in pharmacology both interesting and memorable.

HOW WE ORGANIZED THE BOOK

Pharmacology Essentials is organized from general to specific. Units I and II contain basic information about pharmacology. In Unit III, we discuss the problem of drug abuse. In Units IV and V, we discuss drugs that affect microorganisms and those that affect neoplasms. In Units VI through XIV, we give an overview of each body system, then present the drug classifications that act on each of them.

In those chapters covering drug classifications (Chapters 13 to 70), the discussion begins with general information about the classification, usually arranged under these headings:

Actions and Uses

Assessment

Planning and Implementation

Evaluation

When subclassifications or specific drugs within the classification differ from the general classification, we then discuss those differences, using the same four headings where appropriate.

LEARNING AIDS THAT WE'VE PROVIDED

To help you better understand the pharmacology content, we have included five types of learning aids:

Learning Objectives

Introductory drug lists entitled Drugs You Will Learn About in This Chapter

Nursing Alerts

Drug Administration Guidelines

Exercises

Learning Objectives appear at the start of every chapter in the book. Use the Learning Objectives to determine, before reading a chapter, the most important information that you should obtain from your reading. (You might also find it helpful to return to the Learning Objectives after you have finished a chapter, to evaluate your level of understanding of what you have read.)

Beginning with Chapter 19, each chapter includes a drug list entitled Drugs You Will Learn About in This Chapter. This list, found right after the Learning Objectives, introduces you to the drugs that the chapter will cover. It is not an all-inclusive list of drugs in a particular classification; instead, the list serves as an "advance organizer" to help you mentally categorize the drug information that you will read in a chapter.

Throughout the book, we have also included Nursing Alerts. Nursing Alerts highlight information that is critical to the safe administration of medications.

In Unit II, we include boxed highlights entitled Drug Administration Guidelines. Drug Administration Guidelines provide step-by-step instructions to guide you safely through the administration of various types of medications by different routes.

At the end of each chapter, you will find one or more Exercises. These Exercises fall into three categories:

Case Studies

Mental Aerobics

Learning Activities

Case Studies typically present brief patient scenarios and ask you to apply information that you have learned in the chapter to address them. Mental Aerobics challenge you to apply chapter content in such a way as to strengthen your ability to solve problems in pharmacology. Learning Activities include assignments, directed research, role playing, games, surveys, and even poetry; we have created these activities to reinforce or expand your knowledge of the chapter's content.

Pharmacology Essentials also includes an array of figures, tables, and boxes to highlight and clarify important information. In addition, we define important new terms where we first use them in the text, and we include those same terms and definitions in a Glossary at the end of the book.

As an additional learning aid, we have also written the *Student Study Guide to Accompany Eckler and Fair's Pharmacology Essentials.* In it, you will find exercises, a variety of different types of questions, activities, and even games to help you identify important information and lock it into your memory. The *Student Study Guide* also includes tear-out versions of the Drug Administration Guidelines from the textbook. Use these tear-out Guidelines to check yourself and your classmates on your mastery of drug administration techniques.

STUDY TIPS

Students often complain that pharmacology is a difficult subject, and it *can* be. Invariably, those students who find pharmacology difficult are those who try to *memorize* information about individual drugs rather than *use drug classifications* to focus their studies.

Study Tip 1: *Learn first about each drug classification, then about each drug.* If you learn the basic information about a classification, you have already learned the same information about all of the drugs in that classification! After that, all you need to learn about each specific drug is the ways in which it differs from the classification.

Study Tip 2: *Never cram for this course.* If you cram, you will quickly become confused and overwhelmed. Instead, review the Learning Objectives and Drugs You Will Learn About in This Chapter. Then read the chapter. Next, reread the chapter and highlight or underline important points. Then, review the Learning Objectives again to evaluate your level of learning. Next, complete the Exercises at the end of the chapter. Finally, just before taking a test, review the information that you highlighted and any additional notes you may have taken.

If you follow these tips, you should be able to complete your pharmacology course successfully. More important, however, you will retain the information not just long enough to ace your tests but for the long term—for the state boards and beyond. Best wishes for a successful pharmacology course!

JODY A. LAMBRIGHT ECKLER, RN, BSN
JUDY M. STIMMEL FAIR, RN, MEd

TO THE INSTRUCTOR

Our goal in writing *Pharmacology Essentials* is to present basic information about pharmacology in such a manner as to facilitate learning and promote the student's success in safely administering medications.

BASIC THEMES

There are several important themes to the book. First, we present general knowledge before specific knowledge. Second, we use a drug classification approach to teaching pharmacology. Third, we *apply* information on pharmacological actions to the care of patients. Fourth, throughout the book, we encourage learners to build on knowledge that they have acquired previously. Finally, from beginning to end, we emphasize the responsibility of nurses in educating patients and caregivers about prescribed medications. We encourage students to see that they are learning not just a collection of facts, but information that is vital to the patient's safety.

HOW THE BOOK IS STRUCTURED

Pharmacology Essentials is divided into 14 units. We have written the text in such a way as to enable you to follow your own sequence in teaching the content. After the first two units, you can present units—and even chapters—in any order.

Unit I contains basic information that is important for orienting learners to the use of medications in holistic patient care. Among other topics, it includes the legislation for the manufacture and testing of medications, for truth in the marketing of medications, and for the distribution, preparation, and administration of medications. It also describes basic formulas, the primary systems used for the measurement of drugs, the methods of converting from one measurement system to another, and the methods of dosage calculation; this coverage eliminates the need for a separate mathematics course and textbook.

In Unit II, we help the learner relate the steps of the nursing process to medication administration. We also present techniques of safe medication administration in an orderly, step-by-step fashion, highlighting these techniques in special Drug Administration Guidelines. Of particular note, the unit includes intravenous therapy techniques (Chapter 9), because many states in the United States have proposed or enacted legislation permitting Licensed Practical Nurses, Licensed Vocational Nurses, and paramedics to start, monitor, and discontinue some intravenous medications. The unit concludes with a chapter covering differences in the ways in which pediatric and geriatric patients accept and metabolize medications. This chapter also describes the modifications in technique necessary for safe drug administration to pediatric and geriatric patients.

Unit III deals with drug abuse, including differences in drug tolerance and the factors affecting habituation, dependency, and withdrawal. In this unit, we also emphasize the hazards of the misuse of medications.

Unit IV covers drugs that affect microorganisms. We present this content early in the book for two reasons. First, microorganisms affect every body system. Second, many learners are already somewhat familiar with the drugs used to prevent or treat infections, and their inclusion early in the book instills a sense of confidence in students that they *can* learn pharmacology.

Unit V presents drugs that affect neoplasms. Again, we cover this content early in the book because neoplasms involve all body systems. We include radiation therapy (Chapter 26) in this unit because even though nurses do not administer radioactive substances or insert radioactive implants or other devices for radiation delivery, they often attend or assist with these procedures. Also, nurses are responsible for the care of patients during their treatment with radioactive elements and are responsible for the safety of people who may be exposed to the radiation.

In Units VI through XIV, we cover the drug classifications that affect particular body systems. Each of these units begins with a brief review of anatomy and physiology related to the drug classifications in the unit. In the chapters that follow, we present the specific drug classifications that affect the body system.

HOW THE CHAPTERS ARE STRUCTURED

To help learners focus on the information to be absorbed, each chapter in the book begins with Learning Objectives. Beginning with Chapter 19, each chapter also includes a drug list entitled Drugs You Will Learn About in This Chapter. Together, these pedagogical aids serve as "advance organizers" to help students anticipate and categorize the important information that they will read in the chapter.

In those chapters covering drug classifications (Chapters 13 to 70), the discussion begins with general information about the classification, usually arranged under these headings:

Actions and Uses

Assessment

Planning and Implementation

Evaluation

When subclassifications or specific drugs within the classification differ from the general classification, we then discuss those differences, using the same four headings where appropriate.

At the end of each chapter, we provide one or more Exercises. These Exercises fall into three categories:

Case Studies

Mental Aerobics

Learning Activities

Case Studies typically present brief patient scenarios and ask students to apply information that they have just learned in the chapter to address them. Mental Aerobics challenge students to apply chapter content in such a way as to strengthen their ability to solve problems in pharmacology. Learning Activities include assignments, directed research, role playing, games, surveys, and even poetry; we have created these activities to reinforce or expand the student's knowledge of the chapter's content.

Throughout the book, we also include Nursing Alerts. Nursing Alerts highlight information that is critical to the safe administration of medications.

In Unit II, we include boxed highlights entitled Drug Administration Guidelines. Drug Administration Guidelines provide step-by-step instructions to guide students safely through the administration of various types of medications by different routes.

Pharmacology Essentials also includes an array of figures, tables, and boxes to highlight and clarify important information. In addition, we define important new terms where we first use them in the text, and we include those same terms and definitions in a Glossary at the end of the book. Where applicable, we have provided cross-references to help you and your students locate related content.

COMPANION PUBLICATIONS

Two companion publications are available to accompany *Pharmacology Essentials:* a *Student Study Guide* and an *Instructor's Manual.*

In the *Student Study Guide to Accompany Eckler and Fair's Pharmacology Essentials,* we use a variety of exercises, different types of questions, activities, and games to help students identify and retain important information. Answers are included to provide positive reinforcement or to indicate the need for review or assistance. The *Student Study Guide* also includes tear-out versions of the Drug Administration Guidelines from the textbook. Students can use these tear-out Guidelines to check themselves or one another on their mastery of drug administration techniques. You can also use them in grading students on their drug administration techniques.

The *Instructor's Manual to Accompany Eckler and Fair's Pharmacology Essentials* provides related test questions and answers to accompany each chapter of the text. For the new instructor, this resource eliminates the need to create an entire bank of test questions. For the seasoned educator, it will serve as a source of new test questions for supplementing or updating existing test banks.

We believe that *Pharmacology Essentials* and its companion publications are unique resources for teaching basic pharmacology. It is our hope that they will facilitate learning and promote the success of your students in the safe administration of medications.

JODY A. LAMBRIGHT ECKLER, RN, BSN
JUDY M. STIMMEL FAIR, RN, MEd

CONTENTS

UNIT ONE

INTRODUCTION TO PHARMACOLOGY

There are many ways to treat a person with a disease or illness. The different approaches are referred to as therapeutic methods. Successful treatment of a person usually requires a combination of methods. A few examples of therapeutic methods are

1. Drug therapy: treatment with medicinal drugs.
2. Diet therapy: encouraging the consumption or the avoidance of certain foods.
3. Physiotherapy: treatment with natural physical forces, such as heat, light, water, or exercise.
4. Psychotherapy: use of mental processes, such as knowledge and understanding, suggestion, analysis, or hypnosis, to treat medical problems.

You will be using this text to assist you in your study of treatment with drugs. This subject is called *pharmacology*. Pharmacology is a science that deals with the study of chemicals and their preparations, actions, and effects on living tissues.

Drugs are chemical substances that exert an effect on living tissues. The effect may be good or bad. The drugs a physician prescribes for their effect on a person with a disease or illness are often referred to as medicines or prescriptions. To obtain these drugs, a person must contact a physician or other professional licensed to write prescriptions, such as a physician's assistant, nurse practitioner, or chiropractor. The prescription must then be taken to a pharmacy, where a specially licensed person, a *pharmacist,* dispenses the product. Other drugs do not require a prescription for purchase and consumption. These are referred to as patent medicines, nonprescription drugs, or over-the-counter drugs. These are displayed on shelves at the local drugstore, grocery, or carry-out.

Other chemicals that we often fail to recognize as drugs are the nicotine in cigarettes and the alcohol sold for social or recreational consumption. These are sometimes referred to as social drugs.

Some drugs, such as heroin, are illegal to possess at any time. Other drugs are legal to possess, but individuals may be abusing them or using them for illegal purposes. Some examples are narcotic pain relievers, such as morphine; tranquilizers, such as diazepam (Valium); sleeping pills, such as haloperidol (Haldol); and other types of drugs.

Poisons are also chemicals that have an effect on living tissues. Other chemicals are often required to counteract the effects of the poisons on tissues.

All of this is part of the science of pharmacology, and it involves a much broader concept than many may consider when they hear the name.

HISTORY AND TRENDS IN PHARMACOLOGY

LEARNING OBJECTIVES

After studying this chapter, you should be able to:

1. Define pharmacology.

2. Briefly discuss historical uses of chemicals.

3. List at least four pharmaceutical discoveries of the 20th century.

4. List the four sources of drugs.

5. Discuss the role of the nurse in incorporating the pharmacological aspects of patient care into the nursing process.

6. List at least six points of teaching to facilitate patient education regarding the medication regimen.

Pharmacology is one of the oldest sciences. The history of primitive cultures reveals that people first used plants for nourishment. However, they sometimes became ill and even died after eating certain plants. By trial and error, they began to recognize which plants provided nourishment, which were poisonous, and which could be used for healing. Herbal remedies for illnesses afflicting both humans and animals are part of every cultural heritage. Some of this information became general knowledge; other times, the information was kept secret and was known only to the witch doctors and wise men or women of the community. Chemists and other researchers for drug companies are still exploring the possibilities of using these chemicals in modern medicines.

Folklore also contains descriptions of poisons that were used to hunt. By smearing the chemicals on the ends of their arrowheads and spears, natives were able to stun, paralyze, or kill their prey. This was useful in obtaining food or in defending themselves from their enemies.

Included in the history of many cultures are references to the use of stimulants, tranquilizers, or mood-altering drugs to escape the troubles and realities of life. There are frequent descriptions of the preparation of alcohol from the fermentation of carbohydrate foods, such as grapes (wine), rice (sake), and potatoes (vodka). Coffee, teas, chocolate, tobaccos, opium, marijuana, and other substances have long been used both legally and illegally.

It can be interesting to read of the various cultures and the discoveries made in each era.

Until the 19th century, drugs were crude preparations composed of multiple ingredients. The development of the "scientific method of inquiry" allowed experimentation and investigation, which were carefully documented. Advances in other sciences, such as chemistry, botany, and physiology, permitted new discoveries about the actions of substances in the body. Active ingredients of substances could now be isolated.

Researchers of this era identified these basic problems of pharmacology:

- The dose and effect relationships.
- The processes involved in absorption, distribution, transformation, and excretion of drugs.
- The localization of the site of action of drugs.
- The mechanisms of drug action.
- The relationship between the chemical's structure and the biological activity of substances.

Some important discoveries of the 19th century included anesthetics, such as ether and chloroform; analgesics, such as morphine and codeine; and antipyretic agents, such as acetylsalicylic acid (aspirin). The many scientific discoveries led to the building of large-scale drug manufacturing plants, which made new and convenient dosage forms and more palatable forms of drugs in accurate doses. The first of the national pharmacopeias of drugs appeared. These references contain standards of acceptability for drug preparations marketed for use in the United States.

The 20th century was one of great progress in pharmacology and medicine in general. There has probably been more progress in the past 50 years than in all the preceding years. Some of this progress was made because of new knowledge of the causes of disease. This led to the development of serums, vaccines, antitoxins, antibiotics, and other advances in the field of immunology. Production of synthetic drug preparations was another major advance. Pharmacists became recognized as professionals. Professional organizations were strengthened, and their work improved. Legislation was promoted to control experimentation, manufacture, and sale of food, drugs, and cosmetics. Some of the major discoveries of this era include the following:

Early 1900s: Phenobarbital, a sedative-hypnotic, was sometimes used as an anticonvulsant. This was followed by many other barbiturates. Quinidine was introduced to decrease atrial fibrillation.

1921: Drs. Banting and Best of Toronto, Canada, discovered insulin, which dramatically changed the prognosis for diabetics.

1930s: Sulfa drugs were used as anti-infectives. Many of the sulfonamide derivatives are still in use today. Phenytoin began the era of treatment for epileptic seizures.

1940s: Penicillin, discovered by Fleming, was introduced into the United States and used to treat infection. Cortisone was first used in medicine.

1950s: Many advances were made in medicines for use in psychiatry, with tremendous effects on the care of those with mental illness. Phenothiazines, benzodiazepines, minor tranquilizers, and antipsychotic agents were introduced.

1960s through 1990s: The industry "snowballed" with major advances in chemicals used for infection, hypertension, psychiatric disorders, ulcers, cancer, and most other illnesses.

DRUG SOURCES

The chemicals used in the manufacture of drugs are derived from four sources.

ANIMALS Secretions or hormones are often extracted from the glands of pigs, sheep, and cattle to replace hormones in humans (example: thyroid hormones and insulin).

VEGETABLES AND PLANTS Roots, bark, sap, leaves, flowers, and seeds from plants are sources of chemicals for drugs (example: digitalis is prepared from the purple foxglove flower; the dried leaves of the plant are used to treat arrhythmias and congestive heart failure).

Alkaloids (alkaline substances) in plants have a bitter taste and powerful physiological activity (example: atropine and scopolamine, which are belladonna alkaloids from the deadly nightshade plant).

Glycosides are compounds in plants that contain carbohydrate (example: digitalis).

Resins are substances from plants that are soluble in alcohol (example: cascara).

Gums are secretions of plants (example: bulk-type laxatives that absorb water).

Oils are viscous and sometimes greasy substances obtained from plants (example: castor oil or aromatic oils, such as oil of wintergreen).

MINERALS Chemicals extracted from metallic and nonmetallic mineral sources include acids, bases, and salts found in food (example: dilute hydrochloric acid, calcium, potassium chloride).

SYNTHETICS Most drugs used today are synthetically produced. Synthesis is a process of making a compound by alteration of other compounds or elements (example: steroids, sulfas, meperidine).

NURSING ROLE IN PHARMACOLOGY

Early physicians controlled all medications received by patients. They often did not share information with the patients or the nurse giving care to them. The physician was often considered to be "all wise," and the nurse and caregivers were to follow orders without question. A frequent response to patients' questions was "You'll have to ask the doctor."

In time, the role of nurses in society changed, nursing education became more formal and science oriented, and nurses asked more questions of the physician. Physicians eventually accepted the nurses' level of knowledge and allowed them to assume increased responsibilities. One of the first medical functions delegated to nurses was the administration of medications.

An increase in responsibility implies that one has the level of knowledge necessary to perform that responsibility. Nurses had to learn about these medications. Eventually, it came to be expected that they would have knowledge of the drug's action, therapeutic effects, and possible adverse effects. Today, nurses must counsel their patients about their medications and how to manage them for optimal effect. This teaching role has been expanded to include poison control, nonmedical use of drugs, drug abuse, and addiction because it is important to promote health and prevent drug-related complications.

It has been said that there are four levels of nursing care. The nurse's function is different at each level, and each level requires knowledge of pharmacology. These functions are as follows:

1. Prevention of problems in healthy persons: Nursing care at this level often takes place in public health, occupational health, and physicians' offices. The nurse attempts to educate and prevent illness. Much of the teaching is aimed at avoiding drug hazards and adverse effects.

2. Early detection of problems in healthy persons: Nurses assess for problems of drug dependence, toxic effects or adverse reactions, and detrimental effects of exposure to chemicals.

3. Care for patients with acute needs: Care of the patient with acute illness is often complex and usually occurs in an institutional setting. Nursing care includes administering medications. Patients are often receiving many drugs and may experience complex interactions. Nurses must assess for the therapeutic responses to the treatments being used and the adverse effects. They work with the physicians to revise the medication regimen and teach the patients about the regimen, anticipated side effects, and other related information.

4. Rehabilitation and resumption of normal living for recovering patients: The nursing focus is patient education. Nurses assist patients to resume control of their lives and maximize their health potential. Referral to community health agencies before discharge from acute-care facilities provides continuity of care. These community health nurses and others reinforce teaching received in acute-care settings and teach patients to manage their drug regimens as well as other aspects of self-care.

Today's nurses apply knowledge and skills from many fields, such as the physical and social sciences, to help the patient develop and implement a plan of care that will achieve optimal therapeutic effects. However, patients are no longer passive. They often take an active role in determining their therapy, and nurses act as patient-advocates for those too weak to do so. As uses of drugs expand to alleviate suffering and prolong life, nurses are facing many situations that involve a value judgment related to the quality of life compared with the quantity of life. This requires knowledge of ethics and law pertaining to nursing roles. Nursing remains not only a science but also an art.

NURSING PROCESS

Nursing process is a systematic method of identifying and solving the actual and potential problems individuals may experience during the course of an illness or disease. Just as the nursing process is the framework for all nursing functions, it is also the framework for administration of pharmacological agents. When using the nursing process to assess for problems or potential problems to be included in the individual's plan of care, consider the information listed in the drug information sources regarding adverse effects, drug interactions, and nursing implications.

Nursing process is A PIE divided into four parts. Each of the parts is applicable to the administration of drugs.

A = Assessment

Assessment of the patient is always important because the data obtained influence nursing decisions. There are two parts to every assessment:

1. In *objective* assessment, the nurse obtains data by physical assessment of the patient, such as by monitoring the vital signs, weighing the patient, and assessing skin color and condition. Objective assessment data also include results of diagnostic tests, such as x-ray studies and blood tests.

2. In *subjective* assessment, the patient or family supplies data, such as allergy history, occupation, and complaints.

Assessment not only provides an initial data base but is ongoing throughout the course of treatment.

P = Planning

Planning involves sorting and analyzing the data to develop the plan of care. The nurse defines the problems, sets the goals, and lists the interventions to meet the goals. Planning the patient teaching to prepare for discharge is included in this part.

I = Implementation

Implementation is carrying out the plan of care. It includes preparation and administration of drugs, assessment of vital signs, and patient teaching.

E = Evaluation

Evaluation is deciding how the patient is responding to the interventions in relation to the stated goals and expected outcomes. For example, is the patient still in pain 1 hour after the analgesic was administered? Does assessment of the vital signs need to be repeated? Is the patient lethargic? Is the plan still relevant, or does it need to be revised? It is important to remember that the nursing process is continuous, and the plan must be revised as the patient's condition improves or deteriorates.

PATIENT TEACHING

Health education, or patient education, is an area of care that has undergone a dramatic change in recent years. Formerly, the patient was given only that information which the physician thought should be given. Often it was believed that if a patient knew too much about the possible problems that could occur from an illness or the treatment, he would refuse the treatment or would worry too much and not get well. Therefore, the only information that was shared was first approved by the physician. Literature was not available in a language that could be understood by the average patient, so even if the patient was resourceful enough to search for information, it just was not available. In fact, physicians and pharmacists were required to know Latin, and early prescriptions and medical literature were written in this ancient language.

Today, in contrast to that era, patient teaching is recognized as one of the most important roles of the physician, nurse, and pharmacist. This responsibility carries legal implications for those who fail to provide and document education. It is now generally believed that the more a patient understands about the condition and its causes, symptoms, treatments, and prognosis, the more responsible he may be. All significant caregivers should be included in the teaching because it is often necessary to review and repeat instructions, especially when one is ill or under stress. This must also be documented.

When patient teaching is considered in relation to pharmacology, the best one can say is that the days when the physician was the only one who knew anything about the patient's medications are long gone. Too many possible problems can occur with today's medications to allow the patient and the family to be ignorant of them. After all, the sooner the physician is made aware of a problem, the sooner steps can be taken to correct it. In addition, many of the problems can be prevented just by making the patient and significant caregivers aware of the potential. For example, some of the main causes of medication failure are taking the medication at the wrong time; taking the wrong dose; omitting doses; taking outdated medications; and taking medications by the wrong method, such as crushing pills that are enteric coated. Other causes are not reading or not understanding directions or warnings and stopping the drug before the therapy is completed. Most of these problems can be prevented by proper patient teaching.

NURSING ALERT

▼▼▼▼▼▼▼▼▼▼▼▼▼▼▼▼▼▼▼▼▼▼▼▼▼▼▼▼▼▼▼▼▼▼▼▼▼

For the patient to learn the information and follow through with the medication or treatment as directed, the information must be recognized as important and personally relevant. Finding out what the patient believes to be important is a key issue in any teaching success.

▲▲▲▲▲▲▲▲▲▲▲▲▲▲▲▲▲▲▲▲▲▲▲▲▲▲▲▲▲▲▲▲▲▲▲▲▲

In teaching a patient or the patient's family about medications, the same principles apply as with other types of teaching. Some teaching may be spontaneous, as when a patient asks a question, but all thorough teaching begins with a plan. Using the nursing process format, begin assessment by gathering data about the patient's level of understanding of the subject. For all teaching, use a vocabulary easily understood by the patient. Outline the plan to ensure that all key points are covered.

Give information in short sessions that consider the complexity of the material and the patient's state of comfort and attention span. When anxiety or pain is at a high level, the ability to concentrate on details is limited. Teaching times must also be scheduled around the patient's other therapies or activities.

Provide written materials whenever possible. This provides the patient with the opportunity to review the materials as many times as desired.

At each teaching session, allow some time for review of material previously presented and for the patient's questions.

Reinforce key points by repeating them. Ask the patient to explain the information to you as a way of evaluating understanding. If there are misconceptions, it will be apparent. Be sure your plan is individualized. Include information on the condition being treated; how the medication should be taken (for example, before meals, with food, or at bedtime); the likely side effects of the medication; any special precautions to observe in taking the medication (for example, take pulse before taking medication; avoid aspirin; avoid sunlight); any potential drug interactions with other medications the patient is taking (antibiotics decrease the effectiveness of birth control pills); and the actions to be taken in response to a drug interaction, such as to omit the next dose or call the physician.

If you are teaching a skill, such as injection technique, practice times must be scheduled. Document all teaching sessions and summarize the information discussed, demonstrated, or practiced.

If the information presented is complex or lengthy, such as diabetic teaching, you may wish to refer the patient to a community resource for follow-up after discharge. Questions often arise after the patient leaves the controlled environment of the hospital. If the patient is experiencing difficulties and no resources are available, the medication is often omitted or taken incorrectly.

Finally, remember that everyone makes decisions on the basis of personal attitudes or beliefs. No matter how well you teach a subject, once the patient is in the home environment, he is free to choose to follow the prescribed treatment, alter it, or discontinue it.

E X E R C I S E S

LEARNING ACTIVITIES

1. Research an article on folklore that discusses the use of a plant as a remedy for an ailment. Report to the class with your findings.

2. Use an encyclopedia to research a pharmaceutical discovery that occurred during the year of your birth. Write a report and share it with your class.

practice times
Document all teaching sessions
Sumerize information discussed

PHARMACODYNAMICS AND PHARMACOKINETICS

LEARNING OBJECTIVES

After studying this chapter, you should be able to:

1. Define **pharmacokinetics.**

2. List the four processes by which drugs are used by the body.

3. Define **pharmacodynamics.**

4. Distinguish between local and systemic sites of action.

5. Define **drug effects.**

6. List at least four factors that affect pharmacodynamics and pharmacokinetics.

To understand the actions of a drug, the nurse must first thoroughly understand how a drug is used by the body and how it changes the behavior of the body. These two basic processes are vital to the study of pharmacology.

The first of these processes is *pharmacokinetics*. Pharmacokinetics is defined as the use of a drug by the body. To use the drug, the body follows four steps: absorption, distribution, biotransformation, and excretion.

The second process is *pharmacodynamics*. Pharmacodynamics is defined as the study of a drug's actions and the effects it has on the body. The actions of a drug are depression, stimulation, irritation, and demulcence. Drug effects include cumulation, addition or summation, synergism or potentiation, antagonism, tolerance, adverse reaction, anaphylaxis, idiosyncratic effects, and addiction. In addition, the two major sites of drug action are local and systemic.

PHARMACOKINETICS

Absorption

The first step of drug use is absorption. This is the passage of the drug from the outside of the body to the bloodstream. There are many ways in which the drug may enter the bloodstream. The method used depends on the drug and on the route of administration of the drug chosen.

If a drug is ingested, it passes into the digestive system and goes through all or part of the digestive processes. This means the drug must survive these processes to be effective. Many drugs are absorbed into the bloodstream from the stomach or the small intestine through the villi by a combination of osmosis, active transport, filtration, and diffusion. Some drugs are absorbed at different areas of the digestive tract. For example, some are placed under the tongue and are absorbed into the bloodstream through the delicate mucous membranes there.

If a drug is inhaled, it passes into the bloodstream by way of the alveoli, again by processes similar to drug ingestion, such as diffusion and active transport.

If a drug is applied topically to the skin or mucous membranes, it is absorbed through the tiny capillaries there.

If a drug is injected into subcutaneous or muscular tissue, it is absorbed into the bloodstream through the capillaries near the site of injection.

If a drug is administered intravenously, this eliminates the need for the body to absorb the drug because it has been placed directly into the bloodstream. Therefore, the intravenous route of administration is the fastest acting.

For the drug to be absorbed from its site of administration, a good blood supply must be present at that site. For example, if a drug is injected into muscular tissue, capillaries must be present and in good working order, or the drug will simply not reach the blood-stream. For the drug that is inhaled, capillaries of the alveoli must be working adequately to ensure absorption. Once a drug has reached the bloodstream, it is said to be free or unbound, meaning it is available for use by the body.

Many factors can affect the blood supply of an area, including edema, infection, congestion of the blood vessels, poor circulation to the area, poor pumping ability of the heart, or pressure. If a patient has one of these factors existing, the physician may use a different route of administration to overcome the problem. The nurse can help ensure that the patient is receiving adequate effects from the drug by observing for any of these risk factors.

Distribution

Once the drug reaches the bloodstream, it must then progress to its particular site of action. Beginning students may ask how a drug "knows" where to go. You must understand the chemical nature of drugs to fully comprehend how drugs can have actions on specific parts of the body.

A drug does not stay free or unbound in the bloodstream. There are actually up to three forms of the drug in the body: a portion that stays unbound; a portion that binds with a protein (most commonly albumin); and with some drugs, a portion that binds with fat (called lipid soluble). The proportions of these forms of the drug stay relatively stable. The body releases some of the protein-bound or lipid-bound drug to replace the portion of the free or unbound drug that has left the bloodstream. Generally, the protein-bound drug is released more quickly than the lipid-bound drug. Therefore, lipid-soluble drugs tend to have longer lasting effects.

As the free drug is circulating in the bloodstream, it comes in contact with chemicals to which it is attracted. These are referred to as *receptors*. A place on the receptor becomes attached to the drug. This is called the *receptor site*.

Sometimes a drug will fit the receptor site exactly and have a strong attachment to it. Once the drug and the receptor have attached, the drug elicits a response from the receptor. The receptor is said to be stimulated. The drug is then called an *agonist*.

With other receptors, the drug may attach strongly but not elicit a response. However, it does prevent other chemicals from reacting with the receptor simply because it is in the way. The drug is then called an *antagonist*.

With still other receptors, the drug may attach with only a weak bond. It elicits a weak response from the receptor and often prevents other reactions from

occurring with that receptor and any other chemical. The drug is then called a *partial agonist*.

For the drug to reach the receptors, it must be circulated through the bloodstream. An area or tissue of the body that has a good blood supply will have an increased supply of the drug. The drug will then have more opportunity to attach to receptors in that part of the body. An area or tissue that has less blood traveling to it will have a decreased supply of the drug and less action by the drug.

Some tissues require special transport activities for the drug to enter them. Central nervous system tissue is affected only by certain drugs. This is because the drug must pass the *blood-brain barrier*. This is not a place in the body but rather a chemical barrier. Only certain drugs will pass through the placenta to a fetus. This is because of the *placental barrier*. Again, we are not naming a specific tissue, but rather the inability of many drugs to interact with chemicals from the placenta.

Biotransformation

Biotransformation is also called metabolism. It is the process by which the drug is detoxified (turned into harmless substances). This is done primarily by the liver through the use of enzymes and chemical reactions. It is important, therefore, for a patient receiving medication to have adequate liver function. Without biotransformation, the drug continues to have its effect on the body and eventually harms the body.

Pharmacologists measure the speed by which the body biotransforms a drug. A *half-life* is the amount of time it takes for the body to inactivate half of the available drug. This information is used in determining the proper dosage and dosage intervals for specific drugs.

Excretion

A drug is eliminated from the body through excretion. This may be through respiration, perspiration, or defecation. Most often, excretion is through the kidneys. Good kidney function is vital for the proper elimination of drugs. If the drug or its transformed substances are not eliminated from the body, they build up and cause harm.

To ensure optimal kidney function in the hospitalized or bedridden patient, the nurse should encourage activity to the patient's tolerance. This stimulates circulation through the kidneys and excretion of the drug and waste products.

If a patient has impaired kidney function, it is the duty of the nurse to bring this to the attention of the physician if it is not already known. The dosage, the route, and even the drug itself may have to be changed.

PHARMACODYNAMICS

Drug Actions

When a drug attaches to a receptor at the receptor site, it then acts on that receptor to elicit a physiological response. That physiological response is said to be the drug's action. The four major drug actions are depression, stimulation, irritation, and demulcence.

① Depression

When a drug depresses, it lowers or lessens activity in some body part. Commonly, this is respiratory depression, cardiac depression, nervous system depression, motor depression (mostly affecting the involuntary muscles), mental depression, and excretory (or glandular) depression.

If a drug produces respiratory depression, the nurse notes a slowing of the respiratory rate. It is the responsibility of the nurse to observe respirations closely for any patient receiving a respiratory depressant drug. In general, if a patient's respirations are below 12 per minute, the next dose of the drug should be withheld until the physician can be notified. Often, the dosage or the drug itself needs to be altered.

If a drug produces cardiac depression, the nurse notes a slowing of the pulse. With extreme bradycardia, irregular rhythm (arrhythmia) may also be noted. Again, the nurse notifies the physician immediately on noticing the decline in the pulse rate. In general, if a patient's pulse is below 60 per minute, the physician may change the dosage or the drug.

If a drug produces nervous system depression, the nurse notes slowed speech and response to questions, slowed reaction to reflex stimulation, lethargy, and drowsiness. It is the responsibility of the nurse to protect the patient's safety. With slower reactions and drowsiness, the patient could easily fall. Discourage the patient from driving an automobile, operating hazardous machinery, or doing any activity that requires mental alertness. Allow time for the patient to answer questions without trying to answer for her.

If a drug produces motor depression, encourage the patient to remain active to discourage immobility complications. Primarily, however, the effects of motor depression are seen on the involuntary muscles, including respiratory muscles and muscles of organs such as the bladder.

Drugs that can produce mental depression cause a feeling of emotional dispiritedness. Patients experiencing this action should inform the physician immediately because mental depression is uncomfortable and can lead to suicidal thoughts and behaviors. The nurse assesses the patient carefully for any signs of this and reports it.

Exocrine or glandular depression can envelop a wide range of sites of action. Glands are located throughout the body, including in the stomach, skin, blood vessels, organs, breasts, and many other sites. Each of these glands secretes a substance that produces an action somewhere in the body. If this secretion is depressed by the drug, the action does not take place or is lessened. Therefore, the exact action of the drug depends on which gland is affected.

② Stimulation

Drugs that stimulate increase the function or activity of a part of the body. The sites of action are the same as for depression: respiratory, cardiac, nervous, motor, mental, and excretory. The action would be the opposite of depression. Respirations are increased; pulse is increased and often bounding; the patient feels nervous and cannot sleep, may be agitated, and is alert; and glandular functions throughout the body are increased. The nurse is responsible for observing these actions and reporting any dangerous levels or behaviors.

③ Irritation

Drugs that act by irritation are primarily applied to skin or mucous membranes. These drugs produce symptoms of inflammation at that site. These symptoms include redness, swelling, warmth, pain, and a change in normal functioning of the part. Although these symptoms are generally thought of as pathological, they can be useful in some circumstances. A common example is the irritant laxative. This drug acts directly on the mucosa of the intestine and produces an emptying of the bowel. The nurse needs to be aware of excessive irritation from the drug as exhibited by excessive action of the drug, pain or cramping, or decreased circulation to a part due to swelling.

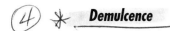

④ ✳ Demulcence

A drug that produces demulcence acts by soothing that part of the body. Demulcents are applied to skin or mucous membranes to relieve symptoms of irritation.

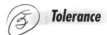

⑤ Tolerance

When a patient has tolerance to a drug, the effects are lessened. This is not in response to the presence of another drug, but rather, it is a response to the continual presence of the drug. The body "gets used to" the drug and no longer reacts to it with the same power. Often, the dosage of the drug must be increased to achieve the same therapeutic effects. Drug abusers also find themselves victim to tolerance and must increase the dosage of the drug they are abusing to achieve the same effects they wish.

✳ Drug Effects

Drug effects result from the actions of the drug. Some effects, however, are changed because of other effects of the drug or effects of another drug or food taken simultaneously.

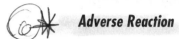

⑥ ✳ Adverse Reaction

Adverse reactions are effects that are not the desired drug effect and are unpleasant or even harmful. All drugs have the potential to produce adverse reactions, and they can happen at any time during drug therapy. Some patients mistakenly believe that if they have not had a reaction to a drug before, because they have taken it many times, they will not have a reaction this time. The nurse needs to educate the patient about the dangers of drug therapy and to always be alert to changes in the drug effect.

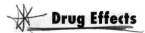

① Cumulation

Some drugs remain in the body longer than others do. If balanced amounts of the drug are not excreted from the body as new amounts are absorbed, the effects of the drug increase and eventually reach toxic (poisonous) levels.

Adverse reactions are to be reported. The Food and Drug Administration (FDA) wants nurses to report any serious reactions they note in their patients. The FDA requests reports even if you are unsure whether the reaction was due to a specific drug. The type of drug reaction the FDA wants to hear about is one that (1) was life-threatening, (2) caused death, (3) caused disability, (4) caused a hospital stay or a longer hospital stay, or (5) did not produce the expected therapeutic response. Your pharmacist should have the form to use for filing the report.

② Addition or Summation

Additive or summative effects are best explained by comparing them with simple arithmetic. When you add 1 plus 1, you expect to get 2. When the effects of one drug are added to the effects of another drug, you can estimate the combined effect by simply adding the separate effects of the two drugs. This, then, is an additive effect.

The Joint Commission on Accreditation of Healthcare Organizations (JCAHO) also regulates reporting of adverse reactions. In addition to those required by the FDA, JCAHO requires reactions to be reported (1) if the drug needed to be discontinued because of the reaction or (2) when another drug was used to treat the adverse reaction.

③ Synergism or Potentiation

Synergistic or potentiated effects go beyond simple arithmetic. When the effects of one drug are added to the effects of another drug, the combined effect is greater than would be expected by simply adding the two. The combined effect is boosted by using the two drugs together. We say that one drug potentiates the other.

Reporting adverse reactions helps your patients in the long run by increasing the knowledge base of practitioners everywhere. The physicians and nurses responsible for giving the medications will be able to adjust their care accordingly.

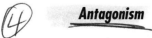

④ Antagonism

Antagonistic effects of one drug counteract the effects of another drug. This effect can be viewed as the opposite of potentiation or addition. Instead of greater effects, the drug produces less than expected results because of the presence of the second drug.

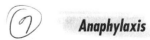

⑦ Anaphylaxis

Anaphylaxis is an extreme hypersensitivity to a drug and is an emergency situation. It produces sudden and severe symptoms, including a drop in blood pressure, pallor, cyanosis, respiratory distress, seizures, collapse, coma, and even death. Anaphylaxis is also referred to as anaphylactic shock because of the symptoms. Anaphylaxis may be fatal within minutes, or it may be preceded by a skin rash, hives, or itching (with or without the rash or hives). Therefore, the nurse should withhold the next dose of a drug when the patient has these symptoms and immediately notify the physician. In most cases, the drug will be discontinued and an appropriate substitution made.

Idiosyncratic Effects

Idiosyncratic effects are effects that are not expected or desired but are highly individualized. Nearly every person will react to some substance differently from others in the population. These may also be called paradoxical effects.

Addiction

Addiction is covered thoroughly in Chapter 10.

Sites of Action

Local

Drugs that act locally are not absorbed into the bloodstream. They produce their actions and effects at the site where they are applied. Drugs with local effect include those applied to the skin and mucous membranes, inhaled to come into contact with mucous membranes of the respiratory system, inserted to come into contact with mucous membranes of the digestive tract or reproductive tract, or injected to come into contact with subcutaneous tissue under the skin.

Drugs that act locally can have systemic effects, however, if they are absorbed into the bloodstream.

Systemic

Drugs that act systemically can have effects throughout the body because they are absorbed into the bloodstream and distributed. Which areas are affected by a specific drug depend on the receptors to which that drug is attracted. The drug can also have one effect in one area of the body and a different effect elsewhere. The nurse needs to be aware of the systemic actions and effects of drugs to adequately prepare and protect the patient.

E X E R C I S E S

MENTAL AEROBICS

Look up each of the following drugs in a reliable drug information resource (see Chapter 3 for some examples). You may need some help using the reference book at first. Look for what types of information are given. What are the subheadings? Are actions listed? Are adverse reactions given? Are there any drugs that are potentiated by the drug? Are any drugs listed that are antagonistic? Does the reference book explain the pharmacokinetics of the drug? How is it absorbed? Where is it biotransformed? How is it distributed, and to where? By what method is it excreted? Does anything interfere with any of these processes?

1. meperidine (Demerol)
2. doxycycline (Vibramycin)
3. phenelzine (Nardil)
4. aspirin
5. acetaminophen (Tylenol)
6. furosemide (Lasix)

SOURCES OF DRUG INFORMATION

LEARNING OBJECTIVES

After studying this chapter, you should be able to:

1. List the five areas of concern that have standards regulated by legislation.

2. Distinguish the difference between chemical, generic, official, and trade names.

3. Discuss the meaning of the term "drug classifications."

4. List at least five sources of drug information.

DRUG STANDARDS

Standards are our way of measuring something. In our society, we have come to expect a certain standard of quality with any given product. Our expectations are probably even greater when it comes to our medicines. When we go to the cabinet to get a drug, we expect that each pill in the container will be composed of the same substances. We also expect the same potency and thereby the same degree of safety with each pill in the container.

In primitive societies, information about potions and preparations for cures was passed from one generation to another by word of mouth. Medicine men and witches had "apprentices" who learned their secrets by watching and by preparing their remedies under the watchful eye and direct supervision of these mentors. Preparations were not purified, and there were no methods for measuring strength or potency.

Today's technology provides many sophisticated means of extracting and purifying chemicals, measuring chemicals and ingredients, and analyzing the chemical composition of the finished product. Our society has established standards for drug quality and enabled the government to enforce them through legislation regarding the properties of drugs. There are regulations concerning the purity, potency or strength, bioavailability, efficacy, and safety or toxicity of drugs.

Purity

A pure drug is one that contains only one specific chemical. There are few substances sold that would meet this criterion. Most products are a combination of ingredients that include fillers, dyes, solvents, buffers, and waxes. These additional ingredients are necessary to give form to pills and capsules, to make products more palatable, and to enhance or inhibit the absorption process. In addition, drugs are not prepared in a completely sterile environment. Dusts and other contaminants from the environment may get into the product. Government standards of purity specify the type and concentration of substances that are allowed to be present in the drug.

Potency

The potency or strength of a drug depends on the concentration of the active ingredient in the preparation. When the active ingredients are known, the potency is measured by chemical analysis. When this technique is used, the amounts of the ingredients are reflected in grams, milligrams, micrograms, or other appropriate unit of weight measurement. When the active ingredients are unknown, potency is measured by testing in laboratory animals, and dosages are often reflected in units. One unit must always be equal to another. Some drugs whose dosages are still reflected in units are injectable penicillin and many of the hormones, such as insulin, and heparin.

Bioavailability

Bioavailability is the degree that a drug can be absorbed and transported to the site of its action. This property depends on the size and structure of the chemical particles, how soluble they are, and how they polarize with other particles. Bioavailability is measured by the concentration of the drug in blood or tissue at a specific time after administration.

Efficacy

The efficacy of a drug is its ability to produce a desired chemical change in the body. This is a less objective quality than the others because there are many variables in individual responses. Clinical trials are used to compare the response of individuals receiving the drug with those given a placebo, but the data must be interpreted by individuals who make value judgments, which may be somewhat subjective.

Safety and Toxicity

Safety and toxicity are opposite properties. They are determined by recording the type and number of adverse or undesirable effects that occur in individuals after a drug is administered. Safety and toxicity are tested to a certain degree on animals before a product is marketed, but many adverse effects, such as birth defects or cancer, may not be apparent until years later.

All chemicals have some toxic effects. The difference between dosages that produce desirable effects and those that produce toxic effects is considered the margin of safety. The dosages that fall within the margin of safety are called therapeutic dosages. Whenever use of a drug is considered, the desired therapeutic effects must be compared with the potential for adverse or toxic effects before it is decided whether the drug is appropriate for a given individual.

DRUG NOMENCLATURE

Drug nomenclature is a system that attempts to classify drugs. However, drugs have more than one name, which can be confusing for all involved. The exact spelling of the drug name is crucial to obtaining and administering the ordered drug.

Chemical Name

The chemical name of a drug describes the drug's composition with the actual labeling of the structure of its atoms and molecules. It is accompanied by a diagram of the chemical structure of the drug. This name is of most meaning to the chemist.

Generic or Nonproprietary Name

The generic or nonproprietary name (sometimes called the common name) is the name given a drug when it is first proposed by a company to be approved for use. The generic name for a proposed drug is provided by the United States Adopted Names (USAN) Council. It is never capitalized, and it is much simpler than the chemical name. The generic name may be used in all countries by any manufacturer. Patients may wish to ask the physician to prescribe their medications using the generic name because drugs prescribed in this manner are usually less costly.

Official Name

Since 1962, federal legislation mandates that the United States Food and Drug Administration (FDA) give one official name to each drug approved for human use in the United States. This has decreased the confusion that was caused by several names being given to the same drug. Listings of official names of drugs are found in official drug reference books, such as the United States Pharmacopeia and National Formulary (USP-NF).

Drugs with the same generic and official names must have the same chemical name and structure, regardless of who manufactures them.

Trade Name, Trademark, Brand Name, and Proprietary Name

Several other names, such as trade name, trademark, brand name, and proprietary name, are used interchangeably in pharmacology to identify drugs manufactured by different companies. These names are followed by the symbol ®, which indicates that the name is registered and its use is restricted to the owner of the drug, who is usually the manufacturer of the product. In other words, trade names identify a particular company's product. Trade names are easier to pronounce, spell, and remember. The first letter of a trade name is capitalized. Trade names are derived from some property of the drug's chemical composition.

Because of similarities in names, there is more confusion and potential for error when the trade name is used. Two drugs with similar trade names might be used for two entirely different purposes. For example, the drug Benadryl (an antihistamine) sounds very much like the drug Benuryl (a uricosuric), and unless the names of these two drugs are written carefully, the letters of one could be mistaken for the letters of the other. However, if the generic names (diphenhydramine hydrochloride and probenecid) are used, the similarities vanish.

DRUG CLASSIFICATION

Drug classifications or categories are ways of grouping or arranging drugs according to their similarities. There are several different ways to do this, which may be confusing when you first see one drug listed in more than one classification. However, as your knowledge of pharmacology increases, you will see that classifications are a tremendous help in learning and remembering the similarities and differences of drugs.

One way of classifying drugs is according to body systems, such as drugs that affect the circulatory system, drugs that affect the digestive system, and so on. Each classification also includes subclassifications of drugs that affect the same system but in a different manner. For example, drugs that affect the circulatory system include antihypertensives, antiarrhythmics, vasodilators, and others. Each of these classifications also has subclasses of drugs that cause the same or similar effect but do so by acting in a different manner.

Knowledge of basic drug classifications, correlated with basic knowledge of human anatomy and physiology, helps us to locate and remember specific drug information more quickly.

REFERENCES

Many references contain information on drugs. The resources are directed at individuals who function in a variety of ways.

PHARMACOPEIA–NATIONAL FORMULARY OF THE UNITED STATES OF AMERICA (USP-NF) This reference relates to standardization of drugs. In previous centuries, drug purity and potency varied from batch to batch and from manufacturer to manufacturer. By the establishment of an authoritative reference that defined the standards of purity as well as the methods that must be used to determine purity,

it was guaranteed that drug products made by different manufacturers or even in different batches within the same company are uniform in purity and potency.

In 1906, the Food, Drug, and Cosmetic Act designated the United States Pharmacopeia (USP) the official compendium of the United States. This book was combined with the National Formulary (NF) in 1980. The USP-NF is revised every 5 years, with supplements published more frequently. It contains little or no medical or nursing information, so it is more useful to pharmacists than to other health care professionals. For this reason, it is kept in pharmacies and usually not found anywhere else. Its standards have been adopted by the Food and Drug Administration (FDA) as the official standards for manufacture and quality control of medications in the United States.

UNITED STATES ADOPTED NAMES (USAN) COUNCIL This committee is responsible for producing simple and useful nonproprietary or generic names for drugs. The FDA now accepts the adopted generic name as the official name for a drug.

USP DICTIONARY OF DRUG NAMES This is a compiled listing of about 20,000 drug names. It includes the USAN name, a pronunciation guide, the graphic and molecular formula, the chemical and brand names, the manufacturer, and the therapeutic category or classification.

AMERICAN HOSPITAL FORMULARY SERVICE The American Society of Hospital Pharmacists annually publishes a two-volume set of references with four supplements. It contains information on most drugs available in the United States.

PHYSICIANS' DESK REFERENCE (PDR) The preceding publications are extremely valuable for manufacturers and to pharmacists but are of little use to the average physician or health care worker. Physicians, nurses, and others frequently refer to the PDR as an authoritative reference. The PDR is published annually, with several supplements yearly.

The PDR is divided into several sections that include information on the manufacturers of the products listed; emergency phone numbers for the manufacturers; product names listed alphabetically by trade names; a product classification index; a generic and chemical name index; a product identification section, which has color pictures of the products in actual size; and a product information section, which lists actions, uses, side effects, routes of administration, dose, contraindications to use, composition of the drug, and how the drug is supplied. The PDR also includes information on drugs used as diagnostic test agents and lists poison control centers and their telephone numbers.

Although this book is complete, it contains so much information that one cannot easily use it as a "quick" reference. Also, beginning health care professionals often complain that the language is complicated and that they lack the expertise to "sort out" what is really important.

NONPRESCRIPTION PHYSICIANS' DESK REFERENCE (PDR) This book contains a listing similar to the PDR, but for commonly used nonprescription drugs. It is much smaller than the PDR, is published annually, and is less complicated in its language. Its value lies in the fact that individuals often self-medicate for minor illnesses while taking prescribed medications for chronic illnesses. Many of the prescription and nonprescription drugs interact, causing altered effects and side effects of either of the drugs.

PACKAGE BROCHURES OR INSERTS These are available on request from the pharmacy filling the prescription for an individual. They contain excerpts of material from the PDR, put into somewhat simplified language. Caregivers should encourage patients to request this information from their pharmacist, to read it, and to question the pharmacist or their physician about information they do not understand.

MEDICATION CARDS These are produced by various authors and publishing companies in an index card format. They are designed to be used as a quick reference in assorted health care settings. Most of these products include an index of generic and trade names, classification of the drug, actions and uses, side effects, contraindications, drug interactions, and nursing interventions.

MISCELLANEOUS There are a variety of textbooks and other references written at different levels of depth and thoroughness. Individuals who administer medications should browse for a reference that meets their needs so they can be safe practitioners without wasting a lot of time searching for and translating information.

E X E R C I S E S

LEARNING ACTIVITIES

1. Choose one of the listed sources of drug information (or any other source) and bring it to class. Explain to the group the type of information to be found in the reference and how to use that particular reference to locate information on a drug that you have chosen.

2. Select a drug. Research and report to the class the chemical name (include the diagram of the chemical structure of the drug), the generic name, the official name, and the trade name of the drug.

3. Select a drug with a trade name that sounds like one of those presented by a classmate in activity 2. Present the same information for the "sound-alike drug" and emphasize the differences between the two.

DRUG LEGISLATION

LEARNING OBJECTIVES

After studying this chapter, you should be able to:

1. List the four levels of governmental drug legislation and control.

2. List at least three functions of the Food, Drug, and Cosmetic Act.

3. Discuss at least three functions of the Controlled Substances Act.

4. Define "controlled substance schedules."

Historically, it has been documented that some members of each society have chosen to abuse the chemicals that were used therapeutically for illnesses among the people of that society. Therefore, it became necessary for governing members of the society to establish regulations controlling the use of those substances. Many of the first restrictions were in the form of religious rituals. Chemicals affecting the central nervous system were often reserved for use in religious ceremonies, where the effects of the chemicals were looked on as mystical experiences.

Today, some religious denominations continue to prohibit the use of alcohol among their members. Congregations of many denominations have taken public stands against the social use and abuse of drugs and alcohol.

Many societies have enacted legislation to protect the consumer and the patient. This became important because of the vast amounts of money spent by companies on advertising and promotional campaigns—information about a product's positive effects was widely publicized in an effort to increase sales; information regarding drug effects, adverse effects, drug interactions, and other precautions was suppressed or given minimal coverage by the media. Now, information about the drug's negative effects is more available to enable the consumer to make an informed choice regarding the value of a particular therapy.

Currently, there are many controls on the use of addictive substances. Some of these controls are in the form of governmental legislation, which ranges from international, national, state or provincial, to local legislation. Local restrictions are generally more stringent than those of the larger agencies, because each agency adds specific details to the regulation yet must still comply with the restrictions of the larger agency. Individual institutions also impose restrictions or regulations on some substances.

INTERNATIONAL CONTROLS

The World Health Organization (WHO) of the United Nations (UN) provides technical assistance and promotes research in the areas of drug abuse. Many nations voluntarily participate and cooperate with each other to control drug traffic, but there are no international judicial groups to enforce this control.

NATIONAL CONTROLS

The severity of drug enforcement laws varies with each country, as do the penalties for violations of these laws. Many countries are more strict than the United States and impose long prison sentences and even death for possession of drugs and participation in drug traffic.

United States Controls

In the United States, federal legislation began with the *1906 Food, Drug, and Cosmetic Act,* which was concerned with the purity of food, designated national standards for drugs (United States Pharmacopeia–National Formulary), and empowered the federal

Table 4–1. Federal Drug Legislation

1906 Federal Food, Drug, and Cosmetic Act	Began federal legislation Concerned with purity of food Designated national standards for drugs Empowered the federal government to enforce regulations
1914 Harrison Narcotic Act	First narcotic control act Denoted many habit-forming drugs as "narcotics" Established regulations for import, manufacture, sale, and use
1938 Federal Food, Drug, and Cosmetic Act (revision)	Required animal toxicology tests to determine safety of drugs Labeling of drug contents required Label must state whether drug is habit forming
1945 Federal Food, Drug, and Cosmetic Act (amendment)	Food and Drug Administration (FDA) testing of each batch of drug Government inspection and supervision of drug production
1952 Durham-Humphrey Amendment	Distinguished between prescription and over-the-counter drugs Established procedures governing prescription orders and refills Required licensure to distribute or dispense medications
1962 Kefauver-Harris Amendment	Registration/inspection of drug firms Truth in advertising Drug safety
1970 Comprehensive Abuse Prevention and Control Act (Controlled Substances Act)	Composite law (repealed 50 previous drug laws since 1914) Established 5 classes of habit-forming drugs Established government programs to promote prevention and treatment of drug dependence Illegal to possess controlled substance without prescription Required detailed records of dispensing Organized the Drug Enforcement Agency to enforce act

government with enforcement of regulations. Since that time, many other acts and laws have extended the federal drug controls (Table 4–1). Some of these important changes are as follows.

1914 HARRISON NARCOTIC ACT This law is historically significant because it was the first narcotic control act passed by any nation. It classified many of the habit-forming drugs as "narcotics" and regulated their importation, manufacture, sale, and use.

1938 FEDERAL FOOD, DRUG, AND COSMETIC ACT This act revised the 1906 law by adding more requirements related to the safety of drugs. New drugs had to be approved by the government as safe before sale between states; animal toxicology tests determined safety. Labeling of drug contents was now legislated, and this labeling was not to be false or misleading. The label was required to specify whether the drug contained alcohol or atropine, for example, and also to state whether the drug was habit forming. Many other requirements and frequent revisions followed.

1945 FEDERAL FOOD, DRUG, AND COSMETIC ACT (AMENDMENT) This amendment provided for certification of certain drugs through testing by the Food and Drug Administration (FDA) of each batch produced. This opened the door for government inspection and supervision of drug production.

1952 DURHAM-HUMPHREY AMENDMENT This amendment distinguished between prescription and over-the-counter (OTC) drugs. It also specified procedures governing distribution of prescription drugs by written, oral, or telephone orders. Refilling of written and oral prescriptions was legalized, as long as the original prescription authorized the refill. It also required health professionals to be licensed to distribute or dispense medications.

During the 1950s, several widely publicized incidents involving drugs made the public more aware of the potential problems associated with consumption of medications. The Salk vaccine was rushed into production in an attempt to stall the polio epidemic. However, after more than 200 cases of permanent paralysis resulted, it was determined that the virus in the vaccine was not as weak (attenuated) as it should have been. Another drug, called thalidomide, was widely used in Europe as an antiemetic and sedative to curb the nausea and vomiting of pregnancy. It was later proved to be teratogenic (causes birth defects) when numerous infants were born without arms or legs, a condition called phocomelia.

1962 KEFAUVER-HARRIS AMENDMENT This amendment attempted to provide assurance of safety and effectiveness of drugs. It required registration of drug manufacturing firms, with inspection of firms at least every 2 years.

Among the controls enacted by this amendment, drugs must be withdrawn from the market if a question of safety arises. There must be truth in advertising, and side effects must be reported and listed. Official names for drugs must be published by the FDA. Drugs must be tested and certified by the government as safe before marketing.

1970 COMPREHENSIVE DRUG ABUSE PREVENTION AND CONTROL ACT (CONTROLLED SUBSTANCES ACT) This is a composite law that repealed almost 50 other laws written since the 1914 Harrison Narcotic Act. It outlined strict controls on the manufacturing and distribution of habit-forming drugs. Five classes of drugs were established on the basis of their potential for abuse and dependence. The law also required the establishment of government programs to promote prevention and treatment of drug dependence. It made it illegal to possess controlled substances without prescription and required detailed records of drugs dispensed. The Drug Enforcement Agency (DEA) was organized under the Department of Justice to enforce the act.

Practitioners must apply for a certificate of registration from the DEA if they wish to administer, prescribe, or dispense a controlled substance. Certification is valid for a period of 3 years and must be maintained and available for official inspection at the registered location (Table 4–2).

State Controls

The state governments must comply with federal regulations when they make their own regulations. Each state regulates whether the sale of alcohol is private or by agency, and it establishes the legal age of consumption. It details regulations concerning storage and dispensing of controlled substances, such as specifying the number of locks on narcotic storage in hospitals, the number of persons who may have access to these areas, the type of information required on drug records, and which drugs must be "signed out." The state also regulates the frequency of inspection of institutions.

State law also determines who may legally prescribe medications. The state practice act governing the particular profession specifies the minimum educational and licensure requirements of its members. For example, physicians and dentists may legally write prescriptions for medications for humans. Veterinarians may write certain types of prescriptions for use in animals. Other specialists may have specific limited privileges. Some states permit nurse practitioners to write prescriptions for antibiotics, cold and allergy medications, and others. Podiatrists may write prescriptions to treat conditions of the feet only.

Local Controls

Local governments frequently have ordinances or laws governing the sale of tobacco and alcohol. For example, in some states, liquor is purchased only in a store that sells liquor exclusively. In other states, beer and wine may be purchased at a gas station or grocery store. Some states sell liquor every day, and others forbid sale on Sunday.

Table 4–2. Classification Schedules of Controlled Substances

	I OR C-I	II OR C-II	III OR C-III	IV OR C-IV	V OR C-V
Potential for abuse	High	High	High but less than I or II	Low	Low compared with IV
Accepted medical use in the United States	None (research only)	Accepted	Accepted	Accepted	Accepted
Safety	Lack of accepted safety	May lead to severe psychological and physical dependence	May lead to moderate or low psychological and physical dependence	Limited psychological or physical dependence compared with III	Limited psychological and physical abuse compared with IV
Examples	Lysergic acid diethylamide (LSD), marijuana, peyote, heroin, hashish	Some barbiturates, amphetamines, morphine, meperidine, methadone, oxycodone hydrochloride, codeine	Opium, tinctures, glutethimide, thiopental sodium	Phenobarbital, chloral hydrate, diazepam, alprazolam, hydroxyzine hydrochloride	Antitussives and antidiarrheals with codeine, diphenoxylate hydrochloride with atropine sulfate

Institution Controls

Institutions establish controls or policies regarding what they believe to be safety practices within their institution. These often concern renewal of orders, standing orders, and dispensing methods for drugs. All policies must conform with international, federal, state, and local regulations.

Individual Controls

Individual controls originate from personal beliefs of the physician, the patient, and the patient's family. They may relate to religious beliefs or beliefs about personal health and nutrition. They are the final control that determines whether a patient will take a drug and whether it will be taken appropriately.

For example, some individuals believe that alcohol use is unacceptable; others find no problem with social use or even use for medicinal purposes. There are also those who seek medical advice but then rely on religious beliefs and prayer to heal the body or mind. Some patients believe and trust in their physician and follow all medical advice in detail and without question. Others evaluate what they are told and make decisions as to the merits of a particular regimen. They may obtain their prescriptions but never take the medicine.

LABELING REGULATIONS

Manufacturers are required to include certain information on the package, the insert or brochure, or the label. The name and business address of the manufacturer and the lot number of the drug batch must be included in the event that someone needs to make contact regarding the product or a specific batch of the product. The label must designate the official name or the generic name of all drugs contained in the product. The kind and proportion of specific ingredients must be included. All information must be accurate and not false or misleading in any manner. Recommended dosages and frequency of use must be clearly stated. The product must be safe for use when recommendations are followed. Specific directions for use, contraindications, and special warnings for children and persons with certain disease conditions must be included. If the drug is unsafe for self-medication, the label must state **"Caution: Federal law prohibits dispensing without a prescription."** If the drug is habit forming, a warning to this effect is also mandated.

Federal regulations require that labels on individual prescription bottles include the name, address, and telephone number of the pharmacy filling the prescription. This is usually preprinted on a label. Additional information is usually typed on the label to avoid any possible error in interpreting a handwritten message. This information includes the prescription number; the name of the person for whom it is prescribed; specific directions as to the number of pills, tablets, or capsules that are to be taken as one "dose"; and the number of times per day the dose is to be taken. The route of administration is included on the label. The name of the drug is listed as ordered by the physician. If a generic drug is substituted, the label must state so and give the generic name of the drug. The date filled, the pharmacist's initials or name, and the number of refills allowed must be on the label. The physician's name and, if the drug is a controlled substance, the physician's DEA number are listed. In addition, specific precautions are included, such as "Do not take with food," or "Take with food or milk," or "Avoid consumption of alcohol when taking this medication." State regulations may also require other information, such as the lot number or expiration date of the drug and the name of the manufacturer.

E X E R C I S E S

LEARNING ACTIVITIES

1. Using the classification schedules of controlled substances, identify additional drugs for each classification.

2. If you have begun clinical nursing experience, review your patient's medications for those that are controlled substances. Identify the schedule to which the drug belongs. Also list the drug classification to which it belongs and explain the reason for administration to your patient.

THE MEDICATION ORDER AND RECORD

LEARNING OBJECTIVES

After studying this chapter, you should be able to:

1. List the types of medication orders.

2. Interpret a prescription or order.

3. State legal requirements for a medication order.

4. Identify dosage strength in an order.

5. Identify dosage form in an order.

6. Differentiate total volume of the container from dosage strength in an order.

MEDICATION ORDERS

A physician can order medications in many different ways: by written orders, verbal orders, prescriptions, standing orders, stat orders, and single orders.

Written Orders

In an institution, the most common way for the physician to order medications is with a written order. It is considered to be the safest method because there is less chance for misunderstanding, as long as the order is written legibly and care is taken in reading it.

The physician writes the name of the drug to be given (either generic or trade name), the dosage to be given, the route to be used, and the frequency of administration. For example, an order may read

Lasix 40 mg PO bid

This order means the nurse is to administer 40 milligrams of the drug Lasix by mouth twice a day. Another example is

Demerol 50 mg IM q4h prn

This order means the nurse is to administer 50 milligrams of the drug Demerol by intramuscular injection every 4 hours as needed.

As you can see, many abbreviations are commonly used in writing medication orders. The nurse must be able to interpret these abbreviations easily. A listing of common abbreviations used in drug administration appears in Table 5–1.

Once an order has been written, the nurse or the medical secretary must transcribe the order onto worksheets used by the administering nurse. We discuss types of these worksheets in the Medication Records section of this chapter.

NURSING ALERT

Errors are easily made during transcription. To prevent these errors before the medication goes to the patient, several safeguards are used. The person transcribing the order should not be interrupted and should check the work three times. The transcription should be checked again by another person before it goes to the administering nurse. The administering nurse is responsible for checking medication orders before the drug is given.

Verbal Orders

At times, it is necessary for a physician to give an order verbally without writing it down immediately. Examples include emergency or stat drugs and telephone orders. Because of the greater possibility of error due to misunderstanding of a verbal order, many

Table 5–1. Abbreviations Used with Drug Administration

āā	of each
Abd	abdomen
a.c.	before meals
amt	amount
aq	aqueous (water, solution)
ax	axillary
bid	twice a day
BP	blood pressure
C.	Celsius
c̄	with
cap	capsule
cc	cubic centimeter
DC or dc	discontinue
dr	dram
elix	elixir
et	and
F.	Fahrenheit
Fe	iron
GI	gastrointestinal
Gm, gm, g, or G	gram

Table 5–1. Abbreviations Used with Drug Administration *Continued*

gr	grain
gtt, gtts	drops or drops
GU	genitourinary
H_2O	water
hs	hour of sleep (at bedtime)
hypo	hypodermic injection
ID	intradermal
I & O	intake and output measurement
IM	intramuscular injection
irrig	irrigation
IV	intravenous
L	liter
LLQ	left lower quadrant
LUQ	left upper quadrant
m	minims
M or m	meter
NPO	nothing by mouth
NS	normal saline
O.D.	right eye
O.S.	left eye

Table continued on following page

Table 5-1. Abbreviations Used with Drug Administration *Continued*

os	mouth
O.U.	both eyes
P	pulse
p.c.	after meals
prn	as needed
pt	patient or pint
qd	every day
qh	every hour
qid	every 4 hours
qod	every other day
q2h	every 2 hours (different numbers can be inserted)
R	respirations
RLQ	right lower quadrant
RUQ	right upper quadrant
Rx	prescription (take thou)
s̄	without
SC or SQ	subcutaneous
SL	sublingual
s̄s̄	one half
spec	specimen

Table 5-1. Abbreviations Used with Drug Administration *Continued*

SS	soap suds
stat	immediately (implies emergency)
T	temperature
tab	tablet
tbsp	tablespoon
tsp	teaspoon
tid	three times a day
tr or tinct	tincture
wt	weight

facilities do not allow verbal orders except in emergencies. The physician must then write the order as soon as possible, within at least 24 hours.

N U R S I N G   A L E R T
▼▼▼▼▼▼▼▼▼▼▼▼▼▼▼▼▼▼▼▼▼▼▼▼▼▼▼▼▼▼

If you are given a verbal order, always repeat the order back to the physician slowly to be sure you have understood. Ask for confirmation that you have repeated the order correctly.

▲▲▲▲▲▲▲▲▲▲▲▲▲▲▲▲▲▲▲▲▲▲▲▲▲▲▲▲▲▲

The nurse often needs to write the order on the proper form in the patient's chart. To indicate that this was a verbal order, it should be written as follows:

Demerol 50 mg IM now and q4h prn.
V.O. Dr. John Smith/A. Wright, LPN.

This type of notation indicates that the order was given verbally (V.O. = verbal order), names the physician who gave the order, and names the nurse who received the order. The physician must then cosign the order, indicating that this is indeed the order as it was given.

Prescriptions

Prescriptions are given often in the office setting and on discharge from a facility. In the broader definition of the term, any prescribed medication comes in the form of a prescription, but the common use of the word refers to a slip of paper on which the physician's order is written.

Prescriptions are often preprinted and made into a tear-off pad. The physician needs to fill in only the essential elements of the order. A prescription order must contain four parts to be accurately filled by a pharmacist:

1. Superscription, which is simply the ℞ appearing at the beginning of every prescription. This is an abbreviation for recipe or *recipere,* which stands for "take thou."

2. Inscription. This line contains the name of the drug, the dosage strength, and the drug form.

3. Subscription. This line begins with either the symbol # or with N, which stands for number. Following is the number of tablets, milliliters, or other appropriate directions to the pharmacist explaining the amount to be dispensed.

4. Signature, beginning with the abbreviation Sig. The signature is actually a line containing directions to the patient about how to use the medication. For example, the physician may write "take one tablet three times a day." However, the physician generally uses appropriate abbreviations, which may be interpreted for the patient by the pharmacist.

The prescription is then signed by the physician. In addition, the physician's DEA number needs to appear on the form. The Drug Enforcement Agency (DEA) assigns a number to each physician as a control device for prescription drugs. The patient's name, address, and possibly age are also written on the form. The prescription must be dated. Prescriptions cannot be refilled after 1 year even if refills remain on the bottle.

Many prescriptions have extra features for convenience. For example, there may be a box, which the physician need only check to indicate the number of refills allowed. A preprinted line may state "Dispense as written," which prevents the pharmacist from filling the prescription with generic drugs. The physician's name and address may also be preprinted on the pad.

N U R S I N G   A L E R T
▼▼▼▼▼▼▼▼▼▼▼▼▼▼▼▼▼▼▼▼▼▼▼▼▼▼▼▼▼▼▼▼▼▼▼▼

Nurses are not permitted to fill prescriptions and in most states cannot write prescriptions of any type.

▲▲▲▲▲▲▲▲▲▲▲▲▲▲▲▲▲▲▲▲▲▲▲▲▲▲▲▲▲▲▲▲▲▲▲▲

The nurse can, however, ensure that the patient knows all pertinent information about the prescribed medications, that the patient has transportation to a pharmacy or someone to pick up the prescription, and that the patient has the financial means to obtain the medication.

Standing Orders

Standing orders are prewritten and signed by the physician to be used by the nurse when needed. These are generally orders that apply to all patients universally. For example, the physician may order a mild analgesic such as acetaminophen for patients who complain of a headache while in the facility.

Standing orders can be useful, eliminating the need to call the physician for every problem. They are a convenience for both the physician and the nurse. However, standing orders can be dangerous if the nurse applies them to patients who have a contraindication for a particular medication. For example, acetaminophen is usually not used for patients with liver dysfunction. To prevent this problem, many facilities do not allow standing orders. If your facility does permit them, be sure to consult a standard drug reference about the medication, even if you believe it to be a mild drug.

In another form of standing orders, a medication is ordered to be given at a particular time interval until it is specifically discontinued. For example, the physician may order Demerol 25 mg IM q4h prn. This means the nurse is to continue giving the drug as it is needed until it is discontinued. To prevent some particularly dangerous drugs from being continued because they were forgotten, some facilities place restrictions on medications. Commonly, narcotics must be specifically reordered every 1, 2, or 3 days or they are automatically discontinued. Antibiotics are generally discontinued automatically after 5 or 10 days. If a patient goes to surgery, all of the medications must be reordered after surgery. Anticoagulants must often be ordered one dose at a time. As the nurse responsible for drug administration, you must be familiar with your facility's policies.

Stat and Single Orders

Stat and single orders are similar in that they are given on a one-time only basis. However, the stat order relates to the nurse that the dosage must be given immediately and implies some urgency. Types of medications that may be ordered in single dosages include anticoagulants, analgesics, some anthelmintics (medications given for some types of worms), preoperative medications, and others. Stat orders may be for any type of drug needed in an emergency: anticonvulsants, antiarrhythmics, antianginals, anti-asthmatics, and many more.

COMPONENTS OF MEDICATION ORDERS

All orders, no matter in what form they are given, must contain the same vital elements. The order must list the name of the patient, the name and signature of the physician, the date ordered and possibly the date to be discontinued, the name of the drug, the dosage strength, the dosage form, the amount to be given at each dose, the time interval between dosages, and the route of administration. If there are special instructions for the patient or the nurse, these must also appear in the order.

MEDICATION RECORDS

There are two main ways to organize the administration and recording of medications: the drug card method and the drug administration record method.

The Card Method

In this method, the order is transcribed onto small cards, one card for each medication. Once transcribed, the cards are placed in special slots according to the predetermined administration times. For example, all drugs to be given at 8 AM are together, all 9 AM drugs are together, and so on, regardless of the patient who will receive them. In this way, a single nurse can be responsible for administering medications to several patients. The nurse must be careful, however, to read the name on each card to prevent giving drugs to the wrong patient.

When using the card method, the nurse can take the individual cards into the patient's room when administering drugs. The card can be consulted before the drug is given. After administration, the card is put into a special slot for medications that have already been given. The nurse must then record the administration of the drug on a separate sheet.

The Drug Administration Record Method

The drug administration record (DAR) is a form that lists all the medications for a single patient regardless

of the time the drug is to be given. All of the patient's medications have been transcribed onto the DAR. If the transcriber runs out of space for the medications on one DAR, a second is used, but both forms must clearly state the existence of the other. The DAR provides the nurse with a quick overview of all the patient's medications, allowing easier reference for drug interactions. The nurse must carefully read the time listed on the DAR to prevent giving a medication at the wrong time.

The nurse may take the DAR into the patient's room to refer to before administering the drug. Recording of the administration of the drug is usually done directly on the DAR. The nurse initials the time at which the drug was given and signs the DAR at a designated place. For medications given prn, the time of administration must also be written in.

E X E R C I S E S

CASE STUDIES

1. A physician orders a drug to be given immediately. What type of order is this? What abbreviation would the nurse expect to see in the order?

2. A drug is ordered to be given q6h prn. When would you give the next dose if it is given at 12 noon?

3. What is missing from the following order: erythromycin 250 mg q8h?

MENTAL AEROBICS

1. Observe a nurse administering medications to several patients in the hospital or nursing home. Note the process used for transcription. How often did the nurse check the orders? What method of drug recording was used?

2. Observe a nurse administering medications at a physician's office. How did the nurse obtain the drug order? What method of drug recording was used? What other differences did you note between administration of drugs at a care facility and administration at the physician's office? Look closely for prescriptions given to patients at both facilities so you can become familiar with this type of drug order as well.

CHAPTER 6

DOSAGE CALCULATION

LEARNING OBJECTIVES

After studying this chapter, you should be able to:

1. Solve problems using common fractions.

2. Find the percentage of a given quantity.

3. Solve problems using proportions.

4. Read and write Roman numerals correctly.

5. Define metric terms of measurement.

6. Define terms used in metric, apothecary, and household measures.

7. Convert measurements of weight and volume in metric, apothecary, and household systems.

8. Calculate intravenous (IV) flow rates.

When determining the dosage to give a patient, the physician considers many factors. This chapter explores several of these factors and the mathematics and systems of measurement the nurse must use to correctly administer drugs.

FACTORS OF DRUG DOSAGES

Although drugs are used in our bodies in the same way, not all drugs are used at the same rate by different people. Absorption, distribution, biotransformation, and excretion are affected by many factors.

The person's age is a major factor. As we age, our body systems do not function at the same level of efficiency as they once did. When we are infants, our body systems have not yet begun functioning at top form. The age factor is more fully explored in Chapter 11.

Weight is another factor that alters the amount of drug needed to achieve the same effect. The larger the body, the more dilute the drug will be. Therefore, the physician needs to order larger dosages for larger people. In addition, many drugs bind with the fat in a body. The higher the body fat content, the more the drug will bind in the body. This leaves less free drug in the system to perform its actions.

The sex of the patient also alters the rate at which drugs are used. In general, men have larger body mass than women do. In addition, the metabolism rates of men and women are different. Compare the normal rates of the heart for men and women. You will see that men usually have a slower pulse. This alone will alter the use of a drug.

If a patient has a disease process other than the one being treated, this, too, can alter the body's use of medications. Some diseases affecting the heart, blood vessels, liver, kidney, or bowel affect different parts of the pharmacokinetics of drugs.

If a patient is receiving additional drugs, these can alter the dosage needed for *both* medications. The physician needs to consider the possibility of drug interactions, additive effects, synergism or potentiation, and antagonism effects of the multiple drugs.

Food alters the pharmacokinetics of drugs. Some foods hasten the rate of use, while others slow the rate. For example, tetracycline antibiotics are absorbed less efficiently by the body if the person drinks or eats dairy products while taking this drug.

The route chosen also determines what dosage is ordered. In general, doses of drugs administered orally are larger than injectable drug doses. Intravenous drugs are given at the lowest dosage.

Some persons will simply respond to a drug differently from most other people. For this person, it may be necessary to give a dose that is higher or lower than the customary amount. This is unusual, however, and the physician can simply choose to order a different drug instead.

SYSTEMS OF MEASUREMENT

Several systems of measurement are used in ordering medications. Because of this, you must be familiar with each system of measurement and the methods for converting from one system to another. Conversion is necessary when the drug is ordered in units of one system, but the drug is provided from the pharmacy in units of another system.

Metric System

The metric system is becoming the most commonly used system of measurement. It is a simple system based on a factor of 10 and is widely recognized around the world, making communication with other caregivers more accurate.

The basic units of measurement in the metric system are the gram, the meter, and the liter. The gram is used to measure the weight of dry substances, the meter is used to measure length, and the liter is used to measure liquids.

The metric system can be seen as a scale, starting in the middle at zero and reaching in both directions, both smaller and larger. The nomenclature of the weights and measures is as follows:

kilo = one thousand

hecto = one hundred

deca = ten

gram, meter, or liter = one

deci = one tenth

centi = one hundredth

milli = one thousandth

micro = one millionth

Therefore, the metric system of weight measurement includes kilograms, hectograms, decagrams, grams, decigrams, centigrams, milligrams, and micrograms. The metric system of liquid measure includes kiloliters, hectoliters, decaliters, liters, deciliters, centiliters, milliliters, and microliters. One additional unit of measurement is the cubic centimeter (cc). It is equal to the milliliter. The metric system of length measurement includes kilometers, hectometers, decameters, meters, decimeters, centimeters, millimeters, and micrometers.

As a nurse, you will primarily be using kilograms, grams, and milligrams for weight; kilometers, meters, centimeters, and millimeters for length; and kiloliters, liters, and milliliters for liquids. This

Table 6–1. Numerical Expression of the Metric System

NAME	NUMERICAL EXPRESSION
Kilo- (gram, liter, meter)	1000
Gram, liter, or meter	1
Centi- (gram, meter)	0.01
Milli- (gram, liter, meter)	0.001

decreases the number of equivalences you must learn. You also need to know the abbreviations for these units. See Appendix B for abbreviations of all the units of measurement.

When converting from one measurement within the system to another, use the prefixes to help you remember the size of the unit. A kilometer, for example, is 1000 meters. A centimeter is one hundredth of a meter. A millimeter is one thousandth of a meter.

There are 1000 liters in 1 kiloliter. There are 1000 milliliters in 1 liter. A gram is larger than a milligram by 1000-fold, but there are 1000 grams in a kilogram.

Because the metric system is based on 10, the measures can be expressed decimally (Table 6–1). To convert, you need only move the decimal point the appropriate number of spaces. For example, if a drug is supplied in 500-mg tablets, how many grams is this? Because milligrams are three decimal places from zero, you need to move the decimal point three spaces. But what direction? You must determine whether milligrams are larger or smaller than grams. By looking at Table 6–1, you can see it is smaller. Therefore, your answer will be a number that is smaller than the original. So the answer here is 0.500 g or, much simpler, 0.5 g.

Let's try another one. Your order involves 2.5 kL. You need to know how many liters this is. You must move the decimal point three spaces, but this time the number in your answer should be larger. Therefore, the answer is 2500 L.

Household Measurements

The household system of measurement is an imprecise method of measurement. Therefore, many physicians are changing the way they prescribe medications. However, you may still see some of the more common units used in medication orders.

The household system uses teaspoons, tablespoons, drops, fluid ounces, cups, pints, quarts, and gallons to measure liquid:

There are 60 drops in 1 teaspoon.

There are 3 teaspoons in 1 tablespoon.

2 tablespoons equal 1 fluid ounce.

16 tablespoons or 8 fluid ounces are in 1 cup of liquid.

There are 2 cups in 1 pint, 2 pints in 1 quart, and 4 quarts in 1 gallon.

Pounds and ounces measure weight. There are 16 ounces to a pound. These ounces are sometimes called avoirdupois ounces to differentiate them from fluid ounces.

Inches, feet, and yards are measures of length. There are 12 inches in a foot and 3 feet in a yard.

Apothecary System

An apothecary is a pharmacist. Therefore, the apothecary system is the method of measurement that was once used widely by pharmacists to measure medications. It has gradually been replaced by the metric system, but you may still see some of the more common units used in medication orders. The units most often used include the grain, dram, fluid dram, and minim.

In liquid measure, there are 60 minims in a fluid dram. For measuring weight, there are 60 grains in a dram. Other units of measurement in the apothecary system are generally no longer used for medications.

ROMAN NUMERALS In the apothecary system, Roman numerals are used after the name of the unit of measurement. Roman numerals you should become familiar with include

I	1
V	5
X	10
L	50
C	100
D	500
M	1000

Only these symbols are used to make all numbers. You must remember the following rules to make other numbers:

1. When you wish to add value to a number, add the appropriate symbol or symbols to the right of that Roman numeral. For example, VI is 5 + 1 or 6.

2. When you wish to decrease the value of a number, place the appropriate symbol to the left of that Roman numeral. For example, IV is 5 − 1 or 4.

3. Never add more than one symbol to the left. For example, IX is 9. To make 8, you must add to the right, VIII.

When indicating the amount of an apothecary unit, the Roman numerals are used in lowercase. Therefore, if 6 grains of a medication are ordered, it is written "grains vi." If the amount wanted is less than 1, this is written by use of a fraction and not decimals, as was the case in the metric system. Examples are drams 1/2, grains 1/100.

CONVERSION METHODS

As you might expect, there will be times when you need to convert from one system of measurement to another. This requires you to know the equivalencies listed in Appendix A. Once you know these equivalencies, you then need to know what formula to use to convert the ordered medication.

Ratio-Proportion

To fully use all methods of measurement, you must know how to convert one measurement to another by using mathematical equations. These equations are made up of different parts. The first part is called a ratio.

A ratio is a pair of numbers that indicate a relationship between two items. For example, if there are 3 male patients and 1 female patient in intensive care, then we could say that the ratio of males to females is 3:1. In pharmacology, if there are 50 m in 1 cc of liquid, then we can write the ratio as 50:1.

See whether you can determine the following ratios:

a. There are 5 cats sold in a pet store for every dog.
b. There are 5 m of medicine in 2 cc of liquid.
c. 37 of every 100 men wore a blue tie.
d. There are 2.2 pounds in every kilogram.

The answers to these problems are (a) 5:1; (b) 5:2; (c) 37:100; (d) 2.2:1.

The next part of the mathematical equations you will be using for medications is called a proportion. A proportion represents a relationship between two ratios. The ratios are equal. For example, if you want to double a cookie recipe, you would use a proportion. If there are supposed to be 2 cups of sugar in 1 batch of cookies, then there will be 4 cups of sugar in 2 batches of cookies. The proportion can be written 2:1 as 4:2. This is read "2 is to 1 as 4 is to 2." Often, you see the symbol :: used to represent as. Therefore, the proportion will look like 2:1 :: 4:2. Another example is the gasoline and oil mixture needed for two-cycle engines such as lawnmowers. If you need to add 1 ounce of oil to a quart of gasoline, then you would need to add 4 ounces of oil to a gallon (or 4 quarts) of gasoline. The proportion would look like 1:1 :: 4:4.

It is also possible to write a ratio or proportion by using a line under the first number and third number, such as

$$\frac{2}{1} \sim \frac{4}{2}$$

This is read the same as previously, 2 is to 1 as 4 is to 2. Here, the symbol for as is ~.

It follows that if you know three of the numbers of a proportion, you can mathematically determine the fourth. In many of the examples, you were probably able to do this "in your head" without realizing what equation you were using to arrive at the answer. Let's take one of these easier problems to work through an equation. Don't get frustrated because you already know the answer. We will be using numbers soon that you won't be able to work out "in your head."

Let's take the problem 2:1 :: 4:2, but we don't know what number is in the place where 4 will appear:

$$2:1 :: x:2$$

We use x to indicate a number we do not yet know. To calculate this problem, you must identify the "means" and the "extremes." The means of the equation are the inner two numbers, in this case, 1 and x. The extremes of the equation are the outer two numbers, in this case, 2 and 2. See whether you can identify the means and extremes of the following equations:

a. 5:10 :: 25:x
b. 14:7 :: x:49
c. 50:1 :: 75:x

The answers to these equations are (a) means, 10 and 25; extremes, 5 and x; (b) means, 7 and x; extremes, 14 and 49; (c) means, 1 and 75; extremes, 50 and x.

In a proportion, when you multiply the means together and multiply the extremes together, the answers are equal. Let's try it. Remember our problem, 2:1 :: 4:2. Multiply the means together, and you will find $1 \times 4 = 4$. Multiply the extremes together, and you will find $2 \times 2 = 4$. The answers are equal. As long as the ratios are equal, the products of the means and the extremes are equal.

How does this help us when we don't know one of the numbers? Let's use our same problem, 2:1 :: x:2. Multiply the means and you will find 1(x). Multiply the extremes and you will find 2×2. This can be expressed as

$$1(x) = 2 \times 2$$

We then satisfy as much of the problem as we can. Therefore, it can be expressed as 1(x) = 4. In this case, it is easy to see that the answer is going to be 4, but it won't be that easy in many problems. You will need to divide the product of the extremes by the number qualifying x. So that the value of the proportion is not changed, you must divide both sides of the equation equally. In this case, it is written

$$\frac{1(x)}{1} = \frac{4}{1}$$

or 1 divided by 1 multiplied by x is equal to 4 divided by 1. Once you calculate both division problems, your answer will read 1x or just x = 4.

Now that we worked through a simple problem to establish the rules, let's try something a little more difficult.

$$14:7 :: x:49$$

The first step is to multiply the means and the extremes and write them as equalities.

$$7(x) = 14 \times 49$$

The next step is to satisfy as much of the equation as you can. Because 14 times 49 equals 686,

$$7(x) = 686$$

The next step is to divide both sides of the equation by a number that leaves only a single x on the one side, in this case, 7.

$$\frac{7x}{7} = \frac{686}{7}$$

Because 7 divided by 7 equals 1, and 686 divided by 7 equals 98, the answer is

$$x = 98$$

Just to test this out, why don't you put the answer back into the proportion and see whether it is correct?

Let's try a pharmacology problem. The physician has ordered 90 mg of a medication. It has been supplied to you by the pharmacy in a liquid at a ratio of 3 m in every 2 mL. How many milliliters will you need to give the patient?

We find two ratios in the problem, and they have to equal each other. The first is 3 mg:2 mL, and the second is 90 mg:x mL. Therefore, the problem is

$$3:2 :: 90:x$$

$$2 \times 90 = 3(x)$$

$$180 = 3(x)$$

$$\frac{180}{3} = \frac{3(x)}{3}$$

$$60 = x$$

So you will give the patient 60 mL. In case you forgot whether the answer was in milliliters or milligrams, look back at the original problem. Which did we not yet know then? It was milliliters.

Try a few more on your own:

a. The physician orders 75 mg of medication. It is supplied as 50 mg in every milliliter. How many milliliters will you give?
b. The order reads to give 180 mg. The medication is supplied as 90 mg in every 5 mL. How many milliliters will you give?
c. The order reads to give 1000 mg. The medication is supplied as 250 mg per tablet. How many tablets will you give?

The answers to these problems are (a) 1.5 mL; (b) 10 mL; (c) 4 tablets.

Using ratios and proportions helps you convert from one system of measurement to another. When you need to do this, the appropriate equivalency that you have learned will be one of the ratios you use in the equation. The other ratio will be your unknown. See whether you can decide which equivalency to use for each of the following, and then write the equation.

a. The physician ordered 10 mg of a medication. It is supplied in grains. How many grains should you give?
b. The physician ordered 5 ounces of a liquid nutritional supplement. The supplement is supplied in cc. How many cc should you give?
c. Your drug reference book states a medication should be given at 30 mg per kilogram of body weight. Your patient's body weight is listed in pounds at 135. How many kilograms does your patient weigh? How many milligrams should the patient receive?
d. The physician orders a medication in teaspoons. The medication is supplied in milliliters. If the order is for 2.5 teaspoons, how many milliliters should you give?

Answers:

a. 60 mg:1 gr :: 10 mg:x gr
$$1 \times 10 = 60x$$
$$10 = 60x$$
$$\frac{10}{60} = \frac{60x}{60}$$
$$\frac{10}{60} = x$$
$$\frac{1}{6} = x$$

Did you remember grains are in fractions and not decimal points?

b. 5 oz:x cc :: 1 oz:30 cc
$$1x = 5 \times 30$$
$$x = 150 \text{ cc}$$
c. 2.2 lb:1 kg :: 135 lb:x kg
$$1 \times 135 = 2.2x$$
$$135 = 2.2x$$
$$\frac{135}{2.2} = \frac{2.2x}{2.2}$$
$$61.4 = x$$
$$30 \text{ mg} \times 61.4 \text{ kg} = x \text{ mg}$$
$$1842 \text{ mg} = x$$
d. 1 tsp:5 mL :: 2.5 tsp:x mL
$$5 \times 2.5 = 1x$$
$$12.5 = x$$

FRACTIONS AND DECIMALS

Because many medications are ordered or supplied in terms of fractions and decimals, you must be familiar with mathematical rules applying to these.

Fractions

When adding fractions, check first to see whether the bottom number (denominator) is the same. If it is, then you need only add the two top numbers (numerators) to achieve the answer. For example:

a. $\dfrac{1}{2} + \dfrac{3}{2}$

b. $\dfrac{5}{8} + \dfrac{7}{8}$

The answers are (a) 4/2; (b) 12/8.

Whenever the numerator is a higher number than the denominator, you can reduce the fraction to a more readily understood number. You do this by dividing the denominator into the numerator. Therefore, answer (a) becomes 2 and answer (b) becomes 1 and 4/8.

If both the numerator and the denominator can be divided by the same number evenly, then the fraction can be reduced again. This time, we see that 4 and 8 can both be divided by 2 evenly. Therefore, answer (b) becomes 1 and 1/2.

If the denominators of two fractions you wish to add are not the same, then you must determine a "common denominator." This means you must find two fractions that have the same denominator and then add them.

To find the common denominator, a simple method is to multiply the two denominators together. Then the numerators must be altered so they represent fractions that are equal in value to the original fractions. This can be achieved by multiplying each numerator by the same number as the denominator below it was multiplied by.

Let's look at an example. You want to add 1/2 and 2/3. To determine a common denominator, multiply the denominators together: $2 \times 3 = 6$. To determine a fraction equal to the original for 1/2, multiply the numerator (1) by the same number you had to use to change 2 into a 6. This number was 3. So we see that 1/2 is equal in value to 3/6. A fraction that is equal to 2/3 using our common denominator is found by multiplying 2 by the same number you had to use to change the 3 into a 6. This number was 2. So 2/3 is equal in value to 4/6. Now our problem has changed to $3/6 + 4/6$. With equal denominators, it is a simple matter to add $3 + 4$ and find our answer is 7/6. Reduce the fraction, and the answer is now 1 and 1/6.

Try the following addition problems:

a. $5/8 + 9/5$
b. $3/4 + 7/9$
c. $3/100 + 5/75$

The answers to these are (a) 97/40 or 2 and 17/40; (b) 55/36 or 1 and 19/36; (c) 725/7500 or 29/300.

If you need to subtract fractions, check first to see whether the denominators are the same. If they are, then simply subtract the numerators. If they are not, then you must find a common denominator and determine fractions of equal value to the original fractions. Then you can subtract the numerators. Try the following:

a. $7/10 - 3/8$
b. $3/4 - 1/4$
c. $7/100 - 1/25$

The answers to these are (a) 26/80 or 13/40; (b) 2/4 or 1/2; (c) 75/2500 or 3/100.

If you want to multiply two fractions, you need to multiply the two numerators together and then the two denominators together. Try these:

a. $2/4 \times 7/8$
b. $5/9 \times 98$
c. $7/100 \times 50$

The answers to these are (a) 14/32 or 7/16; (b) 490/9 or 54 and 4/9 (Did you remember that all whole numbers have a denominator of 1?); (c) 350/100 or 3 and 1/2.

When you want to divide fractions, you must invert the second fraction and then proceed by multiplying. For example,

$$\frac{1}{2} \div \frac{3}{8}$$

Invert the second fraction to 8/3, then multiply the two fractions:

$$\tfrac{1}{2} \times \tfrac{8}{3} = \tfrac{8}{6} \text{ or } 1\tfrac{1}{3}$$

Try these division problems:

a. 7/8 divided by 3/5
b. 1/100 divided by 60
c. 1/2 divided by 7/50

The answers are (a) 35/24 or 1 and 11/24; (b) 1/6000; (c) 50/14 or 3 and 4/7.

Fractions can be handled in a ratio-proportion problem by applying the mathematical rules. Try the following problems.

a. The physician ordered gr 1/2 of a medication. It is supplied in milligrams. How many milligrams should you give the patient?
b. The physician ordered gr 1/100 of a medication. It is supplied in a vial marked 2.5 mg per 5 mL. How much should you give the patient?
c. The physician ordered 12 1/2 ounces of liquid nutritional supplement. The supplement is supplied in cc. How many cc should you give?

Answers:

a. 60 mg:1 gr :: x mg:gr 1/2
$$60 \times 1/2 = 1x$$
$$30 = x$$
b. 60 mg:1 gr :: x mg:gr 1/1000
$$60 \times 1/100 = 1x$$
$$0.6 \text{ mg} = x$$

Did you remember milligrams use decimals and not fractions?

0.6 mg:x mL :: 2.5 mg:5 mL
$$0.6 \times 5 = 2.5x$$
$$3.0 = 2.5x$$

$$\frac{3.0}{2.5} = \frac{2.5x}{2.5}$$
$$1.2 = x$$

c. 12 1/2 oz:x cc :: 1 oz:30 cc
$$12\ 1/2 \times 30 = 1x$$
$$375 = x$$

Decimals

When you must use decimals to obtain a correct medication dosage, use the following rules.

If you need to add two decimals together, remember to keep the decimal points aligned. If the two numbers do not have the same number of decimal places, you can add zeroes to the right of the last decimal place until they do. For example,

$$\begin{array}{r} 3.75 \\ + \ 4.5 \\ \hline \end{array}$$

Add a zero to the right of the 5. Now the problem is

$$\begin{array}{r} 3.75 \\ + \ 4.50 \\ \hline 8.25 \end{array}$$

Subtraction of decimals is done in the same way.

If you need to multiply numbers that have decimal places, you do not need to align the decimal points. Simply multiply the two numbers as though the decimal points were not there. When you have achieved the answer, count how many *total* decimal places are in the original numbers. Mark your decimal point in the answer the same number of places to the left of the last digit.

Try these:

a. 6.7×5
b. 8.95×2.1
c. 127.32×8.666

Answers:

a.
$$\begin{array}{r} 6.7 \\ 5 \\ \hline 33.5 \end{array}$$

There is one decimal place in the original numbers, so the decimal point in the answer is one space to the left of the last digit.

b.
$$\begin{array}{r} 8.95 \\ 2.1 \\ \hline 18.795 \end{array}$$

c.
$$\begin{array}{r} 127.32 \\ 8.666 \\ \hline 1103.35510 \end{array}$$

It is unnecessary to keep zeroes at the end of a decimal number, so this answer becomes 1103.3551.

When you divide decimal numbers, you need to eliminate the decimal point from the divisor (the number you are dividing by). To do this, though, you need to move the decimal point in the dividend (the number you are to divide) the same number of spaces. If necessary, add zeroes to the right of the decimal.

Try the following:

a. 5 divided by 1.25
b. 6 divided by 2.2
c. 3.8 divided by 1.2
d. 12.575 divided by 5.5

Answers:

a. $1.25\overline{)5.00}$ $125\overline{)500}$ $125\overline{)500}^{\ 4}$

b. $2.2\overline{)6.0}$ $22\overline{)60}$ $22\overline{)60.00}^{\ 2.73}$

c. $1.2\overline{)3.8}$ $12\overline{)38}$ $12\overline{)38.00}^{\ 3.17}$

d. $5.5\overline{)12.575}$ $55\overline{)125.75}$ $55\overline{)125.75}^{\ 2.286}$

Decimal numbers are used often in medications. Ask your supervisor or consult the hospital policy book to determine directions for rounding off.

PERCENTAGES

The term percent is often written by the symbol %. To indicate a certain percentage of something is to indicate a certain number of parts of the whole item. One hundred percent (100%) of an item is the entire item. Ten percent (10%) of the item is 10 parts of the 100 parts that make up the whole item. Fifty percent (50%) is 50 parts of the 100 parts that make up the whole item.

Percentages can be written with the % sign, or they can be changed to fractions. Recall that in fractions, the number written above the line is called the numerator, and the number written below the line is called the denominator. If a typewriter or computer is used to write the fraction, a slant line is used; the numerator (N) is the number to the left of the line, and the denominator (D) is the number to the right of the line (N/D). The denominator indicates the number of parts into which a whole item has been divided. For example, if a whole item is divided into 10 parts, the fraction indicating this would be 10/10. We said previously that the % sign indicates that the item is divided into 100 parts; therefore, in changing a percentage to a fraction, the denominator is 100. For example, 10% is changed to 10/100, 50% is changed to 50/100.

In pharmacology, percentages are used to indicate the strength of a solution. Again, 100% indicates the whole or "full-strength" solution; therefore, a 10% solution is 10 of 100 parts of the solution. A 50% solution is 50 of 100 parts of the solution.

To find the percentage of a solution, the following formula can be used in a fractional equation or in a ratio-proportion problem:

D = desired percentage

H = parts "on hand" (which is 100)

V = volume desired (total)

X = unknown amount of solution

EXAMPLE The physician ordered: Give 200 mL of 50% Ensure q8h per nasogastric tube feeding.

How much water should be mixed with the Ensure to make 200 mL of a 50% solution?

Fractional Equation

$$D/H \times V = X$$
$$50/100 \times 200/1 = X$$
$$100 \text{ mL} = X$$

The total amount of solution – amount of tube feeding = amount of water to be added.

200 mL – 100 mL Ensure = 100 mL water
100 mL water and 100 mL Ensure mixed together make
200 mL of 50% solution.

Ratio-Proportion

$$H:V :: D:X$$
$$100:200 :: 50:X$$
$$200 \times 50 = 100 \times X$$
$$10,000 = 100X$$
$$100 = X$$

The total amount of solution – amount of tube feeding = amount of water to be added.

200 mL – 100 mL Ensure = 100 mL water
100 mL water and 100 mL Ensure mixed together make
200 mL of 50% solution.

a. Work the same problem to find a 75% solution.

b. Find a 30% solution.

Answers:

a. 150 mL Ensure and 50 mL water.
b. 60 mL Ensure and 140 mL water.

Percentages can also be written as decimals. To do this, omit the % sign and insert a decimal point two places to the left of the last number. Remember, percentage indicates 100 parts to the whole; therefore, the decimal number is expressed as hundredths. For example, 10% can be written .10 or .1, and 15% can be written .15.

NOTE In pharmacology, a zero is inserted in front of the decimal point to avoid any error that might result from someone's not seeing the decimal point and interpreting the order to be a whole number instead of a decimal or fraction of a whole number. If someone did not see the decimal point and misinterpreted the number .1 as 1, the error would be 10 times the dose ordered! Therefore, 10% would actually be written 0.1; 50%, 0.5; 15%, 0.15; and so on.

Orders for intravenous (IV) solutions may be written in percentages or as decimals. For example, the physician may order the following: Give 1000 mL dextrose 5% in water IV for 8 hours. This could also be written as 1000 mL dextrose .05 in water. There is no mathematical problem to compute to mix the solution because the manufacturer does this for us under aseptic conditions and labels the bottle or bag of solution accordingly. The nurse need only read the label accurately.

E X E R C I S E S

Write the following percentages as decimals and the decimals as percentages.

a. 20%
b. 45%
c. 0.33
d. 0.75

Answers:

a. 0.2
b. 0.45
c. 33%
d. 75%

CALCULATION OF INTRAVENOUS FLOW RATES

When an intravenous (IV) solution is ordered, the physician specifies the amount of solution to be given and the rate of flow or the number of hours the solution is to flow. One of the nurse's responsibilities is to monitor the flow rate. To do this, the nurse does not wait an entire hour to verify whether the ordered amount has infused but calculates the IV rate, adjusts the flow regulator, and monitors the infusion rate frequently.

When an IV solution is being infused by gravity (that is, no infusion pump is being used), if the nurse's calculations are correct and the patient remains in basically the same position, the rate of infusion should remain stable. However, if the patient changes from a lying to a sitting or standing position, the distance from the infusion site to the infusion container changes. This alters the gravitational pressure and may change the flow rate. The rate may then have to be readjusted. If an infusion pump is being used, the pump automatically adjusts for the difference in gravity and maintains the rate as ordered.

There are several formulas for calculating IV flow rates, which may involve one or more steps. The basic one-step formula is as follows:

$$\frac{\text{amount of fluid} \times \text{drop factor}}{\text{hours to administer} \times \text{minutes per hour}} = \text{drops (gtt) per minute}$$

The number of drops per milliliter that an administration set will deliver is called the drop factor. The drop factor is determined by the manufacturer and is printed on the box containing the infusion administration set. Macrodrip sets contain 10 to 20 gtt/mL, and microdrip or minidrip sets contain 60 gtt/mL. To verify the number to use in the equation, consult the box.

EXAMPLE The physician ordered 1000 mL 5% dextrose in water (D/W) to be infused IV in 10 hours.

Calculate the infusion rate in drops per minute. The drop factor is 12.

$$\frac{1000 \text{ mL} \times 12 \text{ gtt/mL}}{10\text{h} \times 60\text{min}} = ?\text{gtt/min}$$

$$\frac{1000 \times 12}{10 \times 60} = ?$$

$$\frac{12000}{600} = ?$$

$$\frac{1200}{60} = 20$$

The infusion rate is 20 gtt/min.

EXAMPLE The physician ordered 500 mL of 0.9% sodium chloride (NaCl) to run at 50 mL/h. (The drop factor is 10.)

$$\frac{500 \times 10}{? \times 60} = ? \text{ gtt/min}$$

Although this problem is set up in the same manner as the preceding example, it must be worked in two steps because there are two unknowns.

Step 1

$$\frac{500 \text{ mL}}{50 \text{ mL/h}} = 10 \text{ h to administer}$$

Step 2

$$\frac{500 \times 10}{10 \times 60} = 8.33 \text{ gtt/min}$$

(round off) = 8 gtt/min

PROBLEM The physician ordered 500 mL of 5% dextrose in 0.9% NaCl to be infused at 50 mL/h. (Drop factor is 60 gtt/mL.) How many drops per minute should be infused? How many hours will it take to infuse the 500 mL? Be sure to show your work.

Answers 50 gtt/min; 10 h.

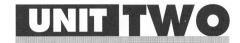

UNIT TWO

DRUG ADMINISTRATION

The administration of medications follows the steps of the nursing process, just as other nursing actions do. The four steps, as they relate to medications, are discussed with examples of each.

There are many ways to prepare medications and various routes by which medication can be administered. The form given to the drug and the route by which it is administered influence the efficacy of the drug. In general, the routes can be classified as enteral, parenteral, and percutaneous. Enteral refers to the gastrointestinal tract and includes the oral and nasogastric routes. Parenteral technically refers to all routes outside the gastrointestinal tract; but in actual practice, it is understood to mean the intravenous, subcutaneous, and intramuscular routes of administration. Percutaneous means application of medica-

tion to the skin and mucous membranes for absorption. This route includes topical applications to the skin; sublingual and buccal preparations (because they bypass the stomach); and instillations into the eyes, ears, nose, throat, lungs, bladder, vagina, and rectum. Preparation forms commonly used for each route are discussed in the appropriate chapters.

Age also greatly influences how a medication is administered. We discuss how normal growth and development affect the administration and dosages of medications in children and offer administration guidelines to follow. In the same way, normal growth and development affect the administration and dosages of medications as we become older. Guidelines are offered for the administration of drugs to the elderly.

THE NURSING PROCESS IN DRUG ADMINISTRATION

[handwritten annotation: Special emphasis on — documented need of med. — current & past medication use — presc. OTC, street — known allergies — response to med.]

LEARNING OBJECTIVES

After studying this chapter, you should be able to:

1. State the rationale for basic knowledge of a drug before administration.

2. State common safety measures used in the administration of drugs.

3. State the five rights.

DRUG ADMINISTRATION

The administration of medications must be performed carefully to avoid errors and prevent harm to the patient. The principles of drug administration can be learned by using the steps of the nursing process. You should become familiar with using the nursing process as a study technique to internalize the problem-solving steps it involves.

ASSESSMENT You must be familiar with the purpose of the drug to be given. Without this knowledge, you will not be able to evaluate its effectiveness. The same logic accounts for the need to know and anticipate common side effects. Any nursing implications that are indicated for this drug must be common knowledge to the nurse, or errors of omission will occur in the patient's care. Knowledge of the usual route of administration prevents errors as well. It is not possible for a human being to know all of this information about every drug. Any drugs unfamiliar to you need to be looked up in a reliable reference book. Having no knowledge of drugs would cause the nurse

to take excessive amounts of time to give drugs to the patients.

Assess the patient before giving the drug. This is to establish baseline data for each assessment and to prevent the patient from receiving a drug that would be inappropriate. Specific assessments to be performed are dictated by the results expected from the drug and its common side effects. Some assessment data that may be indicated include

- Vital signs, weight, breath sounds, bowel sounds, and capillary refill time
- Level of consciousness
- The patient's complaints and allergies
- Other drugs the patient is taking (including both prescription and over-the-counter)
- The patient's daily schedule when at home

A review of chart information from all sources is also warranted, including the physician's and consultants' examination findings, laboratory study results, x-ray results, therapy notes, medical history, family medical history, other illnesses, and even the patient's occupation.

Just before preparing a medication for a patient, assess the drug itself. If a liquid medication has become cloudy, changed color, or developed a sediment or a precipitate, do not use this preparation. Return it to the pharmacy and obtain a new bottle.

PLANNING The planning step of the nursing process in the administration of drugs includes setting goals and the nursing steps to be taken. This may include expected outcomes of patient teaching related to medications, related nursing care to encourage the effects of the drug, and planning the materials needed for administration of the drug.

You may be required to give medications to a large number of patients. To best use the time available, give medications last to the patients who require the most time. This avoids making all the other patients late for their drugs.

Be sure to prepare medications in a well-lit area. If your plan of action requires you to prepare the medications next to the bed in dim light, change your plan.

Many drugs can upset the gastrointestinal (GI) system. Based on your knowledge of this common side effect, you may need to give the drug with or immediately after food. However, some medications are best taken on an empty stomach. For example, although iron preparations often upset the GI system, they are best absorbed on an empty stomach. So the disadvantages of interrupted absorption must be weighed against GI upset. Check with a physician for specific orders in these cases.

Some medications have a particularly bad taste. This can be minimized by sucking on ice, or the drug can be mixed with food or drink. You will need to decide which is most appropriate for each patient.

Some drugs can damage or discolor the teeth if the drug comes into contact with the teeth. Plan to dilute the medication and have the patient drink the drug through a straw. Tell the patient not to "swish" the drug around in the mouth because this would defeat the purpose of the straw. This means that you must plan not only nursing action but materials needed and patient teaching as well.

If a dropper or syringe is to be used to give oral medications, plan to use each for only one medication. Using a dropper or syringe for more than one drug causes a mixing of drugs, which could bind to form unknown substances.

Determine whether drugs that are to be given at the same time are compatible. This includes not only oral drugs but drugs given by other routes and even liquid nutritive substitutes often given by nasogastric or gastrostomy tube. Check with the pharmacist if you are unsure.

IMPLEMENTATION Implementation includes prepar-
▲▲▲▲▲▲▲▲▲▲▲▲▲▲▲ ing, administering, and teaching about drugs. Never give a medication without an order. Prescription as well as over-the-counter drugs are illegal if given by a nurse without a physician's order. In some states, certain advanced-degree nurses do have limited ability to prescribe medication. You will need to be familiar with your state's Nurse Practice Act.

Medications are kept locked, and only an authorized person should have the key. If too many people have access to a medication cupboard or cart, accountability is lost.

To ensure that you are following the order correctly, several safeguards are used. These safeguards take the form of standard procedures and are aimed at maintaining the five rights. The five rights are

- Right drug   *Right documentation*
- Right dose
- Right route
- Right time
- Right patient

Most drug errors are committed because one of these rights was a wrong.

Some resources now include a sixth right, the right documentation. This right does not prevent an error from being committed because documentation of drug administration *always* occurs after the drug has been given. However, it will ensure that the nurse has correctly informed other health care workers that the dose was given.

The nurse who will administer the drugs should check the transcribed order with the original written by the physician. Documentation errors may occur in transcribing the order from the original to the medication record or card. If this happens and the nurse does not check her records, the wrong drug, dose, route, or time may be used. The error would be both the transcribing nurse's and the administering nurse's responsibility.

If you note any changes in established orders, this, too, must be checked against the original. If the transcribed order is unusual in any way, for example, if you must use more than 2 tablets or capsules to administer the written dosage, check the record with the original.

While preparing medications for administration, check the medication record or card three times before giving the medicine. Read the order when getting the container from storage, again before dispensing the drug, and once more before returning the container to storage. This reduces errors before the medication is delivered to the patient.

If preparation of a drug requires a dosage calculation, always have another nurse check your math. Minor errors in mathematics can be major errors in pharmacology. See Chapter 6 for dosage calculations.

If you are unsure of any part of an order because it is difficult to read, unfamiliar, or just different from the norm, do not give the drug until you verify the order with the original and, if necessary, with the physician.

Always follow guidelines for universal precautions. Before the actual preparation of medications, always wash your hands. Wear gloves if you will come in contact with mucous membranes. Throughout the procedure, maintain medical asepsis with each step. This prevents contamination and the necessity of wasting the medication.

Never pour capsules or tablets into your hand. This breaks aseptic technique. Instead, pour them into the top of the bottle. If you pour too many by mistake, they will have to be thrown away if they have touched your hand. Tablets poured into the top of the bottle can be returned to that bottle. Medications that have been dropped must also be thrown away.

In planning your time, remember that most drugs can be given from 1/2 hour before the ordered time to 1/2 hour after the ordered time. Within these strict limits, this is not considered a drug error. However, medications that are ordered "stat" or immediately, preoperative medications, and medications that are to be taken before testing or laboratory studies must be given exactly on time. Make these drugs a top priority.

While preparing medications, allow absolutely no interruptions. This could cause errors by diverting attention. In reverse, never talk to a nurse who is preparing medications or you could be the cause of an error.

For the same reason, do not stop in the midst of preparing medication unless a true emergency exists. If you must stop and leave the medications, secure them so they cannot be taken by an unauthorized person. These medications will need to be destroyed after you return. Consult your facility policy manual for the method and witnesses to be used. Follow facility policy to account for and replace these "wasted" medications.

Never give medications that were prepared by someone else. If that person made a mistake in preparation, it is that person's responsibility. You would have no way of knowing what drug you are actually giving. If you give the medication, the error then becomes your responsibility.

If you cannot read a label on a container or the label has been removed, do not use any medication from that container. Send the container back to the pharmacy. A new supply will be needed for the patient. To prevent a label from becoming unreadable, pour liquid medications from the side of the bottle.

When pouring liquid medications, read the amount at eye level. This does not mean to hold the medication cup up to you. It means to bring your eyes down to the level of the medication cup. This is because the medication cup must be placed on a flat surface. In the air, it may be held just slightly crooked, and thus you would read a falsely high or falsely low dosage. Read the measurement of the liquid at the bottom of the meniscus. The meniscus is the top level of the liquid. Because of surface tension, however, the edges will "stick" slightly and "ride up" the medication cup's sides. If you read the amount at the sides, this would be a falsely high level (Fig. 7–1).

Never crush long-acting, sustained-release, timed-release, or enteric coated medications or pellets from a capsule. These types of drugs are prepared in these ways to serve specialized purposes. Long-acting, sustained-release, and timed-release medications

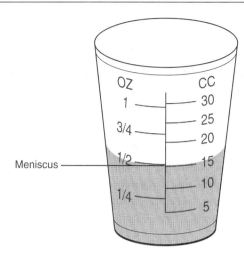

Figure 7–1. Glass and plastic medicine cups or spoons are calibrated in apothecary, metric, and household scales for the use of measuring liquid medications. Volume is read at the lowest level of the meniscus or the bottom of the concave surface.

and pellets from a capsule are meant to dissolve slowly and thereby provide slower absorption, distribution, and biotransformation of the drug. By crushing these forms, you are eliminating this aspect of their action, and the patient will receive the full dose immediately. This could cause symptoms of toxicity or even overdose. Be alert for any drugs that have the following abbreviations: LA (long-acting), SR (sustained-release), or TR (timed-release). Enteric-coated medications have been treated so they will not dissolve until they reach a lower portion of the digestive tract, generally the small intestine, because they cause GI distress if they dissolve in the stomach. Therefore, if you crush the enteric coated drug, you could easily be causing the patient unnecessary discomfort.

For similar reasons, do not open a capsule without a specific order to do so. A common way of ordering a drug in capsule form to be opened is by calling it "sprinkles." This indicates the drug is to be sprinkled over a substance, usually food.

When using individually packaged medications, or unit-dose systems, do not remove the medication from its package until you are at the patient's bedside. You can open the package directly into the patient's hand if the patient is alert. Many slightly disoriented patients will take their medication more easily if it is presented to them in a medication cup.

If you have made an error and poured or dispensed the wrong medication or the wrong amount of medication, do not return it to its container. This safeguard prevents accidental mixing of drugs.

Do not transfer a drug from one container to another; only a pharmacist is legally permitted to do this. You can administer only one dose at a time, not dispense a prescription, not even samples at a physician's office.

If a drug needs to be refrigerated, protected from light, or protected from heat, it must be returned to its proper storage immediately. If a drug has been accidently left out, it must be considered deteriorated and must be destroyed.

While transporting a drug to the patient, keep the medication card or record with it to avoid confusion. This allows you to identify both the drug and the patient when necessary. Keep caps on needles when transporting them to a patient to prevent accidents.

Medications must remain in your sight at all times. If you are using a cart, it must be locked if it will leave your line of vision. This is obviously necessary in administering injections because you will need to pull a curtain or shut the door to protect the patient's privacy. Locking the medication cart is also necessary if you must enter an isolation room where the door must be closed.

Before giving the drug to the patient, check the identification band against your medication record or card. Repeat this procedure no matter how many times you have given this person care or medications. If your facility does not have identification bands for the patients, a picture of the patient should be displayed on the medication record. If you are at all unsure, ask another nurse for confirmation. Never ask a patient, Are you Mr. Thomas? If the patient is confused, he may answer yes even though he is Mr. Janowitz. You may ask an alert patient, What is your name, please?

Screen the patient for privacy, if necessary, and position appropriately for administration.

Any time a patient questions any aspect of his drug, always check it out. The patients are often right because they are familiar with their medications. If patient questions a tablet of a different size or color, or states that another nurse just gave him that drug, or acts surprised because "the doctor said this drug would be changed," always check before the patient takes the drug.

If a patient refuses a drug, a drug has been delayed, or an error has occurred, report the incident to the charge nurse immediately. Do not wait until you are finished passing to all of your patients. The charge nurse will want to notify the physician, or it may be your responsibility to do so. The physician can then make a decision about further orders based on all the information.

Remember, patients do have the right to refuse any and all treatment, and this includes medication. As a nurse, it is your responsibility to explain the purpose of and need for a medication. You can encourage your patient to comply with the drug regimen, but you cannot force compliance.

Once you have given an oral drug to the patient, be sure the medication has been swallowed. Do not leave the room until you are sure. In some cases, a patient

may pretend to take a medication and then collect the tablets or capsules until there is enough to reach a lethal dose. Or a patient may not want the physician to know about noncompliance.

Do not leave any medication at the patient's bedside without a specific order to do so. If a patient asks to take the drug later and suggests that you leave it with him, inform him that you will come back later with the medication when it will be more convenient for him. This is a common request by patients who receive medications at mealtimes. If the patient consistently makes the same request, mark a note on the medication record so other nurses passing medications will have advance warning.

If a patient has a nasogastric or gastrostomy tube feeding, do not mix the medications with the feeding. Instead, the proper procedure is to disconnect the tubing from the feeding and administer the drug. Then reconnect the feeding. Medications that are mixed with a tube feeding cannot be accurately charted for time of delivery. Slow administration may alter the action of the drug. Do not forget to include any liquids you used during administration in the intake and output tally.

In most cases, after you have given the patient an oral medication, offer a drink of liquid. Do not give liquid or food, however, after an expectorant type of cough syrup. The substance may "rinse" away some of the syrup and disrupt its effectiveness.

After administration:

- Remove gloves if you are wearing them
- Reposition the patient, if necessary or if desired
- Secure the patient as ordered or as necessitated by the medication

For example, side rails should be maintained if the drug will cause sedation. Inform patients of any special precautions, such as remaining in bed or requesting assistance for ambulation. Secure signal cords within the patient's reach. Wash your hands before leaving the room.

Record the administration of any drug immediately after giving it. This eliminates any memory errors later on and prevents other nurses from administering the same dose over again.

EVALUATION The evaluation step of the administra-
▲▲▲▲▲▲▲▲▲ tion of drugs includes checking for positive effects. Note any relief of symptoms. For example, ask a patient given a medication for nausea or pain about relief of these symptoms 1/2 to 1 hour after administration. This is evidence that the drug is working.

Also check for any side effects, either expected or unexpected. If you determine that a patient has a symptom indicative of an adverse drug reaction, do not give the drug, see that the physician is called, and chart the reason that the drug was withheld. Any adverse reaction may indicate that the patient could have a more severe reaction with additional doses. For example, many antibiotics cause a rash in sensitive persons. If additional doses are administered, the patient may go into anaphylactic shock, a life-threatening condition.

Compare all results of your evaluations with the baseline information you gathered in the assessment step of the process. Therefore, any assessments that are recommended for a drug are also evaluations for that drug. Notify the charge nurse and the physician of any changes in the patient's status. Chart the patient's response to all drugs in your nurse's notes.

EXERCISES

MENTAL AEROBICS

1. What are the four steps of the process of administration of drugs?

2. If a drug is being used to improve breathing, what assessments and evaluations would you expect to perform for that patient?

3. Your patient has a nasogastric tube feeding presently filled with liquid nutritional supplement. You must administer medications to the patient. What procedure would you follow, and what precautions would you take?

① Assessment
Planning
Implementation
Evaluation

② B/P - respirations - relief

③ Disconnect tube feeding
Include any liquid intake
you give on I & O. sheet.

Precautions) remove gloves
Reposition patient
Secure patient as ordered.

ENTERAL ADMINISTRATION

LEARNING OBJECTIVES

After studying this chapter, you should be able to:

1. Define the enteral route of medication administration.

2. List two reasons for administration of medication through a feeding tube.

3. Discuss the difference between tablets, capsules, lozenges, elixirs, gels, and suspensions.

4. Discuss appropriate methods of administration of medications by the enteral route.

5. Discuss which oral forms may be altered for administration.

6. Describe the correct methods of altering the form of tablets and capsules for administration.

ROUTES OF ADMINISTRATION

There are many ways to prepare medications and various routes by which medication can be administered. The Drug Administration Guidelines describe the preparation of all medications.

The form given to the drug and the route by which it is administered influence the efficacy of the drug. In general, the routes can be classified as enteral, parenteral, and percutaneous. Enteral refers to the gastrointestinal tract and includes the oral and nasogastric routes. Parenteral technically refers to all routes outside the gastrointestinal tract; but in actual practice, it is understood to mean the intravenous, subcutaneous, and intramuscular routes of administration. Percutaneous means application of medica-

tion to the skin and mucous membranes for absorption. This route includes

- Topical applications to the skin
- Sublingual and buccal preparations (because they bypass the stomach)
- Instillations into the eyes, ears, nose, throat, lungs, bladder, vagina, and rectum.

Preparation forms commonly used for each route are discussed in the appropriate chapters.

DRUG ADMINISTRATION GUIDELINES

Preparation of All Medications

1. Retrieve the medication order (medication administration record [MAR], card, per institutional policy) and bring it to the medication station.
2. Check appropriate references if you are unfamiliar with the ordered medication.
3. Wash hands.
4. Assemble equipment.
5. **Concentrate** on the procedure.
6. Read the order, noting all details: date, expiration date, patient, drug, time/frequency, route, dose.

REMEMBER THE FIVE RIGHTS:
- **Right drug**
- **Right patient**
- **Right time**
- **Right route**
- **Right dose**

7. Check calculations. Follow institutional policy about verification of calculations with other personnel.
8. Read the label three times:
   a. Before pouring
   b. After pouring
   c. As you return the medication to its storage place
9. **Never** use an unlabeled medication.
10. Chart medication immediately **after** administration.
(Right documentation is the sixth right.)

ENTERAL ADMINISTRATION

ORAL ADMINISTRATION The simplest route is the oral route. This does not imply that no problems are encountered when this route is used; rather, it is usually more convenient, economical, and safer than some of the other routes. Drugs administered orally or "per os" (PO) are subject to the actions of the gastrointestinal tract, which include peristalsis and secretions. Vomiting, diarrhea, and constipation influence the length of time that medications remain in the tract. Acids and other digestive enzymes break down the medication form and sometimes even destroy its action. The presence or absence of food in the tract influences breakdown and absorption of drugs.

In the event of a major error or accidental or intentional overdose, drugs may be removed from the gastrointestinal tract by inducing vomiting, lavage (washing out the stomach), or speeding peristalsis with cathartics. If intervention occurs within a short time of ingestion, serious consequences are sometimes avoided.

NASOGASTRIC AND GASTRIC ADMINISTRATION

If the patient is comatose or has difficulty swallowing, medications may be administered through a feeding tube, such as a nasogastric (ng) tube, gastrostomy tube (g-tube), or jejunostomy tube (j-tube).

MEDICATION FORMS

Solid Forms

TABLETS Tablets are dried, powdered forms of drugs that are compressed into round disks. They are not meant to be cut into parts to obtain partial doses unless they are "scored" with indented lines, which facilitates cutting or breaking them into identical halves or fourths (Fig. 8–1). Tablets are easily dis-

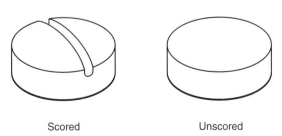

Scored   Unscored

Figure 8-1. The indented line or "scoring" at the center of some tablets facilitates cutting or breaking them into halves or fourths for partial doses. Unscored tablets are not meant to be broken into partial doses.

solved and are sometimes crushed into powder and mixed with small amounts of food or liquid to facilitate administration to someone who has difficulty swallowing them in their whole form.

Some tablets are given special coatings that delay the digestion of the tablet. These are sometimes called extentabs or are said to have an enteric coating. The enteric coating protects the stomach from irritation by causing the tablet to be dissolved farther down the digestive tract. This may also be done to allow the drug to be released over a longer time. Enteric coated tablets should not be crushed or cut because this action destroys the effectiveness of the coating.

CAPSULES Capsules are small, cylinder-shaped containers that hold a dry powder or granules. The containers are made of gelatin and constructed of two pieces that fit together at the center. The capsules come in a variety of sizes. Some capsules are called gelcaps. These are one-piece capsules that contain liquid medication and do not come apart at the center. Pharmaceutical companies sometimes prepare drugs in this manner to delay the absorption and extend the action of the medication. Some of the granules inside are coated so that as the gelatin capsule dissolves, some granules begin to dissolve immediately and some do not. These products are often called spansules.

Another reason for preparing medications in this form is to mask an unpleasant odor or taste. Empty capsules are often purchased by the pharmacist or other individuals, and the capsule is filled after the drug has been purchased.

A safety issue is apparent with capsules. There have been instances when capsules have been opened and the contents altered, causing injury or death to those who consumed the altered product. For this reason, capsules are becoming a less popular form of medication, and manufacturers have responded with the introduction of a new form called a caplet. The caplet is shaped like a capsule but cannot be altered by separating it into two parts.

LOZENGES Lozenges are flat disks that contain a drug in a pleasantly flavored base. Lozenges are placed in the mouth and sucked to slowly release the drug. A common example is a cough drop or throat lozenge.

Liquid Forms

ELIXIRS Liquids prepared with alcohol, sugar, and a pleasantly scented substance are called elixirs. These preparations are manufactured for medications that are unpleasant to taste or as an alternative form for those who have difficulty swallowing solids. Cough medicines are often prepared as elixirs.

N U R S I N G   A L E R T

Because elixirs contain alcohol, do not administer elixirs to patients who cannot have alcohol.

GELS Gels are suspensions of larger particles that do not dissolve in water. They are often ordered when the pharynx, esophagus, or stomach is to be coated to prevent irritation. Antacids are commonly prepared in this manner.

SUSPENSIONS Solid particles of a drug that do not dissolve when mixed in a liquid are called suspensions. When the bottle is allowed to sit, the solids settle to the bottom of the bottle and the liquid rises to the top. Suspensions *must always be shaken* until the solid particles are evenly distributed throughout the liquid. If this step is omitted, the dose poured would not contain the ordered amount of the drug. The dose must be poured and administered immediately or the particles will once again settle to the bottom of the container.

ORAL ADMINISTRATION

The preparation and administration of oral medications are detailed in the Drug Administration Guidelines.

In hospitals and nursing homes, solid forms of oral medication, such as tablets, capsules, and caplets, may come from the pharmacy in individually labeled packages called unit doses, which are ready for dispensing. The manufacturer, lot number, expiration date, generic and trade names, and dosage are included on the label just as they are on a large bottle of medication. Unit-dose medications may be taken to the patient and administered directly from the package into the patient's hand. Bottled tablets and capsules are transferred into the lid of the container and then into a medicine cup. Care is taken not to touch the medication for reasons of hygiene and also to prevent the oils and moisture on the hands from affecting the medication.

If the patient is unable to swallow a solid form, sometimes the form may be altered. A tablet may be

DRUG ADMINISTRATION GUIDELINES

Preparation and Administration of Oral Medications

1. Check the physician's order.
2. Wash hands.
3. Assemble medication bottle and soufflé cup or plastic medication cup.
4. Check the label and calculate the dosage.
5. If the medication is in tablet or capsule form, pour into cap of bottle to count correct number, then into soufflé cup. Do not touch the drug with your hands. A unit dose may be placed into the cup without removing the tablet or capsule from the bubble package.
6. If the medication is in liquid form:

   - Shake before pouring, if the drug is a suspension.
   - Remove cap and place top side down on table.
   - Identify mark for desired dose with thumbnail.
   - Place cup on a flat surface at eye level.
   - Pour dose. Remember to read the dose at the lowest point of the meniscus.
   - Wipe off the neck of the bottle with a paper towel and replace cap.

7. Recheck the order, remembering **the five rights.**
8. Identify the patient and obtain necessary assessment data in relation to medications to be given.
9. Explain the procedure to the patient and review medications.
10. Obtain a sufficient quantity of fresh water to allow the patient to swallow the medications.
11. Verify that the patient has swallowed the medication.
12. Record administration on MAR per institutional policy **(sixth right).**

altered by placing it in a mortar or between two soufflé cups and crushing it with a pestle (Fig. 8–2). The powdered drug may then be mixed with a small amount of food, such as pudding or applesauce.

N U R S I N G   A L E R T

Enteric coated tablets may not be prepared in this manner because crushing destroys the advantage of the enteric coating.

A capsule may be opened and the contents mixed with a small amount of food if the drug is not a long-acting

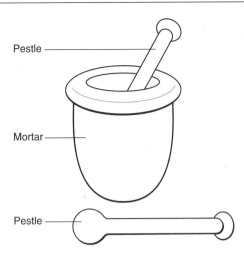

Figure 8–2. When patients are unable to swallow a solid form, a mortar and pestle are used to alter the form. The tablet is placed in the mortar and crushed with the pestle. The powdered drug may them be mixed with a small amount of food.

type or if it is not in capsule form to prevent gastrointestinal irritation.

N U R S I N G   A L E R T

Consult the pharmacist if there is any question about the appropriateness of altering the form of the ordered medication.

If altering the form will alter the action, the physician needs to be notified of the difficulty with administration. The physician may then wish to order an alternative form of the medication.

Liquid medications for oral use are administered in a glass or plastic medicine cup calibrated in apothecary, metric, and household scales (see Fig. 7–1). Use the scale that corresponds with the physician's order. Pour liquids with the label side of the bottle in the palm of the hand. This prevents medication from dripping down the side of the bottle and damaging the label (Fig. 8–3). Place the cup on the counter and pour. Volume is read at the meniscus or lowest point of the concave surface of the liquid.

Oral syringes or medicine droppers may be used to administer liquids directly into the mouth of children and some adults. Various sizes are available, so read the package or look at the device to be certain the calibrations are appropriate for the dosage ordered. The medication may be withdrawn directly from the bottle into the syringe or dropper if the opening of the bottle is large enough. Use a new syringe each time.

The alternative method is to pour the medication into a medicine cup and withdraw it from there with a new syringe. Small amounts of medication remain in the medicine cup, so always check the dosage after it is in the syringe or dropper.

It is difficult and dangerous to swallow a solid or liquid when lying down, so place the patient in an upright position if it is permitted. If not, modify position according to the physician's orders. Have a full glass of liquid available and encourage the patient to take a sip to moisten the mouth and throat. Offer the patient assistance as necessary to remove the drug from the package or cup, place it in the mouth, and drink the liquid. Tablets and capsules should be placed at the back of the tongue. If the head is tilted slightly back, tablets go down the throat more easily. Tipping the head slightly forward facilitates swallowing capsules because they are light and float. Unless a special circumstance requires limitation of intake, encourage the patient to drink a minimum of 90 mL of liquid. This facilitates carrying the medication to the stomach and assists with dissolving the medication.

Never leave the patient until the medication has been swallowed. If the patient is a child or a confused or mentally ill person, check the mouth to verify that the medication has been swallowed.

Never leave medications with the patient unless there is a specific order to do so. Some drugs, such as antacids or nitroglycerin, may be ordered to be left at the bedside. If so, instruct the patient to notify you of the time of dose, the reason for use, and whether relief was obtained.

Liquid medications may be administered to infants with a nipple. Dose must be measured with a dropper or syringe first, then placed into the nipple for the infant to suck. Hold the infant in a football hold with the head slightly elevated. Ascertain that the infant is

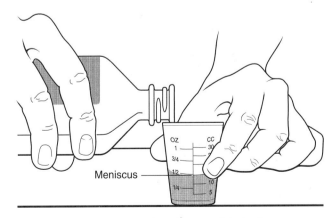

Figure 8–3. Pouring liquid medications label side up prevents the medication from dripping down the label side and damaging the instructions on the label.

awake and able to suck. Insert the nipple into the mouth and tip it forward so the medication fills the nipple. After the infant has sucked the medication, follow with water or formula.

NASOGASTRIC AND GASTRIC ADMINISTRATION

Whenever possible, liquid forms of drugs are used for instillation through feeding tubes (Fig. 8–4). If liquid forms are not available from the pharmacy, verify whether the tablet or capsule form may be altered. Crush the tablet or open the capsule, dissolve the contents in at least 1 ounce of water, and administer the entire amount through the tube.

Always elevate the head of the bed at least 30 degrees when either a nasogastric or gastrostomy tube is in place. This allows gravity to facilitate the passage of the liquid through the gastrointestinal tract and helps prevent reflux of the liquid up the esophagus and into the airway, where it may be aspirated.

Wear gloves according to universal precautions. If there is pressure in the gastrointestinal tract, gastric secretions may spill from the tube when it is unclamped.

Always check for correct placement of the tube before instillation of the liquid. If the nasogastric tube is not in correct position, the liquid may be aspirated into the lung, where it can cause pneumonia or death. If the gastrostomy tube is not in correct position, the liquid may be instilled directly into the duodenum, where it can cause dumping syndrome.

Medications may be instilled by gravity, with use of the barrel of an Asepto or other type of large syringe as a funnel. The height of the syringe and tubing determines the amount of pressure in the syringe. Position them in one hand and elevate them above the patient's head. Pour liquids with the other hand. Solution should flow slowly. Lower the syringe to slow the flow.

Medications administered through these tubes should always be followed by at least 50 mL of water to flush the tube and prevent clogging. Tubing should be clamped immediately after instillation to prevent air from entering the tubing and causing gastric distention and flatulence.

If continuous feedings are ordered, reconnect the feeding tube to the tubing from the pump (Fig. 8–5). If gastric suction has been ordered, keep the tube clamped and secured. Do not reattach the suction for at least 30 minutes to allow the medication to be absorbed or passed into the intestine. See the Drug Administration Guidelines for administration of medication by the nasogastric or gastric route.

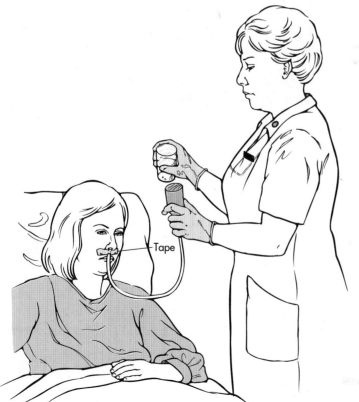

Figure 8–4. Always check for correct placement of the nasogastric tube before instillation of liquid medication for intermittent feedings.

Tape

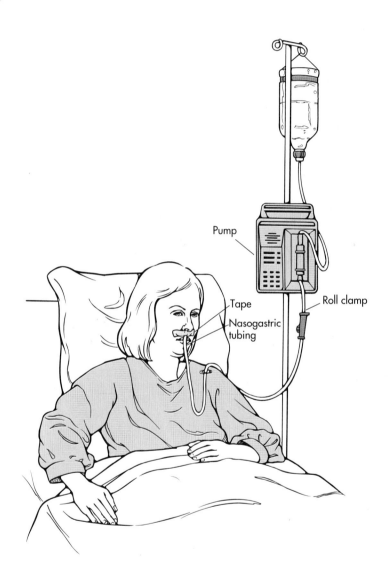

Figure 8-5. A continuous nasogastric tube feeding is done by use of a pump, rather than by manual feeding through a funnel or syringe barrel.

DRUG ADMINISTRATION GUIDELINES

Administration of Medications by the Nasogastric or Gastric Route

1. Check the order.
2. Wash hands and assemble equipment.
3. Prepare the medication, remembering **the five rights.** Medications must be in a liquid or powdered form. If the medication is available only as a tablet, it must be crushed into a powder. **Do not crush enteric coated tablets or timed-release capsules!** If the medication is available as a capsule, the gelatin parts must be pulled apart and the contents used. Powdered forms of drugs should be dissolved in at least 1 ounce 30 mL of water.
4. Identify the patient.
5. Screen the patient and position with the head elevated.
6. Put gloves on.
7. Disconnect the tube from the suction machine or the feeding pump; if the tube is not connected to suction or a pump, unclamp the end.
8. Check the nasogastric tube for correct placement in the stomach:

Method a: Use a syringe to inject 5 to 10 mL of air (up to 5 mL for a child) into the tube while listening with a stethoscope placed over the stomach area. The air will make a gurgling sound as it escapes into the stomach. Withdraw the amount of air inserted.

Method b: Use a syringe to aspirate stomach contents. If nothing returns, use an alternative method to assess.

Method c: Place the unclamped end of the nasogastric tube next to the ear. If the tube has been misplaced or displaced into the lung, breath sounds may be heard. The tube must be removed and properly reinserted before any instillation!

9. Check the gastrostomy tube for correct placement in the stomach by checking orders for type and placement of tube.

• If tubing has markings, a piece of tape may be wrapped at the level where the tube should remain.

• If the tubing is held in place with a catheter balloon, apply gentle traction until resistance is felt.

• Some gastrostomy tubes are sutured in place.

10. Using the nondominant hand to clamp the tubing, insert the barrel of the syringe into the tubing with the other hand.
11. Using the dominant hand, pour the medication into the syringe.
12. Unclamp the tubing and elevate the tubing and syringe until the solution begins to flow slowly by gravity.
13. With the dominant hand, slowly add the ordered amount of water to the syringe (at least 50 mL) and allow it to flow by gravity to flush the tubing.

DRUG ADMINISTRATION GUIDELINES

Administration of Medications by the Nasogastric or Gastric Route *Continued*

14. Clamp the tubing when finished or reconnect to the tubing from the pump. If it is to be connected to suction, wait 20 minutes before reconnecting the tubing.
15. Chart the time, drug, amount of solution, and signature **(sixth right).**

E X E R C I S E S

LEARNING ACTIVITIES

Using the Guidelines and the appropriate administration equipment, practice enteral administration techniques until you feel comfortable with them. Then ask a classmate to use the Guidelines to critique your technique. When you are ready, ask your instructor to verify that your technique is appropriate.

PARENTERAL ADMINISTRATION

LEARNING OBJECTIVES

After studying this chapter, you should be able to:

1. Define the parenteral route of medication administration.

2. Discuss the difference between ampules and vials.

3. Name the parts of a syringe, indicating which need to remain sterile during preparation and administration of medications by the parenteral route.

4. Explain how needles and syringes are sized and calibrated.

5. Select an appropriately sized and calibrated needle and syringe for administration by the parenteral route when given an example of a physician's order.

6. Demonstrate the correct procedure for preparing subcutaneous, intramuscular, and intradermal injections.

7. Discuss the rationale for use of the Z-track method of intramuscular injection.

8. Identify the appropriate sites of administration of subcutaneous and intramuscular injections.

9. Correctly describe the techniques of administration of subcutaneous and intramuscular injections.

10. Discuss methods to reduce the pain of the injection.

11. Demonstrate the correct procedure for preparing intravenous solutions for administration.

12. Correctly describe the techniques of administration of intravenous solutions and discontinuing the administration.

Parenteral drug routes that are frequently used by medical personnel include the subcutaneous (SC or sometimes called SQ), intramuscular (IM), intravenous (IV), and intradermal (ID) routes. Physicians sometimes administer drugs by other parenteral routes, which include intra-arterial, intracardiac, and intra-articular (into a joint).

When the patient's condition requires it, the physician may choose to surgically insert a central venous catheter. The central venous catheter is inserted into the superior vena cava and sutured in place. Hickman and Broviac catheters are types of this device. Their main advantage is that the patient is spared frequent venipunctures. They are usually made with several lumens or "ports" from which blood samples can be obtained, blood and nutritional supplements as well as other IV solutions can be infused, and central venous pressure can be monitored.

Special catheters are sometimes surgically implanted into an artery by the physician. These are usually used to administer high concentrations of chemotherapeutic drugs. Chemotherapy medications are also administered by other special routes. Intrapleural (into the pleural cavity), intraperitoneal (into the peritoneal cavity), and intrathecal (into the cerebrospinal fluid) are a few. Infusion ports or reservoirs are sometimes implanted subcutaneously by surgical methods. Nurses who have received special training may administer medications into these devices, which dispense medication over a set period of time, such as 2 to 4 weeks.

The Nurse Practice Act of each state addresses the role of the nurse practicing within that state. In addition, institutional regulations specify the type and amount of education required to administer medications. For example, in some states, licensed practical/vocational nurses are permitted to start IV lines; in other states, they are not. Even if the Nurse Practice Act permits it, the institution may require an additional medication course beyond that required by the Board of Licensure. Some institutions, especially in specialty areas, require periodic proficiency tests relating to drugs and sometimes mathematical calculations. Nurses must know and abide by the limitations placed on them by their practice act and their employing institutions.

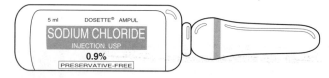

Figure 9–1. Ampules are sealed glass containers holding a single dose of powdered or liquid medication.

PREPARATION FORMS

Ampules and Vials

Small glass containers are manufactured to hold drugs in powdered or liquid form to be used for injection into the body. If the drug is in powdered form, the proper diluent must be added into the container to

DRUG ADMINISTRATION GUIDELINES

Reconstitution of a Sterile Powder

1. Read the literature accompanying the vial of sterile powder.
2. Assemble the injection equipment and sterile diluent specified by the manufacturer.
3. Maintain principles of aseptic technique throughout the procedure.
4. Uncap the needle and pull back the plunger, drawing in the amount of air equal to the volume of ordered diluent.
5. Cleanse the rubber stopper of the vial of sterile diluent with an antiseptic swab.
6. With the vial of diluent sitting on the counter, insert the needle through the rubber stopper and inject the air.
7. Leaving the needle in the vial, pick up and invert the vial.
8. Aspirate the ordered amount of diluent and withdraw the needle from the vial.
9. Cleanse the rubber stopper of the vial of sterile powder with an antiseptic swab.
10. Insert the needle into the vial of sterile powder, inject the diluent, and remove the needle.
11. Mix thoroughly and ascertain that the powder is completely dissolved. Consult the accompanying literature for a description of the expected color and clarity of the reconstituted product.
12. If the entire volume of reconstituted product will not be used in one dose, the vial must be labeled with the following: date, time of reconstitution, volume and type of diluent added, concentration of drug, expiration date and time, and name of the person reconstituting the drug.
13. Store the unused portion according to the manufacturer's instructions.

DRUG ADMINISTRATION GUIDELINES

Removal of a Medication from an Ampule

1. Check the physician's order.
2. Calculate the ordered dose of medication.
3. Assemble the injection equipment.
4. Maintain principles of aseptic technique throughout the procedure.
5. Tap the ampule to displace the medication from the top portion of the ampule.
6. Cover the neck of the ampule with a sterile 2 × 2 pad to protect the fingers, and break the top of the ampule at the neck.
7. Remove the needle from the syringe and replace it with a filter needle.
8. Insert the needle into the ampule and withdraw the ordered volume of medication.
9. Recheck the physician's order to verify the dosage.
10. Remove the filter needle and replace it with an appropriately sized needle for the ordered route and site.

reconstitute the drug into a liquid form before injection (see Drug Administration Guidelines). Drugs that are unstable in solution are often packaged in this manner. Ampules are sealed glass containers holding a single dose of a drug (Fig. 9–1). The top must be broken off at the "neck" to gain access to the drug (see Drug Administration Guidelines). Vials have rubber stoppers that seal them closed. They may also have a metal or plastic cap that must be removed to expose the rubber stopper. The needle of the syringe is used to puncture the stopper and gain access to the drug within (see Drug Administration Guidelines). Vials may be single-dose or multiple-dose containers.

Mix-O-Vials

These glass containers have two compartments. The lower compartment contains the powdered drug (solute), and the upper compartment contains the liquid solvent or diluent that will be used to produce the solution. There is a rubber "cork" between the chambers to keep them separate. The vial is closed with a

DRUG ADMINISTRATION GUIDELINES

Removal of Liquid from a Vial

1. Check the physician's order for the prescribed dose of medication.
2. Calculate the correct dose of medication.
3. Assemble the equipment.
4. Maintain principles of aseptic technique throughout the procedure.
5. Cleanse the rubber stopper of the vial with an antiseptic swab.
6. Uncap the needle and pull back the plunger, drawing in the amount of air equal to the volume of medication.
7. Insert the needle through the rubber stopper and inject air.
8. Aspirate the ordered volume of medication into the syringe.
9. Remove the needle from the vial.
10. Change needles if the drug is caustic or the needle tip may be dulled.
11. Recheck the order.

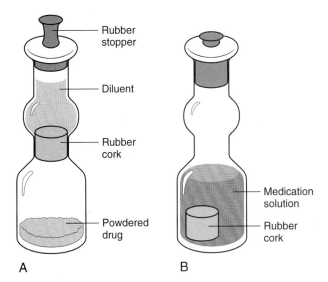

Figure 9–2. *A.* A mix-o-vial has a rubber stopper at one end. The solvent or diluent (liquid) and solute (powdered drug) are separated by a rubber "cork." *B.* When pressure is applied to the rubber stopper, the cork is forced out, allowing the solvent and solute to mix.

rubber stopper that protrudes from the end of the vial. When the drug is to be administered, pressure is placed on the rubber stopper on the end of the vial. This causes the cork to be forced down into the lower chamber and allows the liquid from the upper chamber to flow into the lower chamber and mix with the powder (Fig. 9–2A). The vial is rotated or lightly shaken until the solute is completely mixed with the solvent (Fig. 9–2B). The solution should now be clear,

although it may have color, depending on the drug. A needle and syringe are used to puncture the stopper and gain access to the drug, just as is done with any other vial.

Intravenous Fluids

Intravenous (IV) solutions are available in vacuum-sealed glass bottles or plastic bags that vary in size from 50-mL to 1000-mL capacity. There are many types of solutions available and also various concentrations of those solutions.

ADMINISTRATION

Injection Equipment

SYRINGES In the past, syringes were manufactured of glass, cleaned after use, and resterilized for repeated use. Because of the risk of transferring diseases such as acquired immunodeficiency syndrome (AIDS) and hepatitis, which may cause death, today's syringes are most commonly manufactured of plastic and disposed of after a single use. The syringe has three parts:

1. the barrel, which is the outer portion marked with calibrations for measurement of the drug volume;
2. the plunger, which is the cylinder that fits into the barrel and is used to draw up and eject the drug from the barrel; and
3. The tip, which is the part that connects into the needle (Fig. 9–3).

There are two types of tips:

- The plain tip pushes into the end of the needle.
- The Luer-Lok tip pushes into, twists, and locks into the end of the needle.

Needles are less likely to loosen and leak medication from syringes with Luer-Lok tips.

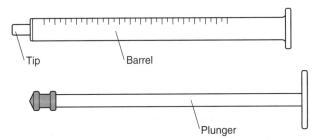

Figure 9–3. The syringe is composed of the barrel, the plunger, and the tip.

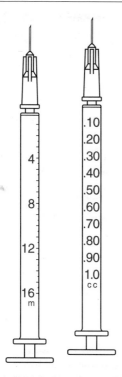

Figure 9–4. Most syringes have two scales of calibration. One side is calibrated in cubic centimeters (cc), the other is marked in minims (m). This tuberculin syringe shows both calibrations.

The most commonly used syringes are calibrated in 1, 3, or 5 cc/mL, but larger syringes are available in 10, 20, or 50 cc/mL calibrations (1 cc = 1 mL). There are two scales of calibration on most syringes (Fig. 9–4). One side of the barrel is calibrated in minims. Each line on the scale represents 1 minim (m), with a longer line representing every fifth minim. Numbers are placed only at the longer lines; 15 or 16 m equal 1 cc. The other side of the barrel is calibrated in cubic centimeters (cc). Each small line represents 0.1 cc; a longer line and a number at each fifth mark indicate 0.5 cc, or a longer line and a number at each tenth mark indicate 1 cc.

The tuberculin syringe has a 1-cc capacity. Each small line represents 0.01 cc. There are 100 lines on the scale. Every fifth line is a longer line, but there are no numbers until the twentieth line, which represents 0.2 cc (20/100 or 2/10). Numbers indicate 0.2, 0.4, 0.6, 0.8, and 1 cc. The other side of the barrel is often calibrated in minims (15 to 16 m = 1 cc). The tuberculin syringe is used to measure small amounts of drugs, such as pediatric doses, immunizing agents, or proteins used for skin testing for allergens.

Insulin strength is measured in units. Insulin is most commonly available in U-100 concentrations. This means that each ml/cc contains 100 units. The label on the vial states the concentration. The syringe used for administration must be an insulin syringe that is calibrated in units (Fig. 9–5). It should also state on the syringe that it is to be used with U-100 insulin only (Fig. 9–6). Always compare the label on the vial with the marking on the syringe. Use of an inappropriate syringe could result in an error in dosage. Insulin syringes are manufactured in 1-cc sizes, with each short line on the scale representing 2 units. Every fifth line is longer and represents 10 units, with 100 units or 1-cc capacity. If the dose ordered is less than 50 units, a special "low-dose" syringe may be used. This syringe is also labeled for use with U-100 insulin only, but it has a 0.5-cc capacity. The advantage is that calibrations are easier to read because each small line represents 1 unit, with a larger line and a number indicating each 5 units. Capacity is 50 units of U-100 insulin. Insulin is administered according to the Drug Administration Guidelines.

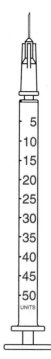

Figure 9–5. Insulin syringes are calibrated in units to correspond to insulin strength. This is a low-dose (0.5-cc) insulin syringe.

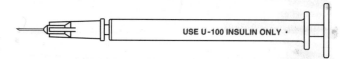

Figure 9–6. The syringe is marked with the insulin strength that should be used.

Smaller # Bigger hole (handwritten)

DRUG ADMINISTRATION GUIDELINES

Preparation and Administration of Insulin

1. Check the physician's order.

2. Maintain asepsis throughout the procedure and follow Guidelines for Administration of a Subcutaneous Injection.

3. Assemble the equipment. The label on the insulin vial will state the concentration in units. The insulin syringe must be marked to be used with the same concentration of insulin (usually U-100). If the syringe is not preassembled, choose a 25- to 28-gauge 1/2- to 5/8-inch needle.

4. Check the expiration date on the vial. Discard if outdated.

5. Check color of insulin. Modified insulins appear cloudy or milky white. Other insulins are clear.

6. Vials of modified insulin suspensions should be rotated or rolled between the palms of the hands to mix. Do not shake vial.

7. Cleanse the rubber stopper of the vial with an antiseptic swab.

8. Pull the plunger back to the number of units equal to the amount of insulin ordered. No calculations are required when the proper syringe is used.

9. Insert the needle into the vial and inject air.

10. With the needle still in the vial, invert the vial, withdraw the ordered number of units of insulin, and remove the needle from the vial.

11. Remove all air bubbles and recheck the physician's order.

12. Check the patient's medication administration record to verify the site of the last injection to rotate injection sites. See Figure 9–12 for appropriate sites.

13. Administer insulin into subcutaneous tissue at a 45-degree angle, or at a 90-degree angle if the patient is obese.

14. Withdraw the needle and press the skin. Do not rub, because rubbing may alter the absorption rate.

PREFILLED SYRINGES Some manufacturers prepare medication in a sterile disposable cartridge with an attached needle of the appropriate size for injection. The cartridge contains the amount of drug required for administration of an average dose of the medication and is labeled with the name, dose, and volume of drug. A special reusable cartridge holder must be used to administer the drug (Fig. 9–7). Each manufacturer has its own type. Some commonly used brands are Tubex and Carpuject. Once the drug is given, the medication cartridge is carefully placed in a sharps container for disposal, and the holder is reused for the next patient.

NEEDLES

A needle has three parts: *Bevel & Palmaap.* (handwritten)

1. the hub, which is a hollow, funnel-shaped area that fits over a plain-tip syringe or twists and locks into a Luer-Lok syringe;

2. the shaft, a hollow tube of various lengths to carry the medication to various depths in the tissue; and

3. the bevel, which is the angle at the tip (Fig. 9–8).

On piercing the skin, the bevel is held up so the point at the tip pierces the skin first.

Needles are manufactured in various gauges. Needle gauge is the diameter of the hole through the needle. A larger gauge must be used for a thicker (more viscous) liquid to enable the molecules to pass through the needle. A smaller gauge causes less discomfort to the patient, so you will want to use the smallest appropriate gauge possible. A confusing but important fact to remember about gauge is that smaller numbers indicate a larger gauge, and larger numbers indicate a smaller or finer gauge. For example, an 18-gauge needle is used to administer blood because it is viscous, and a 27- or 28-gauge needle is used to administer insulin because it is a watery liquid (Fig. 9–9).

When a standard steel needle is used for intravenous (IV) administration, there is considerable irritation to the vein, which often causes phlebitis (inflammation of the vein), puncture through the vein, or leakage of IV fluid into the extravascular space. The extremity must be immobilized to minimize these problems. This causes additional discomfort to the patient.

Special needles have been manufactured to decrease irritation. An IV catheter, or intracath, is designed with a special needle to puncture the skin and vein. There is a plastic or Teflon-coated tube over the needle shaft, except for the tip. After the venipuncture is made, the tube is threaded into the vein and then the needle is removed. The tube is plugged for intermittent infusion (called a heparin lock, prn lock, or med lock) or connected to a standard IV administration set. The tubing of the administration set is taped securely to the extremity (Fig. 9–10). Because these catheters are less irritating to the vein than the steel needles are, the extremity is not usually immobilized, and the site may remain intact for several days. Consult institutional policy for directions about the length of time an IV catheter may remain in the same site.

A scalp-vein needle or "butterfly" is a short steel needle with plastic "wings" that are grasped and folded back as a handle during insertion into the vein. The wings are then taped flat against the skin to

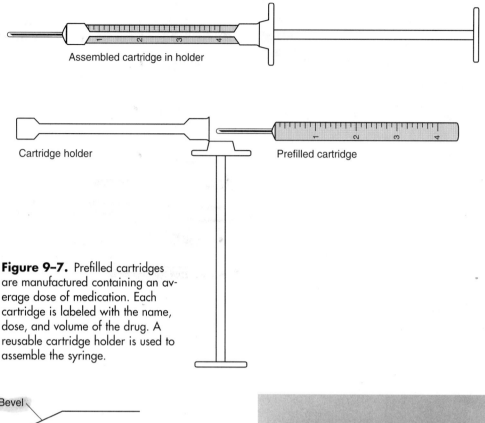

Assembled cartridge in holder

Cartridge holder   Prefilled cartridge

Figure 9–7. Prefilled cartridges are manufactured containing an average dose of medication. Each cartridge is labeled with the name, dose, and volume of the drug. A reusable cartridge holder is used to assemble the syringe.

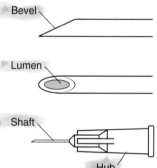

Bevel

Lumen

Shaft

Hub

Figure 9–8. The needle is composed of the hub, the shaft, and the bevel. The medication comes out through the lumen.

secure the needle in the vein. Attached to the needle, beyond the wings, is a 4- to 6-inch length of plastic tubing with an adapter on the end (Fig. 9–11). This can be connected to a standard IV administration set, or it can be plugged and taped to the skin to be used for intermittent infusions. The scalp-vein needles are primarily used with infants and children.

Needles and syringes are packaged and sterilized in plastic or paper wrappers. Examine the wrapper before opening it to check for factors that would cause the contents to become contaminated. Verify that the wrapper is intact, without tears or punctures. Look for water rings or other signs that moisture has come in contact with the wrapper. If sterility is in question, discard the package and obtain a new one.

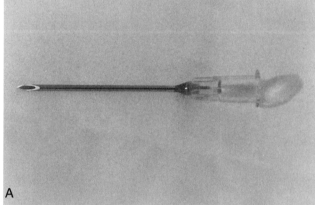

A

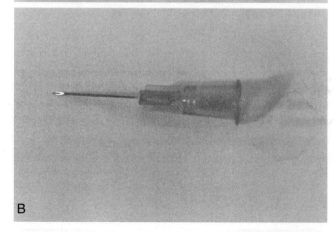

B

Figure 9–9. Smaller numbers indicate a larger gauge, and larger numbers indicate a smaller or finer gauge. A. An 18-gauge needle has a larger diameter and is used to administer viscous materials. B. This 25-gauge needle is used to administer watery liquids. (Photos by Roger W. Fair.)

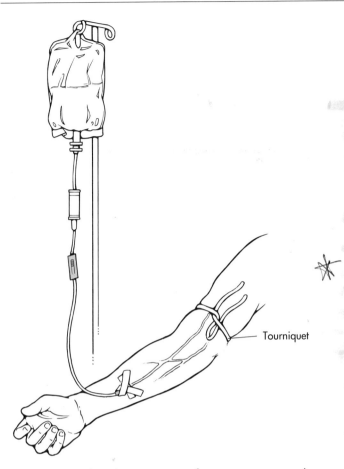

Figure 9–10. The administration set for an intravenous catheter is taped securely to the extremity.

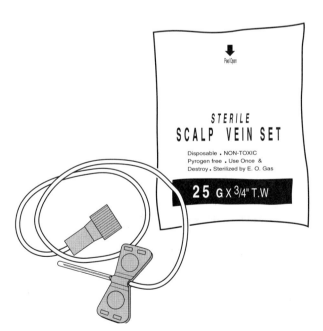

Figure 9–11. A scalp-vein needle or "butterfly" is a short steel needle with plastic "wings" that are folded back as a handle during insertion into the vein. Beyond the wings is a 4- to 6-inch length of plastic tubing with an adapter on the end. This adapter can be connected to a standard intravenous administration set or be used for intermittent infusions.

Identifying information is printed on the wrapper. The type of syringe and the volume it will hold are indicated. If a needle is already attached, the length and gauge are stated. There is an expiration date printed on it. Discard if the expiration date has passed because sterility will be in question. Needles are also packaged separately, and the same information applies to them.

Choose the syringe according to the <u>volume</u> of solution to be administered and the <u>type</u> of medication to be administered. Obviously, if you are ordered to give 3 cc of solution, a 1-cc syringe is not appropriate. Insulin is administered only with an insulin syringe. Pediatric doses and immunizations are administered with a tuberculin syringe.

Choose the needle size and length according to the viscosity of the solution and the route of administration. Thicker solutions require a larger gauge, and smaller gauges cause less discomfort. Remember that the larger gauges have the smaller numbers! Use smaller gauge needles for infants, young children, the frail, and some elderly.

You must also consider the muscle mass and fat deposits of the patient when choosing needle length. For example, an obese patient may require a longer needle to reach the muscle; an infant, child, or thin or frail person will require a shorter needle. In general, you can use a 1/2- to 5/8-inch needle for intradermal (ID) injections, 1/2- to 1-inch needle for subcutaneous (SC) injections, 1 1/2- to 2 1/2-inch needle for intramuscular (IM) injections, and 1/2- to 2-inch needle (or intracath) for IV infusions.

Administration Techniques

In preparing medications for administration by the parenteral route, aseptic technique must be followed. The contents of the ampule, vial, or IV bag or bottle are prepared by the manufacturer under aseptic conditions. Their sterility must be maintained throughout the process of preparing and administering the injection. One part of this process is to use only sterile equipment throughout the procedure.

Initially, all syringes, needles, and IV administration sets are sterile. If any item is contaminated, it must be discarded, and the procedure must be begun again with new equipment.

Syringes may be handled only by the barrel and the tip of the plunger. The wrapper is peeled back to remove the syringe. The tip of the barrel must not be touched. The syringe is held in one hand until the needle is attached and secured. The needle is never touched. The wrapper of the needle is peeled back to expose the hub, which is attached to the tip of the barrel and secured in place. The wrapper is then removed from the needle cap.

After removal of the top seal, the rubber stopper on the end of a vial must be cleansed with alcohol or other disinfectant before insertion of the needle. Follow institutional policy for the type of disinfectant. The shaft of the needle must never be touched. Draw the medication into the syringe following the Drug Administration Guidelines for removal of a medication from an ampule and for removal of a liquid from a vial. Discard all empty ampules and vials in sharps containers to prevent others from being cut.

In addition to asepsis during parenteral injections, care must be taken to protect the caregiver and others from contamination or injury from the equipment used for the injection. This is done by observing universal precautions for items contaminated with blood or body fluids. These precautions involve wearing gloves to protect the hands from contact with blood or body fluids. To give an SC, IM, or ID injection, glove the hand you will be using to cleanse the patient's skin before and after the injection because sometimes blood oozes from the injection site until it is covered with an adhesive bandage.

All injection sites must be cleansed with disinfectant and friction according to institutional policy. Start at the site of injection and cleanse in a circular motion from the center outward. Do not touch the site of the intended puncture after cleansing. Inject the medication according to the Drug Administration Guidelines for SC, IM, or ID injection.

Dispose of all needles and syringes in a sharps container labeled with a biohazard label immediately after use. Needles should not be recapped, bent, or manipulated. In the event that a needle must be recapped until it can be properly disposed of, the one-hand scoop technique must be used. Place the cap on a solid surface and, using one hand only, insert the needle into the cap and lift it up. Then, carefully secure the cap in place by pushing the cap against a firm surface. As soon as feasible, dispose of the entire unit in a sharps container. Dispose of bandages, gloves, and any other items contaminated with blood or drainage in a bag labeled with a biohazard label.

INJECTION SITES

Subcutaneous Injections

The subcutaneous (SC) route is usually appropriate for small doses (0.5 to 1 mL) of water-soluble drugs.

Oil-based or other types of drugs that may be irritating to tissues are best given by the intramuscular (IM) route. Drugs administered by the SC route are absorbed more slowly than those given by IM or intravenous (IV) routes and, therefore, give a more sustained action. The Drug Administration Guidelines describe subcutaneous injection.

Persons with peripheral vascular disease, patients with congestive heart failure with edema, those in terminal stages of illness, and some other patients may not be able to absorb SC injections appropriately. If the patient does not respond as expected to the injection, do not hesitate to discuss the situation with the supervisor or the physician.

DRUG ADMINISTRATION GUIDELINES

Administration of a Subcutaneous Injection

1. Check the medication order.
2. Wash hands.
3. Prepare the medication following aseptic technique and remembering **the five rights.**
4. Screen the patient.
5. Choose the administration site and position the patient. Give no more than 1 mL per site.
6. Glove nondominant hand.
7. Cleanse the site with an antiseptic swab. Cleanse from site outward, using a circular motion.
8. Grasp skin by bunching or spreading.
9. Insert the needle quickly, with bevel up, at a 45-degree angle (90-degree angle if the patient is obese).
10. Aspirate for blood to verify whether a blood vessel has been penetrated. If blood is aspirated, remove the needle, explain to the patient, return to the medication station, and begin again with step 1. (Do not aspirate when administering heparin.)
11. Inject the medication slowly and steadily.
12. Remove the needle quickly.
13. Using your gloved hand and an antiseptic swab, apply gentle pressure or massage the area according to the procedure for the medication given. Do not massage the site of a heparin injection.
14. **Do not recap needle!** If it is absolutely necessary to recap the needle, use the one-hand scoop method.
15. Remove glove by peeling it off, enclosing contaminated swab within the glove.
16. Secure the patient.
17. Dispose of the syringe in an appropriate sharps container.
18. Dispose of the glove in a waste container labeled with a biohazard label.
19. Wash hands.
20. Chart medication given, time, dose, route, site, and your name **(sixth right).**

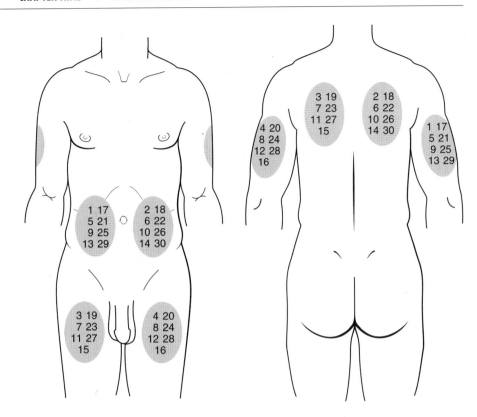

Figure 9–12. Suitable sites for subcutaneous injections include the posterior arms, anterior thighs, upper abdomen, and upper back.

There are many suitable sites for SC injections, such as the upper (posterior) arms, anterior thighs, upper abdomen, and back between the scapulae (Fig. 9–12). Sites must be rotated for the medication to be absorbed properly. Avoid scarred or edematous areas.

The patient's size and the amount of adipose tissue influence the thickness of the subcutaneous layer. Needle length and angle of insertion must vary accordingly. In general, the tissue is stretched taut, and a 1/2- to 5/8-inch needle is inserted at a 45-degree angle. If the patient is thin, pinch up the tissue and insert the needle at a 90-degree angle. If the patient is obese, a 1-inch needle may be used; insert the needle at a 90-degree angle without pinching the tissue. If the patient is thin, the upper abdomen is the best site because subcutaneous tissue remains there after it is lost from the peripheral sites. If the patient does not seem to have adequate subcutaneous tissue, discuss the dosage and route with the physician because the drug will be absorbed more rapidly than expected if the injection is actually being given into the muscle.

HYPODERMOCLYSIS OR "CLYSIS" Hypodermoclysis is a method of infusing larger amounts of solution into subcutaneous tissues. Large-volume solution containers are connected to special Y-type administration sets. Long needles are used to facilitate propping

and securing of the needles to the sites. To divide the dose, two parallel sites, such as the anterior or lateral thighs or scapula areas, are selected for infusion (Fig. 9–13). Sometimes an enzyme called hyaluronidase (Wydase) is ordered to be injected into the tubing to facilitate absorption of the fluids being administered.

Infuse solutions at the rate ordered by the physician. Check sites at least once an hour. If tissue at the sites becomes cool, pale, or hard, slow or discontinue the infusion rate.

Clysis is sometimes used to prevent or treat dehydration. Although not ordered frequently, it may sometimes provide a source of hydration to semicomatose or comatose patients in nursing homes or private homes where qualified nursing staff are not available to properly monitor IV solutions. See the Drug Administration Guidelines for administration and discontinuation of hypodermoclysis.

Intramuscular Injections

Because of the increased blood supply to the muscles, IM injections are absorbed more rapidly than SC injections are. Muscle tissue can tolerate more irritation than SC tissue can, so larger volumes of drugs can be injected at one time (1 to 3 mL, or even 1 to 5 mL *in special cases* if the patient has large muscle mass).

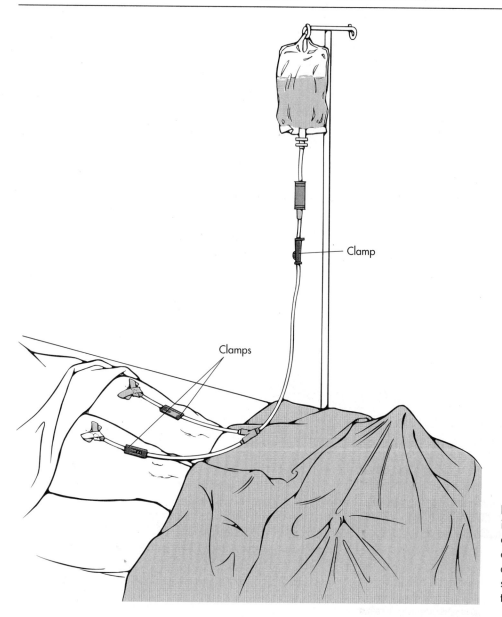

Figure 9–13. Hypodermoclysis is a method of infusing larger amounts of solution into subcutaneous tissues. Two parallel sites, such as the anterior or lateral thighs or scapula areas, are used to divide the dose.

Drugs that have an oil base or are irritating to tissues can often be given safely by the IM route.

Appropriate sites for IM injections are the deltoid muscle of the upper arm, the gluteus medius muscle in the dorsogluteal and ventrogluteal sites, the vastus lateralis muscle of the lateral thigh, and the rectus femoris muscle of the anterior thigh. See the Drug Administration Guidelines for locating the deltoid, gluteal, vastus lateralis, and rectus femoris injection sites.

The thigh is the recommended site for infants and small children because their gluteus medius muscle is not well enough developed to protect the nerve and arteries in the gluteal area. Drug absorption is also the most rapid from this site.

A needle of 1 1/2 to 2 1/2 inches is generally appropriate, but the size of the patient must always be considered. Infants, small children, the elderly, and emaciated patients may require a shorter needle, and those who are obese or have a large muscle mass may require a slightly longer needle. Manufacturers of some of the drugs that are irritating to tissues may also recommend a longer needle for administration of their product.

To minimize discomfort when an IM injection is given, the muscle should be relaxed. Position patients comfortably in a reclining position, if possible (except for injection into the deltoid). To relax the gluteus medius muscle, position the patient prone with the toes pointing inward. Tissues are either stretched taut

DRUG ADMINISTRATION GUIDELINES

Hypodermoclysis Administration

1. Check the order.
2. Wash hands.
3. Assemble the solution bag or bottle, administration tubing set, and needles using aseptic technique.
4. Hang the bag or bottle on an IV pole, flush the tubing, and transport to the patient's room.
5. Screen the patient.
6. Choose the sites and position the patient. Commonly used sites are under the breasts, upper surfaces of the thighs, and subscapular region of the back.
7. Glove nondominant hand.
8. Cleanse the site with an antiseptic swab. Cleanse from site outward, using a circular motion.
9. Grasp skin by bunching or spreading.
10. Insert the needle quickly at a 45-degree angle (90-degree angle if the patient is obese).
11. Support the needle with a cotton ball, if necessary, and tape securely.
12. Repeat steps 8, 9, 10, and 11 for the other site. Give 1/2 volume in each site.
13. Remove the glove by peeling it off.
14. Adjust the flow clamp to ordered flow rate.
15. Secure the patient.
16. Wash hands.
17. Chart name and volume of solution hung, time started, sites of administration, and your name (**sixth right**).
18. Check flow rate and administration sites frequently (at least hourly).

Always check with the pharmacist or other appropriate resource to verify whether drugs are chemically compatible. Also, the total volume of the combined drugs may not exceed that which is appropriate for the chosen site. Refer to the Drug Administration Guidelines for locating the gluteal, deltoid, vastus lateralis, and rectus femoris injection sites. See Box 9–1 for Z-track method of intramuscular injection.

No more than 3cc/muscle

Intradermal or Intracutaneous Injection

Drugs administered by the intradermal (ID) route (see Drug Administration Guidelines) are those used to test sensitivity to allergens or the tuberculin bacillus. For an inflammatory reaction to be observed, sites must be lightly pigmented and relatively free of hair. The medial aspect of the lower arm and the upper back are usually appropriate sites.

Tuberculin syringes are used to measure the small amounts of medication used for these tests. Short, fine-gauge needles are used to minimize irritation to the area (1/2-inch, 27- or 28-gauge). After the skin is cleansed, it is allowed to dry or is wiped dry with a sterile swab. This prevents the alcohol from irritating the tissue and interfering with the test. Hold the skin

or pinched if the patient is an infant, a child, or thin. The needle is injected at a 90-degree angle. Hand movement for insertion of the needle is rapid and dart-like, which also minimizes discomfort. The Drug Administration Guidelines describe intramuscular injection.

Manufacturers may also recommend a special Z-track technique for administration of irritating drugs or drugs such as iron, which may leak to the surface and permanently stain the skin (Box 9–1).

MIXING DRUGS IN THE SAME SYRINGE Sometimes the physician orders two or more medications to be given intramuscularly at the same time. To minimize discomfort to the patient, you may wish to combine these drugs into a single injection. This may be done as described in the Drug Administration Guidelines if the drugs are compatible with each other. Some drugs cannot be mixed together because they react chemically and cause a precipitate to form.

DRUG ADMINISTRATION GUIDELINES

Discontinuation of a Hypodermoclysis Infusion

1. Wash hands.
2. Screen the patient.
3. Close the flow clamps on the administration set.
4. Glove nondominant hand.
5. Remove the needle and apply gentle pressure to the site with an antiseptic swab.
6. Use one-hand scoop method to recap needle.
7. Apply adhesive bandage to site (and antiseptic ointment per institutional policy).
8. Repeat steps 5, 6, and 7 for the other site.
9. Remove the glove by peeling it off, enclosing contaminated swabs within glove.
10. Secure the patient.
11. Carefully remove capped needles and dispose of in an appropriate sharps container.
12. Dispose of bag and administration tubing in an appropriate container.
13. Wash hands.
14. Document time discontinued and description of sites (**sixth right**).

D R U G   A D M I N I S T R A T I O N   G U I D E L I N E S

Locating the Deltoid Injection Site

The deltoid muscle is used frequently because it is accessible with the patient in many positions. It should not be used if the drug being injected is irritating to tissues or slow to absorb. The site cannot be used for repeated injections or large amounts of medication.

   1. Identify the area by drawing an imaginary line across the arm in the area of the axilla. This is the lower border of the area. The upper border is the lower edge of the acromion process. The lateral borders are imaginary lines one third and two thirds of the way around the outer lateral aspect of the arm.

   2. Picture an upside-down triangle with the base at the upper border and the tip at the center of the lower border. The area to be used for injection falls within the triangle. This avoids the major bones, blood vessels, and nerves in the area.

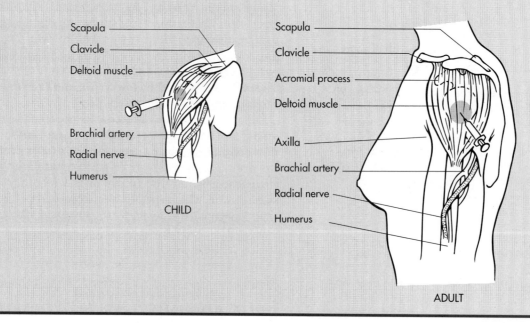

CHILD

ADULT

---

taut and insert the needle with the bevel up, at a 10- to 15-degree angle. This angle is nearly parallel to the skin. As the drug is injected, a raised wheal is produced. A wheal is a blister-like area that is white in the center. If the wheal is not produced, the injection may have been into the subcutaneous tissue, and the test will not be valid. If multiple injections are given (as in allergy testing), make a record of sites and solutions to determine which substances caused any reactions. Sites are "read" for reactions in 48 to 72 hours.

Intravenous Infusion

During infusion through the IV route, the correct type and the correct concentration of solution are just as important as administration of the correct medication. Other drugs are sometimes added to IV solutions and administered with the solution. A medication label indicating the drug, dose, time added, and initials of the person adding the drug must then be applied to the IV bottle. Some drugs are added by the pharmacist; others are added by the nurse at time of administration.

   Glass bottles are sealed with a rubber stopper that is covered by various types of rubber or metal disks and caps, depending on the manufacturer. These outer caps and disks must be removed at time of use to expose the rubber stopper. The IV administration set (tubing and connectors) must be inserted at time of administration. The "spiked" or pointed end is grasped at the drip chamber behind the phalange and inserted through the rubber stopper in the area marked. IV bottles must have an air vent to allow the air to displace the solution in the bottle. The pressure of the air allows the solution to flow out of the bottle. In some types of bottles, this vent is a sterile needle inserted into the rubber stopper in the area indicated. Other manufacturers place the air vent on the side of the administration set near the spike. The bottle is hung upside down by a metal wire that hangs on a hook on the IV pole on or next to the patient's bed. The other end of the tubing is connected to a needle or catheter in the patient's vein. A clamp on the tubing regulates the rate of flow of the solution. The height of the IV pole also influences the rate of flow. The pole is elevated to increase the gravitational pull on the solution and speed the rate of flow. Lowering the pole decreases the rate of flow (Fig. 9–14).

The manufacturer protects plastic IV bags by sealing them within another tough plastic bag. The outer bag is removed immediately before use. The inner bag often feels wet from condensation from the outer bag.

Examine the inner bag carefully to be certain the moisture is not caused by a puncture or other damage that has contaminated the contents. Never use a damaged bag. The spike of the administration set must be grasped at the drip chamber behind the phalange and carefully inserted into the portal to avoid damage to the bag. An internal seal is broken by the spike, which allows the solution to flow into the drip chamber and tubing. The bag is hung upside down on the IV pole by a plastic loop on the end of the bag. The height of the pole and the flow clamp control the rate of infusion, just as with the glass bottles.

D R U G   A D M I N I S T R A T I O N   G U I D E L I N E S

Locating Gluteal Injection Sites

Dorsogluteal Site (uses the gluteus medius muscle)
Note: The dorsogluteal site should not be used in children younger than 3 years because the muscles are not developed enough to protect the major blood vessels in this area and the sciatic nerve.

1. Direct/assist the patient to assume a prone position, if possible.

2. Direct the patient to assume a toe-in position because this helps to relax the muscle.

3. Identify the site by locating the crest of the ilium with one hand. Visually divide the buttock into four equal quadrants bounded on the top by the iliac crest, the bottom by the crease below the buttock, the medial aspect by the sacrum, and the lateral aspect by the greater trochanter of the femur.

Draw an imaginary line from the posterior superior iliac spine to the greater trochanter. Injections can be given anywhere above and to the outside of the diagonal line.

Ventrogluteal Site (uses the gluteus medius muscle)

1. The patient may be positioned prone, supine, or side-lying.

2. Identify the site by placing the palm of the hand on the lateral hip over the greater trochanter and spreading the index and middle fingers. One finger should be on the anterior superior iliac spine and the other on the iliac crest.

Injections can be given in the V area formed between the index and middle fingers. There are no major nerves or blood vessels in this area, so it may be safely used for children or adults.

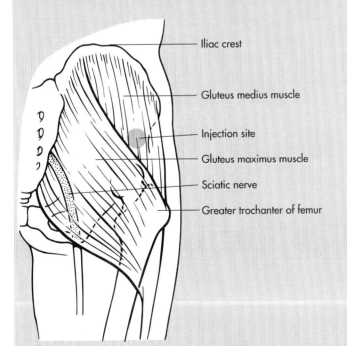

Iliac crest
Gluteus medius muscle
Injection site
Gluteus maximus muscle
Sciatic nerve
Greater trochanter of femur

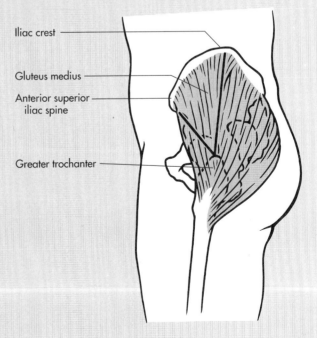

Iliac crest
Gluteus medius
Anterior superior iliac spine
Greater trochanter

D R U G   A D M I N I S T R A T I O N   G U I D E L I N E S

Locating the Vastus Lateralis and Rectus Femoris Injection Sites

Vastus Lateralis Site

The vastus lateralis muscle is used frequently in infants and children but can also be used in adults. It is free of major nerves and blood vessels.

1. Position the patient in a recumbent or in a sitting position.

2. Identify the site by drawing an imaginary rectangle on the lateral middle third of the thigh. This is the area onehand's breadth above the knee and one hand's breadth below the greater trochanter.

Rectus Femoris Site

The rectus femoris muscle is medial to the vastus lateralis muscle. It is identified in the same manner, but on the anterior middle third of the thigh. It is easily used by the patient for self-injection of medications. This site is close to the sciatic nerve and major blood vessels, so use caution in locating the site.

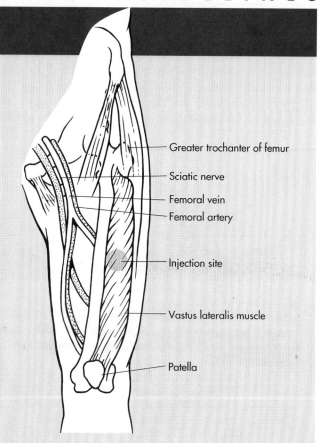

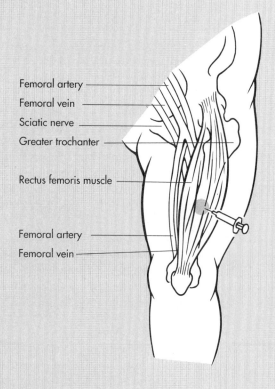

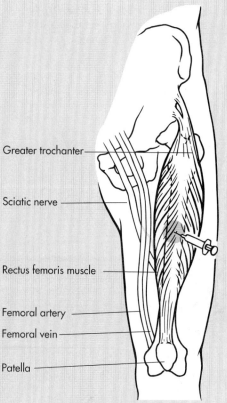

DRUG ADMINISTRATION GUIDELINES

Administration of Intramuscular Injections

1. Check the medication order.
2. Wash hands.
3. Prepare the medication following aseptic technique and remembering **the five rights.**
4. Screen the patient.
5. Choose the administration site and position the patient. (Give less than 5 mL in each site.)
6. Glove nondominant hand.
7. Cleanse the site with an antiseptic swab. Cleanse from site outward, using a circular motion.
8. Grasp skin by bunching or spreading.
9. Insert the needle quickly with dart-like action and at a 90-degree angle (45-degree angle if the patient is very thin).
10. Aspirate for blood to verify whether a blood vessel has been penetrated. If blood is aspirated, remove the needle, explain to the patient, return to the medication station, and begin again with step 1.
11. Inject the medication slowly and steadily.
12. Remove the needle quickly.
13. Using your gloved hand and an antiseptic swab, apply gentle pressure or massage the area according to the procedure for the medication given.
14. **Do not recap needle!** If it is absolutely necessary to recap the needle, use the one-hand scoop method.
15. Remove glove by peeling it off, enclosing contaminated swab within the glove.
16. Secure the patient.
17. Dispose of the syringe in an appropriate sharps container.
18. Dispose of the glove in a waste container labeled with a biohazard label.
19. Wash hands.
20. Chart medication given, time, dose, route, site, and your name **(sixth right).**

Whether a glass bottle or a plastic bag system is used, another important consideration in determining the rate of flow is the drip chamber on the administration set. Manufacturers design these to deliver a set number of drops per cubic centimeter or milliliter. Some chambers are referred to as macrochambers. These deliver 10, 15, or 20 gtt/mL. Others are referred to as microchambers and deliver as much as 60 gtt/mL. It is *essential*, therefore, to read the information on the box that has been provided by the manufacturer. Failure to do so can result in a massive fluid overload to the circulatory system, a failure to hydrate the patient in the ordered number of hours, or a medication overdose or underdose.

Sometimes two bottles or bags of solution are run into the same vein. This is called a tandem setup or an intravenous piggyback (IVPB) (Fig. 9–15). The first bottle or bag hung is called the primary IV infusion. The secondary bottle or bag is connected into the primary tubing or "line" by means of a special secondary tubing and another needle or special needleless connector. The secondary tubing has its own drip chamber and a flow clamp to control the rate of infusion. This IVPB setup allows intermittent infusion of drugs or other solutions without requiring the patient to have a new venipuncture each time. For example, an IV antibiotic ordered every 6 hours would require four venipunctures in a 24-hour period. By using an IVPB, only one venipuncture is required to start the primary IV infusion. At the ordered time, the IVPB is suspended from the pole and connected to the primary line; the clamp is opened and adjusted to the proper rate of flow. The secondary container must be suspended higher than the primary container for it to flow. A special hook is used to lower the primary container a few inches. This stops the flow of the primary container until the secondary bag or bottle empties. The primary bag or bottle then resumes its flow automatically. The rate of flow of the secondary IV infusion should be set according to the physician's order. This may differ from the ordered rate of flow for the primary IV infusion.

In certain situations, such as when elderly or children are receiving IV solutions, a volume-control device such as a Buretrol or Volutrol is placed between the bottle or bag and the regular administration set (Fig. 9–16). A clamp allows a specified amount of solution to enter the volume-control device. The rate of flow is then regulated by a clamp between the device and the patient. When the volume-control device empties, a nurse must then refill it by releasing the clamp between the device and the bottle or bag. For example, the physician orders 250 mL of a solution to be infused in a 5-hour period. A specified amount, such as 100 mL, is allowed to flow into the device, then the clamp is closed. This prevents movement of the patient or other factors from altering the flow rate and permitting the entire container to empty within a short time. Even if the flow rate is altered, only the limited amount of solution would be permitted to enter the vein. This is an important safety factor in preventing circulatory overload in the patient.

Many institutions require the use of infusion pumps to control the safety of IV infusions. Some infusion devices monitor the rate of IV flow by sounding an alarm when the drip rate falls above or below the parameters set on the device. Others control the rate of flow in various ways, such as by stretching or putting pressure on the IV tubing. If the device is unable to maintain the flow as set, an alarm sounds.

Follow manufacturers' instructions with all types of infusion pumps to set them up correctly. Tub-

Box 9–1. Z-Track Method of Intramuscular Injection

1. Check the medication order.

2. Wash hands.

3. Prepare the medication following aseptic technique and remembering the five rights.

4. Add 0.2 cc of air to the syringe to ensure that the drug will clear the needle.

5. Change the needle if the drug is one that will stain skin. Use a needle long enough to inject **deep** IM (2–3 inches).

6. Screen the patient and choose the site. **Use only large muscle mass!**

7. Glove nondominant hand.

8. Cleanse the area with an antiseptic swab, from site outward, using a circular motion.

9. Stretch the skin to one side approximately 1 inch and hold it in place while giving the injection.

10. Insert the needle at a 90-degree angle, using dart-like action.

11. Aspirate to verify whether a blood vessel has been penetrated. If blood is aspirated, remove the needle, explain to the patient, return to the medication area, and begin again with step 1.

12. Slowly inject the medication and the 0.2 cc of air.

13. Wait 10 seconds before removing the needle.

14. Remove the needle and allow the skin to return to normal position.

15. **Do not massage site!** Apply gentle pressure if necessary.

16. Dispose of syringe and needle in an appropriate sharps container.

17. Peel glove off, enclosing contaminated swab inside.

18. Secure the patient.

19. Chart medication, dose, site, route and method, time, and your name **(sixth right).**

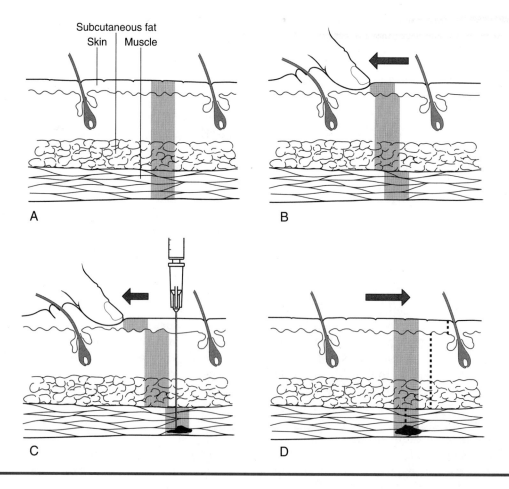

Subcutaneous fat
Skin | Muscle

A

B

C

D

DRUG ADMINISTRATION GUIDELINES

Mixing Two Medications in the Same Syringe

1. Check compatibility of the drugs to be mixed.
2. Calculate the volume of medications required for the prescribed dose.
3. Ascertain that the combined volume is appropriate for injection in one site and appropriate for the ordered route.
4. Assemble the injection equipment.
5. Maintain principles of aseptic technique throughout the procedure.
6. Cleanse the rubber stoppers of both vials with an antiseptic swab.
7. Uncap the needle and pull back the plunger, drawing in the amount of air equal to the volume of the first ordered drug.
8. Insert needle into the vial of that first ordered drug, inject the air, and withdraw the needle.
9. Pull back the plunger, drawing in the amount of air equal to the volume of the second ordered drug.
10. Insert the needle into the second vial and inject the air.
11. Leaving the needle in the vial, invert the vial, withdraw the ordered amount of medication, and withdraw the needle from the vial.
12. Verify with the physician's order that the volume of drug in the syringe is appropriate.
13. Reinsert the needle into the first vial, **carefully** withdraw the volume of the first ordered drug, and remove the needle.
14. Verify with the physician's order that the volume of drug in the syringe is appropriate.
15. Change the needle as it is dulled by repeated puncturing of the rubber stoppers.

ings must be threaded through certain pathways within the pump, and flow rates must be programmed into the device. Larger infusion pumps are mounted on the IV pole and connected to an electrical outlet for power. The unit contains a battery that automatically activates if the power source is disconnected. The pole is mounted on a base with wheels to facilitate ambulation and transportation of the patient.

Another type of pump, called a syringe pump, is capable of injecting small doses of drugs into the IV tubing by putting pressure on the plunger of the prefilled syringe contained inside the pump. This type of pump is sometimes used to deliver intermittent doses of insulin throughout the day or narcotic analgesics. If the drug is an analgesic, the term PCA (patient-controlled analgesia) is often used. This system allows the patient to self-administer a preset amount of medication when needed. Safety devices built into the pump prevent dosing too frequently and therefore prevent an overdose. The individual dose and the dose per hour are programmed into the pump by the pharmacist, according to the physician's order. Syringe pumps are small battery-operated devices that are placed in bed beside the patient or worn on a belt or halter arrangement to facilitate ambulation.

Although this type of device gives an alert patient control over the medication, it is important for you to check with the patient at regular intervals to assess the effects of the medication. Is the pain controlled? Is the patient too drowsy? Are the vital signs remaining stable? Relinquishing control of the dosing time to the patient does not relieve the nurse of the responsibility to monitor the effects and adverse effects of the medication.

The contents of the IV bag or bottle and the IV administration sets are prepared by the manufacturer under aseptic conditions. The stopper on the end of an IV bottle must also be cleansed with disinfectant before insertion of the spike. IV bags have a cap protecting the port that must be removed before insertion of the spike. Never touch the shaft of the intracath or needle and the end of the IV tubing.

To maintain universal precautions, glove both hands during IV injection technique; the chance of contamination of the hands is great because of the amount of manipulation of equipment involved in the procedure. Whenever the chance of splatter exists, as with IV procedures, also wear glasses or goggles. In some cases, protective lab coats or aprons that are impervious to liquids are worn to protect the clothing. The injection site must be cleansed in the same manner as described previously.

Intravenous Injection

Infants have such small peripheral vessels that a scalp vein is often chosen as the IV site. These veins often dilate as the infant cries, which facilitates location of the vessel and insertion of the needle. In addition, it is easier to secure the needle at the site, and the infant does not have to be immobilized as much as when an arm vein is chosen. In adults and larger children, IV solutions and medications are usually administered into a peripheral vein in the arm or hand.

To facilitate an IV injection, first distend the chosen vessel by blocking venous flow from the area. Apply a tourniquet to the arm above the chosen site. If the vein does not distend rapidly, ask the patient to hang the

D R U G   A D M I N I S T R A T I O N   G U I D E L I N E S

Administration of Medication by the Intradermal Route

1. Check the order.
2. Wash hands.
3. Prepare the medication in a tuberculin syringe, with 26- to 28-gauge 3/8- to 1/2-inch needle, following aseptic technique and remembering **the five rights.** Doses are **always** small volumes of approximately 0.1 cc.
4. Screen the patient.
5. Select the site or sites and position the patient. **In tuberculin testing, the anterior forearm is the desired site.**
6. Glove nondominant hand.
7. Cleanse the area or areas with an antiseptic swab from the site outward, using a circular motion. **Allow to air dry.**
8. Insert the needle at a 15-degree angle with the bevel up.
9. Inject the medication slowly into the dermis. A wheal forms if the injection has been done properly. Remove the needle quickly.

10. Dispose of the syringe in an appropriate sharps container.
11. Chart the time, drug, concentration, amount, site, and your signature **(sixth right).**
12. In performing allergy testing, repeat steps 1 to 11 with each allergen ordered to be tested. Make a diagram indicating the sites of injection and number each site to correspond with the allergen injected.
13. Read sites at the ordered time (usually 48 to 72 hours after injection). A metric ruler must be used. Read in a good light. Measure diameter of area of erythema in millimeters and record. Palpate and measure area of induration in millimeters and record. Readings are recorded for each site numbered on the diagram. **In tuberculin testing, only the area of induration is recorded.**

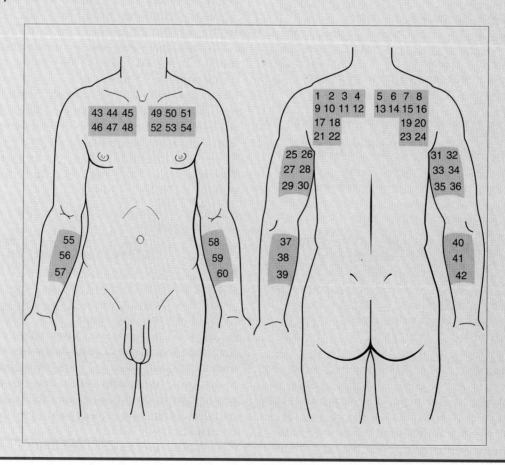

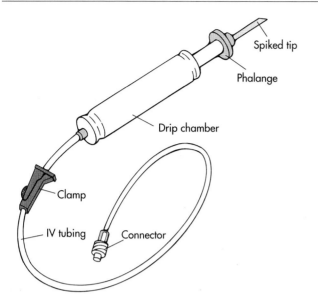

Figure 9–14. An intravenous administration set.

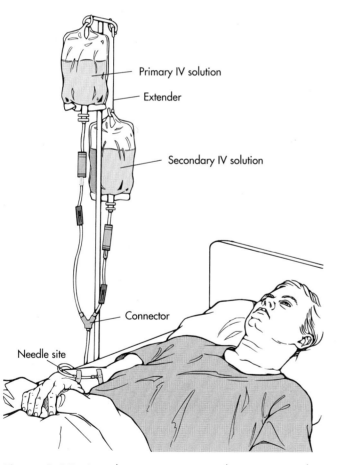

Figure 9–15. A tandem intravenous setup has primary and secondary bottles or bags connected into the same tubing. This prevents multiple venipunctures while still allowing intermittent infusions.

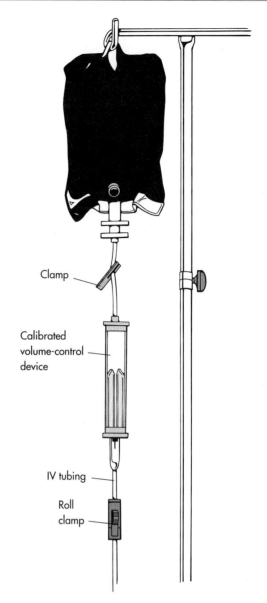

Figure 9–16. Intravenous administration set with calibrated volume-control device.

limb down in a dependent position or to flex and extend the fingers (alternately make a fist and relax it). If the vein still does not distend, a warm moist cloth can be applied to the area for a few minutes, or the area can be gently "slapped." If these efforts do not work, another site may be chosen.

When the chosen vein is sufficiently dilated, cleanse the area and insert a needle or intracath of sufficient length (1/2 to 2 inches) to deliver the solution or medication. Hold the skin taut and insert the needle with the bevel up, at an angle parallel to the skin and pointed toward the heart. Make the puncture next to the vein, then sideways and forward into the vein. This is to prevent puncturing all the way through both walls of the vein.

DRUG ADMINISTRATION GUIDELINES

Administration of Intravenous Fluids

1. Verify the physician's order.
2. Wash hands.
3. Assemble the equipment.
4. Maintain aseptic technique throughout the procedure.
5. Close the clamp on the solution administration set.
6. Insert the spike of the solution administration set into the bag or bottle.
7. Pump the drip chamber to fill it.
8. Open the clamp on the solution administration set to flush the tubing.
9. Close the clamp.
10. Transport the equipment to the patient's bedside.
11. Identify the patient. **Remember the five rights.**
12. Screen the patient.
13. Position the patient for comfort.
14. Select the IV site and place a tourniquet on the extremity above the site.
15. Open the dressing kit, tear the tape, and so on.
16. Put on gloves and protective eyewear.
17. Cleanse the site in a circular motion from the site outward, using an antiseptic swab or solution according to institutional policy.
18. Open the intracath and turn the bevel up.
19. Hold the skin taut; puncture the skin next to the vein and then into the vein.
20. Verify venous return by pulling back approximately 1/2 inch on the needle stylet.
21. Carefully thread the intracath into the vein.
22. Remove the sterile cover from the end of the solution administration set.
23. Remove the needle stylet from the intracath, place it on the overbed table out of the patient's way, and quickly connect the solution administration set to the hub of the intracath.
24. Release the tourniquet.
25. Open the flow valve and observe the site. If there are no problems with the flow or the site, slow the flow.
26. Apply antibiotic and sterile dressing according to institutional policy and secure the tubing with tape.
27. Peel one glove off.
28. Adjust the flow clamp to provide the ordered rate of flow.
29. Secure the patient.
30. Dispose of the needle stylet in an appropriate sharps container; dispose of any contaminated swabs, second glove, and other items in an appropriate container; wash hands.
31. Chart amount and type of solution, site of administration, and time begun **(sixth right).**
32. Monitor at least every hour for appropriate rate and signs of complications; document same.

If the solution is to be administered by infusion pump or monitor, connect the setup to this device between steps 9 and 10; turn the pump on and program flow rate at step 25.

If a syringe and needle are being used to withdraw blood or to administer medication, pulling back on the plunger will aspirate blood into the syringe if the needle is properly placed in the vein. If so, release the tourniquet and proceed.

"IV push" medications are usually administered slowly in a period of a few minutes. Most of them have specific requirements for administration. Consult institutional policies to verify educational requirements to administer them, and always check appropriate resources for technical information. This is important with all medications, but it is critical with IV drugs because of their rapid action. Use a watch with a second hand to monitor the administration time to guarantee accuracy.

Many medications are too toxic or too irritating to the vein to be given by push and must be diluted and administered in a longer time. Check drug resources to determine the appropriate solution for dilution. Solutions are prepared in an IV bag or bottle labeled with the drug, dose, and time. The person preparing the solution signs or initials the label. The contents may then be infused through an IV administration tubing attached to the needle or intracath.

To give an infusion through an intracath, make the venipuncture and attach the IV administration set to the hub. Hold it in place with one hand while releasing the clamp with the other hand to begin the flow of solution. If the solution flows freely, regulate the rate according to the physician's order, and secure the catheter and tubing to the limb.

IV sites are protected by an occlusive dressing or disinfectant or antibiotic ointment. Follow institutional policy in all aspects of these procedures. Instruct patients not to handle IV sites and to notify the caregiver if the IV site becomes edematous or painful. See the Drug Administration Guidelines for administration of IV fluids.

Monitor all IV infusions at least every hour to assess for problems. Problems that frequently occur are inaccurate infusion rates, kinks in the tubing, infiltration of fluids into the tissues surrounding the vein, circulatory overload, and thrombus formation.

Sometimes the physician orders a very slow rate of IV infusion to keep the vein open in case of an emergency or to intermittently infuse IV drugs. This is called a KVO (keep vein open) rate or TKO (to keep open). Suggested rate of flow for KVO is usually 10 mL/h.

When an IV is discontinued, immediately dispose of the needle or intracath in a sharps container. Dispose of tubing, occlusive dressings, bandages, gloves, and any other items contaminated with blood or drainage in a bag labeled with a biohazard label. See the Drug Administration Guidelines for discontinuation of an IV infusion.

DRUG ADMINISTRATION GUIDELINES

Discontinuation of an Intravenous Infusion

1. Check the order.
2. Assemble the equipment.
3. Identify the patient.
4. Screen the patient.
5. Don gloves.
6. Stop the IV pump, if present, and clamp the IV tubing.
7. Hold the needle or intracath securely while removing the tape or sterile transparent dressing.
8. Hold a dry gauze pad at the insertion site with one hand while slowly withdrawing the needle or intracath with the other hand, keeping it parallel to the extremity until it is completely removed.
9. As soon as the tip is visible, apply pressure to the insertion site with the dry gauze sponge and elevate the extremity to stop bleeding from the vein.
10. When you are certain there is no bleeding, apply an adhesive bandage or gauze and antibiotic ointment to the site. (Follow institutional policy.)
11. Dispose of equipment following universal precautions.
12. Chart time, amount of solution infused, and signature. In nurse's notes, document appearance of the infusion site **(sixth right).**

E X E R C I S E S

LEARNING ACTIVITIES

Using the Guidelines and the appropriate administration equipment, practice parenteral administration techniques until you feel comfortable with them. Then ask a classmate to use the Guidelines to critique your techniques. When you are ready, ask your instructor to verify that your techniques are appropriate.

General + Purpose of Med.
cure = antibiotic
Treat = chemotherapy
diagnose - IVP dye
relieve - Calamine & Analgesia.
prevent - immunization programs

Enteral
Oral simplest, more convenient
Solids & Liquids
access swallowing reflex.
- suitable position
- adequate flds
- modify swallowing problems

PERCUTANEOUS ADMINISTRATION

LEARNING OBJECTIVES

After studying this chapter, you should be able to:

1. Define the percutaneous route of medication administration.

2. Describe the difference between inunctions, creams, ointments, liniments, and lotions.

3. Explain the mode of action of sublingual and buccal medications.

4. Demonstrate appropriate techniques for preparation and administration of percutaneous (topical) medications by inhalation, direct application, irrigation, instillation, and insertion.

The percutaneous (topical) route involves the application of medication to the skin or mucous membranes. This route is used in an effort to prevent or to lessen systemic adverse effects that may occur. However, patients can still experience adverse effects from these products, just as they may from other forms of drugs. Always check physicians' orders and pharmacists' directions carefully.

PREPARATION FORMS

The percutaneous route includes

• The application of lotions, creams, ointments, powders, or patches to the skin
• The application of moist, medicated compresses to the skin
• The instillation of solutions into the eye, ear, nose, mouth, vagina, rectum, or bladder

• The use of aerosol to deliver liquids or gases to the lungs

The concentration (strength) of these preparations is an important part of the dosing information. In general, you will note that ophthalmic (eye) preparations and otic (ear) preparations are weak concentrations and are often ordered in 1%, 2%, or 3% strengths or as fractions of 1%, such as 0.25% or 0.5%.

Skin

Inunctions

Xylocaine

Inunctions are medicated substances that are massaged or rubbed into the skin to produce localized external effects. Systemic effects may be noted from some of these also.

Creams

Cream preparations have a "creamy" colored appearance. They are packaged in tubes or jars. Creams are frequently ordered to soothe burns or rashes. The base is generally nongreasy and can be removed with water. *Kenalog*

Ointments

Drugs prepared in an oily lanolin or petroleum base are ointments. They usually cannot be removed with water. This form is often ordered for antibiotics to be applied directly into a wound.

Liniments

Drugs are sometimes manufactured in a mixture with soap, oil, alcohol, or water, which is massaged or rubbed into the skin. The friction of the massage helps produce heat to the skin by increasing circulation to the area. Liniments are used to relieve muscle and joint pain. *AT 39*

Lotions

Lotions are aqueous (water-based) preparations that contain suspended particles. They *must always be shaken* before use to redistribute the particles throughout the liquid. Lotions have several purposes. Some lotions soothe rashes or irritation and are just patted onto the skin. Others have an astringent or drawing action and may be stroked on the skin. *Calamine*

Dermal Patches

Manufacturers are now preparing drugs in patches that look like adhesive bandages of various sizes and shapes. Heart medications, hormones, antigens for skin testing for allergens, and drugs to prevent "seasickness" and vomiting are now being dispensed in this form. *nitro patch – Nicoderm*

Wet Dressings/Irrigations

Chemicals are sometimes mixed with water or normal saline and applied as wet dressings or compresses to the skin or as irrigations to the vagina, bladder, eyes, or ears. Their strength is determined by the amount of solution with which they are prepared. They are always ordered by their strength, such as, 1%, 3%, or 10%. It is important to verify the strength of a solution because tissue damage may result if an improper strength is used.

Medicated Powders

Medications are sometimes prepared in a talc base to cool, dry, or protect areas. *Goldbond*

Sublingual and Buccal Preparations

Medications administered by the sublingual (SL) or buccal routes are dissolved and absorbed into the circulation by the blood vessels in the area. These drugs give a systemic effect as they pass directly into the circulatory system.

Ophthalmic Preparations

Medications should be labeled "ophthalmic" if they are to be used in the eye. They are always sterile and are prepared in dilute concentrations. Eye medications may be in the form of drops, ointments, or irrigations. These are always in individual-use containers to prevent cross-contamination to another person.

Otic Preparations

Medications to be used in the ear must be labeled "otic." Antibiotics and agents for cerumen removal are often prepared in solutions for use in the ear.

Nasal Preparations

Nose Drops and Nasal Sprays

Nose drops and nasal sprays are used to relieve temporary conditions of the nose. These are always in individual-use containers. Nasal sprays are often more effective than drops because they contact a larger area of the mucosa without being wasted by draining down the throat as drops do (Fig. 10–1).

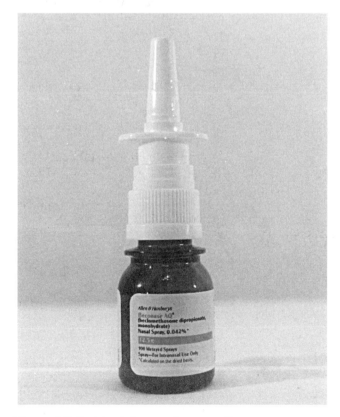

Figure 10-1. Nasal drops and sprays relieve temporary conditions of the nose. (Photo by Roger W. Fair.)

Inhalation Devices

Inhalers and Nebulizers

Nebulizers are devices used to spray medication into the throat. Aerosols use air or oxygen under pressure to deliver the medication deep into the respiratory passages. The manufacturer's instructions for cleaning should be followed carefully.

Metered dose inhalers (MDI) are pressurized aerosol devices used to apply medication directly to the bronchial smooth muscles. The valve delivers the same (metered) dose each time it is pressed (Fig. 10–2).

Vaginal Medications

Several types of vaginal medications are prescribed for a variety of gynecological disorders. There are creams, suppositories, and irrigations (douches) manufactured to treat vaginal infections. Hormones are sometimes administered as vaginal creams. Suppositories are drugs that are prepared in an oily or creamy base that solidifies into a firm shape; cocoa butter is frequently used as the base. Suppositories are inserted into body openings such as the vagina, rectum, and urethra. They are manufactured in various shapes, but the end to be inserted is usually

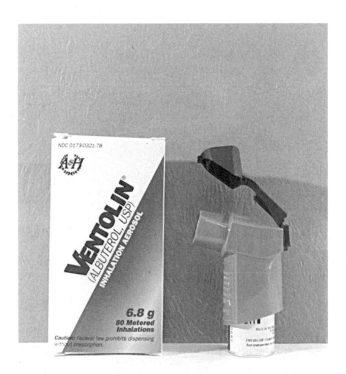

Figure 10–2. Metered dose inhalers apply medication directly to the bronchial smooth muscles by pressurized aerosol. (Photo by Roger W. Fair.)

rounded to facilitate insertion. At body temperature, the base melts and allows the medication to contact the mucous membranes of the passage, where it produces a localized or systemic effect. For example, sulfa drugs are sometimes prepared as a vaginal cream or as suppositories for use in the localized treatment of vaginal infections.

In addition to these prescription drugs, a variety of nonprescription products available at the drug store or supermarket are frequently administered into the vagina. Spermicidal chemicals are prepared as creams, jellies, foams, and sponges.

Many types of commercially prepared douche products are available. Diluted vinegar and baking soda, common household products, are frequently used as irrigations.

Bladder Irrigations and Instillations

Sterile water, sterile normal saline, disinfectants, and chemotherapeutic drugs are sometimes instilled into the bladder. The procedure may be ordered to remove clots or debris or to treat an infection or cancer. Disinfectants or chemotherapeutic drugs are occasionally prepared as urethral suppositories.

Rectal Medications

Suppositories

Patients who are vomiting, are comatose, or have difficulty swallowing oral medications may sometimes receive them by rectal suppository with systemic effects similar to those caused by oral administration. Examples are antipyretics, antiemetics, and analgesics. Suppositories are also ordered for localized effects, such as to stimulate peristalsis of the lower gastrointestinal tract to cause defecation.

Medicated Enemas

In some instances, medication is ordered to be given as an enema. This form is often ordered to be given in preparation for bowel surgery.

ADMINISTRATION

Skin

Medications to be applied to the skin should never be touched directly with the hand. Always use a swab, tongue blade, or gloves to handle them to prevent absorption by the skin of the hands and resultant side effects. Check orders for cleansing of the area before application of the next dose. Chemical irritation may result from build-up of residue at the site of application.

Some solutions, such as povidone-iodine, potassium permanganate, and silver nitrate, will stain skin, flooring, cloth, and almost anything else. Other solutions, such as sodium hypochlorite (Dakin's solution), will bleach cloth and flooring. Take care to protect the surrounding area from spills, and be careful to contain the drainage from the area being treated. Obtain specific directions from the physician about the type of dressing required.

Know what color the solution is supposed to be. Some chemicals change color, indicating a chemical breakdown into a different substance, and must not be used. You must be knowledgeable of solutions, just as you are of any other medication you are administering.

call Dr. if patch falls off

Medication Patches

Dermal or transdermal patches can be applied to areas of intact skin that are free of hair. The patch must be maintained securely against the skin for proper absorption to occur. Carefully follow directions regarding the site. Sites are to be rotated daily. The chest, flank, and upper arms are frequently used because they are easily reached by the patient. Develop a rotation schedule to avoid skin irritation. Institutions often have policies requiring the nurse to date and initial the patch with a pen after it is applied.

Some patches can be worn during bathing or showering; others should be removed if they become wet. Skin must be cleansed before application of a patch and after removal of a patch. Take care during application and removal to avoid contact of the fingers with the medicated surface, because the drug can also be absorbed by the skin of the person applying the patch. Teach patients to wrap and dispose of patches carefully to avoid accidental overdose by children or pets who may find the discarded patch and handle or chew on it.

Patch Testing for Allergens

The antigens are placed on the patient's skin and occluded with nonabsorbent, hypoallergenic tape. The back, arms, and thighs are frequently used as test sites. Careful recording of the antigen (allergen) used and the patch site is imperative to interpretation of the results.

Instruct patients not to get the patch sites wet. If severe burning or itching occurs, they should remove the patch and wash the area, taking care not to disturb the surrounding patches. Teach them to immediately report to the physician or the emergency room the occurrence of any symptoms that may indicate anaphylaxis, such as tightness or swelling of the tongue or throat, tightness in the chest, breathing difficulty, severe hives, or rash.

Patches are usually left in place for 48 hours, left open to the air for 15 minutes, and then "read." Redness and swelling indicate allergy to the specific antigen used at that site.

Medicated Powders

Before applying medicated powders, first cleanse the area and carefully dry it. Shake the powder from the container gently, then spread it smoothly over the area with a glove or swab. Always take care to protect the patient's and care giver's respiratory passages from inhalation of the powder.

Sublingual and Buccal Medications

Sublingual (SL) medications are placed under the tongue, and buccal medications are placed between the cheek and the molars. The mucous membranes of the mouth must be moist for the drug to dissolve and be absorbed. If the person is dehydrated or has been mouth breathing, the mouth may be rinsed before administration of the drug.

Ophthalmic Preparations

If there are excessive secretions or crusting, carefully cleanse these before administration of ophthalmic preparations.

Never touch the eye with the dropper or the tip of the medication tube because this contaminates the applicator and may also scratch the cornea. Wear a glove on the hand used to touch the eyelid to protect from contact with tears or secretions, in accord with universal precautions (Fig. 10–3).

Some drops dilate or constrict the pupil and affect vision. Ointments cause blurring of vision. Teach patients to avoid hazardous activities after use. To avoid systemic effects, apply gentle pressure with a cotton ball at the inner canthus of the eye for 1 to 2 minutes after instilling drops. This prevents passage of the drops through the nasolacrimal duct into the nose, with resultant absorption into the systemic circulation by the nasal mucosa.

If more than one type of drop is ordered, wait 5 minutes between medications. If drops and ointment are ordered at the same time, instill drops before ointments, because ointments are oil based and the drops would just run off the eye.

Significant abbreviations to know for interpretation of the physician's order are

OD = right eye

OS = left eye

OU = both eyes

See the Drug Administration Guidelines for the methods of instilling eye drops or ointment.

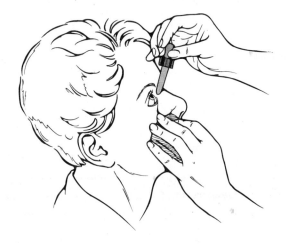

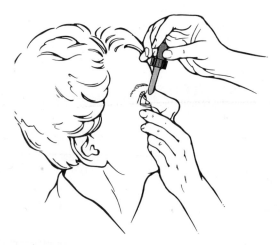

Figure 10–3. In administering ophthalmic preparations, never touch the eye with the dropper or tip of the medication tube because this causes contamination and may scratch the cornea.

DRUG ADMINISTRATION GUIDELINES

Administration of Eye Drops or Ointment

1. Verify the physician's order.
2. Wash hands.
3. Assemble the medication, a cotton ball, and a glove.
4. Identify the patient. **Remember the five rights.**
5. Screen the patient and place in a sitting position or elevate the head of the bed 45 degrees, if permitted.
6. Put the glove on.
7. Cleanse the eye to remove crusting, if necessary.
8. Have the patient look upward.
9. Using the gloved hand, apply gentle traction to facial tissue below the lower lid to expose the conjunctival sac.
10. Using the other hand, instill the eye drops into the sac. **Do not touch the eye with the dropper.**
11. Using the gloved hand and a cotton ball, apply gentle pressure to the bone at the inner canthus of the eye for 1 to 2 minutes to prevent/minimize systemic absorption through the nasal mucosa.
12. Peel glove off and dispose of in an appropriate container.
13. Wash hands.
14. Chart time, medication, number of drops, which eye, and your name **(sixth right).**

If more than one type of eye drop is ordered to be given, wait 5 minutes and follow above steps for each type.

For *eye ointment,* follow steps 1 through 9.

15. Using the other hand, gently squeeze the ointment in a strip into the sac from the inner to the outer canthus. **Do not touch the eye with the tip.**
16. Ask the patient to close the eye and roll it around to disperse the medication.

Continue with step 12.

Otic Preparations

Warm ear medications before instillation to prevent nausea or dizziness. Ear medications are never shared with other patients. Do not allow the dropper to touch the ear. Follow universal precautions by wearing a glove on the hand used to straighten the ear canal.

To prevent loss of the medication, have the patient remain on the side with the medicated ear up for approximately 10 minutes after administration. Place cotton *loosely* in the ear, if ordered. *Never* occlude the ear with a firm plug. See the Drug Administration Guidelines for administration of ear drops.

DRUG ADMINISTRATION GUIDELINES

Administration of Ear Drops

1. Verify the physician's order.
2. Wash hands.
3. Identify the patient. **Remember the five rights.**
4. Screen the patient and position so the affected ear is up.
5. Glove one hand.
6. Using an otoscope, assess for earwax. If irrigation is necessary, obtain the physician's order.
7. **Child younger than 3 years:** restrain; turn head to appropriate side; with gloved hand, pull ear lobe down and back. **Adult/child older than 3 years:** turn head to appropriate side; with gloved hand, pull ear lobe up and back.
8. Do not allow the dropper tip to touch the ear.
9. The patient should remain in that position for a few minutes.
10. If the physician orders, apply a piece of cotton **loosely** in the outer canal. **Do not occlude tightly!**
11. Peel glove off and dispose of properly.
12. Wash hands.
13. Chart time, medication, number of drops, which ear, and your name **(sixth right).**

If ear drops are ordered for both ears, repeat steps for the other ear.

Nasal Preparations

Teach patients to gently blow the nose before administration to clear the passages of excess mucus. Nasal decongestant preparations should be used only for 1 to 2 weeks. If symptoms are not relieved in that time, the physician should be consulted. Prolonged use can result in the "rebound phenomenon," in which the symptoms recur worse than ever. See the Drug Administration Guidelines for nose drops and nasal sprays.

Metered Dose Inhalers

The metered dose inhaler (MDI) has directions in the package; teach patients to follow them carefully. If the patient is unable to coordinate compression of the valve releasing the medication and inhalation, a device called an extender can be purchased. When the valve is pushed, the measured dose of medication is trapped in another chamber, from which the patient inhales it. Follow the manufacturer's instructions for cleaning the device.

Medications used in the respiratory tract should never have an oily base. Oil-based products could cause a lipid pneumonia.

Note: Patients frequently do not follow prescription orders about frequency of dosing with nasal and

DRUG ADMINISTRATION GUIDELINES

Administration of Nose Drops

1. Verify the order.
2. Wash hands.
3. Identify the patient. **Remember the five rights.**
4. Screen the patient.
5. If the patient is an adult or older child, have the patient gently blow the nose.
6. Have the patient lie down on the back with the head over the edge of the bed. Position and restrain infants and young children.
7. Hold the dropper above the nostril and instill the ordered number of drops. **Do not touch the nose with the dropper.** Repeat in second nostril, if ordered.
8. Have patient remain in this position for several minutes to allow drops to remain in contact with the mucosa.
9. Have tissues available, because the nose may drip when the patient sits up.
10. Wash hands.
11. Chart time, medication, number of drops, which naris or nares, and your name **(sixth right).**

DRUG ADMINISTRATION GUIDELINES

Administration of Nasal Sprays

1. Verify the order.
2. Wash hands.
3. Identify the patient. **Remember the five rights.**
4. Screen the patient.
5. Position upright.
6. Have the patient gently blow the nose.
7. Have the patient block one naris by pressing on the side of the nose.
8. Shake the bottle.
9. Insert the tip of the bottle into the naris and ask the patient to inhale while squeezing the bottle the ordered number of times.
10. Repeat with the other naris if ordered.
11. The patient should have a tissue ready in case the nose drips. Caution not to blow the nose for a few minutes unless it is absolutely necessary.
12. Wash hands.
13. Chart time, drug, number of sprays, which naris or nares, and your name **(sixth right).**

inhalation preparations. Emphasize that these medications, like all others, can have serious side effects when they are not taken as directed. See the Drug Administration Guidelines for medication administration through metered dose inhalers and by inhalation nebulizer.

Vaginal Medications

Availability of these products tends to lead the consumer to believe that there are no consequences to the use of these products, which is far from true. Allergic reactions can occur and cause severe burning, itching, and swelling. Bleeding may follow the friction of intercourse. Too frequent douching destroys the normal flora of the vaginal tract, and fungal infections can occur. Self-medication sometimes delays effective treatment, as in the case of bacterial and parasitic infections and sexually transmitted diseases (STDs), which require specific drug therapy. This delay may be enough time to allow the organisms to travel up the mucous membrane of the vagina to infect the cervix, uterus, fallopian tubes, and even the pelvic tissues themselves. This results in pelvic inflammatory dis-

DRUG ADMINISTRATION GUIDELINES

Medication Administration Through Metered Dose Inhalers

1. Verify the order.
2. Wash hands.
3. Identify the patient. **Remember the five rights.**
4. Screen the patient.
5. Encourage an upright position, if possible.
6. Follow the directions provided with the patient's inhaler.
7. If the medication is a suspension, shake the inhaler.
8. Have the patient open the mouth.
9. If the patient is using an extender, place it in the patient's mouth with the lips around it; if no extender is used, hold the inhaler 2 to 4 inches away from the patient's open mouth.
10. Have the patient inhale as deeply as possible for about 10 seconds while the valve on the inhaler is compressed.
11. Have the patient hold breath as long as is comfortable, then slowly exhale.
12. Repeat in 2 to 3 minutes, if ordered.
13. Secure the patient.
14. Wash hands.
15. Chart time, medication, number of puffs, and your name **(sixth right).**

DRUG ADMINISTRATION GUIDELINES

Medication Administration by Inhalation Nebulizer

1. Verify the order.
2. Wash hands.
3. Identify the patient. **Remember the five rights.**
4. Screen the patient.
5. Position the patient in a sitting position.
6. Put gloves on.
7. Add the prescribed amount of medication and diluent to the nebulizer.
8. Encourage the patient to purse lips and exhale.
9. Have the patient place mouthpiece in mouth with the lips around it but *not* completely sealed.
10. Have the patient inhale a deep breath while the nebulizer is activated.
11. Have the patient exhale slowly through pursed lips.
12. Wait approximately 1 minute to allow the medication to distribute and act in the bronchial tree, then repeat steps 8 to 11 until the nebulizer is empty.
13. Reposition the patient.
14. Cleanse equipment according to directions provided by the manufacturer.
15. Peel gloves off and dispose of properly.
16. Wash hands.
17. Chart time, medication, diluent, length of treatment, and your name **(sixth right).**

ease (PID), which can cause pain and sterility, or necessitates major surgery to free adhesions and bowel obstructions. In addition, sexual partners may also become infected and suffer serious consequences.

This is valuable information to convey to the patient, in addition to the proper techniques for each type of treatment. See the Drug Administration Guidelines for administration of a vaginal douche and vaginal medications. Also teach the appropriate hygienic measures to prevent transmission of infection to the bladder, the eyes, or the sexual partner.

Bladder Irrigations and Instillations

A Foley catheter is necessary for both bladder irrigations and instillations. The main difference between the procedures is that in an irrigation, the solution flows back out of the catheter immediately; with an instillation, the solution is trapped in the bladder by clamping the Foley catheter for an ordered time, usually about 20 minutes. If the patient becomes uncomfortable, release the clamp immediately, even if the ordered amount of time has not yet elapsed.

Maintenance of aseptic technique is critical to prevention of (or control of) bladder infections. See the Drug Administration Guidelines for administration of medication into the bladder.

Rectal Medications

Rectal Suppositories

Because suppositories melt when warm, they are often found in the refrigerator. They come in jars or in individually packaged and labeled unit-dose forms. If

DRUG ADMINISTRATION GUIDELINES

Administration of a Vaginal Douche

1. Verify the order.
2. Assemble the equipment.
3. Identify the patient. **Remember the five rights.**
4. Have the patient void.
5. If the solution is not already prepared, add the ordered amount of medication and diluent to the douche bag and suspend the bag from an IV pole approximately 12 inches above the hips.
6. If permitted, transfer the patient to the tub room; position in a semireclining position. If not permitted, screen the patient, glove, and place the patient on a bedpan in a semi-reclining position.
7. Glove, if not already done.
8. Release the clamp and allow a small amount of solution to flow over the vulva.
9. With one gloved hand, gently separate the labia.
10. With the other gloved hand, gently insert the nozzle 2 to 3 inches inward and downward, following the curve of the vagina. Gently rotate the nozzle to facilitate insertion.
11. With first gloved hand, hold the labia together around the nozzle to allow the vagina to fill with solution while the other hand gently rotates the nozzle.
12. Release the labia at intervals to allow the solution to flow out and prevent discomfort to the patient.
13. Remove the nozzle when the douche bag is empty.
14. Elevate the patient's head to facilitate drainage of the solution into the bedpan, or ask the patient to sit upright in the bathtub.
15. Equipment can be rinsed and hung to dry while the patient is sitting.
16. Gently pat the labia dry.
17. Remove the bedpan and empty it, or assist the patient from the tub and cleanse the tub.
18. Peel gloves off and dispose of properly.
19. Chart time, solution, amount, consistency of drainage, and your name **(sixth right).**

DRUG ADMINISTRATION GUIDELINES

Administration of Vaginal Medications

1. Verify the order.
2. Wash hands.
3. Identify the patient. **Remember the five rights.**
4. Screen the patient and place in dorsal recumbent position.
5. Don gloves.
6. Fill the applicator with the ordered amount of cream, foam, jelly, or suppository.
7. With one gloved hand, gently separate the labia.
8. With the other gloved hand, gently insert the applicator downward and inward 2 to 3 inches. Rotate the applicator, if necessary, to facilitate insertion.
9. Push the plunger to deposit the medication.
10. Gently withdraw the applicator and peel one glove over the end of it.
11. Apply a perineal pad to the patient.
12. Peel second glove off.
13. Secure the patient. The patient should remain recumbent for at least 30 minutes, if possible, to prevent medication from draining out.
14. Dispose of the applicator, if appropriate; or glove and rinse and dry the applicator and store in bedside stand with the medication.
15. Wash hands.
16. Chart time, medication, dose, and your name. Note any drainage color and amount **(sixth right).**

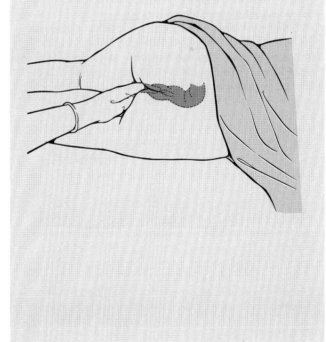

the suppository becomes soft before the package is opened for administration, it may be held under cold running water or placed on ice until it hardens again. At the bedside, screen the patient for privacy and position on the side with the upper leg flexed. Apply a nonsterile glove in compliance with universal precau-

DRUG ADMINISTRATION GUIDELINES

Administration of Medication into the Bladder

1. Check the order.
2. Wash hands and assemble the equipment.
3. Prepare the medication using aseptic technique and remembering **the five rights.**
4. Identify the patient.
5. Screen the patient and position (recumbent if catheter is in place; dorsal recumbent for insertion of urethral suppository or if catheter must be inserted before bladder instillation).
6. **To insert suppository:** Request that the patient empty the bladder. Don sterile gloves and cleanse the periurethral area as you would to insert a catheter. Lubricate the tip of the suppository and gently insert it into the urethra. Remove gloves and wash hands.

Instruct the patient to remain in recumbent position and not to void for at least 30 minutes.
7. **To instill solution into the bladder:** Catheterize the patient with use of aseptic technique. If the catheter is already in place, don sterile gloves and disconnect the catheter from the tubing. Place the tubing between fingers of nondominant hand. Maintain sterility of end of tubing! Insert the barrel of the syringe into the end of the catheter and hold with nondominant hand. Use dominant hand to pour medication into the syringe. Elevate the tubing and syringe slightly to allow the solution to flow into the bladder slowly by gravity. Clamp the tubing immediately and remove the syringe. Reconnect the tubing to maintain sterility. Remove gloves and wash hands.

Instruct the patient to remain in bed for the ordered amount of time and instruct the patient regarding ordered position. It is sometimes necessary to instruct the patient to rotate positions at timed intervals to allow the medication to contact all parts of the bladder. Inform the patient of the amount of time the catheter is to remain clamped. Inform the patient to report any discomfort, because the catheter may have to be unclamped before the intended time. After the ordered interval, unclamp the catheter and allow the solution to drain. Wash hands.
8. Chart the time, drug, route of administration, and signature. Note procedure in nurse's notes also, and document whether the patient was directed to rotate position and how the patient tolerated the procedure **(sixth right).**

DRUG ADMINISTRATION GUIDELINES

Administration of Rectal Suppositories

1. Check the order.
2. Encourage the patient to defecate before the insertion of any suppository ordered for any reason other than to cause defecation.
3. Wash hands.
4. Assemble medication, gloves, and lubricant, remembering **the five rights.**
5. Identify the patient.
6. Screen the patient and place in Sims' left lateral position, if possible.
7. Glove dominant hand.
8. Lubricate the suppository.
9. Insert the suppository while the patient exhales (to prevent contraction of the sphincter during insertion). Guide the suppository with end of the index finger until it is beyond the internal sphincter (1 to 1 1/2 inches beyond the orifice).
10. Direct the patient to remain in bed for at least 20 minutes to allow absorption of the medication. If the medication is to cause defecation, request that the patient try to defecate 30 to 60 minutes after insertion.
11. Chart the time, drug, route, and signature. In nurse's notes, document the results of the medication **(sixth right).**

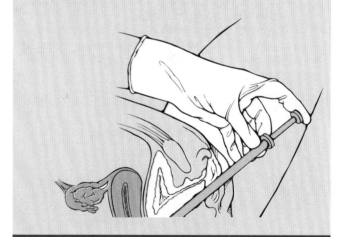

tions. Open the package, lubricate the suppository with a small amount of water-soluble lubricant, and insert it about an inch beyond the internal sphincter of the anus.

The patient should remain in bed for 15 to 20 minutes to allow the suppository to melt and begin action. In infants and young children, gently hold the buttocks together for 15 to 20 minutes to prevent expulsion before melting.

See the Drug Administration Guidelines for administration of rectal suppositories.

Medicated Enemas

The pharmacist prepares the medication as a solution, labels the contents, and includes directions for dilution if this is necessary before administration. Some of these solutions are refrigerated until time of use and must be warmed before administration. The entire container can be placed in a basin of warm water for approximately 10 to 20 minutes.

Encourage the patient to defecate, if possible, before administration because presence of stool in the bowel interferes with absorption.

Pour the warmed solution into a disposable enema bag. Screen the patient for privacy and position and drape the patient in a Sims' left lateral position, unless otherwise ordered. Apply gloves in accord with universal precautions. Administer the enema following appropriate procedure. Encourage the patient to hold the solution for 20 to 30 minutes, if possible, before defecating and releasing the unabsorbed solution.

E X E R C I S E S

LEARNING ACTIVITIES

Using the Guidelines and the appropriate administration equipment, practice percutaneous/local administration techniques until you feel comfortable with them. Then ask a classmate to use the Guidelines to critique your techniques. When you are ready, ask your instructor to verify that your techniques are appropriate.

ADMINISTRATION TO CHILDREN AND THE ELDERLY

LEARNING OBJECTIVES

After studying this chapter, you should be able to:

1. List growth and development factors that alter administration of drugs to children.

2. List growth and development factors that alter administration of drugs to the elderly.

3. Discuss factors that alter dosages for children.

4. Discuss factors that alter dosages for the elderly.

5. Compute the amount of drug to be administered per pound or per kilogram of body weight.

6. Compute the safe amount using Young's, Clark's, or Fried's rule for pediatric dosages.

7. State under which circumstances each dosage calculation formula is most accurate.

8. State common sites of intravenous and intramuscular drug administration for pediatric patients.

9. State common methods of administration of medications for pediatric patients.

10. State common methods of administration of medications for the elderly.

The administration of medications must be altered to meet the special needs of the person. One of the factors that must be considered in planning techniques to use is the age of the patient. Both children and the elderly require special attention.

CHILDREN

ASSESSMENT When deciding how to approach a child who has been prescribed a medication, you must first know the child's age. You would not approach an infant in the same manner as you would a teenager, nor a toddler the same as a school-age child. Determine what the child already knows about medication and how to take it. The parents are an excellent source of this information. Other staff members will also be able to explain techniques they have tried with this child and how successful each was.

PLANNING AND IMPLEMENTATION Many oral medications ordered for children are in a liquid form. If the child is an infant, allow the baby to suck the medication from a medicine dropper or syringe (without the needle!). Syringes as well as some droppers are calibrated for easy measuring. Place the dispenser in the side of the infant's mouth. If you place it on the tongue, the infant is likely to spit it back out because of the protrusion reflex, which causes the tongue to be "stuck out." Thus, the medicine will roll back out the mouth and onto the chin. Immediately after the instillation of the medicine, you may wish to introduce a pacifier or nipple to encourage the infant to swallow.

Other oral medications may be in tablet form. Check with the pharmacy for a liquid form of the drug. If it does not exist, ask whether this tablet can be crushed or dissolved in liquid. Some should not. Examples of forms of drugs that should not be crushed or dissolved include enteric coated tablets, long-acting or timed-release medications, and certain capsules.

If alteration of the drug form is not contraindicated, you may mix the medication with foods or liquids. Be cautious about using this strategy, however, because the child may begin to refuse that food if you use the same one every time. An alternative is to follow the crushed medication with a "chaser" of the child's choice.

Other special devices may be available for use. Special spoons that allow accurate measurement as well as dispensing of the medication can save steps and provide some continuity with methods used at home. A drinking glass with a pill holder built into the inside lip can teach a child how to swallow pills without chewing as the tablet slips into her mouth as she drinks.

Ear drops are administered in much the same manner as for adults, with one notable exception. The pinna of the ear is pulled *down* and back for children. An easy way to remember which way to pull on the ear is by remembering the other word for adult—grown*up*. Therefore, you pull up for grownups and down for children.

Some medications may be administered to children by rectal suppository. Again, the procedure is much the same as for an adult. However, when instilling a rectal suppository in small children, be sure to use your little finger. Hold the buttocks together until the child's urge to expel the suppository is gone, normally 20 to 30 minutes.

Another major way medications are administered to children is by injection. Most commonly, you will be using the subcutaneous or intramuscular route. The subcutaneous route is much the same as for adults. Needles used for intramuscular injections are not usually longer than 5/8 inch for infants and 1 inch for older children. Most often you will use between 25 and 27 gauge, although the medication itself may dictate a larger gauge.

When choosing a site for the intramuscular injection, you should know your patient's level of development. If the child is not yet walking, the muscles in the buttocks will not be well formed. Therefore, the thigh muscles are most often used. This site includes either the vastus lateralis or the rectus femoris muscle.

The vastus lateralis muscle may be located by placing one of your hands above the knee and your other hand below the greater trochanter. In many infants, you will be able to visualize the contours of the muscle between your two hands and slightly to the side. In infants with a heavy layer of subcutaneous fat, you may need to feel for the muscle at this site. To find the rectus femoris muscle, proceed in the same manner, except this muscle is on the top of the thigh rather than on the side. For older children, these same sites or the gluteus medius muscle of the buttocks may be used, as previously explained with adult administration.

Just before you are to give any injection, explain to the child what will be done. Never "surprise" a child, but do not tell the child more than a minute or two ahead of time. Without any warning, you are depriving the child of the chance to cooperate with you, but

warning of the "shot" too far in advance merely adds to the pain of anticipation.

Explain to the child that the injection will hurt. *Never lie* to a child because you will never be believed again. Let her know it is all right to cry or say ouch or otherwise express pain, but warn her she must hold very still.

Take adequate numbers of other staff members with you to act as holders. Explain to the child that the holders will help her stay still so there will not be any extra hurt. Laying across legs ensures that the child stays still but prevents damage to the muscles from "grabbing."

Keep the syringe and needle out of sight as long as possible, but do not let a child's behavior delay the injection. Simply assist the patient to stay still and give the injection quickly. This will not prolong the anticipatory stage.

Talk to the child throughout the injection, assuring the child that it is almost over and, finally, that it is over. You may elicit more cooperation by having a contest to see which one of you can holler ouch the loudest. The child almost always wins. Talking directly into the child's ear in a therapeutic voice can also calm your patient. It matters less what you say than how you say it. Remain calm, deepen your voice, and talk continuously.

As soon as the injection is over, encourage a hug from the parents or offer one yourself if the family is absent. It is possible the child will reject the administrator of the pain. One of the holders may then provide comfort.

A bandage may be applied if bleeding occurs after an injection. Many children see this as a safeguard against something vital they need leaking out. However, try pressure with a cotton ball first because many children are sensitive to the adhesive on bandages.

Rewards can also be used. Many facilities offer stickers, bandages with cartoon characters, or small toys. Be sure any reward you give is appropriate to the age of the child. Small parts could be aspirated if they are placed in the mouth.

Sometimes children must have an intravenous (IV) line started. This requires an injection, and a portion of the line must remain intact in the vein. If you are to assist with an IV injection for a child, you will need to hold the child carefully. Devices such as a papoose board are sometimes used to keep the child secure, but you still need to hold the head, arm, or leg.

Another of your responsibilities is comfort. Therapeutic communication and voice are again used as for the intramuscular injection. Again, do not allow the child's behavior to delay the IV injection.

The most common IV site in an infant is a scalp vein. In older children, the same sites are used as in adults. If a sandbag or other device must be used to protect the site, be sure to weigh the device before its application.

This allows you to keep an accurate record of the child's weight, which is vital in administering fluids.

Protective shields may also be used to protect the IV site from prying fingers. You may also anchor the IV line away from the child's fingers or kicking legs. However, never attach the line to the bed or bed rails because the IV will then be pulled out when the child is moved.

A controller, such as a Buretrol brand controller or an electrical pump, is usually used for children to prevent the instillation of a large amount of fluid in a short time. Children are more sensitive to smaller fluid imbalances because of the relatively smaller amount of body fluids.

EVALUATION After the medication has been adminis-
▲▲▲▲▲▲▲▲▲▲ tered, you are not finished. You need to evaluate how well the procedure went, for you as well as for the child. Evaluate the level of compliance with requests. Is there another approach that may work better for this child?

Could the length of anticipation be shortened next time without compromising the child's cooperation? Do you need more or less holders for the next injection? With some children, the more people helping, the more secure the child feels. Other children feel threatened by a crowd of strangers.

Evaluate the injection site periodically for swelling, redness, or bruising. Is ice needed to decrease pain and swelling? Do you need an order for this in your institution?

After an IV line has been established, check the site often for signs or symptoms of infiltration (skin feels cold, swelling) or infection (skin feels warm, swelling, redness). Know and check the rate and solution often and report any errors immediately.

THE ELDERLY

ASSESSMENT When caring for an older adult, be aware
▲▲▲▲▲▲▲▲▲▲ of the person's status and abilities. Treating all senior adults alike is as much a mistake as treating all children or all middle adults the same. Again, talking with the family and with other staff members helps you in assessing and planning techniques to use. However, with senior adults, do not forget the option of talking with the patient. The elderly patient has no doubt been taking medication of some type for many years (even if only an aspirin now and then) and will be able to make suggestions to ease drug administration.

Assess your patient for any disabilities, such as arthritis, poor vision, poor hearing, swallowing difficulties, or faulty memory. Any of these can affect how drugs are taken at home. Self-injection may be difficult if arthritis or poor vision interferes with drawing up or administration. Poor hearing and faulty memory can lead to misunderstandings about drugs, their schedules, or other instructions.

Also, as with any patient, be sure to check through the entire drug regimen for any drug interactions. This is especially important in the elderly for two reasons: (1) on average, there is a higher number of drugs prescribed at this age, and (2) drug side effects and toxic effects occur earlier, as explained later. Do not forget to ask about nonprescription medications the patient may take occasionally. Be sure the physician is aware of all drugs the patient is taking (Table 11–1).

Work with your patient to find a drug schedule that will work with her lifestyle. If the schedule is difficult, is complicated, or interrupts personal daily routine too much, there is a high likelihood with any patient, elderly or not, that the schedule will not be followed.

PLANNING AND IMPLEMENTATION After you and the
▲▲▲▲▲▲▲▲▲▲▲▲▲▲▲▲▲▲▲▲▲▲▲▲▲▲▲▲ patient have decided on the drug regimen, techniques can be used to help your patient remember to take the medications on time. Calendars can be written out and dates crossed off if medications are a once-a-day or twice-a-day event. Pill organizers are available with individual slots for each day of the week, or even several slots for different time periods each day. Some organizers even have alarms that alert the patient if the box has not been opened by the next scheduled medication time.

A written schedule helps the patient to remember what the schedule is supposed to be next week or even next month. With busy daily lives, medications are often not a top priority.

If your patient is not capable of administering the medications alone, arrangements may be made to have a home health nurse visit. If finances or insurance constrictions prohibit this (for example, Medicare does not currently pay for this type of service), a family member, friend, or neighbor may be taught how to administer the medication. It must be emphasized to volunteers that this is a permanent job. They cannot take a day off unless more than one person shares the responsibility. Nevertheless, this may make the difference between a senior adult's remaining independent and in her own home or needing to be placed into a nursing facility.

Intravenous insertion can be more difficult in the elderly because of fragile skin and the fragile sclerotic veins. Both the skin and the veins are more easily damaged, and bruising is more likely. Choose a smaller needle gauge and protect the IV site carefully once it is established. Holding the vein steady with the noninserting thumb may also ease insertion.

Table 11–1. Common Medications Used by Seniors

CLASSIFICATION	COMMON EXAMPLE
Antianginals	nitroglycerin
Antiarrhythmics	cardiac glycosides (digoxin)
Anticoagulants	warfarin (Coumadin)
Antiglaucoma agents	timolol (Timoptic)
Antigout agents	probenecid (Benemid)
Antihypertensives	captopril (Capoten)
Aspirin	(Bufferin)
Bronchodilators	albuterol (Ventolin)
Calcium channel blockers	verapamil (Calan)
Diuretics	furosemide (Lasix)
Electrolytes	potassium chloride (K-TAB)
Hypoglycemics	chlorpropamide (Diabinese)
Insulin	regular (Humulin R)
Laxatives	magnesium salts (milk of magnesia)
Lipid-lowering agents	cholestyramine (Questran)
Nonsteroidal anti-inflammatory drugs (NSAIDs)	ibuprofen (Motrin)
Sedatives	diphenhydramine (Sominex)

EVALUATION Continually evaluate the patient for increased drug effects, side effects, and toxic effects. In addition to those specific to the drugs being administered, confusion, lack of motivation or energy, and even depression can be flags to the nurse of drug interactions or overdose.

Periodically evaluate the drug regimen to ensure that it is being followed correctly. In case of any daily routine changes, help the patient to establish new schedules as needed.

Always ask patients each time you see them for the names of any and all drugs they are taking. Even though you may see her regularly, the patient may have started using a new over-the-counter medication or visited another physician.

AGE-RELATED DOSAGES

Dosages for children and for seniors are both decreased, and for some of the same reasons (Table 11–2). Children are of a lower weight than adults, which means they require less of a drug for the same effect. In addition, their metabolism is at a different rate but much less efficient than an adult's. Many of the major body systems involved in absorption, distribution, biotransformation, and excretion are not yet mature. The digestive (including the liver), circulatory, urinary, and respiratory systems have not reached their full function. As a result, medications are not absorbed as well, are not distributed as quickly or efficiently, are not detoxified as soon, and are not excreted as fast as in an adult. This can produce increased side effects and toxic effects.

There are several ways to calculate the correct dose for a child. As a nurse, it is your responsibility to check that the order is correct for a specific child under your care. Specific formulas for each drug can be obtained from drug inserts, the *Physician's Desk Reference,* or any good reference book. An example of one of these formulas is

Give 30 mg/kg/day in 3 divided doses.

Translated, this formula means to determine the child's weight in kilograms and multiply that number by 30. This gives you the daily total dose. The formula goes on to indicate that this total dose must be divided by three. This, then, gives you the dose to be given every 8 hours.

Another option for checking a child's dosage is to use Fried's, Young's, or Clark's rule. These formulas allow you to quickly calculate the dosage on the basis of information you already have. Fried's rule is based on the child's age in months. Therefore, it is best used for infants. You can use the simple rule that if you tend to state the child's age in months, you would use Fried's

Table 11–2. Age-Related Drug Administration Rationales

CHILDREN	SENIORS
Rationales for Decreased Age-Related Dosages	
Immature body systems	Degeneration of body systems
Circulatory	Circulatory
Digestive	Digestive
Urinary	Urinary
Respiratory	Respiratory
Less weight	Less activity
Inefficient metabolism	Decreased metabolism
Less body fluids	Less body fluids
Rationales for Special Age-Related Techniques	
Stage of growth and development	Degeneration of neurological tissue
Confusion	Confusion
Limited understanding	Limited understanding
Limited abilities	Limited abilities

(handwritten: Know This Side)

formula. For instance, we usually say a child is 6 months old or 18 months old, rather than 1/2 year or 1 and 1/2 years old; but we generally say a child is 2 or 3 and 1/2 years old rather than 24 or 42 months old. For children whose age is measured in months, follow Fried's formula:

$$\frac{\text{age in months} \times \text{average adult dose}}{150} = \text{infant's dose}$$

Young's rule is based on the child's age in years. For the child whose age we generally measure in years (e.g., 2 or 3 and 1/2 years old), use Young's formula:

$$\frac{\text{age in years} \times \text{average adult dose}}{\text{age in years} + 12} = \text{child's dose}$$

Clark's rule is generally the most accurate of the three formulas because it is based on the child's weight rather than age. Children of course come in all sizes, just like adults. It is possible to have one 4-year-old who weighs 30 pounds and another 4-year-old who weighs 60 pounds. By use of a formula based on age, both children would receive the same dosage of medication. Clark's formula makes the dosage more individualized:

$$\frac{\text{child's weight in pounds} \times \text{average adult dose}}{150} = \text{child's dose}$$

Body changes as we age mean that dosages for seniors should also be adjusted. Absorption is slowed because of slower digestive motility and commonly overextended abdominal blood vessels (from congestive heart failure, for example). Distribution is slowed because of malnutrition, slowed circulation, slowed metabolism, decreased body fluids, decreased skeletal muscle tissue, and increased body fat. Biotransformation and excretion are affected by degeneration of the liver and kidneys. As a result, given the same dose as previously administered all through the middle years, an elderly person will have a higher amount of unbound drug in the body. This will produce increased drug effects, side effects, and toxicity effects. Most drug references list separate dosages for the elderly as part of the basic information.

E X E R C I S E S

CASE STUDIES

1. J. M. is 4 years old. He has been prescribed a medication that has an average adult dose of 120 mg. How much should J. M. receive? How does your answer change if J. M. is only 6 months old? What if J. M. weighs 22 pounds? What techniques would you use to administer an oral drug to J. M.? An IM?

2. T. C. is 83 years old. What changes in body function would alter the dosage of medications? What techniques would you possibly need to use?

UNIT THREE

DRUG ABUSE

The misuse and abuse of drugs are a major problem in our society. One cannot pick up a newspaper without reading some reference to drug abuse, trafficking, and addiction. Some of the drugs are ones seen every day in the health care profession because they have legitimate medical uses. Others are street drugs that have no other use.

Despite all the information available on the subject, many people are still confused by the problem. We discuss some simple definitions and general symptoms of the misuse and abuse of drugs. We also highlight some general symptoms of withdrawal from drugs.

In this unit, several drugs or groups of drugs become the focus of a chapter. These include alcohol, the opiates, hallucinogens, amphetamines and barbiturates, cocaine or crack, and "glue sniffing." The main emphasis of each chapter is on the symptoms and complications of the use of the specific drug and the treatments used when the drug is abused.

We also look at some of the psychosocial aspects of drug abuse. How does the abuser become an abuser? What type of person becomes an abuser? Could you become an abuser? How does our society actually encourage or discourage the use of drugs?

DEPENDENCY, ADDICTION, HABITUATION, AND WITHDRAWAL

Abuse & misuse

LEARNING OBJECTIVES

After studying this chapter, you should be able to:

1. Define drug abuse.

2. Distinguish among drug dependency, addiction, and habituation.

3. Relate symptoms and clues indicative of general drug use /abuse.

4. List at least four symptoms of drug withdrawal.

Drug abuse is a disease that kills or permanently incapacitates millions of people every year. It has been estimated that between 70% and 90% of all children of high-school age have tried at least one drug at least once. The current use of drugs in the United States is now higher than in any other developed country.

Just what is drug abuse? Drug abuse is the use of any drug not prescribed by a physician or the improper or excessive use of a drug. But wait! you say. If that is the definition, have I abused drugs the last time I took too many aspirins for a headache that would not go away, or took a second dose of a cold remedy before I was supposed to because the cold was so bad? The answer is yes, that *is* drug abuse. You should not be doing these things, especially as a health care provider.

In our society, when we say drug abuse, we generally have something else in mind. More often, we are thinking of drug dependency. Drug dependency is the physical or psychological need to use drugs to achieve a sense of well-being or to avoid withdrawal. The use may be continuous or periodic.

Drug addiction, on the other hand, is the compulsive, excessive, or continued use of habit-forming drugs that are harmful to self, society, or both. The addicted person has to have the drug and can become desperate to get it. Drug habit is the term often used synonymously with addiction. A habit is something that has been done often and is difficult to break. As an example, try these two experiments. Cross your arms. Which way did you cross them? Did you know that you probably always cross them just that way? It's a habit. Now try crossing them the other way. Feels uncomfortable, doesn't it? You may have even had a hard time figuring out where to put your arms. That is because habits are hard to break. Try the same experiment with folding your hands. We usually fold our fingers exactly the same way each time—either our right thumb is over the left, or vice versa. Now try folding them the opposite way. Uncomfortable again? That is because you are breaking a habit.

Drug habituation is the frequent use of a drug so that the use becomes a part of the activities of daily (or weekly) living. It is uncomfortable for the person to go without the drug, and it is difficult to break the habit.

One of the reasons that it may be difficult to break a drug habit or dependency is because of withdrawal. Withdrawal is the effect experienced from stopping a drug to which the person was either physiologically or psychologically addicted. The signs and symptoms differ with the drug used.

A person with a drug habit may also experience drug tolerance. An increasingly larger dose of the drug is often required to achieve the original effect, but larger doses may be harmful or even fatal.

Table 12–1 defines special vocabulary words used in the study, treatment, or prevention of drug abuse.

SYMPTOMS OF DRUG USE AND ABUSE

Persons who use and abuse drugs often experience similar effects. These effects can be classified as physical, psychological, or social.

Table 12-1. Special Vocabulary of Drug Abuse Theory

Drug abuse	The use of any drug not prescribed by a physician, or the improper or excessive use of a drug
Drug addiction	The compulsive, excessive, or continued use of habit-forming drugs that are harmful to self, to society, or to both
Drug dependency	The physical or psychological need to use drugs to achieve a sense of well-being or to avoid withdrawal
Drug habit	The frequent use of drugs with difficulty experienced on attempting to stop; often used synonymously with addiction
Drug habituation	Use of a drug so that it becomes a part of the activities of daily (or weekly) living
Drug paraphernalia	Items associated with the use, abuse, distribution, or processing of drugs
Drug tolerance	The need to increase the dose of a drug to achieve the original effect
Withdrawal	The effect experienced from stopping a drug to which the person was either physiologically or psychologically addicted

growth. The person may be lethargic, be ataxic, or slur his words. He may become sick more often, especially at the beginning of the week, when he is first without his drug for the week.

Psychologically, drug users may have a distorted perception of social interactions, meaning that they think someone is being positive toward them when in fact that person is not, or that someone is being negative toward them that is also not the case. The drug user's ability to concentrate is impaired, and memory is shortened. The user is often apathetic about issues that were once important. The ability to organize oneself and one's work is also impaired. The user can no longer be flexible when things do not go exactly as planned. There may even be signs of illogical thinking, so the ability to solve problems is hindered. This last sign is particularly ironic because it is often the drug user's problems that encouraged the use of drugs for an escape in the first place.

The drug user's social performance is altered by the drug habit. Because drug use increases mood swings and irritability, depression, anger, and even defensiveness, the user's popularity is not enhanced. This may cause the drug user to feel the need to take even more drugs or different drugs to escape these new problems. School or work performance drops, including grades or performance at work, promptness, and attendance. Absenteeism becomes a major problem for the employer or school officials. This is especially true on Mondays and Fridays as the drug user tries to lengthen the weekend.

All of these new problems piling up add to the user's feelings of inadequacy. There are feelings of anxiety and over-reactions to situations. Disruptive behaviors may begin, such as sleeping in class or on the job, fighting, and hostility. A disrespect for authority and discipline is shown.

The user becomes even more unpleasant to be around as the manner of dress and cleanliness deteriorate. Once again, this is more common at the beginning of the week, after a long weekend of drug use.

The drug user begins to become isolated. The circle of friends changes. The user is now dependent on those who can supply the drug, and the supplier will be happy to continue to be a "friend" as long as the drugs are purchased. Old friends are ignored as the user becomes more and more wrapped up in the drug world. School-related functions or work social functions are avoided.

Some of the user's behaviors may strike others as "odd." Family members notice anonymous calls and frequent hang-ups. The user may wear outdoor clothing even while indoors, because this provides more hiding places for the drug supply. Family members

Physical symptoms are usually in the form of a change in the normal for that person. This may be a change in weight, in sleeping habits, or in complexion. Teens may demonstrate a slowing or even cessation of may discover secret pockets in clothing, bags, or purses. Dresser drawers, jewelry boxes, or closets may suddenly be kept locked.

Parents often complain that their teen-aged user is not trustworthy. Loved ones of a user may notice a lack of funds, despite allowance or income, or there may be more money than the allowance or wages would account for. They may find the user in odd places. It simply is not normal behavior to sit in a crawl space, the attic, storage areas, closets, or the car for lengthy times.

As the user delves even further into the drug world, there may be evidence of the dangerous world it really is. The user becomes suspicious of everyone. A weapon may be carried to protect the user, guard the drug supply, or obtain drugs or drug money through criminal activities.

Another more obvious clue to drug use is finding drug paraphernalia. This may include glue tubes, solvent residues, aerosol cans, joints, clips, seeds, plant stems, roaches, pills, sugar cubes, syringes and needles, tourniquets, lighters, smoking devices, cigarette makers and papers, unexplained powders, certain chemicals, pills and capsules, straws, razors, or mirrors. You may not even know what all the devices are for.

Drug use usually proceeds slowly. The user does not just wake up one morning and decide to get involved in the underworld. In general, at first, the use is in answer to peer pressure. Few teenagers or adults can withstand the challenge behind the word "chicken." The first use may occur because of a desperate situation, such as the loss of a loved one, severe pain, or divorce. This type of use is irregular and unplanned.

For a time, the use continues to be unplanned, but then the user begins more experimentation. Again, this may be in answer to peer pressure or difficult situations. Once a person has tried one drug, it is much easier to try a second or a third. The user begins planning for times to use drugs. Most often, this is on the weekends. The regular use of drugs then begins.

Eventually, weekends are not enough for the user, and a midweek pick-me-up is needed. It just does not seem possible to make it through a whole week anymore. Amazingly, not until this stage does the user begin having significant behavioral changes. This is a long way down the road of drug addiction before mom, dad, or spouse can tell anything is wrong.

It is a fairly easy step to daily use and possibly trafficking. Many drug users get into selling drugs to finance their own habits. Their entire personality is enveloped by drugs. It is the first thing they think about in the morning and the last thing they think about before going to sleep.

WITHDRAWAL

When a person is denied a drug to which he is addicted, that person will go through withdrawal. These are physical symptoms that can be deadly. The symptoms of withdrawal from alcohol are called delirium tremens (DTs), which is further explained in Chapter 13. Each drug has its own specific symptoms of withdrawal, and these are mentioned in respective chapters.

General symptoms of drug withdrawal, however, can include nervousness, runny nose and sniffling, sweating, bloodshot or puffy eyes, a need to stay in motion, blood pressure and pulse changes, rapid respirations, and possibly death.

The person in withdrawal can become desperate for his next dose of the drug and be willing to do anything to obtain it or the money to buy it. Criminal activities are common. These do not tend to be well thought out or planned in advance. They are generally committed against those who are least able to fight back and who happen to be unlucky enough to be near the addict during withdrawal. This may be a stranger or a loved one. At that moment, it does not matter to the addict.

PLANNING AND INTERVENTION

Treatment of drug abuse is highly variable, depending on the drug or drugs being abused. The patient may need to be hospitalized to maintain life support during withdrawal. Support groups and psychotherapy can be useful interventions as well. The nurse involved in the patient's care is an integral part of the multidisciplinary team. In addition to assessing for the patient's health status, the nurse also needs excellent communication skills to be therapeutic. A review of these skills is advised. At no time should the nurse convey either approval of the drug-abusing behaviors or disapproval of the patient as a person. This is a fine line to draw, and the novice nurse may have difficulty maintaining it.

Prevention is a useful tool in the fight against drug abuse. Many children begin drug experimentation in response to peer pressure. Reversal of the peer pressure directives has been proposed, therefore. This is a slow process and takes many years of diligent work. Interesting alternatives must be presented to the teens. Education must be focused on the effects of drug abuse on the teen *now*, not in the future. The negative effects must be perceived by the teens as negative to them, related to something that is important to them. If the student concentrates for a moment on the events of importance to the teenager, a pattern will be seen. Body image, relationships (girlfriend/boyfriend), athletic ability, and peer relations ("fitting in") are at the top of any teenager's list. Relate negative effects of drugs to these items, and the teens are more likely to listen to you.

Organizations have begun using these themes to sway the general consensus of the age group. SADD (Students Against Drunk Driving) has also used their initials to stand for Student Athletes against Drugged Driving. There are "Just Say No" clubs in many schools as well. DARE (Drug Abuse Resistance Education) groups also concentrate on changing basic attitudes to drugs and alcohol. The nurse can participate with these groups to present factual information about drugs and drug abuse.

Education is an integral part of prevention of drug abuse in other age groups as well. Be sure you explain the possibility of drug abuse to your patients prescribed a drug with this potential. Be clear about what circumstances may cause a person to abuse drugs without consciously wishing do so. Explain to your patients that no one ever started out with a goal to be a drug addict. Each started out slowly, one dose at a time.

Many of your patients may believe that they could not become a drug addict because they are of the wrong age group, or wrong sex, or wrong economic group, or wrong political party. The nurse needs to clearly state that drug abuse crosses all of these boundaries. No one is immune.

The student needs to be aware that the lack of immunity applies to health care workers, too. Because of the availability of drugs and easy access coupled with high-stress work, caregivers are at high risk for drug abuse. The impaired caregiver presents several problems.

The impaired caregiver presents a problem to the patients by acting in ways that would never have been chosen under normal circumstances. No matter how well the caregiver believes the addiction is hidden, errors, misjudgments, and accidents are much more likely to occur if the caregiver is under the influence of a drug or under the influence of withdrawal symptoms. The impaired caregiver may begin to take drugs meant for the patient, and the impaired caregiver takes extra time away from the patient to obtain or use drugs. Obviously, the patient does not receive the care needed.

The impaired caregiver presents a problem to coworkers. Coworkers can not depend on this person to do the duties assigned. They then begin to "take up the slack" and perform more than their fair share of the work. Mistakes that the impaired caregiver makes may have an impact on the practice of the coworkers, increasing their liability. The addiction is then causing extra tension at the workplace, making the job less than enjoyable.

The impaired caregiver also presents a problem to the employer. As the caregiver makes more and more mistakes, the employer's liability also increases. The impaired caregiver is more likely to call off sick, leave early, or come in late. Not only can the employer no longer consider the caregiver reliable, but it becomes expensive to replace the caregiver with other employees so often. The impaired caregiver is more likely than the unimpaired coworkers to need health care for other problems and therefore to use insurance. This presents another financial burden to the employer.

If you believe a coworker is impaired, it is your duty to report your suspicions to the caregiver's immediate supervisor. If your suspicions are not taken seriously, go higher up the management ladder until someone listens to you. The impaired nurse is also to be reported to the state board of nursing.

If you feel uncomfortable about "telling on" your coworker, remember your purpose. You are attempting to ensure the best care for the patients as well as for your coworker.

The impaired caregiver needs to be confronted with evidence of the drug abuse or suspected drug abuse. Often, the worker vigorously denies the charges, but the confrontors need to push for the worker to receive help. It may help to ensure the caregiver that the health care worker who is impaired will not necessarily be fired or lose a professional license.

If you become addicted to drugs at some time during your professional career, it is your duty to recognize the problem and seek help.

The impaired caregiver is entitled to the same treatment and care as any other person with an addiction problem. Some health care workers have a difficult time recognizing this right, somehow believing that health care workers should be held to a higher standard. This only perpetuates the problem. The impaired caregiver does not receive the care needed and remains addicted. Other impaired caregivers are less likely to seek out the help they need.

In addition to the same treatment available to others, the health care worker may be able to receive specialized help. Special programs are sponsored by most state boards of nursing, state medical boards, and other regulatory boards. These programs deal with the specific problems a health care worker faces and offer extra support.

E X E R C I S E S

CASE STUDIES

1. M. H., a 16-year-old boy, is approached by some of his friends to try a drug they are using. What is the

likelihood that M. H. will agree to try a drug, either now or at some point in his teens?

2. M. H. does try the drug. What is the next stage of drug use? At what point are his parents most likely to notice a change in his behavior if he continues use?

3. Ms. R. J.'s boss is concerned about her behavior. She has become inconsistent in her work, is absent more often, and has begun sleeping at work. These types of behaviors are consistent with drug use. Do you think Ms. R. J. is definitely using drugs? Why or why not? What should her boss do?

4. Ms. S. J., age 69 years, is arrested for selling drugs. She has been hospitalized in your facility by the courts for treatment of her drug addiction. When her grown children come to visit, they express disbelief that your patient could possibly be involved in drugs. They cite Ms. S. J.'s age and church affiliation as reasons. What would your best response be to her children?

MENTAL AEROBICS

1. Make a list of at least 10 current songs that contain references to drug use. To get you started, here are some older ones: "Lucy in the Sky with Diamonds" (LSD), "Mellow Yellow" (drug effects), "Cocaine."

2. Make a list of at least 10 movies, television shows, or advertisements that make reference to drug use. Again, to get you started, here are some older ones: anything with Cheech and Chong in it; *Valley of the Dolls;* any alcoholic beverage advertisement; many detective-type television shows, such as the old *Miami Vice* series.

3. Prepare a list of at least 10 reasons people take drugs.

4. Prepare a list of at least one drugless method to achieve each of the same goals listed in number 3.

CHAPTER 13

ALCOHOL ABUSE

General.

LEARNING OBJECTIVES

After studying this chapter, you should be able to:

1. State the disease theory of alcoholism.

2. Relate symptoms and clues indicative of alcohol use and abuse.

3. Relate nursing responsibilities for the patient experiencing alcohol withdrawal.

4. Discuss alcohol abuse rehabilitation.

Alcohol is one of the oldest drugs used—yes, a drug. Because it is legal to use alcohol, many people discount its effects. It has been estimated that about 90% of all high-school seniors have tried alcohol. The statistics tell us there are 1.3 million Americans between the ages of 12 and 17 years with an alcohol dependency, and another 3.3 million have a serious problem but are not yet alcoholics. If you really want to be scared: there are a half-million 9- to 12-year-old alcoholics in this country. None of these numbers includes the millions of Americans 20 years and older who are alcoholics. Alcoholism is now considered to be the third leading health problem in the United States.

The effect of the alcohol is only a portion of the problem. Most alcoholics will die of alcoholism, but this is generally in an accident, such as a motor vehicle accident, a self-induced fire, or an accident in the home.

The study, treatment, and attempted prevention of alcoholism use many of our nation's health care dollars. See Table 12–1 for special vocabulary we use in this chapter relating to alcoholism.

REGULATION

Alcohol is hardly a new drug. Its use is mentioned in the Bible and in Homer's *Iliad*. Even its negative effects have long been understood. In 1919, the Volstead Act was legislated by the U.S. Congress as a result of the Temperance Movement led by the Women's Christian Temperance Union (WCTU). This ushered in the age of Prohibition, moonshining, and speakeasies. Prohibition ended in 1933 because it failed to control alcohol use. However, the WCTU did manage to persuade Congress to keep the portion of the law that required alcohol education in all schools.

Alcohol is still regulated by state laws. In most states, you must be 21 years old to drink, sell, or give away alcoholic beverages. However, we still have not controlled alcohol use.

ALCOHOLISM: THE DISEASE

Alcoholism is a disease. This concept has been met with much resistance. However, alcoholism meets all the criteria of the definition of a disease: it has a cause, it produces signs and symptoms, and it acts in similar ways in each affected person.

In general, the early stages of alcoholism include relief drinking, which is to say the alcoholic drinks to relieve stress. The alcoholic often has repeated drunk driving violations and may be experiencing blackouts. The alcoholic has lost control over the alcohol. Getting "drunk" does not necessarily happen every time a drink is taken. This means that the outcome of each drinking episode cannot be predicted.

As the disease progresses, the alcoholic begins having family problems, employment problems, and financial and legal problems. The usual sense of morals changes with use of alcohol, and the person may therefore act in ways that are uncharacteristic.

Alcohol is not metabolized in the alcoholic in the same way that it is in the normal adult. The brain normally metabolizes alcohol into acetaldehyde (a chemical related to formaldehyde), then to acetic acid, and finally to carbon dioxide and water (Fig. 13–1). In the alcoholic, however, a small amount of the acetaldehyde reacts with the body's normal dopamine to produce THIQ. TIIIQ is a substance found in the

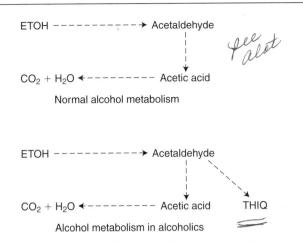

ETOH ----------→ Acetaldehyde

$CO_2 + H_2O$ ◄--------- Acetic acid

Normal alcohol metabolism

ETOH ----------→ Acetaldehyde

$CO_2 + H_2O$ ◄--------- Acetic acid   THIQ

Alcohol metabolism in alcoholics

Figure 13-1. Normal alcohol metabolism and alcohol metabolism in alcoholics. ETOH, ethyl alcohol.

brains of alcoholics and heroin addicts. It is addictive and is related in make-up to the opiates (see Fig. 13-1).

As a result of this knowledge, researchers theorize three different groups of alcoholics. One group contains persons who do not make enough of their own natural endorphins (the substance that helps to make you feel happy and content). When they drink and produce THIQ, they feel "normal" for the first time in their lives. These people tend to become alcoholics early in their adolescence and progress quickly.

The second group have a normal amount of endorphin, and as in most humans, the level is decreased by alcohol use. However, because they make THIQ, they do not notice the lack of endorphins. These alcoholics tend to progress over a long time.

The third group have the normal amount of endorphins, and the level is not affected by alcohol use. Therefore, they are without psychological symptoms. These alcoholics tend to be the easiest to treat because they have enough of their own endorphins and do not have to fight as much depression.

Although much of this theory is backed up by observations, the true cause of alcoholism remains a mystery and the subject of much research.

The level of dependency is another way to group alcoholics. Physical dependence means that physical symptoms of withdrawal result if the subject does not drink. Psychological dependence means that psychological symptoms of withdrawal result if the subject does not drink. Some people believe that if they can go without alcohol for moderate periods, they are not alcoholic. This simply is not true. As an example, the weekend or episodic alcoholic drinks only at specific times and is sober throughout the rest of the week. Although sobriety is maintained each week, come the weekend, drinks are always taken. This is another type of alcoholism.

ASSESSMENT Alcohol is a drug. The excessive use of alcohol, alcoholism, is a disease. It is a disease, however, with many contributing factors, including the alcoholic's genetic make-up and society's attitude toward alcohol.

Alcoholism may be treated. The alcoholic must be persuaded to get help. Treatment, both physical and psychological, is aimed at the person, the family, and the community.

The Person Alcohol affects the body in many different ways. Cardiovascular effects include vasodilatation during drinking or immediately afterward, capillary fragility, and even permanent damage to the heart.

The brain is affected also. Alcohol has a sedative effect. The person feels relaxed and uninhibited. Reaction time is slowed, and speech is slurred. The sense of balance is lost, and the person becomes uncoordinated. The ability to reason correctly is also impaired. During drinking episodes, alcoholics believe they are acting normally. After the episode, they often use denial and rationalization to explain their actions. The alcoholic often feels guilty or anxious, has a low self-esteem, and is unusually sensitive to rejection from others.

N U R S I N G   A L E R T
▼▼▼▼▼▼▼▼▼▼▼▼▼▼▼▼▼▼▼▼▼▼▼▼▼▼▼▼▼▼▼▼

Combined, these feelings can cause depression, suicidal tendencies, and increased drinking episodes.

▲▲▲▲▲▲▲▲▲▲▲▲▲▲▲▲▲▲▲▲▲▲▲▲▲▲▲▲▲▲▲▲

Alcohol also affects the digestive system. The stomach and small intestine are subject to ulcerations caused by alcohol irritation. The blood vessels rise to the surface of the stomach lining, the tissue swells, and excess stomach acid is produced. The alcoholic experiences heartburn, indigestion, and gastritis. An ulcer may then form as the acids begin to eat away at the lining of the stomach or small intestine.

N U R S I N G   A L E R T
▼▼▼▼▼▼▼▼▼▼▼▼▼▼▼▼▼▼▼▼▼▼▼▼▼▼▼▼▼▼▼▼

Ulceration can lead to gastrointestinal tract bleeding, perforation, peritonitis, and death.

▲▲▲▲▲▲▲▲▲▲▲▲▲▲▲▲▲▲▲▲▲▲▲▲▲▲▲▲▲▲▲▲

The pancreas produces enzymes and hormones that are involved in portions of digestion. Alcohol causes the pancreas to overproduce both the enzymes and the hormones in an attempt to use the calories in the alcohol and to digest the alcohol itself. This leads to a high blood sugar level and the development of secondary diabetes.

N U R S I N G   A L E R T

The alcoholic may also experience pancreatitis (inflammation of the pancreas) with nausea, vomiting, and pain.

The liver is also involved in some aspects of digestion as well as in detoxification. It secretes bile, breaks down nutrients into usable forms, stores iron and some vitamins, and breaks down poisons such as alcohol.

N U R S I N G   A L E R T

The use of alcohol causes the liver to swell because it cannot handle the amount of poison being delivered to it. These poisons then build up and cause scarring of the liver cells. This is called cirrhosis.

Once cirrhosis has begun, the liver is even less capable of performing its work. As more and more poisons build up in the bloodstream, the alcoholic becomes jaundiced (has a yellow cast to skin and mucous membranes). Because the liver is scarred and working slowly, blood backs up in the circulatory system instead of flowing smoothly through the liver. This produces high blood pressure, esophageal varices (dilated blood vessels near the surfaces of the esophagus), and ascites (fluid build-up in the abdomen). The build-up of the poisons in the bloodstream also produces confusion and possibly hallucinations. Because the liver is also involved in destroying invading microorganisms, the alcoholic has a lower resistance to infection of all kinds.

In addition to the many effects on the organs of digestion, the alcoholic often suffers from malnutrition as well. The craving for the alcohol is so strong, the alcoholic will drink rather than eat. Although alcohol provides many calories, it does not provide nutrients, so the alcoholic may actually gain weight while becoming more and more malnourished. This is especially true for vitamins B_1 (thiamine), A (retinol), and K. The effects of deficiencies of these vitamins are explained in Chapter 56.

Prolonged alcohol use can also lead to decreased fertility and sexual dysfunction in men. Women often experience menstrual cycle disruptions.

N U R S I N G   A L E R T

Used during pregnancy, alcohol can produce birth defects. One such defect is called fetal alcohol syndrome.

This infant goes through withdrawal after birth because of the removal of alcohol from its system. This withdrawal can be fatal and must be monitored carefully. Medications may be prescribed and emergency or supportive equipment should be kept within easy access. The infant is usually small for gestational age at birth and often has other physical abnormalities, both external and internal. Later, the child may exhibit growth and mental retardation.

N U R S I N G   A L E R T

When alcohol is withdrawn, the alcoholic experiences withdrawal symptoms. These are called delirium tremens (DTs). As the name implies, the alcoholic becomes delirious, with confusion and possibly hallucinations. Severe tremors may even progress into seizures. The alcoholic may have nausea, vomiting, diarrhea, sleeplessness, and hypoglycemia.

The Family The alcoholic is not the only one affected by the disease. The family members also suffer, although they may not be aware of it or acknowledge it.

Many families attempt to ignore the alcoholic's problem. They deny its existence and try to hide it from others. This is often in response to the social view of alcoholism as a moral issue. The family worries about "what the neighbors will think." They try to treat the problem at home, with emotional appeals and broken promises. Lectures, threats, and obstructive actions are met with anger, depression, and perfidy.

Children are often the ones most affected in the alcoholic's family. They have no healthy role models, are not socialized by the family, and often feel guilty, anxious, or "different." They lack a sense of security. Child abuse is prevalent in alcoholic families.

The roles in the alcoholic family often become confused. The alcoholic can be anyone in the family: mother, father, sibling, grandparent. Many times, one or more of the family members takes on the role of enabler. This person becomes overprotective of the alcoholic by offering excuses or taking over the alcoholic's responsibilities. This only allows the alcoholic to continue drinking. It does not encourage the alcoholic to seek help.

Another member of the family might take on the role of Good Samaritan. This is often an older child, who becomes the "model child," gets excellent grades, excels in athletics, or in general is an overachiever. The children who take on this role need to help everyone and find it difficult to say no, even though they actually do not have time for a particular project. These children often go into helping professions, such as physician or nurse. In actuality, the person is angry inside and is attempting to correct the family name and pride.

Another child might take on the role of rebel. Always in trouble, angry and defiant, this child has a better chance of getting help because of high visibility. Indeed, this child may be the catalyst for the whole family to get help.

Some children choose the role of loner. The loner withdraws from everyone and everything. Because she does not cause anyone any trouble, she may be the last to receive help. This allows her time to enter into her own fantasy world and mental illness.

Other children become the family clown. The clown may act immature and is often a comic. This child is attempting to refocus attention away from the alcoholic problem. This is another way of denying the problem.

The Community   Even families are not the only ones affected by the alcoholic. There are other types of "families." At school, the class may act as a pseudo-family. At work, fellow employees may make up a type of family. There may even be social families, such as the bridge club, the golf partners, or the bowling team. All of these people will be affected by the alcoholic. Many of them will take on some of the roles described for the alcoholic's family members.

PLANNING AND IMPLEMENTATION   Treatment of alcoholism is multidisciplinary. Many avenues will be used before the successful one for a patient is found.

First, alcohol must be eliminated from the alcoholic's body. This process is called detoxification. The alcoholic may enter the DTs from detoxification. The drug of choice for delirium tremens is diazepam (Valium). The dose is decreased progressively every day to ensure that the alcoholic does not become addicted to the drug instead of to alcohol. Thiamine may be given to increase the metabolism of the alcohol and to help calm the patient's nerves. Fructose and hormones may also be given to increase alcohol metabolism (see Table 13–1). The alcoholic is given a diet high in protein and nutrients. Appropriate medications are ordered for the vomiting and diarrhea.

The physical treatment of the withdrawing alcoholic is only one small part of the treatment. Psychological help is also necessary. This is provided by a multidisciplinary staff using a therapeutic community. There may be therapy groups, individual sessions, lectures and films, family therapy and education, activities therapy (also called recreational therapy), and aftercare. In most treatment centers, involvement in Alcoholics Anonymous or a similar group is encouraged. Box 13–1 shows the 12 Steps of Alcoholics Anonymous.

The alcoholic may not realize that help is needed, however, and may not understand the effect on others. Another choice the family may use is sometimes referred to as Intervention. Intervention is a session or sessions with the alcoholic and the family and friends. The family and friends then express to the alcoholic how they are affected and why they want the alcoholic to get help. The goal of intervention is to make the alcoholic aware of actions and to express concern for the person. It is not intended as punishment or diagnosis. The interveners must not act alone, but with a counselor and other "family" members. Rules during the session are to remain relaxed, to be honest, and not to attack the alcoholic (Table 13–2). It is best to be prepared and even practice the session

Table 13–1. Medical Control of Delirium Tremens	
Diazepam	To control tremors To prevent seizures
Thiamine	To increase the metabolism of alcohol To calm the patient
Fructose	To increase the metabolism of alcohol
Hormones	To increase the metabolism of alcohol
Antiemetics	To control nausea and vomiting
Antidiarrheals	To control diarrhea

Box 13-1. The Twelve Suggested Steps of Alcoholics Anonymous

1. We admit we are powerless over alcohol—that our lives have become unmanageable.

2. We have come to believe that a Power greater than ourselves can restore us to sanity.

3. We have made a decision to turn our will and our lives over to the care of God as we understand Him.

4. We make a searching and fearless moral inventory of ourselves.

5. We admit to God, to ourselves, and to another human being the exact nature of our wrongs.

6. We are entirely ready to have God remove all these defects of character.

7. We humbly ask Him to remove our shortcomings.

8. We make a list of all persons we have harmed and become willing to make amends to them all.

9. We make direct amends to such people wherever possible, except when to do so would injure them or others.

10. We continue to take personal inventory and when we are wrong promptly admit it.

11. We seek through prayer and meditation to improve our conscious contact with God as we understand Him, praying only for knowledge of His will for us and the power to carry that out.

12. Having had a spiritual awakening as the result of these steps, we try to carry this message to alcoholics and to practice these principles in all our affairs.

Table 13-2. Rules for Intervention

DON'T	DO
Attempt to punish	Relax
Attempt to diagnose	Be honest
Attack	Be prepared, practice
Be alone	Use a counselor
	Express concern

with the counselor before the confrontation with the alcoholic. Intervention is successful in guiding the alcoholic to therapy in about 75% of the cases.

The community can also be involved in eliminating or decreasing alcoholism from our society. Educational programs in the schools are essential to arm young-sters with knowledge. However, because peer pressure is a strong determinant of a child's actions, this peer pressure must be used to decrease alcohol use. One format for this is the Students Against Drunk Driving (SADD). This club combines socialization with alcohol and drug education. They often sponsor "dry" proms or other activities.

Mothers Against Drunk Driving (MADD) is another community organization interested in decreasing alcohol use. MADD is involved in education, sponsors community awareness programs, and even monitors the courts and their actions against drunk drivers.

Even the individual can contribute to the fight against alcohol abuse. Your attitude toward alcohol, drunk driving, comic "drunks," underage drinking, enforcement, and punitive actions can change someone else's attitude, and that person may change someone else's, and so on.

EVALUATION Success of treatment of the alcoholic ▲▲▲▲▲▲▲▲▲▲ may be measured with both short-term and long-term methods. However, in the long run, remember that this is a deadly disease. Because of the many effects alcohol has on the liver, cirrhosis is one of the leading causes of death. The alcoholic generally dies from bacterial infection, excess workload for the circulatory system, hemorrhage (from ruptured esophageal varices or other blood vessels), or accidents related to the perceptual effects.

E X E R C I S E S

CASE STUDIES

1. J.B., age 15 years, is your patient. He was brought into the hospital by his parents because of a "drinking problem." He states that he does not have a problem with alcohol because he only drinks on weekends. What would be your best response to this?

2. J.B. has an intravenous infusion started with fructose and thiamine. What is the purpose of these two drugs?

3. J.B. begins having symptoms of delirium tremens as the alcohol is eliminated from his system. What symptoms would you expect to see? What is the drug of choice for this?

4. After J.B. begins recovering from the DTs, what type of diet might he be on?

5. What psychological care would be offered to J.B.? To his family?

LEARNING ACTIVITIES

1. With permission, attend a meeting of the local Alcoholics Anonymous. Remember, you do not discuss persons you see there.

2. Ask to visit with a probation officer. Ask him or her what percentage of the clients are alcoholics, recovering alcoholics, or family members of alcoholics.

3. Tour a drug and alcohol treatment center.

4. Contact the State Highway Patrol for statistics of alcohol-related traffic accidents and deaths in your area in the last year.

5. Contact your local family court for statistics linking alcohol and domestic violence.

6. Conduct an anonymous survey of your local high school. Ask respondents about their involvement in alcohol and that of their friends. Ask them about their parents' involvement as well.

Alcoholic not in control

OPIATE ABUSE

L E A R N I N G   O B J E C T I V E S

After studying this chapter, you should be able to:

1. List drugs that are opiate based.

2. Relate symptoms and clues indicative of opiate drug use or abuse.

3. Discuss difficulties of opiate withdrawal.

4. Discuss opiate abuse rehabilitation.

Opiates, or opiate derivatives, are prepared from opium. The most common of these include opium, codeine, morphine, and heroin.

These drugs have been used and misused for centuries. We know opium has been around since at least 4000 BC because Homer described its use in the *Odyssey*. Morphine was isolated in 1803, and codeine soon after. Morphine soon became a widely abused drug.

In 1898, the Bayer company advertised a new drug cure for morphine withdrawal that was thought to be nonaddictive. That drug was heroin.

We now know that heroin is a powerful central nervous system depressant, and it is classed as a narcotic. Far from being the nonaddicting cure Bayer thought it to be, heroin produces a level of tolerance so quickly that many addicts must increase their dosage approximately every month to achieve the same effects.

Heroin remains a major abused drug in the United States, and there are more than 500,000 addicts. About half of these addicts are younger than 25 years.

ACTIONS AND USES When heroin is used, it produces mental depression, analgesia, dilated blood vessels, and flushed skin. It depresses the cough reflex, the appetite, and the vital signs.

Some of the opiates have medical uses. For example, morphine is a commonly prescribed analgesic for severe pain. Codeine is found in pain remedies and in cough suppressants. Heroin itself has no accepted medical application and is illegal to possess.

Heroin is generally taken intravenously.

N U R S I N G   A L E R T

Because the drug addict does not have access to a supply of needles and syringes, it is common practice to share these supplies. As a result, heroin addicts are at much greater risk for infection due to blood-borne pathogens, including hepatitis B virus and human immunodeficiency virus (HIV), the causative organism of acquired immunodeficiency syndrome (AIDS).

Other forms of the drug can be taken orally or sniffed into the nasal cavity.

ASSESSMENT When you suspect heroin abuse, be alert for signs of its use, including

- Needle tracks on arms and legs
- Mental depression
- Lack of response to pain
- Flushing
- Signs of withdrawal, such as nasal sniffing, reddened and watery eyes, and nervousness

Be alert for any signs and symptoms that indicate the complications of heroin abuse, such as hepatitis B, positive HIV test results, and signs of malnutrition.

PLANNING AND IMPLEMENTATION The first step of successful intervention is persuading the patient that there is a problem. Many who are caught up in the drug world see drug use as a normal everyday behavior. The desirability of treatment must be presented to the patient in terms important to him or her. This implies that you must know the patient well enough to understand the patient's priorities.

Once the patient has decided on treatment, the physician determines which course to take. Often, it includes detoxification, a term referring to the withdrawal of the drug from the body systems. It is necessary for the patient to be hospitalized for detoxification because withdrawal is painful and dangerous. The physician may order sedatives to be given during the process.

Another possible form of treatment for heroin addiction is methadone replacement therapy. This treatment remains controversial. The theory of this therapy is to replace the heroin in the addict's body with a substance that the body will accept in its place but that is not as addictive. Methadone is an opiate derivative, and therefore it is able to be substituted for the heroin. However, some practitioners believe methadone to be just as addictive and dangerous as heroin, producing an addict who is now reliant on the physician for the next dose of the drug. Other practitioners point to the apparent success of methadone replacement therapy in numerous addicts, who eventually quit both the heroin and the methadone.

The recovering heroin addict requires follow-up psychological care. The same reasons and pressures that were factors of the original addiction are still present unless the patient is taught how to deal with them.

EVALUATION Evaluation of treatment of the heroin ▲▲▲▲▲▲▲▲▲▲ addict is measured in number of days and sometimes hours without the drug. Mental health practitioners often point to the high number of patients who repeatedly become addicted for explaining levels of nurse burnout. Health care workers can be members of support groups that help the worker derive satisfaction from the successes.

E X E R C I S E S

CASE STUDIES

1. Present a case to the class for current practices by the Food and Drug Administration (FDA) for extensive drug testing before marketing. Use the case of heroin as part of your rationale.

2. Mr. J.D. is a client in a walk-in clinic. He asks the nurse what kind of diseases he can get from using heroin. How should the nurse respond?

MENTAL AEROBICS

1. The instructor can arrange a tour of an alcohol and drug treatment center or clinic.

2. Mental health practitioners are an excellent source of guest speakers. Subjects can include the problems of treatment, the usual aspects of treatment, and the types of drugs commonly abused in the area.

Clean needle program is in effect.

HALLUCINOGEN ABUSE

LEARNING OBJECTIVES

After studying this chapter, you should be able to:

1. List drugs that are hallucinogenic.

2. Relate symptoms and clues indicative of hallucinogen use or abuse.

3. Discuss difficulties of hallucinogen withdrawal.

4. Discuss hallucinogen abuse rehabilitation.

Hallucinogens are classed together because of their action. They produce unusual responses from the senses—hallucinations. These effects vary from drug to drug, from user to user, and from dose to dose. The user cannot predict what the effect will be before the use.

MARIJUANA AND HASHISH

Marijuana and hashish both contain the same chemical ingredient, tetrahydrocannabinol (THC). This chemical can stay in the fat in the body up to a month at a time. If, at some time during the month, the user begins to use body fat for energy (for example, goes on a reducing diet or begins strenuous exercise), it is possible for mild effects of the drug to be produced again. This is called a flashback.

Use of marijuana and hashish is estimated to be 20 times more prevalent now than in the "tune-in, turn-on" 1960s. The plants that are raised now are hybrids of the originals, and their THC concentrations are much stronger.

ACTIONS AND USES The user often describes a subjective effect of having stepped outside of oneself. THC causes reaction time to lengthen and reflexes to slow. Memory is impaired, as are logical thinking processes.

With prolonged use, marijuana and hashish can cause delayed puberty, disruptions in the menstrual cycle, and the development of breasts in males (gynecomastia).

In general, both marijuana and hashish are smoked like cigarettes or in a pipe. Many different devices have been developed, and each is supposed to alter the flavor and effect of the drug.

Because these drugs are smoked, you may have already guessed that lung damage is a complication associated with their use. However, you may not have realized that a single "joint" of marijuana or hashish is estimated to have the same damaging effects as an entire pack (20) of tobacco cigarettes. Lung cancer has been associated with smoking marijuana and hashish.

It is also possible for abusers to ingest the drug with food.

ASSESSMENT Frequent users of marijuana or hashish often have a "smokers hack" type of cough, especially on first arising. Listen to breath sounds. Also assess normal progression of growth and development in teenagers, such as menarche, menstrual cycle, and secondary sexual characteristics.

PLANNING AND IMPLEMENTATION Once again, convincing the patient that there is a problem is a major hurdle. Many THC users do not realize the dangers and do not believe the evidence presented. Groups have been formed that promote the legalization of marijuana. These groups are not just teenagers but in fact are more often people in their 30s and 40s, and many are successful business people and professionals.

NURSING ALERT

In addition to the damage to the lungs, marijuana and hashish use has been linked to stillbirths and some congenital fetal defects.

The user also has an increased frequency of infection. This may be related to the lung damage, or it may be related to the lifestyle of the drug abuser.

EVALUATION Quitting smoking of marijuana or hashish is just as difficult as quitting smoking of tobacco. Both are addicting physically and psychologically. Some evidence suggests that the use of marijuana may lead to the use of more potent drugs.

LSD, PCP, STP, SPECIAL K, AND OTHERS

ACTIONS AND USES Lysergic acid diethylamide (LSD), phenylcyclohexyl piperidine (PCP), dimethoxymethamphetamine (STP), ketamine (Special K), and other drugs produce hallucinations.

NURSING ALERT

The user is often unable to detect danger.

Users of these drugs are subject to wide mood swings, paranoia, and panic attacks. Mental confusion is common. Depending on the user's state of mind when taking the drug, these drugs can produce a rush of energy, extreme depression, or even agitated violence. Many can cause the user to become unconscious.

NURSING ALERT

Ketamine (Special K) can cause convulsions in some persons, especially if it is taken in large doses.

Most hallucinogens cause the following effects:

- Lower body temperature
- Chills and sweating
- Irregular respirations
- Nausea and vomiting
- Dilated pupils with light sensitivity

Hallucinogens can be taken orally, sniffed, smoked, and even injected. Each route carries its own complications.

ASSESSMENT If you suspect a patient of using hallucinogens, assess the level of consciousness and orientation. Monitor vital signs frequently. Check for dilated pupils and for nausea.

Documentation of each of these is important. Complete descriptions using the patient's own words when possible are valuable in documenting the orientation. More obvious signs are also possible, such as the smell of smoke on the person's hair and clothing, or even finding the drug itself.

PLANNING AND IMPLEMENTATION Convincing the patient of the need for treatment is often not possible while the influence of the drug is still in effect. You may not be able to communicate because of your patient's disorientation, paranoia, panic, or violence.

NURSING ALERT

Protecting the patient from harm is a priority goal. With the patient's normal response to danger impaired, be alert to any potentially harmful situations or equipment.

The body's ability to maintain its own temperature is also impaired. Take steps to keep the temperature in normal limits. This may include cool baths with sweating or light blankets with chilling.

Dilated pupils make the patient sensitive to light. Keep lights dimmed and drapery closed.

EVALUATION The effects of the drug continue for varied amounts of time, depending on the amount taken, the size of the patient, and how long ago the drug was taken before medical treatment. Continue to evaluate the patient's status by reassessment.

EXERCISES

CASE STUDIES

1. You have been asked to talk to a high-school class about drugs. One of the students asks you why

marijuana is illegal when it is not addicting. How would you respond?

2. Ms. M.R., age 19 years, is brought to the physician's office where you are working. Her companion says she is having a "bad trip." After questioning, it is determined that Ms. M.R. took LSD. What should you assess her for? What actions should you take?

ABUSE OF AMPHETAMINES AND BARBITURATES

LEARNING OBJECTIVES

After studying this chapter, you should be able to:

1. List drugs that are amphetamines.

2. Relate symptoms and clues indicative of amphetamine use or abuse.

3. Discuss difficulties of amphetamine withdrawal.

4. Discuss amphetamine abuse rehabilitation.

5. List drugs that are barbiturates.

6. Relate symptoms and clues indicative of barbiturate use or abuse.

7. Discuss difficulties of barbiturate withdrawal.

8. Discuss barbiturate abuse rehabilitation.

Amphetamines and barbiturates have been called uppers and downers, respectively, because of their effect on the patient's mood. Each has effects on many other aspects as well.

AMPHETAMINES

ACTIONS AND USES Amphetamines are central nervous system (CNS) stimulants, but they stimulate more than mood. All aspects of the CNS are elevated. Heart rate, respirations, blood pressure, and temperature all go up. The mind is hyperalert, causing insomnia. The appetite is suppressed. Pupils are dilated. The patient may have difficulty voiding because the bladder sphincter is contracted. The patient feels energized.

The drug can also cause irritability and tremors, nausea, vomiting, diarrhea, dizziness, headache, and heart palpitations.

Medical Uses Amphetamines may be used to treat chronic fatigue, obesity, narcolepsy, attention deficit in children, and mental depression.

Routes Used Amphetamines are usually taken orally, which makes them highly accessible and easily abused. In fact, amphetamines are one of the most often abused prescription drug classifications.

ASSESSMENT Monitor the patient's level of consciousness and orientation. Brain damage is possible. Amphetamine psychosis is a phenomenon that occurs during amphetamine abuse. It may cause the patient to hallucinate, be afraid of health care workers, or become violent.

NURSING ALERT

Monitor the patient's vital signs frequently. Obtain a baseline reading. Two potential complications of amphetamine use are heart attack and stroke, both of which can occur without warning.

Assess for any tremors; prolonged use of amphetamines can lead to Parkinson's disease. Assess your patient's nutritional status. Amphetamine users are often malnourished as a result of extreme appetite suppression.

PLANNING AND IMPLEMENTATION Maintenance of vital ▲▲▲▲▲▲▲▲▲▲▲▲▲▲▲▲▲▲▲▲▲▲▲▲ body functions is top priority for this patient. Report any deviations of the vital signs immediately.

Encourage your patient to eat high-nutrient foods. The physician may order nutritional supplements. Monitor the patient's weight frequently, at least twice a week. Help your patient avoid caffeine foods and beverages.

You may need to take steps to encourage voiding. If all interventions have failed, the physician may need to order catheterization.

Because of increased physical activity and inability to sleep, encourage the patient to rest. The natural clues to the body have been over-ridden, and the patient may remain active until exhaustion.

Safety is also a nursing concern because the increased activity causes the patient to have impaired judgment. Be alert to dangerous situations.

Psychosocial therapy is also necessary and ordered by the physician. Use therapeutic communication techniques to help the patient develop problem-solving skills.

EVALUATION While amphetamines are being with-▲▲▲▲▲▲▲▲▲▲ drawn from the patient, it is possible for the patient to experience rebound depression and fatigue. Evaluate the patient's mood and energy level.

In evaluating the patient's psychosocial status, be aware of attitudes that indicate increasing ability to problem solve. Document these carefully.

BARBITURATES

ACTIONS AND USES Barbiturates are referred to as ▲▲▲▲▲▲▲▲▲▲▲▲▲▲▲ downers because they slow the body and its processes. The vital signs decrease. The patient becomes lethargic and sleepy. Concentration and coordination are diminished. Speech may be slurred, gait may be ataxic, and the patient may complain of dizziness. The patient's muscles are relaxed.

N U R S I N G   A L E R T
▼▼▼▼▼▼▼▼▼▼▼▼▼▼▼▼▼▼▼▼▼▼▼▼▼▼▼▼▼

The patient may experience depression and even suicidal ideation. This is more pronounced, as are other actions, with the concurrent use of alcohol or other central nervous system (CNS) depressants.

▲▲▲▲▲▲▲▲▲▲▲▲▲▲▲▲▲▲▲▲▲▲▲▲▲▲▲▲▲

Medical Uses Barbiturates are commonly prescribed as sedative-hypnotics for sleep disturbances,

as adjuncts to preoperative medications, as therapy for anxiety, and as part of the treatment of alcohol withdrawal and delirium tremens. Some barbiturates (commonly phenobarbital) are also used as anticonvulsants.

Routes Used Barbiturates that are abused most often are those taken orally. Some of this classification's members are also administered by injection intramuscularly or intravenously by the addict.

ASSESSMENT Safety is a prime consideration while this ▲▲▲▲▲▲▲▲▲▲▲ patient is still under the influence of the drug. Lethargy, drowsiness, ataxia, and dizziness are all factors contributing to accidents. Therefore, be sure to assess the level of consciousness and orientation.

N U R S I N G   A L E R T
▼▼▼▼▼▼▼▼▼▼▼▼▼▼▼▼▼▼▼▼▼▼▼▼▼▼▼▼▼

Monitor the vital signs of the patient known to abuse barbiturates. Sudden withdrawal from this classification can be fatal.

▲▲▲▲▲▲▲▲▲▲▲▲▲▲▲▲▲▲▲▲▲▲▲▲▲▲▲▲▲

Some patients have a productive cough due to the overuse of these drugs. Assess the cough, the production, and breath sounds. Barbiturates can also aggravate pre-existing conditions of the respiratory system.

Note signs of liver damage or dysfunction and anemia. These include skin coloration, activity level, nausea, vomiting and diarrhea, color of urine and stool, and a feeling of being cold.

PLANNING AND IMPLEMENTATION Be sure to supervise ▲▲▲▲▲▲▲▲▲▲▲▲▲▲▲▲▲▲▲▲▲▲▲▲▲▲▲▲▲ all activities that could be harmful, including ambulation, smoking, shaving, and showering. Be sure the patient knows where the call bell is and how to use it. Place side rails in the up position, and put the bed in the lowest position.

During withdrawal from the drug, the prime focus is on the physical well-being of the patient. After withdrawal has been achieved, the patient will feel well enough to concentrate on psychotherapy and patient teaching. The nurse has a responsibility to teach the patient about the drug of abuse. Include in your plan the additive effects of barbiturates with other CNS depressants including alcohol, the dangers of operating machinery or driving while using barbiturates, and the possibility of fetal abnormalities if barbiturates are used during pregnancy. Emphasize long-term effects of the drug on the body, including liver damage.

Understanding the reason the patient began abusing the drug also presents opportunities for intervention. If the drug was used to decrease anxiety, explore with the patient other methods of achieving relaxation, such as relaxation exercises, tapes, activity, and hobbies. If the drug was used to produce sleep for a person with insomnia, discuss methods of inducing sleep without drugs, including a darkened room, white sound devices, and avoidance of caffeine and nicotine or other stimulants. If muscle spasms were the original reason for the use of a barbiturate, investigate the cause of the spasm more thoroughly. The nurse can provide back massage, repositioning, and an explanation of proper body mechanics.

EVALUATION Evaluation of the treatment of barbiturate abuse includes both physical and emotional factors. Stable body functions during and after withdrawal are indicated by vital signs within normal limits; the patient is alert and oriented, and the gait is steady. The patient will need to be able to explain methods to use other than drugs to achieve the same effect that was sought by abuse. Also evaluate the patient's current ability to problem solve.

E X E R C I S E S

CASE STUDIES

1. A patient is admitted for withdrawal from drugs. Amphetamine psychosis is the physician's diagnosis. How would you expect the patient to behave? What actions by the nurse are vital?

2. Your patient is being treated for seizures with a barbiturate. What signs or symptoms would suggest to you that the patient may be abusing the medication?

CHAPTER 17

ABUSE OF COCAINE AND CRACK COCAINE

LEARNING OBJECTIVES

After studying this chapter, you should be able to:

1. State one medical use for cocaine.

2. Relate symptoms and clues indicative of cocaine or crack abuse.

3. Discuss difficulties of cocaine withdrawal.

4. Discuss cocaine or crack abuse rehabilitation.

Cocaine is a potent drug made from the leaves of the cocoa plant found in South America. It is refined into a powder form. This powder is "cut" (meaning that other substances are added to it) to raise the volume of the cocaine and increase profits. It may be cut with innocuous substances, such as baking soda or cornstarch; or it may be cut with highly dangerous substances, such as phenylcyclohexyl piperidine (PCP), anesthetics, or other drugs. Unfortunately, the buyer has no way of knowing with what the cocaine was cut.

Cocaine, or coke, was used regularly at one time in this country by many people. Coca-Cola originally contained cocaine and to this day retains the nickname Coke; of course, the cocaine has now been replaced with caffeine.

Crack is a form of cocaine that has been concentrated. It is sold in rocks, flakes, and chips. It takes its name from the sound it makes in the pipe used to smoke it. When cocaine is concentrated and made into crack, the impurities that were used to cut the cocaine are also concentrated and remain in the rock in a more intense state.

Another form of cocaine abuse is called speedballing. This is a dangerous mixture of cocaine and heroin. The mixture is administered intravenously by the addict. The risk of cocaine overdose is higher with speedballing because of the opiate effects of the heroin.

ACTIONS AND USES Cocaine is a stimulant and a local anesthetic. It produces short-term feelings of enhanced pleasure, but the long-term effect is decreased pleasure and severe depression. The drug can eliminate the survival drives of hunger, sleep, and sex. It may produce feelings of great muscular strength, mental intelligence, euphoria, confidence and power, and indifference to pain. Vital signs are dramatically elevated, and the patient may experience heart palpitations; pupils are dilated. The patient may complain of nausea, vomiting, difficulty sleeping, chronic sore throat or dysphonia, frequent nosebleeds, runny nose, and sinus headaches. Compulsive behaviors may be aggravated, such as licking the lips or shrugging the shoulders. The patient experiences anxiousness, irritability, cramps, hyperactivity, and paranoia. As the initial drug effects wear off, depression develops. The withdrawal from cocaine is said to be a particularly hard-hitting "crash." The patient wishes to avoid the feelings of withdrawal and craves the next dose. Once again, the addict may be irritable, be anxious, and experience decreased appetite or nausea. There may be tremors, insomnia, paranoia, and a feeling of "crawling" on the skin sometimes referred to as coke bugs.

Cocaine restricts blood flow, which makes it difficult for a man to achieve and maintain an erection or for either a man or a woman to experience orgasm. Heavy use can lead to seizures, impotence, liver damage, and chronic depression.

Acute cocaine poisoning occurs when a person takes an overdose of cocaine. This may be due to the tolerance the body develops to the drug with each dose. The addict must increase the dosage each time and yet will never achieve the same "high" that was experienced with the initial dose.

Overdosing may also be accidental. Body packing is a method used to smuggle the drug into the United States. The smuggler swallows or rectally or vaginally inserts balloons or condoms that contain cocaine. If one of the balloons breaks or develops a leak, the smuggler experiences an overdose. Body stuffing is a term sometimes used to describe the panic-swallowing of large quantities of cocaine to avoid arrest. This also leads to overdose.

The symptoms of acute cocaine poisoning include abdominal pain, nausea, vomiting, tachycardia, irregular respirations, seizures, coma, and death.

Medical Uses Cocaine may be used as an anesthetic on mucous membranes, although this practice is decreasing because of the risk for abuse.

Routes Used Cocaine can be inhaled or snorted into nasal passages, injected by mixing with water and administering intravenously, smoked by mixing with tobacco or marijuana cigarettes, swallowed, inserted rectally or vaginally, or used as a bladder irrigant by dissolving in sterile saline. Crack is smoked in a special water pipe so the fumes can be inhaled.

ASSESSMENT Cocaine addicts are usually discovered ▲▲▲▲▲▲▲▲▲▲ because of their intense desire for the next dose of the drug. The cells of the patient's body crave the drug because it replaces dopamine in the brain. The brain stops producing dopamine. Now the patient must have the cocaine just to feel normal.

Craving for cocaine can develop with just one use and can lead to suicidal ideation if the drug is unavailable.

N U R S I N G   A L E R T
▼▼▼▼▼▼▼▼▼▼▼▼▼▼▼▼▼▼▼▼▼▼▼▼▼▼▼▼▼▼▼▼▼

Assessment of vital signs is top priority. Cocaine can cause sudden heart attack, stroke, and seizures. Any of these can cause death.

▲▲▲▲▲▲▲▲▲▲▲▲▲▲▲▲▲▲▲▲▲▲▲▲▲▲▲▲▲▲▲▲▲

Snorting cocaine can also cause ulceration and necrosis of the nasal septum. You may be able to see this destruction even without a nasal speculum.

Assess your patient for signs of chronic sleep deprivation and malnutrition. If the drug was smoked, lung damage may be evidenced by a cough with production of black sputum. If the drug was injected intravenously, assess sites for signs of infection, abscesses, or blood clotting. Intravenous drug users are also more at risk for hepatitis B and acquired immunodeficiency syndrome (AIDS).

PLANNING AND IMPLEMENTATION Detoxification of the
▲▲▲▲▲▲▲▲▲▲▲▲▲▲▲▲▲▲▲▲▲▲▲▲▲▲▲▲▲ cocaine or crack ad-

dict must involve medication. This generally includes antidepressants, amino acids used by the brain to make dopamine (tyrosine and tryptophan), and possibly antiparkinsonian medications. The longer the cocaine was used and the larger the dose, the longer these medications must be continued. The drugs are aimed at decreasing the withdrawal effects, especially cravings.

Inform the patient that if the medications are stopped too soon, the brain will not yet have begun making dopamine on its own again. The cravings will recur, even a year later.

Safety is vital. The patient experiencing a high from cocaine will not recognize danger. The patient experiencing a crash may be suicidal.

High-nutrient foods must be encouraged. The patient cares more about getting the next dose of cocaine than about food.

The patient should be in a facility prepared for emergency measures. Resuscitation may be necessary if cardiac failure, stroke, or seizure occurs.

EVALUATION Treatment of cocaine addiction is long ▲▲▲▲▲▲▲▲▲▲ term and does not lend itself well to immediate evaluation. The physical condition of the patient can be evaluated. The probability of compliance with medication schedules can also be evaluated.

Note the patient's improving ability to problem solve. Also be aware of the possibility of a return of the cravings or the patient's inability to cope with life on the streets.

E X E R C I S E S

CASE STUDIES

1. Ms. O.B. is a patient recovering from cocaine addiction. She asks you how long the cravings will continue. What would be your best response? What medications might the physician prescribe for Ms. O.B. to help with withdrawal?

2. Mr. J.W. is a long-time user of cocaine. He asks you whether cocaine can do any long-term damage. What would be your best response?

Cocaine increases the risk of certain diseases. Which diseases are these, and how might they be transmitted to Mr. J.W.?

3. Ms. C.L. is a patient who uses cocaine. She has not yet decided to stop using the drug. She tells you that she is depressed and that using cocaine helps her to "face life." Using what you now know about the effects of cocaine on the mind and body, how can you respond to Ms. C.L.?

MENTAL AEROBICS

Visit a drug and alcohol treatment or counseling center. With the patient's permission, talk with at least one person who has been using cocaine. Ask what effects were felt, what withdrawal was felt, how the person first began using the drug, and what convinced the person to try to stop using the drug. Share your findings with other students.

GLUE SNIFFING

LEARNING OBJECTIVES

After studying this chapter, you should be able to:

1. Define glue sniffing.

2. Relate symptoms and clues indicative of glue sniffing.

3. List dangers associated with glue sniffing.

4. Discuss drug abuse rehabilitation specific to glue sniffing.

The name given to this particular activity is misleading. It was originated at one time by youngsters who discovered the drug-like effects of inhaling the vapors of such substances as model airplane glue. Glue sniffing has progressed to the point that it has outgrown its name. Innumerable fumes can drug the body to give various types of effects—some pleasant at first, others not. However, the name is retained, or the substances may be referred to as inhalants.

ACTIONS AND USES The actions of the substance in-
▲▲▲▲▲▲▲▲▲▲▲▲▲▲▲ haled depend on the substance. In
 addition to different types of glues, children have experimented with and made popular gasoline, kerosene, paint thinner, lighter fluid, typewriter correction fluid, aerosols, whipping cream gas, and even helium from balloons. This, too, is an incomplete list.

In general, these substances can cause disorientation, decreased coordination, depression, slurred speech, blurred vision and watery eyes, ringing in the ears, nausea and vomiting, violence, stupor, unconsciousness, and death.

NURSING ALERT
▼▼▼▼▼▼▼▼▼▼▼▼▼▼▼▼▼▼▼▼▼▼▼▼▼▼▼▼▼▼▼▼

As you can see from this list, many of the substances are ototoxic, neurotoxic, and central nervous system depressants.

▲▲▲▲▲▲▲▲▲▲▲▲▲▲▲▲▲▲▲▲▲▲▲▲▲▲▲▲▲▲▲▲▲▲

Medical Uses There are no medical uses for these substances. However, because each is a common household product, these substances are readily available to children.

Routes Used To receive the effects of the substance, the user concentrates the fumes in some manner. Often, this is in a paper or plastic bag. Once the substance is in the bag, the opening is kept closed except on inhaling. Long breaths are inhaled and kept in the lungs.

Other products lend themselves well to inhalation directly from the product container, such as aerosol cans.

ASSESSMENT Children who indulge in glue sniffing
▲▲▲▲▲▲▲▲▲▲ are generally younger, in the 10- to 15-year age group, because this type of "drug" is more available to them than other drugs are. This does not preclude glue sniffing in older age groups, however.

In addition to assessing for the symptoms mentioned before, the astute nurse looks for residues on hands, on clothing, around the mouth, and in the immediate interior of the nares. The odor of the substance may also still be on the patient's clothing, or there may have been spillage. If a product container was brought in with the patient, bring this to the attention of the physician immediately. Product containers are often the quickest source of information about the substance.

N U R S I N G   A L E R T

▼▼▼▼▼▼▼▼▼▼▼▼▼▼▼▼▼▼▼▼▼▼▼▼▼▼▼▼▼▼▼

If the vapors have been inhaled for prolonged periods, the patient may have additional symptoms. These may include signs that indicate damage to the brain, liver, kidneys, and bone marrow.

▲▲▲▲▲▲▲▲▲▲▲▲▲▲▲▲▲▲▲▲▲▲▲▲▲▲▲▲▲▲▲

PLANNING AND IMPLEMENTATION Begin planning how
▲▲▲▲▲▲▲▲▲▲▲▲▲▲▲▲▲▲▲▲▲▲▲▲▲ to approach the patient after immediate danger to life is over. Your plan of action must take into account the reason for the glue-sniffing incident. Was it related to a dare or peer pressure? Was this a single use, or was this only one in a series of incidents? The answer to each question will help guide your care.

For example, if this was a single incident, implement teaching programs aimed at the dangers of such behavior. Social responses can be practiced in sheltered situations. Help the patient learn how to say no to as many possible peer relation situations as possible.

If this was not a single incident, the teaching plan is still appropriate, but more intense therapy will no doubt be required.

In either case, the physician may prescribe psychotherapy.

EVALUATION Evaluation of the nursing plan uses the
▲▲▲▲▲▲▲▲▲▲ patient's increasing ability to verbalize understanding. Evaluate, too, the ability to give appropriate answers to situations. Are the answers merely repeated, or are they implementing learned material in a manner that is distinctive to the person?

E X E R C I S E S

MENTAL AEROBICS

Write a short description to explain how you would handle the following situations. Be sure you are using the method that best handles the problem, not the best way to relieve frustration. Discuss your answers in class or with a friend. What other alternatives were there that you did not think of?

1. You arrive home from nursing school tonight and find your 14-year-old inhaling fumes from a bag. What will you do?

2. You find objects to suggest that someone was inhaling fumes of several different substances in your garage: plastic bags with different liquids in them, aerosol cans lying around, cigarette lighters (empty), and the odor of paint thinner in the air. You have two children in your household, and both are in their early teens. What should you do? Are your actions changed if one child is 10 and the other is 17 years old?

3. You find two young children in the city park inhaling the fumes from typewriter correction fluid. What do you do?

UNIT FOUR

DRUGS THAT AFFECT MICROORGANISMS

In this unit, we discuss drugs that affect either microorganisms themselves or the body's response to microorganisms. Before prescribing a drug that will affect a microorganism, the physician must first determine which microbe is present.

In identifying microbes, we use several classifying systems. One classification method is by shape. Coccus (plural, cocci) identifies a bacterium of round or spherical shape. Bacillus (plural, bacilli) is a rod-shaped bacterium. Spirillum (plural, spirilla) describes a spiral or curved bacterium. A second way to differentiate between microbes is by their community, or how they normally group themselves. Combining prefixes to denote this relationship are diplo-, a pair; strept-, a chain; and staphylo-, a cluster. Thus, diplococcus is a pair of spherical microbes. Streptococcus and staphylococcus can be similarly interpreted.

Another method for classifying microbes is according to their staining ability in the laboratory. Gram-positive microbes are those that retain a purple stain. Gram-negative microbes are those that do not. This simple test helps to narrow down the possible microbes quickly. Common gram-positive cocci are *Staphylococcus aureus, Staphylococcus epidermidis, Streptococcus,* and *Enterococcus.* Gram-positive bacilli include *Clostridium, Corynebacterium,* and *Listeria.* One powerful gram-negative coccus is *Neisseria,* the species that causes gonorrhea. There are several common gram-negative bacilli, such as *Escherichia coli, Klebsiella, Proteus, Haemophilus influenzae, Enterobacter,* and *Pseudomonas.*

The organism's need for oxygen is another classification characteristic. Microbes requiring oxygen for life or growth are called aerobes or are said to be aerobic. Anaerobes do not require oxygen (are anaerobic) and often survive best where it does not exist. Staphylococci and streptococci are aerobic; clostridia are anaerobic.

Microorganisms that normally live in or on our bodies in a synergistic (mutually beneficial) relationship are called normal flora. There are many such organisms, but most notable is *E. coli,* which lives in the large bowel.

Other microbes are fungi, viruses, and parasites, such as insects or worms. Each can cause disease or discomfort to the patient.

In Chapter 23, we discuss how our body normally protects itself from microorganisms and how medical science can now augment that protection. We look at the types of immunity possible and some of the most common vaccines and serums. An attempt has been made to provide up-to-date immunization recommendations. However, because new research results are available at a faster and faster pace, it is best for the student to consult a public health department for the latest recommendations and the requirements of the state in which the student lives.

In Chapter 24, we discuss the differences between antiseptics and germicides and give some common examples of each.

CHAPTER 19

ANTIBIOTICS AND RELATED DRUGS

115—170

LEARNING OBJECTIVES

After studying this chapter, you should be able to:

1. Discuss the action and uses of antibiotics and other anti-infectives.

2. List common conditions for which each group of antibiotics are used.

3. Name examples of each group of antibiotics.

4. Discuss adverse reactions to and nursing responsibilities for each group of antibiotics.

5. Prepare an appropriate teaching plan for patients receiving antibiotics.

6. Define antibiotic, bacteria, bactericidal, bacteriostatic, nephrotoxic, and ototoxic.

7. Relate precautions for each type of antibiotic.

8. Demonstrate how to administer antibiotics to patients by use of the nursing process.

DRUGS YOU WILL LEARN ABOUT IN THIS CHAPTER

Penicillins

amoxicillin (Trimox, Amoxil)

amoxicillin with clavulanate potassium (Augmentin)

ampicillin (Polycillin)

bacampicillin (Spectrobid)

carbenicillin (Geopen)

methicillin (Staphcillin)

penicillin G (Penicillin G)

piperacillin (Pipracil)

Cephalosporins

First-Generation

cefazolin (Ancef)

cephalexin (Keflex)

cephalothin (Keflin)

Second-Generation

cefaclor (Ceclor)

cefamandole (Mandol)

cefoxitin (Mefoxin)

Third-Generation

cefixime (Suprax)

cefotaxime (Claforan)

ceftazidime (Fortaz)

ceftriaxone (Rocephin)

cefuroxime (Ceftin)

Macrolides

erythromycin base (ERYC, Ilotycin, PCE)

erythromycin estolate (Ilosone)

erythromycin ethylsuccinate (E.E.S., Pediamycin, E-Mycin)

erythromycin glucceptate (Ilotycin)

erythromycin stearate

erythromycin and sulfisoxazole (Pediazole)

Tetracyclines

demeclocycline (Declomycin)

doxycycline (Vibramycin)

oxytetracycline (Terramycin)

tetracycline (Achromycin)

Aminoglycosides

amikacin (Amikin)

gentamicin (Garamycin)

kanamycin (Kantrex)

streptomycin (Streptomycin)

Sulfonamides

sulfamethoxazole (Gantanol)

sulfamethoxazole and trimethoprim (Bactrim, Septra)

sulfisoxazole (Gantrisin)

Miscellaneous Antibiotics

chloramphenicol (Chloromycetin)

ciprofloxacin (Cipro)

clindamycin (Cleocin)

colistimethate (Coly-Mycin M)

colistin (Coly-Mycin S, Coly-Mycin S Otic)

lincomycin (Lincocin)

neomycin, bacitracin, polymyxin B (Neosporin)

vancomycin (Vancocin)

Other Anti-infectives

methenamine (Mandelamine)

methenamine, azo dye (Azo-Mandelamine)

nitrofurantoin (Furadantin)

nitrofurantoin macrocrystals (Macrodantin)

ACTIONS AND USES Antibiotics are used to fight infec-
▲▲▲▲▲▲▲▲▲▲▲▲▲▲▲ tion by working against specific organisms. They may be either bacteriostatic, which means they prevent growth of the organism, or bact-

ericidal, which means they actively destroy the organism.

Antimicrobial agents use five mechanisms to fight microbes. Some inhibit cell wall synthesis, which in turn causes the cell wall to be destroyed. Others inhibit protein synthesis. A third mechanism changes the microbe's cell wall permeability, which allows substances the microbe needs to escape from the interior of the cell. A fourth mechanism inhibits synthesis of nucleic acid, the genetic material of the microbe (DNA or RNA), which prevents the microbe from reproducing. Last, some antibiotics work by inhibiting the metabolism within the microorganism.

In choosing an antibiotic for a patient, the physician must consider many factors. The type of microbe must be identified by culture. Not all antibiotics work equally well on all microbes. (See Unit IV text for a discussion of types of microbes.)

The physician must also consider whether the antibiotic is bacteriostatic or bactericidal. Antibiotics that are commonly bactericidal include the penicillins, cephalosporins, and aminoglycosides. Bacteriostatic drugs include the tetracyclines, erythromycin, and chloramphenicol. Those patients whose immune response is in some way impaired may not be candidates for use of a drug from the bacteriostatic group, because these agents rely on the patient's immunological system to rid the body of the organism once its growth has stopped. Use of bacteriostatic and bactericidal drugs together often defeats the purpose of the drugs—bactericidals are effective only against actively growing microbes, but the bacteriostatics stop that growth.

Physicians also need to know an antibiotic's ability to penetrate the site of infection. For example, some antibiotics cannot enter the cerebrospinal fluid well; others do not readily pass into soft tissue from the bloodstream. Some antimicrobials are especially good for urinary tract infections, whereas others are most useful in the respiratory system.

Adverse reactions or allergic responses can occur after the first dose, the third dose, the fifteenth dose, or even the last dose—indeed, at any point in the course of drug therapy. As we explore the subgroups of antibiotics, we highlight their specific side effects.

Some adverse reactions are common to many types of antibiotics. When a patient takes an antibiotic, not only are the infectious agents killed, but also some normal flora. When these normal flora are eliminated, their "natural enemies" are allowed to overgrow. These may include bacteria and fungi, which may now begin to produce symptoms of their own, including glossitis (hairy tongue), stomatitis (inflammation of the mouth), diarrhea, and rectal itching. These are called superinfections.

ASSESSMENT As you begin to assess your patient who ▲▲▲▲▲▲▲▲▲▲ has been prescribed an antibiotic, keep three things in mind:

1. Obtain specimens for any ordered culture and sensitivity studies before giving the first dose.
2. Microorganisms grow rapidly.
3. Adverse reactions or allergic reactions can occur at any time during drug therapy.

If your patient is to receive an antibiotic for an infection, the physician often prescribes a broad-spectrum antibiotic (one that is active against a wide range of microbes) before the results of culture and sensitivity studies (C & S) are available. If you were to mistakenly obtain this specimen after the first dose is given, you run the risk of making identification more difficult because so many organisms have now been destroyed.

The culture report identifies the organism found at the site of infection. Sensitivity identifies specific antibiotics as either susceptible or resistant; this actually means that this organism is susceptible or resistant to the drug. The physician is now able to choose the drug that will work best for this patient.

PLANNING AND IMPLEMENTATION Antibiotics are usu-▲▲▲▲▲▲▲▲▲▲▲▲▲▲▲▲▲▲▲▲▲▲▲▲▲▲▲▲▲ ally ordered for 5 to 14 days, but most commonly the physician orders a 10-day supply. If an infection is severe enough or has proved to be somewhat resistant, longer prescriptions are occasionally given. Treatment of some microbial infections requires the patient to take prescribed antibiotics for several months. Some patients who are especially at risk for infection because of debilitating factors will be prescribed antibiotics prophylactically and may take one type or another for the rest of their lives. To prevent the development of resistant strains, the physician alternates between different classes and often requires the patient to remain off the drug for a few days or weeks.

Antibiotics may be used in combination with nursing measures to improve the patient's immune response (such as encouraging intake of dietary protein and vitamin C or fluids), with incision and drainage, with debridement, with irrigation, or with surgery.

Antibiotics are one of the most commonly prescribed drug classifications, but they are also one of the most incorrectly used. A patient being treated with an antibiotic must receive thorough explanation to ensure understanding of the need to take the medicine exactly as prescribed.

Self-treatment is a real danger to the patient and occurs in many different ways because of lack of knowledge. Antibiotics need to be taken in evenly distributed times during the day—not just three times a day or four times a day, but every 8 hours or every 6 hours. This is because the patient needs to establish and maintain a therapeutic blood level. Common reasons for erratic doses include forgetfulness, sleep, or improved symptoms.

Let's look at what happens when antibiotics are taken irregularly. When the first dose of antibiotic is taken, some microbes are killed and growth decreases. These are the microbes that were most susceptible to the drug. The others then begin to reproduce. The next dose of medicine is taken, and a similar response occurs. Now the total number is less than at the beginning. If, however, the patient forgets his medicine or is late with the next dose, these more resistant microbes continue to grow and may eventually outnumber the beginning tally. If a patient is sufficiently erratic in taking his medicine, he may become sicker with a more resistant organism.

In another form of self-treatment, the patient does not finish the medicine. Common reasons given for this include improvement of symptoms and "saving" some for a later date. Although the patient is no longer feeling symptoms, the drug may not have had sufficient time to kill all of the organisms. When the patient is no longer taking the drug, these remaining organisms resume growth until they once again produce symptoms. This patient is likely to state that the medication "didn't work" because he became sick again.

Saving a few capsules of antibiotics for a later date also illustrates another form of self-treatment: self-diagnosis. Without a physician's expertise in diagnosing the infection, the patient cannot know whether this new infection will be susceptible or resistant to the drug. Also, the longer antibiotics are kept on the shelf, the less potent they become.

Parents are often guilty of giving their children medicine prescribed for a sibling. They should do this only with a physician's knowledge and guidance.

As nurses, we must set excellent examples to our patients and our families. Go to your cupboard and clear out all those prescriptions you have been saving for later.

N U R S I N G   A L E R T
▼▼▼▼▼▼▼▼▼▼▼▼▼▼▼▼▼▼▼▼▼▼▼▼▼▼▼▼▼▼▼

Allergic reactions to antibiotics may include a rash or hives. If your patient has symptoms that could indicate an allergy, always withhold the next dose until the physician has been notified. If you do not, your patient may progress to anaphylactic shock.

▲▲▲▲▲▲▲▲▲▲▲▲▲▲▲▲▲▲▲▲▲▲▲▲▲▲▲▲▲▲▲▲

Symptoms include pallor, diaphoresis, drop in blood pressure, and dyspnea. This is an emergency and requires immediate attention. Often, the physician will not prescribe an antibiotic to a child if the parent is allergic to it, because there has been evidence of familial tendencies.

Superinfections are examples of adverse reactions. One nursing measure you can use to reduce the chance of a superinfection (within the confines of the patient's dietary orders) is to encourage the intake of food substances that have been cultured with bacterial colonies, such as buttermilk or yogurt.

Some side effects are related to the route of administration. The oral route is the most common and may be associated with gastrointestinal upset. You may decrease this by having the patient take the medicine with food. Be sure food intake does not affect the absorption or effectiveness of the specific antibiotic.

N U R S I N G   A L E R T
▼▼▼▼▼▼▼▼▼▼▼▼▼▼▼▼▼▼▼▼▼▼▼▼▼▼▼▼▼

The intramuscular (IM) route may be used if the oral or intravenous (IV) route is causing adverse effects. However, IM antibiotics are painful and can be irritating to tissue. Therefore, give the injection deep into large muscles, such as the gluteus medius.

▲▲▲▲▲▲▲▲▲▲▲▲▲▲▲▲▲▲▲▲▲▲▲▲▲▲▲▲▲

The physician may order the injection to be given with a local anesthetic, such as lidocaine or procaine (more about procaine's effects on penicillin later).

If the IV route is being used, know the signs of infiltration (swelling, cold skin, ruddy skin, and possibly a decreased drip rate) as well as the signs of phlebitis (swelling, warmth, redness, and possibly a streak following the vein). To check for the accuracy of the drip rate, use the following formula:

$$\frac{\text{cc ordered} \times \text{drop factor}}{\text{hours} \times 60} = \text{drops per minute}$$

IV antibiotics are given diluted in at least 50 cc of 0.9% sodium chloride (NaCl) or 5% dextrose in water (D5W). Less than this is irritating to the tissue, and some require much more than this. Be sure to flush the IV tubing with either of these two solutions or a similar one between IV antibiotics. This prevents any reactions that might occur if they were to be administered immediately after one another. Change the IV site used for the administration of antibiotics every 2 to 3 days to decrease the chance of phlebitis.

EVALUATION Be prepared for symptoms of infection to
▲▲▲▲▲▲▲▲▲▲ occur quickly in patients, including when

you are assessing them for the effectiveness of the antibiotic. Microbes often double their number each half-hour. Depending on the site, assess for an increase or decrease in redness, warmth, edema, drainage, cough, fever, abnormal breath sounds, or pain.

PENICILLINS (TABLE 19–1)

ACTIONS AND USES Penicillin was the first antibiotic
▲▲▲▲▲▲▲▲▲▲▲▲▲▲▲▲▲ discovered. It therefore takes its logical place at the beginning of the list of antibiotics. Penicillins are now natural or semisynthetic. They are bacteriostatic or bactericidal, depending on the type of

Table 19–1. Common Penicillins and Dosages

GENERIC NAME*	TRADE NAME	DOSE
Amoxicillin	Amoxil, Trimox	Oral: 250–500 mg q8h
Amoxicillin with clavulanate potassium	Augmentin	Oral: 250–500 mg q8h
Ampicillin	Polycillin	Oral: 250–500 mg q6h IM or IV: 1–2 g q3–4h
Bacampicillin	Spectrobid	Oral: 400–800 mg q12h
Carbenicillin	Geopen	Oral: 1–2 tabs q6h IM: 1–2 g q6h IV: 1–2 g 6h
Methicillin	Staphcillin	IM or IV: 1–2 g q4–6h
Penicillin G		Depends on form
Piperacillin	Pipracil	IM or IV: 1.5–4 g q6–12h

*Note the common suffix -cillin.

organism and the distribution of the medication to the site (for example, blood supply). In general, the various forms of penicillin can be effective against many gram-positive organisms, such as streptococcus, staphylococcus, and *Corynebacterium;* several gram-negative organisms, such as *Neisseria* and *Escherichia coli;* and spirochetes as well as some anaerobes.

The semisynthetic forms of penicillin were derived by altering the naturally occurring form of penicillin. These new drugs tend to have a broader spectrum of effectiveness, produce less allergic reactions, and are more likely to have an oral form.

At one time, methicillin was considered the drug of choice for staphylococcal infections. However, in recent years, resistant strains of *Staphylococcus* have appeared. These include methicillin-resistant *S. aureus* (MRSA) and methicillin-resistant *S. epidermidis* (MRSE). For these newer strains, the drug of choice is most often vancomycin.

Some penicillins can cause hyperkalemia, hypernatremia, and seizures.

ASSESSMENT Be aware that penicillin allergy is one of ▲▲▲▲▲▲▲▲▲▲ the most common drug allergies there is. In addition to those assessments already outlined for antibiotics in general, assess the patient's history of allergies. Be alert to any complaints or symptoms that may indicate a current allergic reaction.

PLANNING AND IMPLEMENTATION Give oral penicillins ▲▲▲▲▲▲▲▲▲▲▲▲▲▲▲▲▲▲▲▲▲▲▲▲▲ on an empty stomach for better absorption. To ensure that the stomach is empty, schedule doses 1 hour before meals and 2 hours after meals.

Penicillin G may be given by either the intramuscular (IM) or intravenous (IV) route. IM injection is painful. Therefore, procaine is often added to the solution to decrease the discomfort. Procaine also increases the length of activity of the penicillin G, which tends to be a short-acting drug. Other compounds may also be used for the same purpose. Probenecid, for example, may be given with penicillin or cephalosporins to increase their effectiveness.

EVALUATION Penicillins can interact with several ▲▲▲▲▲▲▲▲▲▲ drugs, including other antibiotics. When given with aminoglycosides, penicillin decreases the effectiveness of the aminoglycoside. Chloramphenicol is antagonistic to penicillin, as are tetracyclines and sulfonamides. The actions of methotrexate are heightened by penicillin.

CEPHALOSPORINS (TABLE 19–2)

ACTIONS AND USES Cephalosporins are chemically re-▲▲▲▲▲▲▲▲▲▲▲▲▲▲▲▲ lated to penicillin. Therefore, they act, and react, in similar ways.

Cephalosporins appear in three subclasses: first-generation, second-generation, and third-generation. Each subsequent generation has been derived by altering the generation that preceded it. This has added to the spectrum of activity for each subclass.

First-generation cephalosporins are generally effective against *Staphylococcus aureus* and *Staphylococcus epidermidis* as well as other gram-positive and gram-negative organisms. Second-generation drugs are effective against more gram-negative organisms than are their first-generation relatives, but they are not effective against *Pseudomonas.* Because of their increased spectrum, the third-generation cephalosporins are also being used to fight severe cases of meningitis. They are effective against more gram-negative organisms than are the second-generation drugs but fewer gram-positive microbes.

Common adverse reactions include nausea or vomiting, possible blood dyscrasias, and toxic effects in the liver.

ASSESSMENT Once again, be aware of the patient's ▲▲▲▲▲▲▲▲▲▲ allergy history. If it includes an allergy to penicillin, notify the physician and observe the patient closely if a cephalosporin is prescribed.

PLANNING AND IMPLEMENTATION Oral cephalosporins ▲▲▲▲▲▲▲▲▲▲▲▲▲▲▲▲▲▲▲▲▲▲▲▲▲ are best taken on an empty stomach, although the patient may experience more nausea or vomiting this way. If this occurs, consult the physician.

Also be aware that this classification can cause false-positive results of urine glucose measurements if Benedict's solution or Clinitest tablets are used. For this reason, alternative methods of testing for glucose in the urine should be used.

EVALUATION Some cephalosporins can cause a disul-▲▲▲▲▲▲▲▲▲▲ firam (Antabuse)–like reaction if they are combined with alcohol intake. This can include severe nausea and vomiting, hypotension, tachycardia, flushing, and even prostration. Cephalosporins also interact with aminoglycosides, colistin, polymyxin B, and vancomycin by increasing the risk of nephrotoxicity. As mentioned previously, probenecid increases the activity of cephalosporins.

Table 19-2. Common Cephalosporins and Dosages

GENERIC NAME*	TRADE NAME	DOSE
Cefaclor	Ceclor	Oral: 250–500 mg q6–8h
Cefamandole	Mandol	IM or IV: 500–1000 mg q4–8h
Cefazolin	Ancef	IM or IV: up to 2 g q6–8h
Cefixime	Suprax	Oral: 400 mg/day
Cefotaxime	Claforan	IM or IV: 1–2 g q6–8h
Cefoxitin	Mefoxin	IM or IV: 1–2 g q6–8h
Ceftazidime	Fortaz	IM or IV: 250–2000 mg 2–3 times daily
Ceftriaxone	Rocephin	IM or IV: 1–2 g q6–8h
Cefuroxime	Ceftin	Oral: 125–500 mg q12h IM or IV: 750–1000 mg q8h
Cephalexin	Keflex	Oral: 250–500 mg q6–8h
Cephalothin	Keflin	IM or IV: 1–2 g q4–6h

*Note the common prefix ceph- or cef-.

MACROLIDES (TABLE 19–3)

Macrolides include the common group of erythromycins. Erythromycin is a nontoxic antibiotic, and for this reason it is the drug of choice when the patient is allergic to penicillin. Although the erythromycins may cause any of the common adverse reactions of antibiotics, the most likely to occur is gastrointestinal (GI) upset.

The various erythromycin salts are effective against many gram-positive organisms and a few gram-negative ones. They may also be useful in treating infections due to *Chlamydia, Mycoplasma, Rickettsia, Treponema, Entamoeba histolytica,* and *Bordetella pertussis.* Erythromycin is the drug of choice against legionnaires' disease.

Although the erythromycins are most effective on an empty stomach, it may be necessary to have the patient take the drug with food if GI upset occurs. Consult the physician.

Erythromycin increases the effectiveness or absorption of several drugs, including carbamazepine (Tegretol), cyclosporine, digitalis, methylprednisolone (Medrol), theophylline, and warfarin (Coumadin).

Table 19–3. Common Macrolides and Doses

GENERIC NAME	TRADE NAME	DOSE
Erythromycin base	ERYC, Ilotycin, PCE	Oral: 250–500 mg q6–8h
Erythromycin estolate	Ilosone	Same as above
Erythromycin stearate		Same as above
Erythromycin ethylsuccinate	E.E.S., Pediamycin	Oral: 400–800 mg q6–8h
Erythromycin gluceptate	Ilotycin	IV: 1–4 g/day
Erythromycin ophthalmic	Ilotycin	0.5% ointment

Table 19-4. Common Tetracyclines and Doses

GENERIC NAME*	TRADE NAME	DOSE
Demeclocycline	Declomycin	Oral: 150 mg q6h or 300 mg q12h
Doxycycline	Vibramycin	Oral: 50–100 mg q12h IV: 100–200 mg q24h
Oxytetracycline	Terramycin	Oral: 250–500 mg q6h IM: 250 mg q24h or 100–150 mg q8–12h
Tetracycline	Achromycin	Oral: 250–1000 mg q6–12h IM or IV: 250–500 mg q12h

*Note common suffix -cycline.

TETRACYCLINES (TABLE 19–4)

Tetracyclines were the first group of broad-spectrum antibiotics and are commonly given orally. Tetracyclines are useful against most bacteria, although some have developed resistance now. This group may be prescribed for infections due to *Rickettsia, Chlamydia, Mycoplasma, Mycobacterium,* spirochetes, and *Balantidium.* They are also often given for infection due to *Propionibacterium acnes,* the cause of acne vulgaris. They cause many of the adverse reactions of general antibiotics as well as photosensitivity, gastrointestinal upset, and staining of the permanent teeth if they are given to children younger than 8 years or to the mother during pregnancy.

Be especially aware of the possible side effects of this group when they are prescribed to teenage girls. They are often reluctant to admit to the possibility of pregnancy, and many enjoy sun-bathing as a pastime.

Tetracyclines interact with iron supplements, which decreases the effectiveness of both. Milk or milk products decrease the absorption of the tetracyclines. With concomitant use of aminoglycosides, tetracyclines decrease the effectiveness of the aminoglycoside

Antacids, anticonvulsants, and local-acting antidiarrheals all decrease the effectiveness of tetracycline. Tetracyclines increase the activity of anti-coagulants.

AMINOGLYCOSIDES (TABLE 19–5)

Aminoglycosides are an effective, although often dangerous, group of antibiotics. All of these drugs are nephrotoxic, meaning that they will attack and destroy renal tissue.

The aminoglycosides are also neurotoxic. This effect is expressed as muscle paralysis and even apnea. Ototoxic effects are the mildest symptoms of neurotoxicity with these drugs.

Various aminoglycosides are used for tuberculosis, endocarditis, tularemia, other serious infections, and even the plague. They are effective against many gram-negative bacteria, including many species of *Pseudomonas.* Kanamycin, given orally, may be used to reduce the presence of normal flora before bowel surgery or to lower the blood urea nitrogen (BUN) concentration in some cases.

Among the aminoglycosides are oral, topical, oph-

Table 19-5. Common Aminoglycosides and Doses

GENERIC NAME*	TRADE NAME	DOSE
Amikacin	Amikin	IM or IV: 15 mg/kg/day in 2–3 evenly spaced, divided doses
Gentamicin	Garamycin	IM or IV: 3–5 mg/kg/day in 3 evenly spaced, divided doses
Kanamycin	Kantrex	IM or IV: 15 mg/kg/day in 2–3 evenly spaced, divided doses
Streptomycin		IM: 1 g q12–24h

*Note common suffix -mycin or -cin.

thalmic, nebulization, intramuscular, and intravenous preparations.

Be alert to changes in the output and any complaints of back or flank pain as well as any signs of renal failure. These could indicate renal tissue damage. Also be alert for and report any complaints of tinnitus, vertigo, weakness, or changes in the respiratory rate, which may indicate neurotoxic injury.

The adverse effects of the aminoglycosides may be enhanced if they are given in combination with other drugs, such as amphotericin B (Fungizone) or cephalothin (Keflin), both of which increase the risk of nephrotoxic effects. Ototoxic injury is more likely if aminoglycosides are given with the loop diuretics, such as furosemide (Lasix), or with dimenhydrinate (Dramamine). Other symptoms of neurotoxicity, such as respiratory paralysis, may be caused by concurrent use with peripheral muscle relaxants, such as succinylcholine (Anectine). The aminoglycosides can increase the effectiveness of anticoagulants, leading to dangerous hemorrhages. However, the effectiveness of digitalis and some penicillins is decreased by the aminoglycosides.

MISCELLANEOUS ANTIBIOTICS

Ciprofloxacin (Cipro) is a quinolone antibiotic. A broad-spectrum agent, it is used against both gram-positive and gram-negative organisms for infections of the lower respiratory tract, soft tissue, bones and joints, and urinary tract; it is also used in the treatment of infectious diarrheas. Ciprofloxacin works against the infectious agents by interfering with the synthesis of DNA, making it impossible for the organism to reproduce.

Ciprofloxacin is not recommended for use in children because it can cause lesions in the bones, leading to an impaired gait. Cautious use is also recommended for persons taking theophylline because this mixture can prove fatal. Tell the patient to avoid caffeine, because ciprofloxacin increases the effects of the caffeine.

Although ciprofloxacin has proved to be a useful antibiotic, still be aware of the many possible adverse reactions associated with its use. It has been known to cause convulsions, crystalluria, photosensitivity, liver dysfunction, and blood dyscrasias. Other less serious effects can include gastrointestinal distress, abdominal pain, headache, restlessness, and a rash.

The usual oral dose is 250 to 750 mg every 12 hours. Ciprofloxacin can also be given intravenously (IV) at a rate of 200 to 400 mg every 12 hours. The IV solution should be given slowly in a period of 60 minutes.

The nurse can decrease the chance of crystalluria in the patient using ciprofloxacin by encouraging foods that cause an acidic urine. The physician may prescribe acidifying agents.

Coly-Mycin is a drug similar to the aminoglycosides. It, too, is ototoxic. This drug is given parenterally as colistimethate (Coly-Mycin M) by either the intramuscular (IM) or IV route. Colistin, another form of the drug, may be given as ear drops (Coly-Mycin S Otic) or orally (Coly-Mycin S). Coly-Mycin can be used against *Pseudomonas* and is possibly effective with infections caused by *Escherichia coli.*

Lincomycin (Lincocin) and clindamycin (Cleocin) are closely related broad-spectrum antibiotics used for severe infections due to staphylococci, streptococci, pneumococci *(Streptococcus pneumoniae), Clostridium,* and *Corynebacterium diphtheriae.* They may also be used if the patient is allergic to penicillin.

Lincomycin and clindamycin should not be given if the patient has colitis or similar bowel diseases. Further, they may initiate life-threatening cases of colitis in anyone, and it may become necessary to treat the colitis with vancomycin. Other adverse reactions include serious blood dyscrasias. Both of these drugs are available in oral, IM, IV, or topical forms.

Vancomycin (Vancocin) is often the drug of choice for methicillin-resistant *Staphylococcus aureus* (MRSA) and methicillin-resistant *Staphylococcus epidermidis* (MRSE). It may also be used for other severe staphylococcal infections and when the patient is allergic to penicillin, cephalosporins, and erythromycins, although it may also cause allergic reactions. Vancomycin is both nephrotoxic and ototoxic. The drug may be given orally or IV, although this may lead to phlebitis. Never give vancomycin IM because this can lead to necrosis of the muscle tissue. The concurrent use of cephalosporins and vancomycin increases the risk of nephrotoxic effects.

Chloramphenicol (Chloromycetin) is a toxic antibiotic normally reserved for infections that do not respond to other antibiotics. Susceptible organisms can include *Haemophilus influenzae, Salmonella typhi, Rickettsia,* and *Chlamydia.* Chloramphenicol can cause serious blood dyscrasias and even cardiovascular collapse. Therefore, assess blood pressure and pulse frequently and advise the patients they will need frequent blood studies to ensure they are not having adverse reactions. Chloramphenicol should not be given IM.

Chloramphenicol interacts with barbiturates by increasing their effectiveness; at the same time, the effectiveness of chloramphenicol is decreased. It also increases the effectiveness of dicumarol, phenytoin (Dilantin), and oral hypoglycemics. Chloramphenicol, a bacteriostatic agent, and bactericidal agents such as penicillin are considered to be antagonistic.

Another common antibiotic given to children is Pediazole. This medication contains erythromycin and sulfisoxazole (a sulfonamide) and is given orally.

Table 19–6. Common Sulfonamides and Doses

GENERIC NAME	TRADE NAME	DOSE
Sulfamethoxazole	Gantanol	Oral: 1 g q8–12h
Sulfamethoxazole and trimethoprim (another antibacterial agent)	Bactrim, Septra	Oral 1 tab q12h IV: 5–10 mg/kg of sulfamethoxazole with 25–50 mg/kg of trimethoprim in evenly spaced, divided doses q6–12h
Sulfisoxazole	Gantrisin	Oral: 600 mg–2 g q4–6h

It is most often used for otitis media caused by *H. influenzae.*

Many antibiotics are available as over-the-counter preparations in a topical form. A common example is Neosporin, which contains neomycin, polymyxin B, and bacitracin. It may be used as a first-aid remedy applied to the skin. The physician may also order this drug as a genitourinary tract irrigant or for ophthalmic administration. Neomycin may be given in oral or rectal form to reduce normal flora before bowel surgery and to lower the blood urea nitrogen (BUN) concentration.

SULFONAMIDES (TABLE 19–6)

ACTIONS AND USES Sulfonamides are not strictly antibiotics, although they are antibacterial. These drugs are commonly used for genitourinary tract infections, skin and soft tissue infections, and burns. They are effective against *Escherichia coli, Klebsiella, Staphylococcus aureus, Proteus,* and *Enterobacter.* The most common adverse reactions include skin rash and gastrointestinal upset.

Sulfonamides may also be associated with rare fatalities caused by Stevens-Johnson syndrome, blood dyscrasias, liver toxicity, and neurotoxic effects. When given in the presence of a low intake of fluids or acidic urine, sulfa drugs may lead to crystalluria, which in turn may lead to the formation of renal calculi.

ASSESSMENT In addition to those assessments previously mentioned for antibiotic therapy in general, assess the client's fluid intake to determine adequacy. Also check the medical history for any liver dysfunction or abnormal results of blood cell studies.

PLANNING AND IMPLEMENTATION Since a common nursing intervention for urinary tract infections is to encourage acidifying of foods and liquids, be aware of any order for a sulfonamide. This nursing intervention is contraindicated with sulfonamides because of the chance of crystalluria. Physicians may even order sodium bicarbonate to alkalinize the urine in some cases. Also be especially aware of the patient's intake of fluids to ensure adequate hydration, changes in the vital signs (especially the respirations), muscle weakness, tinnitus, or vertigo. Sulfonamides may also cause allergic reactions, so withhold the next dose of the drug if a rash develops.

Sulfonamides interact with several other medications. They increase the actions of anticoagulants, diuretics, and oral hypoglycemics. Sulfa drugs decrease the effectiveness of or are antagonistic to digoxin, aminobenzoic acid (PABA, a drug used to treat fibrosis), and procaine. The side effects of several drugs are increased when they are used with sulfonamides, for example, phenytoin (Dilantin), aspirin, and nonsteroidal anti-inflammatory drugs (NSAIDs). Concurrent use with methenamine (Mandelamine), a urinary antiseptic, increases the chances of crystalluria.

OTHER ANTI-INFECTIVES

Methenamine (Mandelamine) is a combination drug that exhibits antiseptic activity in the urinary tract. Primary side effects include nausea and vomiting. Methenamine may also be ordered in a combination with azo dye (a urinary analgesic) and is then called Azo-Mandelamine.

Methenamine should be used in the presence of acidic urine; therefore, encourage acidifying of foods and fluids. The physician may order an acidifying agent with methenamine, such as ammonium chloride. Azo dye turns the urine red-orange; warn the patient of this before it happens.

Nitrofurantoin (Furadantin and its relative Macrodantin) is an effective anti-infective for the urinary system. It causes the urine to be dark in color; issue this warning to the patient to prevent any fear. Nitrofurantoin may also cause gastrointestinal upset and may be given with meals if this occurs.

E X E R C I S E S

CASE STUDIES

1. Ms. S.J. has been diagnosed with pneumonia. She has been prescribed procaine penicillin G IM, which is being given on a twice-a-day schedule. Today, as you are about to give Ms. S.J. her injection, she comments that she did not sleep well last night from all the itching. She points out to you a pinpoint rash on many exposed areas of her body. What should your next action be?

After conference with the physician, you have been ordered to give Keflex orally instead of the procaine penicillin G injections. What are your responsibilities?

2. Mr. N.H. has strep throat. His physician has ordered ERYC orally. What patient teaching should you do for him?

3. T.M., a 15-year-old girl, has acne. Her physician ordered Vibramycin orally to treat the problem. Given T.M.'s age and sex, what patient teaching should she receive?

4. Ms. C.H. is your patient, with a diagnosis of a staph infection. The physician ordered amikacin orally. What should your assessment of this patient include? How could you involve Ms. C.H. in her own care?

The staph infection Ms. C.H. has is now diagnosed as methicillin-resistant *Staphylococcus aureus* (MRSA). The physician changes her antibiotic order to vancomycin IV. What additional assessments should you be making?

5. Mr. J.O. has been diagnosed with a urinary tract infection, with the organism as yet undetermined. The following orders have been written for Mr. J.O.: culture and sensitivity of urine, intake and output, Bactrim orally, sodium bicarbonate orally. Which of these orders should be carried out first? What is the purpose of the sodium bicarbonate? Why is an accurate record of intake and output important? What patient teaching is necessary because Mr. J.O. has been placed on Bactrim?

The nurse was ready to give the Bactrim to Mr. J.O. She discovered the medication supplied by the pharmacy is labeled Septra. What should she do?

In addition to his previous orders, Mr. J.O. is also prescribed Azo-Mandelamine. What additional responsibilities does the nurse have?

6. Mr. S.D. has been prescribed procaine penicillin G IM. As the nurse begins to prepare the medication, he discovers the order reads procaine penicillin G 100,000 U IM. The label reads procaine penicillin G 2,000,000 U. Directions on the label read: Add 18 mL of sterile water to obtain 20 mL of solution. How much solution should the nurse administer to Mr. S.D.?

While Mr. S.D. is receiving penicillin, what observations should the nurse make to evaluate the effectiveness of the medication?

MENTAL AEROBICS

1. Using a *Physician's Desk Reference* or similar reference book, research the precautions and usual dosages of the following: ampicillin, amoxicillin, methicillin, penicillin G, cephalexin, cephalothin, cefaclor, ceftriaxone, cefuroxime, cefixime, Ilosone, Pediazole, doxycycline, gentamicin, amikacin, colistin, vancomycin, chloramphenicol, sulfisoxazole, methenamine, nitrofurantoin.

2. Write an appropriate care plan for a patient receiving gentamicin. Be sure to include at least five nursing diagnoses, with an appropriate goal, one assessment, and one action for each of the diagnoses.

CHAPTER 20

ANTIFUNGAL DRUGS

LEARNING OBJECTIVES

After studying this chapter, you should be able to:

1. Discuss the action of and adverse reactions to antifungal drugs and nursing responsibilities appropriate for patients receiving them.

2. List common conditions for which antifungal drugs are used.

3. Name examples of antifungal drugs.

4. Prepare an appropriate teaching plan for patients receiving antifungal drugs.

DRUGS YOU WILL LEARN ABOUT IN THIS CHAPTER

Topical Antifungals

clotrimazole (Gyne-Lotrimin, Lotrimin, Mycelex)

miconazole (Micatin, Monistat)

ketoconazole (Nizoral)

nystatin (Mycostatin)

tolnaftate (Dr. Scholl's Athlete's Foot Powder, Tinactin)

naftifine (Naftin)

oxiconazole (Oxistat)

amphotericin B (Fungizone)

Systemic Antifungals

miconazole (Micatin, Monistat)

amphotericin B (Fungizone IV)

ketoconazole (Nizoral)

griseofulvin (Fulvicin)

nystatin (Mycostatin)

ACTIONS AND USES A fungus is a plant with no color or chlorophyll. Some fungi can attack the human body. This is called a mycotic infection. The nurse may also see the diagnosis candidiasis, which is an infection caused by the organism *Candida*. This type of mycotic infection is also called moniliasis or yeast infection by the layman.

Medications used to treat fungal or mycotic infections are called antifungals. These medications may be fungicidal or fungistatic. A fungicidal drug is capable of killing the fungus. A fungistatic drug only reduces the growth of the fungus, allowing the body's own defenses to work against it. Some antifungals are also classified as antibiotics because of their action on other organisms.

The majority of antifungal medications are used topically on the skin or mucous membranes. Some work systemically and are given orally or parenterally.

Most topical antifungal agents are used for tinea pedis (athlete's foot), tinea cruris (jock itch), tinea corporis (fungal infection of the body, most often ringworm), tinea versicolor (causes yellowing of the skin), tinea capitis (ringworm of the scalp), tinea barbae (fungal infection of the bearded portion of the neck and face, sometimes called barber's itch), and other dermal fungal infections.

ASSESSMENT When a patient is prescribed an antifungal, assess the area of involvement for signs and symptoms. Accurately document the size of the area, color, and presence of inflammation. Some systemic fungal infections require other as-

125

sessment techniques, depending on the location. For example, a respiratory fungal infection requires assessment of breath sounds and other respiratory functions.

PLANNING AND IMPLEMENTATION When the antifungal is ordered to be administered topically, teach the patient how to apply the medication. First, show the patient the correct method.

N U R S I N G   A L E R T

Be sure to wear gloves to prevent the drug from contacting your own skin.

Be sure the patient sees the amount of medication you apply. Some patients are likely to apply only a thin layer, thinking that this is more economical and saves the drug. Instead, the infection will not be adequately treated, and the patient will incur additional expense for a new drug. Other patients tend to apply thick layers of the drug. Some persons believe that if a given amount will help the infection, a larger amount will cause a cure faster. This, too, is erroneous. The patient only wastes the medication.

After application of the topical medication, do not use an occlusive dressing unless the physician orders it. Occlusive dressings are more likely to cause irritation.

Have the patient apply the next dose with your supervision. Offer advice and instruction as needed. This step may need to be repeated several times before the patient can perform the procedure correctly. By this method, you will be sure the patient is proficient before going home. (Tell me, I forget. Show me, I remember. Involve me, I learn.— Benjamin Franklin.)

If the medication is in another form, be sure the patient knows how and where to apply it. For example, where does a vaginal suppository go? Some patients think all suppositories are rectal.

EVALUATION Carefully evaluate the signs and symptoms you documented originally. Is there any sign of improvement? Is the area smaller? Is there less inflammation? Does the patient perceive changes, such as less itching?

Also look for irritation. If any occurs, or if the condition does not improve, report your findings to the physician. If the patient goes home with the medication, be sure to teach what symptoms to report.

Systemic antifungals are more likely to cause systemic adverse reactions. A common one is bone marrow depression. Monitor laboratory findings frequently. Systemic adverse reactions are possible with topical antifungals as well.

TOPICAL ANTIFUNGAL DRUGS

Clotrimazole

ACTION AND USES Clotrimazole (Mycelex, Lotrimin, Gyne-Lotrimin) is active against dermal infections from several classes of fungi, including *Candida*. In strength, it is considered equal to griseofulvin, tolnaftate, amphotericin B, and nystatin.

Some patients may experience stinging and burning, inflammation, blistering and peeling of the skin, urticaria, and pruritus. On occasion, patients have experienced nausea and vomiting from systemic effects. If clotrimazole is given as a vaginal tablet, be aware of the possibility of vaginal irritation.

ASSESSMENT In addition to the normal integumentary assessments, also monitor results of liver function tests. The physician should order a baseline test and periodic repetitions.

PLANNING AND IMPLEMENTATION Clotrimazole can be administered as a troche, cream, lotion, solution, vaginal cream, or vaginal tablet.

The troche is normally ordered for oral candidiasis and is allowed to melt fully in the mouth. The cream is massaged into the affected skin twice a day. Relief with this route is expected within 1 week. A vaginal tablet is inserted once a day for 7 days. Some tablets are now a larger dose (500 mg) and are to be inserted once only. Vaginal cream is inserted with an applicator once a day for 1 to 2 weeks.

Be sure the patient is aware of the need to continue taking the medication until ordered to stop. If irritation develops, the patient must contact the physician to determine the next step.

EVALUATION Evaluation is the same as described for antifungals in general. A troche is more likely to cause systemic effects.

Miconazole

Miconazole (Monistat, Micatin) is available as a topical preparation for dermal infections. The most common side effect is a skin irritation. Miconazole may be ordered in various forms, including cream, lotion, vaginal cream, and vaginal suppository. Creams and lotions are normally applied in the morning and evening. Vaginal route dosages depend on the agent used.

Ketoconazole

Ketoconazole (Nizoral) is available in a cream form for dermal fungal infections and for seborrheic dermatitis. The most common adverse reactions are skin irritation with pruritus and stinging. The patient should apply the cream once daily for 2 weeks. If the cream is ordered for treatment of seborrhea, the usual dose is twice a day for 4 weeks.

N U R S I N G   A L E R T

Be sure to check for allergies before applying ketoconazole. The cream contains a sulfite. Asthmatic patients are especially susceptible to this type of allergy.

Nystatin

Nystatin (Mycostatin) is available topically as a cream, powder, ointment, or vaginal suppository. Normally used to treat candidiasis, nystatin is also an antibiotic. Adverse reactions are rare from this medication. When nystatin is used as a cream or ointment, the patient should apply the medication twice a day. The powder is applied either twice or three times a day. Vaginal suppositories or tablets are inserted by use of an applicator once a day for 2 weeks. Warn the patient not to stop using the medication even if the signs or symptoms stop or during menses.

Tolnaftate

As one of the trade names implies (Dr. Scholl's Athlete's Foot Powder, Tinactin), this medication is given for tinea pedis. It is available as a powder, spray, cream, or lotion.

Naftifine

Naftifine (Naftin) is available as a cream or gel. It is used for dermal fungal infections, but never on mucous membranes. The most common side effect is skin irritation. The cream is normally applied once a day, the gel twice a day.

Oxiconazole

Oxiconazole (Oxistat) is a cream applied once a day for 2 weeks. If it is ordered for tinea pedis, the order will generally continue for 1 month. Skin irritation is the most likely adverse reaction.

Amphotericin B

As a topical agent, amphotericin B (Fungizone) is available as a cream, lotion, or ointment. It is most often used to treat candidiasis, but it is also an antibiotic. Skin or mucous membrane irritation is the most likely adverse reaction. Warn the patient that this drug can discolor the skin and fabrics. The cream and lotion can be removed from fabrics with soap and water, but the ointment requires cleaning fluid. This topical antifungal is normally applied between two and four times a day.

SYSTEMIC ANTIFUNGAL DRUGS

Miconazole

ACTIONS AND USES Miconazole intravenous (IV) (Micatin, Monistat) is used to treat severe systemic fungal infections, coccidioidomycosis (valley fever), candidiasis, and others. Because it is given intravenously, it can cause some systemic adverse reactions. Observe the patient carefully for each of the following: gastrointestinal upset, drowsiness, pruritus or rash, phlebitis, fever and chills, flushing, blood dyscrasias, and hyperlipidemia. An allergic reaction to miconazole may have serious results, including cardiopulmonary arrest.

ASSESSMENT In addition to symptomatic assessments, ▲▲▲▲▲▲▲▲▲▲ monitor the serum electrolyte, complete blood count, and serum lipid laboratory values. Report any changes to the physician.

PLANNING AND IMPLEMENTATION Miconazole IV is ▲▲▲▲▲▲▲▲▲▲▲▲▲▲▲▲▲▲▲▲▲▲▲▲▲▲ available as a solution of 10 mg/mL. The normal dose is 200 to 3600 mg in three divided doses. The medication is delivered by slow infusion. It is best if no more than 200 mg is given in a 2-hour period. The solution may be instilled with normal saline or 5% dextrose.

This solution can also be administered intrathecally or as a bladder instillation.

EVALUATION In addition to evaluating for improve-▲▲▲▲▲▲▲▲▲▲ ment of symptoms, look for potential adverse reactions. Some medications are also known to interact with miconazole IV. When given with miconazole, anticoagulants may have an increased effect. Severe hypoglycemia is a potential when miconazole and oral hypoglycemics are given together. Rifampin (an antitubercular) can decrease the effects of miconazole. When miconazole is given with either phenytoin or carbamazepine (both anticonvulsants), the actions of both drugs can be altered.

Amphotericin B

ACTIONS AND USES Amphotericin B (Fungizone IV) is ▲▲▲▲▲▲▲▲▲▲▲▲▲▲▲▲ used systemically for potentially fatal, severe infections. These can include coccidioidomycosis, candidiasis, histoplasmosis, aspergillosis, and others.

N U R S I N G   A L E R T
▼▼▼▼▼▼▼▼▼▼▼▼▼▼▼▼▼▼▼▼▼▼▼▼▼▼▼▼▼▼▼▼

Unfortunately, adverse reactions will be common and can be dangerous. If the solution extravasates, the patient will experience sloughing. Thrombophlebitis is also common.

▲▲▲▲▲▲▲▲▲▲▲▲▲▲▲▲▲▲▲▲▲▲▲▲▲▲▲▲▲▲▲▲

The patient may complain of headache, gastrointestinal upset, or chills. The patient may have a fever, abdominal cramping or generalized pain, tinnitus, vertigo, or blurred vision. There may be development of a rash, flushing, signs of liver failure, blood dyscrasias, toxic renal effects, electrolyte imbalances, acidosis, cardiac arrhythmias, and altered blood pressure (either up or down).

ASSESSMENT Add assessment for symptoms to your ▲▲▲▲▲▲▲▲▲▲ normal routine for this patient. The physician will order frequent laboratory work-ups, notably weekly determinations of blood urea nitrogen (BUN); serum creatinine, serum potassium, and serum magnesium concentrations (and possibly other electrolytes); complete blood count; and liver function tests. Monitor the results of these tests and report abnormalities at once.

PLANNING AND IMPLEMENTATION Amphotericin B IV ▲▲▲▲▲▲▲▲▲▲▲▲▲▲▲▲▲▲▲▲▲▲▲▲▲▲▲▲▲ is given slowly. It should drip for a period of at least 6 hours. The solution should be diluted to no more than 1 mg of amphotericin B to every 10 mL of IV solution. The dosage is normally started at 0.25 mg per kilogram of body weight and gradually increased to 1.0 mg per kilogram daily. This increasing process can take several weeks, and the patient may be taking amphotericin B for several months.

Because the adverse reactions can be so severe, many physicians opt to use other medications in an attempt to lessen these effects. Aspirin, antihistamines, antipyretics, antiemetics, and steroids may be used for this reason.

EVALUATION Monitor the patient for improvement of ▲▲▲▲▲▲▲▲▲▲ symptoms and for any adverse reactions. Continue to monitor laboratory results throughout therapy. If a patient shows signs of toxic renal effects, the drug may be temporarily discontinued until kidney function test results improve. If the patient again shows signs of renal toxic effects after the drug is restarted, the physician will attempt to find another effective medication for the patient.

Also be alert for drug interactions. Because drug therapy with amphotericin is long term, the patient may be prescribed other drugs. The risk of toxic renal injury is increased if amphotericin B is used with antineoplastics or with any other nephrotoxic medication. Hypokalemia is more likely when amphotericin is used with some steroids. The risk of digitalis intoxication is increased when amphotericin is combined with this medication.

Ketoconazole

Given orally as a tablet, ketoconazole (Nizoral) is used for systemic candidiasis, oral thrush, coccidioidomycosis, histoplasmosis, and cutaneous fungal infections that did not clear with the use of topical medications.

N U R S I N G   A L E R T

Be sure the physician orders a baseline liver function test, and monitor repetitions of this test because oral ketoconazole has been associated with fatal hepatitis. Teach the patient what effects to watch for and report.

Other possible adverse reactions include gastrointestinal upset, pruritus, dizziness and drowsiness, headache, photophobia, fever and chills, blood dyscrasias, and severe mental depression.

The dose given orally is usually 200 to 400 mg daily. The dose should be given at least 2 hours apart from any antacids or histamine blockers.

Watch for potential drug interactions. The effects of coumarin and oral hypoglycemics can be increased; both rifampin and isoniazid (antitubercular) can decrease the effects of ketoconazole. When ketoconazole is used with phenytoin (anticonvulsant), the actions of both drugs are altered.

Griseofulvin

ACTIONS AND USES Griseofulvin (Fulvicin) is used for many dermal fungal infections, but it, too, is associated with several adverse reactions. The patient may experience skin rashes or hives, gastrointestinal upset or even bleeding, headache, dizziness, insomnia, or confusion. Griseofulvin is toxic to both the kidney and liver. Blood dyscrasias may develop. Menstrual irregularities can also occur.

N U R S I N G   A L E R T

After assessing for signs and symptoms, evaluate the results of the baseline liver function tests, kidney function tests, and complete blood count. Report any abnormalities to the physician.

Check the patient's history for any hepatic dysfunction, renal dysfunction, or porphyria. A pregnancy test should also be done to ensure that the patient is not now pregnant. Each of these contraindicates the use of griseofulvin.

N U R S I N G   A L E R T

Check the patient's allergies. Those persons allergic to penicillin have an increased risk of an allergy to griseofulvin. Monitor the patient more carefully.

PLANNING AND IMPLEMENTATION Griseofulvin is given orally for 2 weeks to 6 months. The dose is generally 500 to 1000 mg per day.

N U R S I N G   A L E R T

Warn the patient to avoid sunlight. Photosensitivity with severe sunburn is possible.

Pregnancy testing may become necessary during therapy as menstrual irregularities occur. Teach the patient to inform the physician if pregnancy is possible. Teach the patient other methods of birth control if oral contraceptives have been used. The effectiveness of this form of contraception is decreased during griseofulvin therapy.

Implement safety precautions related to dizziness or confusion.

EVALUATION Continue to evaluate signs and symptoms until the medication is stopped. Look for possible adverse reactions. Monitor results of repeated liver and kidney function tests and blood counts.

Look for signs of drug interaction if the patient is using an anticoagulant. The effects of the anticoagulant may be decreased. The effects of griseofulvin may be decreased when it is used with barbiturates.

Also warn the patient not to drink alcohol because the effects will be increased. Alcohol poisoning is possible.

Nystatin

Nystatin (Mycostatin) is available as a systemic in either an oral suspension or tablet form. It is used for oral or intestinal candidiasis. Adverse reactions are rare but can include gastrointestinal upset.

The usual dose for the suspension is 1 mL in each side of the mouth four times a day. Teach the patient to retain the medication in the mouth for as long as possible before swallowing. The usual dose for tablets is 1 to 2 tablets three times a day.

E X E R C I S E S

CASE STUDIES

1. Your patient, Ms. A.W., has been prescribed an antifungal agent topically for a skin infection. She is to apply the medication herself at home. What would be the best method of teaching Ms. A.W. how to apply the medication? How many times would you need to perform the teaching to ensure that she understood?

2. Mrs. W.D. has been ordered a systemic antifungal agent. What important points would you include in her plan of care?

Mrs. W.D. is to go home on the systemic antifungal agent. What teaching will she require?

MENTAL AEROBICS

1. Go to your local pharmacy. Examine the many types of over-the-counter remedies available for athlete's foot or vaginal yeast infections. Read the labels. What teaching is available on the labels? Do you think all patients read these labels before using the products? How does this affect your nursing practice for these patients?

2. Visit a gynecologist's office. Observe during routine and acute-care patient visits. How often were vaginal yeast infections diagnosed? What medications were ordered? What teaching was done for these patients?

ANTIVIRAL DRUGS

LEARNING OBJECTIVES

After studying this chapter, you should be able to:

1. Discuss the action of and adverse reactions to antiviral drugs and nursing responsibilities appropriate for patients receiving them.

2. List common conditions for which antiviral drugs are used.

3. Name examples of antiviral drugs.

4. Prepare an appropriate teaching plan for patients receiving antiviral drugs.

DRUGS YOU WILL LEARN ABOUT IN THIS CHAPTER

acyclovir (Zovirax)

vidarabine (Vira-A)

trifluridine (Viroptic ophthalmic solution 1%)

ganciclovir (Cytovene)

interferon alfa-n[3] (Alferon N injection)

ribavirin (Virazole)

amantadine (Symmetrel)

zidovudine (Retrovir)

The study of viruses has advanced in recent years as scientists struggle to understand the vagaries of this organism class. A virus is so small it is seen only with an electron microscope. It is made of a single strand of DNA or RNA covered by a protein capsule. The virus is a parasite, deriving its nutrients from the host cell.

There are many types of viruses. Some viruses are found on animals (including humans), some are found on plants, and still others are found on bacteria. Only some of the viruses are harmful to people, but they cause some of the most devastating diseases—from acquired immunodeficiency syndrome (AIDS) to the common cold.

The name of the virus or of its class often tells you something about the virus. Enteroviruses, for example, reproduce in the intestinal tract. Herpesviruses cause some type of skin lesion; herpes means "creeping skin disease." Myxoviruses (or paramyxoviruses) are found in or on mucus or need mucus to survive and reproduce; myxo- means mucus. Picornaviruses have a meaning hidden in the name; pico denotes tiny or small, and RNA refers to the strand of RNA in the virus. Rhino-, meaning nose, hints at the disorder rhinovirus causes—the common cold.

ACTIONS AND USES The antiviral drugs work against viruses. Most often, they do this by preventing the virus from entering a host's cell or by prohibiting reproduction of the virus. Virustatic is the term used to denote a substance that stops the growth of viruses. As a result of the rapid increase in knowledge about viruses, we have antiviral drugs for different herpesvirus disorders, cytomegalovirus (CMV) and varicella-zoster virus infections (both of which are related to herpes), influenza type A, and respiratory syncytial virus (RSV) infection. Antiviral drugs can slow the progression of human immunodeficiency virus (HIV) infection into AIDS.

ASSESSMENT Because of the variety of infections possible from different viruses, it is impossible to enumerate them here. Know what type of infection is suspected in the patient and assess for signs and symptoms associated with that diagnosis. Do not ignore assessments that do not seem to confirm the suspected diagnosis, though. It is possible for the patient to have unusual symptoms; or the patient may not have the infection diagnosed, and your assessments could help the physician to give proper care.

PLANNING AND IMPLEMENTATION Just as antibiotics ▲▲▲▲▲▲▲▲▲▲▲▲▲▲▲▲▲▲▲▲▲▲▲▲▲▲▲▲▲▲▲ need to be given at specific times to maintain therapeutic drug levels, so too do antiviral agents. If the patient is left too long between doses, the strongest of the viruses will begin reproduction, which could lead to resistant strains.

For this same reason, teach the patient not to stop taking the drug just because the symptoms have improved or even stopped. Without taking the full prescription of the drug, you cannot be sure of having killed off the virus. Regrowth then occurs. Only the strongest viruses will have survived to this point, so the pursuant infection may be worse than the original and resistant to the medication.

EVALUATION Check your patient carefully for signs of ▲▲▲▲▲▲▲▲▲▲ improvement or regression. If the drug was given as a preventive, carefully assess for any signs of infection anywhere on the body. Look for potential adverse reactions associated with the specific drug.

ACYCLOVIR

ACTIONS AND USES Acyclovir (Zovirax) is an antiviral ▲▲▲▲▲▲▲▲▲▲▲▲▲▲▲▲ drug used for several reasons. It is given to treat genital herpes and to prevent recurrences. It may reduce both the duration of the pain and the lesions themselves. It may also lessen the frequency and severity of recurrences. Given intravenously (IV), acyclovir is used for severe herpes, for herpes simplex encephalitis in persons older than 6 months, and for the immunocompromised patient.

Acyclovir can also be used to treat varicella-zoster virus infection (chickenpox). Children treated correctly with acyclovir generally improve within 3 or 4 days, compared with 3 to 6 days without the medication. Acyclovir also decreases the fever, causes lesions to heal faster, relieves itching, and prevents new lesions after the third day.

Adverse reactions that the patient may experience depend on the route used. If the ointment is applied, the patient may have pain on application, pruritus, or a rash. With oral administration, adverse reactions may be more systemic, including gastrointestinal (GI) upset, headache, dizziness, malaise or fatigue, paresthesia, or rash. When given IV, acyclovir has some potentially dangerous side effects, such as phlebitis, increased blood urea nitrogen (BUN) or serum creatinine concentration, GI upset, itching, and rash. The

central nervous system (CNS) effects of IV acyclovir include lethargy, confusion, tremors, seizures, hallucinations, and coma.

ASSESSMENT Be sure you are aware of the condition for ▲▲▲▲▲▲▲▲▲▲ which acyclovir is being used. Assess the number and appearance as well as the location of lesions. Assess for pain, inflammation, and drainage. Baseline creatinine clearance tests and BUN determinations should be obtained to assess kidney function. Be aware of the patient's immune status. An immunocompromised patient requires special care to remain protected from the environment.

PLANNING AND IMPLEMENTATION On the basis of the ▲▲▲▲▲▲▲▲▲▲▲▲▲▲▲▲▲▲▲▲▲▲▲▲▲▲▲▲▲▲▲ patient's status and the disorder being treated, the physician chooses a route by which acyclovir is to be delivered. The ointment is often used for uncomplicated genital herpes, but the ointment will not decrease recurrences. The oral route is usually used for severe cases of herpes. Uses of the IV route are mentioned earlier.

N U R S I N G   A L E R T
▼▼

Available in both capsules and suspension, oral acyclovir has been associated with carcinogenic effects in laboratory animals and with reproductive effects, such as a decreased sperm count.

▲▲

The normal oral dose for the initial treatment of genital herpes is 200 mg every 4 hours five times a day (or while awake) for 10 days. For the prevention of recurrences, acyclovir is given at 400 mg twice a day for 12 months. Some physicians prefer what is referred to as intermittent therapy. The patient begins taking 200 mg every 4 hours while awake at the earliest sign of a recurrence and continues for 5 days.

If the oral medication is being used for herpes zoster (shingles), the dose is 800 mg every 4 hours while awake for 10 days.

When the IV route is ordered, the medication is given for at least a 1-hour period to reduce the risk of kidney damage. The dose is 5 mg per kilogram of body weight every 8 hours. If the patient is immunocompromised, the schedule is continued for 7 days. If the patient's immune status is normal, the schedule is continued for 5 days. If the IV route is being used for treatment of encephalitis, the dose is 10 mg per kilogram every 8 hours for 10 days.

If the ointment is being used, warn the patient that it may be painful to apply. Ointment is applied every

3 hours six times a day for 7 days. Instruct the patient to cover lesions.

If you are applying the ointment, wear a glove to prevent transmission of the virus. If the patient is applying the ointment, a glove should still be worn to prevent the transfer of the virus to another body site. Wash hands after application and removal of the glove.

▲▲▲▲▲▲▲▲▲▲▲▲▲▲▲▲▲▲▲▲▲▲▲▲▲▲▲▲▲▲▲▲

If acyclovir is given to a child with chickenpox, it must be started within 24 hours of the child's breaking out with the lesions.

Teach your patient about the disorder. For example, genital herpes is a sexually transmitted disease. Therefore, the patient should avoid intercourse while lesions are visible to prevent transmission to others. The medications do not prevent transmission.

Instruct the patient to inform the physician if she becomes pregnant or is breast-feeding a baby. Acyclovir should not be used in these circumstances.

No matter what the disorder being treated, teach the patient not to share the medication with others. This prevents the proper diagnosis of the other person. Encourage the patient to return to the physician if no relief is gained and to inform the physician about any adverse reactions experienced.

EVALUATION To determine the effectiveness of the
▲▲▲▲▲▲▲▲▲▲ medication, compare baseline assessment findings with periodic evaluation results. Does the patient still have symptoms? Are the symptoms as severe? Do the symptoms appear as often?

Evaluate also for any adverse reactions or interactions. Acyclovir increases the half-life of probenecid when they are given together. Periodic kidney function testing should be performed. Check for results of these tests and inform the physician of abnormalities.

VIDARABINE

Vidarabine (Vira-A) is an antiviral that may also be known as adenine arabinoside (ara-A). It is given intravenously (IV) for herpes simplex encephalitis, neonatal herpes simplex, systemic herpes simplex, and herpes zoster in the immunosuppressed patient. The ophthalmic ointment is used for epithelial keratitis and acute keratoconjunctivitis, which arise from a herpes simplex virus infection.

Adverse reactions to the IV formulation of vidarabine can be severe, including blood dyscrasias, liver dysfunction, confusion, and hallucinations. The patient may also experience tremors, dizziness, headache, and gastrointestinal upset. The ophthalmic ointment may lead to tearing, burning, redness, and pain in the eye. The patient may also complain of photophobia.

ASSESSMENT Before initiation of the medication, thor-
▲▲▲▲▲▲▲▲▲▲ oughly assess the patient's condition on the basis of normal assessment findings for the disease. For example, do a neurological examination for a patient with encephalitis. The physician normally orders baseline blood work to include a complete blood count and cell differential.

Be especially alert to signs of fluid overload or cerebral edema, signs of kidney impairment or liver impairment, or a medical history of any of these. Each of these conditions warrants extra caution while the patient is being treated with vidarabine.

PLANNING AND IMPLEMENTATION When vidarabine is
▲▲▲▲▲▲▲▲▲▲▲▲▲▲▲▲▲▲▲▲▲▲▲▲▲▲▲▲▲▲▲▲ ordered to be given IV, give the drug diluted in a 12- to 24-hour period. The dose ordered depends on the disease process being treated. No more than 450 mg should be diluted into 1000 mL of IV fluid. Never mix this drug with blood or other protein or colloidal fluids.

When preparing the drug, shake the vial well before measuring to ensure that you are withdrawing an equalized portion of the drug. The IV fluid into which the drug will be instilled should first be warmed. This encourages the drug to fully dissolve. When the drug is added, mix the solution until it is completely clear. The solution can then be stored for up to 48 hours before use, but do not refrigerate it.

The ophthalmic ointment is a 3% preparation. Instill approximately 1/2 inch into the lower conjunctival sac of the affected eye. The ointment is commonly ordered to be administered five times daily, but be sure at least 3 hours have lapsed since the last dose. Warn the client that vision may be hazy immediately after administration. You may need to adjust the dosage schedule if this interferes excessively with the patient's daily routine.

EVALUATION Throughout drug therapy, frequently re-
▲▲▲▲▲▲▲▲▲▲ peat the assessments you performed before initiating drug therapy, which were adapted to the patient's presenting condition. Compare the results of the assessments with baseline findings to determine whether the medication is being effective. Always be alert for any sign or symptom that may indicate an adverse reaction.

Effectiveness of the drug may be decreased if vidarabine is given in conjunction with allopurinol (an antigout agent). This drug interferes with the metabolism of vidarabine. Check the patient's drug regimen.

TRIFLURIDINE

Trifluridine (Viroptic ophthalmic solution 1%) is also used for epithelial keratitis and keratoconjunctivitis from herpes simplex virus. Commonly, a single drop is ordered to be placed directly onto the cornea every 2 hours during waking hours. No more than nine drops should be administered in a 24-hour period. Caution the patient that the drug may cause burning, stinging, redness, and even edema of the eye.

GANCICLOVIR

ACTIONS AND USES Ganciclovir (Cytovene) is to be
▲▲▲▲▲▲▲▲▲▲▲▲▲▲ used solely in patients with cytomegalovirus (CMV) retinitis who are also immunocompromised. It should be emphasized to the patient that ganciclovir is not a cure. It only slows the progression of the infection.

Ganciclovir is associated with numerous adverse reactions. Some of the most severe include blood dyscrasias, carcinoma, birth defects, and irreversible decreased sperm count. The blood dyscrasia most commonly seen is a lowered white blood cell count. The patient may die of an opportunistic infection if the count goes too low. Other severe adverse reactions can include liver dysfunction, kidney dysfunction, cardiac arrhythmias, hypertension or hypotension, confusion, psychosis, and coma. Your patient may also complain of a headache, dizziness, anxiety, tremors, fever and chills, or gastrointestinal upset. Dyspnea has also been associated with the use of ganciclovir. Skin reactions can include alopecia, rash, pruritus, and urticaria. Because it is administered intravenously (IV), the nurse also needs to watch for phlebitis or pain at the IV site.

ASSESSMENT Be aware of the symptoms the patient is
▲▲▲▲▲▲▲▲▲▲ experiencing. Assess for decreased visual acuity, decreased peripheral vision or other changes in visual field, and photophobia.

N U R S I N G   A L E R T
▼▼▼▼▼▼▼▼▼▼▼▼▼▼▼▼▼▼▼▼▼▼▼▼▼▼▼▼▼▼▼▼

The physician normally orders a baseline complete blood cell count with differential and kidney func-

tion tests. These tests will usually be repeated every 2 weeks throughout drug therapy. Monitor the results and report any changes.

▲▲▲▲▲▲▲▲▲▲▲▲▲▲▲▲▲▲▲▲▲▲▲▲▲▲▲▲▲▲▲▲

Because the use of ganciclovir is contraindicated if the patient is allergic to the related drug acyclovir, check the patient's medical history carefully for this allergy.

PLANNING AND IMPLEMENTATION Ganciclovir is given
▲▲▲▲▲▲▲▲▲▲▲▲▲▲▲▲▲▲▲▲▲▲▲▲▲▲▲▲▲ slowly IV. The usual dose is 5 mg/kg. It should be administered for at least a 1-hour period, no sooner than every 12 hours. This twice-daily schedule is normally maintained for 2 to 3 weeks and then decreased to once a day.

Before administering the drug, reconstitute the drug with sterile water. Never use bacteriostatic water because it will cause a precipitate to form.

N U R S I N G   A L E R T
▼▼▼▼▼▼▼▼▼▼▼▼▼▼▼▼▼▼▼▼▼▼▼▼▼▼▼▼▼▼▼▼

Be sure to wear gloves and protective glasses while mixing or administering this drug. It is highly caustic to the skin and mucous membranes. If accidental contact with skin or mucous membranes does occur, the manufacturer recommends rinsing the area thoroughly with soap and water (clear water for eye exposure). Also be cautious not to inhale the medication and to dispose of the administration equipment in an appropriate container.

▲▲▲▲▲▲▲▲▲▲▲▲▲▲▲▲▲▲▲▲▲▲▲▲▲▲▲▲▲▲▲▲

Do not mix or reconstitute the drug more than 12 hours ahead of the scheduled dose. Do not refrigerate this drug. Excess solution should be disposed of as with any cytotoxic drug. Refer to your facility's policy and procedure manual.

Because ganciclovir has been shown to cause birth defects and possible spermatozoal defects, counsel your patients, both male and female, to avoid causing pregnancy. Teach your patient about available contraception choices.

EVALUATION Evaluate the patient's vision and visual
▲▲▲▲▲▲▲▲▲▲ fields. With the presence of photophobia, evaluate for any evidence of improvement or worsening. Advise the patient that eye examinations should be done at least every 6 weeks after discharge.

Check your patient's drug regimen for any possible drug interactions. If ganciclovir is given with zidovudine, the risk of blood dyscrasias is increased. When ganciclovir is given with either probenecid (an anti-gout medication) or an antineoplastic agent, the toxicity of both drugs is increased. If ganciclovir is given with imipenem-cilastatin (Primaxin, an antibiotic), the patient may experience seizures.

INTERFERON

ACTIONS AND USES Interferon alfa-n³ (Alferon N injection) is used as an antiviral agent in therapy for condylomata acuminata. It is usually reserved for treatment of patients older than 18 years with severe or recurring lesions that did not respond to other treatment.

Interferon can cause serious adverse reactions. It is associated with liver dysfunction, blood dyscrasias, menstrual cycle dysfunction, and serum hormonal level changes. If the patient is pregnant, interferon may cause abortion.

Other side effects include fever, chills and sweating, headache, fatigue and malaise, myalgia or arthralgia (including back pain), gastrointestinal upset, dizziness, depression or insomnia, nasal congestion, and itching.

ASSESSMENT Assess the patient for number and location of lesions. Also look for other symptoms associated with the lesions, such as inflammation.

Before the initiation of interferon therapy, many physicians order baseline liver function tests and complete blood count with differential. A pregnancy test may also be ordered. These tests will be repeated frequently. Monitor the results and report abnormalities.

NURSING ALERT

Ask your patient about allergies. Any allergies to egg proteins, mouse proteins, or neomycin contraindicate the use of this medication.

Extra caution is warranted when interferon is used for patients with debilitating diseases. The drug may cause fever and flu-like symptoms, which may be dangerous for such patients.

Check the patient's history for any coagulation disorders or a history of seizures. Both require extra monitoring while the patient is receiving interferon.

PLANNING AND IMPLEMENTATION The usual dose of interferon is 0.05 mL (or 250,000 IU) per wart twice weekly. The medication is given by intralesional injection with a 30-gauge needle. The injections can be continued for up to 8 weeks.

The nurse responsible for the medication may refrigerate the solution, but do not allow it to freeze. Never shake the solution before drawing up or administration.

Once a brand name of interferon is used, the patient should not change to another brand without the physician's advice and permission. Some manufacturers do not formulate or process the interferon in the same way; thus, the dose or actions of the drug may differ.

NURSING ALERT

Counsel the female patient about contraception because of possible abortion and the changes in the menstrual cycle that would make detection of pregnancy difficult.

EVALUATION Evaluate the number and location of lesions throughout drug therapy. Continue to monitor all laboratory test results and report abnormalities. Check the patient for any signs of adverse reactions.

RIBAVIRIN

ACTIONS AND USES Ribavirin (Virazole) is an aerosolized antiviral agent used most often for infants and young children with severe respiratory syncytial virus (RSV) infection. These children should be hospitalized during use of the drug. Ribavirin is not normally used for adults.

Ribavirin is associated with severe and even fatal adverse effects. Pneumonia or apnea may occur. These and other respiratory dysfunction symptoms are more likely in infants or when the drug is used for adults with chronic obstructive pulmonary disease or asthma. Hypotension or even cardiac arrest may occur as a side effect of ribavirin.

ASSESSMENT Throughout drug therapy, frequently perform a full respiratory assessment of the patient. This should include respiratory rate, rhythm, breath sounds, evidence of respiratory effort, and obvious signs of distress. Cardiovascular assessments should include pulse rate and rhythm, blood pressure, skin color and blanching, and level of consciousness.

If the patient begins to have any signs or symptoms of either respiratory or cardiovascular distress, the physician will order the drug to be stopped immediately. Report any findings that may indicate these reactions and refrain from administering the next dose until the physician has been notified.

▲▲▲▲▲▲▲▲▲▲▲▲▲▲▲▲▲▲▲▲▲▲▲▲▲▲▲▲▲▲▲▲

Check the patient's history for any respiratory disorders. These patients require additional monitoring.

Although ribavirin is not recommended for use with adults, it is still sometimes ordered for an adult in unusual circumstances. A pregnancy test is often ordered before initiation of the drug. Ribavirin is associated with birth defects.

PLANNING AND IMPLEMENTATION The usual dose of
▲▲▲▲▲▲▲▲▲▲▲▲▲▲▲▲▲▲▲▲▲▲▲▲▲▲ ribavirin is 12 to 18 hours of aerosolized medication through an oxygen tent a day for 3 to 7 days. The drug should not be used with a ventilator because it may interfere with the operation of the equipment.

EVALUATION Continue to evaluate the patient's respi-
▲▲▲▲▲▲▲▲▲▲▲ ratory and cardiovascular status. Also check the patient's drug regimen. If ribavirin is given with digitalis, digitalis toxicity is more likely to develop.

AMANTADINE

ACTIONS AND USES Amantadine (Symmetrel) is both
▲▲▲▲▲▲▲▲▲▲▲▲▲▲▲▲ an antiviral agent and an antiparkinsonian agent (see Chapter 36). As an antiviral, amantadine is used to treat or prevent influenza A viral respiratory infection. It is normally reserved for high-risk patients, patients who have been in close contact with another patient with influenza A, patients who are immunocompromised, and health care workers. Influenza vaccination is the method of choice in preventing influenza A. However, amantadine may be used if the vaccine is contraindicated, or it may be used in conjunction with the vaccine to provide protection until the vaccine can take effect.

Amantadine is associated with severe adverse reactions. Cardiovascular effects can include blood dyscrasias, orthostatic hypotension, congestive heart failure, and peripheral edema. Central nervous system effects can include headache, depression or anxiety, confusion or hallucinations, seizures, dizziness, drowsiness, or insomnia. Urinary retention or liver or kidney dysfunction can occur. The patient may experience blurred vision.

ASSESSMENT In addition to assessing for signs and
▲▲▲▲▲▲▲▲▲▲ symptoms of infection, monitor results of baseline liver and kidney function tests and results of complete blood counts with differentials. Report any abnormalities to the physician.

Check the patient's medical history for seizures. The risk of seizures will be increased while the patient is taking amantadine.

PLANNING AND IMPLEMENTATION The usual dose of
▲▲▲▲▲▲▲▲▲▲▲▲▲▲▲▲▲▲▲▲▲▲▲▲▲▲▲▲▲▲▲ amantadine as an antiviral is 200 mg given once a day. Caution the patient not to drive or operate hazardous machinery if drowsiness or blurred vision is experienced. Encourage all patients in at-risk groups to consult their physician about receiving the influenza vaccine. Vaccination is often available at local health departments free or for a nominal fee.

EVALUATION See assessments. Evaluate the patient
▲▲▲▲▲▲▲▲▲▲▲ for signs or symptoms of infection to determine the effectiveness of the drug.

ZIDOVUDINE

ACTIONS AND USES Zidovudine (Retrovir) is an antivi-
▲▲▲▲▲▲▲▲▲▲▲▲▲▲▲▲▲ ral medication formerly known as azidothymidine or AZT. It has been found to be active against human immunodeficiency virus (HIV) but is *not* a cure. Zidovudine is used for HIV-positive patients whose CD4 cell count is 500/mm^3 or less. The patient could be symptomatic or asymptomatic, but immunity is impaired. Zidovudine is also used for children older than 3 years who are HIV-positive and have either symptoms or low CD4 cell counts.

Zidovudine has been found to slow the progression of acquired immunodeficiency syndrome (AIDS) or AIDS-related complex (ARC). It also reduces the patient's risk for development of an opportunistic infection. However, the long-term effects are unknown.

Zidovudine is associated with the possibility of some serious adverse reactions. Blood dyscrasias can develop. Kidney and liver function can be impaired. Nervous system reactions can include asthenia or paresthesia, dizziness, drowsiness or insomnia, headache, and myalgia. The patient may also complain of gastrointestinal upset, malaise, diaphoresis, dyspnea, or a rash.

ASSESSMENT The patient who is HIV-positive must be
▲▲▲▲▲▲▲▲▲▲ carefully monitored by a physician who is experienced with the condition. Frequent CD4 cell counts are necessary to determine the immune status so that safety precautions to prevent infection can be instituted.

N U R S I N G   A L E R T
▼▼▼▼▼▼▼▼▼▼▼▼▼▼▼▼▼▼▼▼▼▼▼▼▼▼▼▼▼▼▼▼

The HIV-positive patient who is receiving zidovudine must have frequent complete blood counts with differential and liver and kidney function tests. Monitor results of all laboratory tests and report abnormalities to the physician.

▲▲▲▲▲▲▲▲▲▲▲▲▲▲▲▲▲▲▲▲▲▲▲▲▲▲▲▲▲▲▲▲

Also perform frequent cephalocaudal assessment of the patient, paying special attention to any symptom that may indicate the presence of an infection. Report findings to the physician.

PLANNING AND IMPLEMENTATION Zidovudine is avail-
▲▲▲▲▲▲▲▲▲▲▲▲▲▲▲▲▲▲▲▲▲▲▲▲▲▲▲▲▲▲▲▲ able as capsules or as syrup to be given orally. It is also available as an intravenous (IV) medication. The usual dose for an adult with symptoms is 200 mg orally every 4 hours, up to 1200 mg a day. This dose is then reduced to 100 mg on the same schedule after 1 month. The asymptomatic adult is started on 100 mg every 4 hours while awake.

If the IV route is to be used, the dose is 1 to 2 mg per kilogram of body weight. The dose is diluted with 5% dextrose injection solution only. Dilute to 4 mg per milliliter or less. You may keep the solution refrigerated up to 48 hours after preparation. The dose is then given in no less than a 1-hour period, every 4 hours, until the oral dose can be started.

Teach your patient not to share medications. Anyone receiving zidovudine should be monitored carefully. By sharing the medication, neither person is receiving needed care.

Be sure the patient understands that zidovudine cannot prevent the transmission of HIV. Sexual contact should be avoided, or a barrier should be used. Counsel the patient about adequate protection.

If CD4 cell counts or complete blood counts become low enough, the patient may need a blood transfusion. The nurse is responsible for monitoring the patient's response to the blood product and reporting any signs or symptoms of a reaction immediately.

EVALUATION Effectiveness of zidovudine is not deter-
▲▲▲▲▲▲▲▲▲▲ mined by survival of the patient. It is determined by increased length of life expected and by absence of opportunistic infections. Continue to monitor all laboratory test results and symptoms of infection. Always evaluate for symptoms of adverse reactions.

Zidovudine may interact with several classes of drugs. The risk of toxicity effect is increased with any drug that is considered nephrotoxic or cytotoxic. Blood dyscrasias are more common if zidovudine is given with probenecid. Other drugs that may interact with zidovudine include aspirin (a nonsteroidal anti-inflammatory drug [NSAID]), acetaminophen (an analgesic and antipyretic), indomethacin (another NSAID), and phenytoin (an anticonvulsant). If these drugs are given with acyclovir, they can cause drowsiness and lethargy.

E X E R C I S E S

CASE STUDIES

1. Your neighbor's child has signs and symptoms of chickenpox. Your neighbor asks you if there is anything that can treat the chickenpox. What would your best advice be as a nurse?

If the child does have the chickenpox, when should treatment be started? If treatment has been delayed, what is the best course of action?

2. Your patient has been prescribed zidovudine prophylactically. What laboratory tests should you monitor? What teaching does your patient require? What evaluation methods will you use to determine effectiveness of the drug?

3. Mr. H.J. has CMV conjunctivitis. He is also HIV-positive. The physician has ordered ganciclovir for the conjunctivitis. Mr. H.J. is relieved and asks you when he can expect the infection to go away. What would your best response be? What safety precautions do you need to institute to protect both Mr. H.J. and yourself? What examination does he need periodically?

MENTAL AEROBICS

1. Visit a clinic where sexually transmitted diseases are treated. What teaching is done for these patients? How many infections were viral? What medications were prescribed?

2. Write a care plan for a patient with AIDS who is receiving zidovudine. Include the important points related to the use of this drug in your care plan.

CHAPTER 22

ANTIPARASITIC DRUGS

LEARNING OBJECTIVES

After studying this chapter, you should be able to:

1. Define anthelmintic, helminthiasis, amebiasis, and amebicide.

2. Discuss the action and uses of antiparasitic drugs.

3. List common conditions for which each group of antiparasitic drugs are used.

4. Name examples of each group of antiparasitic drugs.

5. Discuss adverse reactions to and nursing responsibilities for each group of antiparasitic drugs.

6. Prepare an appropriate teaching plan for patients receiving an antiparasitic drug.

7. Demonstrate how to administer antiparasitic drugs to a patient by use of the nursing process.

DRUGS YOU WILL LEARN ABOUT IN THIS CHAPTER

Antiarthropods

lindane 1% (Kwell) *scabies*

pyrethrins and piperonyl butoxide (RID)

permethrin 1%

Anthelmintics

mebendazole (Vermox)

thiabendazole (Mintezol)

niclosamide (Niclocide)

Antiprotozoals

chloroquine phosphate (Aralen)

metronidazole (Flagyl)

A parasite is a creature that lives off another living thing. It derives its nourishment from the host, often from the blood of the host. Many types of parasites can infest the human body. This chapter deals with medications intended to rid the body of such infestation.

The antiparasitic drugs include the following classes and subclasses:

Antiarthropod agents. Arthropods are insects and include *Pediculus humanus capitis* (head lice), *Pediculus humanus corporis* (body lice), and *Pediculus inguinalis* or *Phthirus pubis* (pubic lice, sometimes called crabs).

Anthelmintics. Helminths are worms, which can be either intestinal or extraintestinal, and include *Enterobius* (pinworms) and *Ascaris* (roundworms) as well as others.

Antiprotozoals (also called protozoacides). These agents work against a class of mostly unicellular animals, including *Entamoeba histolytica, Giardia lamblia, Plasmodium,* and several others. The antiprotozoals can be further subdivided into amebicides (work against amebae) and antimalarials.

ANTIARTHROPODS

Lindane 1%

ACTIONS AND USES Lindane (Kwell) is a pesticide that will kill the adult louse, the larvae, and the ova of *Pediculus humanus capitis, Pediculus* *humanus corporis, Phthirus pubis,* and *Sarcoptes scabiei* (scabies). Lindane is not used as often now as it once was, but it is still one of the most commonly prescribed pediculicides.

N U R S I N G   A L E R T
▼▼▼▼▼▼▼▼▼▼▼▼▼▼▼▼▼▼▼▼▼▼▼▼▼▼▼▼▼▼▼

Although it leaves no residue, the pesticide lindane can cause systemic effects by penetrating through the skin to the bloodstream. Toxic effects may include seizures and other central nervous system (CNS) manifestations. The risk of toxicity is greater in children, the most commonly infested age group.

▲▲▲▲▲▲▲▲▲▲▲▲▲▲▲▲▲▲▲▲▲▲▲▲▲▲▲▲▲▲▲

The signs of CNS stimulation from lindane may be mild (including only dizziness) or severe, although seizures are most often due to misuse of the product. Lindane also crosses into breast milk, although in small amounts. Because of this and the chance of systemic effects, it is not recommended for use with pregnant or lactating women. This patient should contact the physician for advice.

A common side effect from lindane is a skin rash. This does not necessarily indicate an allergic reaction; instead, it relates to the potency of the pesticide.

ASSESSMENT Ascertain the presence of live lice or
▲▲▲▲▲▲▲▲▲▲ "nits" (the ova) or the characteristic primary or secondary lesions of scabies on the patient. Lice are small, gray-white or brown insects with legs on either side of the body. They live on the scalp, body, or pubic region and prefer dark areas. The nits are the eggs of the louse. They are white or light gray and most often are attached to the hair shaft close to the scalp, near or around the ears or back of the neck. You will be able to differentiate between a nit and a piece of dandruff by attempting to remove the speck. A piece of dandruff leaves the hair shaft easily; a nit must be pulled off by use of the fingernail. It is not necessary to see a live louse to know the patient has lice. The presence of nits is diagnostic. School nurses regularly diagnose this problem.

Lice do not necessarily prefer dirty hair or bodies. It is a common misconception that people who have lice are dirty people. Lice are among the most easily contracted disorder, even more so than the common cold. The patient need only share an article of clothing, linen, brush, comb, hat, scarf, barrette, headband, ribbon, or other ornament or article used near the hair. In the case of body lice, any personal possession could transfer the infestation. Pubic lice infestation is considered to be a sexually transmitted disease. Pubic lice can also be contracted from close contact with the infested person.

Scabies produces a characteristic lesion. The primary lesion is a burrow or tunnel under the skin where the female insect lays her eggs. The body attempts to rid itself of this foreign substance and then develops the secondary lesion. The secondary lesion is composed of vesicles and pustules along the initial primary lesion. The patient also complains of extreme itching, especially at night.

Scabies is highly contagious and can easily be passed throughout the patient population and to the health care providers of a facility if proper handwashing and other procedures are not followed.

PLANNING AND IMPLEMENTATION Lindane is available
▲▲▲▲▲▲▲▲▲▲▲▲▲▲▲▲▲▲▲▲▲▲▲▲▲▲▲ as a shampoo, lotion, or cream. When the lotion or cream is to be applied to the skin, be sure to instruct your patient to apply it to dry skin. The patient should apply a thin layer and rub it into the skin well. To ensure that the insect does not simply move to a different part of the body, the entire body should be covered from the neck down to the soles of the feet; it will take approximately 2 ounces of the lotion or cream for most people to follow this guideline. Caution the patient not to use any skin creams, lotions, or ointments while being treated with lindane because this increases the risk of absorption through the skin and systemic effects. Instruct your patient to leave the lotion or cream on for 8 to 12 hours and then wash it off.

If the shampoo is being applied to the scalp, hair, or pubic area, the patient should apply the shampoo to clean, dry hair. If the patient uses hair creams, gels, hairspray, or the like, the hair should be washed and thoroughly dried before lindane shampoo is applied. Use enough of the shampoo to wet the hair entirely. Work it through all areas of the hair and scalp or pubic region. Leave the chemical on for 4 minutes. Add enough water to form a lather and shampoo the hair as normal. Rinse thoroughly and dry the hair.

Be sure your patient understands that the process is not over at this juncture. The next important step is to remove *all* nits. At times, the solution will not have killed every nit. If even one survives and hatches, the patient will be faced with repeating the entire process, so each nit must be searched out in a painstaking process, hair by hair. The nits can be pulled off by using the fingernails. Some manufacturers include a comb to remove the nits. Caution your patient to inspect the hair shaft after the hair has been combed to be sure the nits have indeed been removed.

It is also recommended that all close contacts be

treated simultaneously. Because arthropods are so easily contracted, close contacts may already have the infestation. If they are not treated, the contacts will simply pass the insect back and forth continuously. This can be very frustrating.

N U R S I N G   A L E R T

Whoever is applying the lindane should wear gloves during the procedure. Also be sure not to apply this pesticide to any opened areas. If opened areas are present, consult the physician for advice. Avoid any contact of this chemical with the eyes or mucous membranes. If such contact does occur, flush the area immediately.

Treatment with lindane is normally needed only once. Some physicians recommend retreatment in 7 to 9 days. This is the time required for any nits missed during the removal to hatch. This second treatment is intended to kill the hatchlings before they have a chance to lay eggs of their own.

The patient can also be taught to soak any hair equipment or ornaments in very hot water or in bleach water. Clothing, linens, and other cloth articles that may be contaminated should be washed in hot water and dried on the hot setting of a drier. Items that cannot be washed, such as pillows or stuffed animals, should be placed in a sealed plastic bag for 14 days. Rugs, carpeting, furniture, and car seats should be vacuumed thoroughly.

EVALUATION To be sure the infestation is truly gone, recheck the patient for lice or nits, or scabies, after the treatment has been applied. Most schools now have policies that require all nits to be gone from the hair before the child can return to the school setting.

Perform a second recheck 7 to 9 days after the treatment to ensure that all nits were successfully removed and no new lice or nits are present. With scabies infestation, look for any new primary or secondary lesions.

Also evaluate the patient's understanding of full removal of the infestation from the home and personal belongings. Ask the patient to verbalize the steps that were taken in the home. Provide corrective teaching as necessary.

Look for any signs or symptoms of systemic effects or skin irritation. Be sure the patient has not been overusing the product. Lindane will not ward off a new infestation.

Pyrethrins and Piperonyl Butoxide

Pyrethrins and piperonyl butoxide (RID) is also a pediculicide. It is used for all three types of pediculosis. It leaves no residue, and little of the product is absorbed through the skin, so systemic effects are unlikely.

N U R S I N G   A L E R T

RID is to be used with caution in the person with ragweed allergy. It should not come into contact with eyes or mucous membranes. Caution the patient not to use this product on the eyelashes or eyebrows. If infestation is present in these two areas, the patient should consult the physician.

Like lindane, RID should be applied to dry hair until it is wet or to the dry skin. It should be left on for 10 minutes but no longer. If it remains on longer, the risk of skin irritation is increased greatly. The patient then washes the chemical out (or off) with regular shampoo and water or soap and water. The same procedure for removal of nits and home infestation as described before should be used. This chemical should be used again in 7 to 10 days, but it should never be reused within a 24-hour period.

Permethrin 1%

Permethrin is available as a cream rinse. Unlike the preceding two pediculicides, it does leave a residue, which is to protect the patient from reinfestation for up to 14 days. Permethrin is for head lice and should be applied by the same procedure as for RID. Retreatment should not be necessary but is not contraindicated if new lice are seen.

Permethrin should not be used on infants, pregnant women, or breast-feeding mothers.

N U R S I N G   A L E R T

Permethrin can trigger an asthmatic episode in patients with asthma.

ANTHELMINTICS

Mebendazole

ACTIONS AND USES Mebendazole (Vermox) is a broad-spectrum anthelmintic that inhibits the growth of worms and causes the live worms to be depleted of glucose. It is useful against enterobiasis, ascariasis, or infestations of whipworm or hookworm. The patient may experience abdominal pain and diarrhea as adverse effects of this drug.

ASSESSMENT Assess the patient for signs and symptoms of the suspected infestation. You may be able to see live worms in the stool or in the anal area with certain types of helminths. Stool specimen analysis is ordered by the physician. Review the procedure for obtaining such a specimen. Be sure to keep the specimen warm if transport to the laboratory will be delayed. Otherwise, the worms will die and become more difficult to identify.

Assess female patients of childbearing age for the possibility of pregnancy. This drug is not recommended for use during pregnancy.

PLANNING AND IMPLEMENTATION Mebendazole is provided in chewable form. For pinworms, the recommended dose is 1 tablet once. It does not need to be repeated. If the drug is being used for other types of helminths, the dose is twice a day for 3 days.

Teach the patient (and parents or other family members) good hygiene measures to prevent transmission of the infestation to others. Proper hygiene measures can also prevent self-reinfestation. Caution the patient or parents to keep the patient's hands away from the mouth.

EVALUATION Effectiveness of the medication is determined by absence of symptoms and by repeated stool specimen analysis. Watch the patient for the occurrence of side effects.

Thiabendazole

ACTIONS AND USES Thiabendazole (Mintezol) is primarily used for threadworm infestation and trichinosis. It is considered a secondary drug against enterobiasis, ascariasis, or infestations of whipworm and hookworm. It is believed that thiabendazole may inhibit certain enzymes necessary to the worm's metabolism. It also suppresses both egg and worm growth.

Thiabendazole is associated with numerous adverse reactions. Stevens-Johnson syndrome or erythema multiforme may develop. Other reactions can include drowsiness, dizziness, tinnitus, blurred vision, hypertension, gastric upset, fever, chills, flushing, pruritus, and a drop in blood glucose.

ASSESSMENT See assessment for mebendazole.

PLANNING AND IMPLEMENTATION Thiabendazole is available as chewable tablets or suspension. The dose for most conditions is two doses per day for 2 days. The amount per dose is determined by the patient's weight but is not to exceed 3 g a day.

Caution the patient not to drive or operate hazardous machinery because of possible dizziness, drowsiness, and blurred vision. Also be aware that dizziness may be related to a sudden drop in blood glucose. Monitor the patient's vital signs, especially blood pressure and temperature. Measures to relieve itching may include baking soda baths, antipruritic products, or medication. Consult the physician if the patient is experiencing excessive itching.

EVALUATION See evaluation for mebendazole.

Niclosamide

Niclosamide (Niclocide) is a chewable tablet used to kill tapeworm. The medication kills the worm on contact and loosens the worm's mouth from the bowel wall. The worm may then be passed, or portions of it may be digested in the intestinal tract.

The amount and schedule of the drug depend on the type of worm diagnosed and the age and weight of the patient. Caution the patient to chew the tablet thoroughly with some water. The patient may experience some gastric upset, drowsiness, dizziness, headache, rash, and itching.

The patient is not considered to be cured until stool specimens have been negative for worms and ova (eggs) for at least 3 months.

ANTIPROTOZOALS

Chloroquine Phosphate

ACTIONS AND USES Chloroquine (Aralen) is classified as an amebicide and antimalarial. When used against malaria, it increases the intervals between attacks, stops acute attacks, and suppresses contraction of the disease when endemic areas are entered. In its use against both malaria and amebiasis, the agent interacts with the invasive organism's DNA.

The patient may experience some serious adverse reactions from chloroquine. This drug can produce seizures, tinnitus, nerve deafness, retinal damage, alopecia, skin rash or pigmentation changes of the skin, and gastrointestinal upset.

ASSESSMENT Before the initiation of this drug, the patient should have a baseline complete blood count (CBC) and liver function tests. This drug should be used only with extreme caution in the patient with liver disease or alcoholism. It should not be given concurrently with other drugs that are toxic to the liver.

PLANNING AND IMPLEMENTATION Chloroquine is available as oral tablets or in injectable form. To suppress the occurrence of malaria, an oral form is given at an average dose of 500 mg every week. The oral form can also be used for acute malaria; the dose is 1 g, followed by 500 mg in 6 to 8 hours, followed by 500 mg daily for 2 more days.

The oral form of chloroquine can also be used against amebiasis. This dose is 1 g daily for 2 days, followed by 500 mg daily for 2 to 3 weeks.

The injectable form of chloroquine is used against malaria at a dose of 160 to 200 mg intramuscularly. This dose is repeated in 6 hours if the physician determines it is necessary. The dose is not to exceed 800 mg in a 24-hour period. The goal is to switch the patient to the oral form of the drug as soon as possible.

When the injectable form is used to treat amebiasis, the dose is 160 to 200 mg intramuscularly daily for 10 to 12 days.

N U R S I N G   A L E R T

Throughout therapy, the patient should continue to have frequent CBCs and liver function tests. If results of these tests indicate the presence of adverse reactions, the drug should be discontinued.

EVALUATION Effectiveness of the drug is determined by decreased symptoms, but be alert to adverse reactions.

N U R S I N G   A L E R T

Because the drug can cause retinopathy, check the patient for any abnormal visual phenomena, such as light flashes, streaks, or changes in the visual field.

Evaluate the patient for muscle or reflex weakness. Finally, if the patient is susceptible to psoriasis, watch for a precipitated attack of this skin disorder.

Metronidazole

ACTIONS AND USES Metronidazole (Flagyl) is an amebicide and antitrichomonal agent. It works against *Trichomonas vaginalis, Entamoeba histolytica,* and some anaerobic bacteria. As such, the drug can be prescribed by the physician to patients with amebic dysentery, trichomoniasis with cervicitis, peritonitis, liver abscesses, endometritis or endometrial abscesses, endocarditis, meningitis, septicemia, pneumonia, skin infections, and bone or joint infections.

ASSESSMENT Assess the patient's medical history carefully. Caution is indicated if the patient had or has a history of any central nervous system (CNS) disease or liver disease.

Be careful to obtain all culture and sensitivity specimens before the first dose of the drug. Failure to do so could render the test invalid.

Assess the patient for any signs or symptoms of the disorder suspected. Female patients of childbearing age should have a pregnancy test because the drug is contraindicated during the first trimester of pregnancy.

PLANNING AND IMPLEMENTATION Metronidazole is available in tablet form. Be sure to administer the drug only as directed. If the patient is being treated for trichomoniasis with cervicitis, this is considered a sexually transmitted disease (STD), and the patient's sex partners should be treated at the same time. Contact the local health department for contact follow-up.

EVALUATION Effectiveness of the drug is determined
▲▲▲▲▲▲▲▲▲▲ by decreased symptoms and possibly
repeated culture and sensitivity tests.

If the patient's infection was discovered as a result
of a Pap test, the Pap test should be repeated. The
infection could alter the results of the first test.

Evaluate the patient for any signs of adverse
reactions. The drug must be stopped if seizures,
numbness, tingling, or other signs of neuropathy
develop. Notify the physician immediately.

E X E R C I S E S

CASE STUDIES

1. Imagine you are a school nurse. A child at the
school has nits. The child has two other siblings in
school. Who else should be checked for lice? What
teaching should you do for the family?

The family's physician has recommended permethrin cream rinse. What should you assess the
family's medical history for? What directions for use
should you explain to the child's parents?

2. A patient has been diagnosed with pinworms.
The physician prescribed mebendazole. How should
the patient take these tablets? What teaching should
you do because of the diagnosis and treatment of this
patient?

MENTAL AEROBICS

1. Visit a school that has a school nurse. Follow the
nurse through the daily activities. Review any policies, procedures, handouts, or other teaching materials the nurse has regarding pediculosis.

2. Ask the management of a laboratory that performs stool specimen analysis for helminths if examples of different types of worms are available for
display. Many laboratories will do this for medical
education reasons.

IMMUNIZATIONS

L E A R N I N G   O B J E C T I V E S

After studying this chapter, you should be able to:

1. Define immunity, naturally acquired, artificially acquired, active, passive, serum, vaccine, antitoxin, and gamma globulin.

2. State examples of each type of immunity.

3. Relate general length of immunity for each type.

4. State diseases for which the patient is immunized when receiving MMR, DTP, TOPV, Varivax, or HIB vaccine.

5. Relate the schedule of immunization recommended by the Centers for Disease Control (CDC) for MMR, DTP, TOPV, HIB, Varivax, and hepatitis B vaccines.

6. State examples of diseases for which serums are available.

DRUGS YOU WILL LEARN ABOUT IN THIS CHAPTER

Vaccines

Diphtheria, tetanus, and pertussis (DTP or DTaP)

Diphtheria and tetanus (DT or Td)

Measles, mumps, and rubella (MMR)

Oral poliovirus (OPV)

Trivalent oral poliovirus (TOPV)

Inactivated poliovirus (IPV)

Haemophilus influenzae type b (HIB, Hib-TITER)

Varicella virus vaccine live (Varivax)

Influenza virus

Pneumococcal (Pneumovax)

BCG

Hepatitis B (Heptavax-B)

Rabies virus

Serums

Hepatitis B immune globulin

Tetanus immune globulin (TIG)

Rh_o(D) immune globulin (RhoGAM and MICRhoGAM)

Rabies immune globulin

Immune globulin (Gamastan)

Immune globulin intravenous (Gamimune N IV)

In 1796, only about 200 years ago, Edward Jenner made an exciting and important observation. He noticed that milkmaids who went out into the fields each day to milk the cows often contracted a mild disease called cowpox. This was no great discovery because everyone knew this was one of the hazards of being a milkmaid, and after all, cowpox was mild and they soon recovered. Jenner further noticed that once these milkmaids recovered from cowpox, they never contracted smallpox, a dreaded and often fatal disease in 17th century England. This also was not news, however, because these same milkmaids were often called on to nurse those sick with smallpox. What was notable was what Jenner did with that information. He postulated that if everyone was given cowpox, smallpox would be rid of forever. It was for this reason that Jenner began "immunizing" everyone with cowpox. It was the first successful immunization ever.

Many of you may have a small scar on your upper arm thanks to Jenner. The immunization for smallpox produced a pockmark and gave you immunity to smallpox. The last reported case of smallpox in the United States was in 1949; therefore, this immunization is no longer required by law. If you travel outside the United States, however, you may still be required to have this inoculation because there have been a few reported cases in remote areas (one was in 1978 and one in 1988).

ACTIONS AND USES From this small beginning came ▲▲▲▲▲▲▲▲▲▲▲▲▲▲▲▲ the study of immunology. We now know that substances in your body called antibodies are responsible for immunity. Antibodies are proteins made to fight specific diseases. They are made by your body when an antigen—a foreign protein, such as a virus, bacterium, or toxin—enters your body. Once your body has learned how to make a specific antibody, it does not forget. The next time that same antigen works its way inside the body, the body is ready to fight. That is immunity.

There are different types of immunity. Some immunity is acquired by your body in a natural or nonmedical way. This is simply called naturally acquired immunity. One natural way to acquire immunity is by having the disease yourself. An infant acquires immunity naturally by drinking its mother's colostrum, the first fluid to flow from the breast; colostrum is filled with antibodies.

Some immunity must be acquired by artificial or medical means. We call this artificially acquired immunity. In general, you must receive an injection or possibly drink a solution to receive this immunity.

Passive immunity means your body did not have to do anything to acquire the immunity. You were somehow given antibodies made by another, whether this was another person or an animal.

Active immunity requires your body to make its own antibodies. The body will do this only in the presence of an antigen. Therefore, that antigen must be introduced into your body.

We put these four general terms together to name the four types of immunity. First is naturally acquired active immunity, the simplest type. The antigen enters your body through a nonmedical way, for example, droplets in the air. You become ill with the disease, and your body makes antibodies against that disease. If naturally acquired active immunity is possible with a specific disease, you will not be able to contract that disease again. This type of immunity has an obvious disadvantage—you have to get sick. Although some diseases may be mild, such as cowpox, others run the risk of deformity, disability, or even death. For these diseases, immunologists sought other ways to produce immunity.

The second type of immunity is naturally acquired passive immunity. The most common example of this is an infant's drinking its mother's colostrum. This will protect the child from disease, but because the baby's body did not learn how to make the antibodies for itself, the immunity is short-lasting (only about 6 to 12 months, depending on the disease). Also, the infant's mother must already be immune to the disease. If she does not have immunity to mumps, for example, she cannot pass that immunity to her child.

The third type of immunity is artificially acquired passive immunity. This requires a medical means of transmitting the immunity but does not require the body to make its own antibodies. The inoculation of the body with a serum, which is the part of the blood that contains the antibodies, from a person or animal immune to a specific disease gives temporary immunity to that disease. It is immediately effective. The serum may even be given to a person who has already been exposed to a disease to lessen its effects. However, the body was not taught how to make its own antibodies, so the immunity is short-lasting. An antitoxin is a serum containing a special type of antibody that fights the toxins, or poisons, from a specific antigen. It also produces artificially acquired passive immunity.

The fourth type of immunity is artificially acquired active immunity. This also requires a medical means of transmitting the immunity. This time, however, the body is taught how to make its own antibodies. Remember that this occurs only in the presence of an antigen. Why doesn't the person become sick with the disease, then? A vaccine or toxoid is administered to the person. A vaccine is a solution containing antigens that have been attenuated, which means killed or weakened. Your body cannot detect whether this foreign protein is alive or dead or weak, so it produces the same antibodies regardless. Vaccines may require the administration of boosters, a second or third inoculation of that vaccine at specifically spaced intervals to produce the desired level of immunity. A toxoid is a solution that contains a weakened toxin, or poison, from a specific antigen. It can be administered to produce artificially acquired active immunity because the body produces antibodies in its presence (Table 23–1).

ASSESSMENT As a nurse, you will be administering ▲▲▲▲▲▲▲▲▲▲ vaccines or serums for the purpose of producing immunity. You need to determine whether the patient can safely receive a vaccine or toxoid. Live vaccines should never be given

1. if the person is receiving steroids, radiation, or antineoplastics;
2. if the person has leukemia, acquired immunode-

Table 23–1. Immunity for Common Communicable Diseases

DISEASE	TYPE OF IMMUNITY	AGENT AND SCHEDULE
Rubeola	Naturally acquired passive	Through placenta; lasts approximately 6 mo
	Naturally acquired active	By having the disease; permanent
	Artificially acquired passive	Immune globulin serum; given at time of exposure
	Artificially acquired active	MMR vaccine; usually given at 15 mo
Rubella	Naturally acquired passive	Through placenta; lasts <1 yr
	Naturally acquired active	By having the disease; permanent
	Artificially acquired passive	Immune globulin serum; given at time of exposure
	Artificially acquired active	MMR vaccine; usually given at 15 mo
Chickenpox	Naturally acquired active	By having the disease; permanent
	Artificially acquired passive	Immune globulin serum; given at time of exposure
	Artificially acquired active	Varivax vaccine, usually given at 12 mo in a single dose. Over 13 years, give two doses 4–8 wks apart

Table 23–1. Immunity for Common Communicable Diseases *Continued*

DISEASE	TYPE OF IMMUNITY	AGENT AND SCHEDULE
Mumps	Naturally acquired passive	Through placenta; lasts 6–8 mo
	Naturally acquired active	By having the disease on both sides
	Artificially acquired passive	Immune globulin serum; given at time of exposure
	Artificially acquired active	MMR vaccine; usually given at 15 mo
Pertussis	Naturally acquired active	By having the disease; permanent
	Artificially acquired passive	Immune globulin serum; given at time of exposure
	Artificially acquired active	DTP: at 2, 4, and 6 mo DTaP: at 18 mo and between 4 and 7 y
Diphtheria	Naturally acquired passive	Through placenta; lasts 3–6 mo
	Artificially acquired passive	Diphtheria antitoxin serum; given at time of exposure
	Artificially acquired active	DTP: at 2, 4, and 6 mo DTaP: at 18 mo and between 4 and 7 y Td: every 10 y thereafter

Table 23-1. Immunity for Common Communicable Diseases *Continued*

DISEASE	TYPE OF IMMUNITY	AGENT AND SCHEDULE
Tetanus	Naturally acquired passive	Through placenta; length unknown
	Artifically acquired passive	TIG serum; given within 72 h of injury
	Artificially acquired active	DTP: at 2, 4, and 6 mo DTaP: at 18 mo and between 4 and 7 y Td: every 10 y thereafter

DTP, diphtheria, tetanus, and pertussis; DTaP, diphtheria, tetanus, and acellular pertussis; MMR, measles, mumps, and rubella; Td, tetanus and diphtheria toxoids, adult type; TIG, tetanus immune globulin.

ficiency syndrome (AIDS), a low white blood cell count, or a current infection; or

3. if the person received an immune serum within the last 3 months.

Each of these suppresses the immune system and may allow the antigen, weak though it is, to produce the disease that we are trying to prevent.

Ask whether the patient will be coming into contact with anyone whose immune system is impaired. In this case, although the patient will not be harmed by the vaccine, the immunosuppressed person may be. Live virus vaccines are shed for up to 30 days. This disease may then be contracted by the immunosuppressed person.

Ask about your patient's medical history and medications. Assess for any signs of an infection, such as fever, cough, sore throat, earache, nasal drainage, abnormal breath sounds, or sneezing. Although it is considered safe to give vaccines unless fever or chest congestion is present, any symptom of infection may clue the nurse to other more serious infection symptoms.

Because some vaccines are made in eggs, also assess the person for allergies. Ask whether the patient is allergic to any medications. Certain medications, including neomycin, also contain egg protein. If the patient is allergic to any of these medications, do not give a vaccine made in eggs.

Because some diseases for which we immunize can produce abnormalities in a developing fetus, ask your patient whether she may be pregnant.

Serums and antitoxins may be given during the beginning of a disease to lessen its effects, so the same assessments are not used. However, the patient should still be assessed for allergies because some of these solutions come from animals, such as horse serum or even swine serum.

The physician may decide to test for sensitivity to the solution by injecting a minute dose of the solution intradermally. An allergic patient may exhibit a local reaction, such as a reddened wheal; a systemic reaction includes urticaria, shortness of breath, hypotension, or other symptoms of anaphylactic shock.

Ask the patient or the parents whether the patient has ever had any reactions to this or other vaccines. A history of seizures or a high-pitched scream for a lengthy time after the administration of a vaccine is an adequate reason to withhold a vaccine and consult the physician. A fever, even a high fever, not associated with seizures is no longer considered a reason to withhold a vaccine.

Ask whether the patient has ever had a seizure or has a family history of a seizure. Some vaccines are associated with increased risk of febrile seizures. The patient or parents should be well informed of this risk.

PLANNING AND IMPLEMENTATION Most vaccines are administered by injection to children. Refer to Chapter 11 for guidance. Chapter 11 also provides the student with information on administering a liquid medication to children.

Explain the expected and recommended immunization schedule to the patient. Most states now require specific vaccinations before a child may enter kindergarten. Parents may not understand that it is in the child's best interest to receive the immunizations on time for prevention of disease at younger ages and to lessen the impact of an injection on impressionable minds.

Teach the patient about any adverse reactions that may occur. Many vaccines can produce mild symptoms of the disease for which they produce immunity. Reactions can include fever, myalgia, malaise, irritability, or even a rash. Some vaccines can produce a localized reaction at the injection site, with redness, warmth, swelling, induration, and pain.

Offer possible solutions for the reactions. If a fever occurs, the physician may recommend the use of a nonaspirin antipyretic. Inform the patient or the parents of the appropriate dose for age. For a localized reaction at the injection site, use of the extremity may lessen the duration of the pain. Applications of warmth may decrease the outward symptoms of inflammation. Inform the parents that if a rash does occur, it does not mean the child is contagious.

EVALUATION With some vaccines, it is advisable to
▲▲▲▲▲▲▲▲▲▲ observe the patient for approximately 10
to 15 minutes after administration. Evaluate for any
signs of difficulty breathing, hives, rash, itching, or
fainting.

Most evaluation of vaccines is done by statistical
method. This means that the disease is reported to the
local and state health departments if it occurs. Some
diseases require an investigation by the health department to determine contacts and the source of the
infection. Health department officials will also be able
to supply the family and local physician with the best
plan of action for the patient. Other diseases are kept
only by number for analytical purposes. This helps
practitioners and researchers determine the effectiveness of current vaccines so that they may be compared
with new vaccines as they become available. Health
departments also develop strategies for community
health based on these statistics.

The other portion of vaccine evaluation occurs at the
next visit to the physician's office or clinic. Ask the
patient or family once again about any reactions to
previous vaccinations.

DIPHTHERIA, TETANUS, AND PERTUSSIS VACCINE

ACTIONS AND USES
▲▲▲▲▲▲▲▲▲▲▲▲▲▲▲▲

Diphtheria Diphtheria was a common disease, especially in children. In 1921, there were more than
200,000 cases of diphtheria, and between 5% and 10%
were fatal. With the advent of diphtheria vaccine, only
59 cases of the disease were reported in 1979. As of
that year, because of the lack of cases, diphtheria was
no longer required to be reported. Remember, you do
not produce naturally acquired active immunity to
diphtheria.

Tetanus (Lockjaw) Tetanus has also been greatly
reduced by vaccination. In 1947, there were 560 cases
of tetanus. By 1987, this was down to only 48. Tetanus
is a particularly dangerous disease because it is fatal
in about 20% of cases. It is not possible to have
naturally acquired active immunity to tetanus.

Pertussis (Whooping Cough) Pertussis cases were
once declining. From a high of 265,269 cases in 1934,
we saw the case level drop in the 1970s to approximately 2300 a year. However, since then, there has
been a gradual elevation in the case load. There were
4157 cases in 1989 and more than 5000 in 1993.

Pertussis vaccine has been the focus of much

controversy. There were those researchers who believed it to be responsible for brain damage in some
children. This well-publicized research convinced
many parents not to have their children immunized
against pertussis. It is now believed that the benefits
of the vaccine outweigh the risks. Further information
about these risks follows. Naturally acquired active
immunity is produced after a case of pertussis.

The Vaccines The diphtheria, tetanus, and pertussis
(DTP) vaccination is given to protect against all three
of these diseases. It has been in common use since the
late 1940s. There is an adult version and three
pediatric versions of the vaccine, and the nurse must
be careful to read the label correctly. The adult version
(Td) contains only tetanus and diphtheria toxoids and
is less potent than the child's. The adult does not need
more antigen, and the higher potency is associated
with a higher frequency of adverse reactions. The
adult form is given to patients who are older than 7
years. DTP protects against all three diseases and is
used for the first three doses of the standard immunization schedule. DTaP contains acellular pertussis.
This form is less likely to produce adverse reactions,
although it still produces adequate immune response
when it is given according to directions. It is approved
for use only as the fourth or fifth dose of the standard
immunization series. If a child has had a recognized
adverse reaction to the pertussis portion of this
vaccine, diphtheria and tetanus toxoids (DT) may be
used instead for subsequent doses.

The DTP vaccine commonly causes redness, induration, and tenderness at the site of injection. Inform
the patient or parents of this likelihood. It may also
result in fever, irritability, lack of appetite, and
drowsiness. In fact, fever is so common that many
physicians recommend to their patients that the child
be given an appropriate dose of acetaminophen to
reduce the chance of fever and associated seizures.
Brain damage, however, is no longer considered to be
related to DTP.

ASSESSMENT On presentation of the patient to an office
▲▲▲▲▲▲▲▲▲▲▲ or clinic for immunization, determine
whether DTP can safely be received. The vaccine is
withheld if the child currently has a fever or chest congestion or has had a seizure, unconsciousness, or high-
pitched persistent crying after a DTP vaccination. Consult the physician for the form of vaccine to be used.

PLANNING AND IMPLEMENTATION DTP is given intra-
▲▲▲▲▲▲▲▲▲▲▲▲▲▲▲▲▲▲▲▲▲▲▲▲▲▲▲▲ muscularly at a dose
of 0.5 mL. The recommended schedule is at 2 months,
4 months, 6 months, and 15 to 18 months of age and
once more before school, generally between the ages of

4 and 7 years. If the series is interrupted, it is *not* necessary to start over. The pertussis portion of the vaccine is not yet recommended after the age of 7 years; however, newer research may soon provide for a change in this vaccine. When the patient is to receive only diphtheria and tetanus immunization, DT is given to children younger than 7 years; patients older than 7 years receive Td.

It was a common practice for some time to give lowered doses of DTP to prevent complications. This is not recommended by the ACIP (Immunization Practices Advisory Committee), a division of the U.S. Department of Health and Human Services. If a patient has a possible contraindication to DTP, it is now recommended that he not be given the vaccine; lowered doses did not lessen the possibility of reactions.

Many times, the patient presents with a need for more than one immunization. It has been determined to be safe to give DTP, oral poliovirus vaccine (OPV), *Haemophilus influenzae* type b vaccine (HIB), and measles, mumps, and rubella vaccine (MMR) all at the same time. Encourage patients to have all of these at once if there is any doubt about their return for another visit to the office or clinic.

Sometimes a patient comes to the office after having been exposed to one of the diseases. Persons who have come in contact with a case of diphtheria should be given the diphtheria vaccine if they have not had a booster in the last 5 years. The diphtheria serum is from horse serum and is associated with many reactions; therefore, it is not usually given.

Persons who have received a wound are evaluated for their need for tetanus prophylaxis. The tetanus vaccine is given if

1. the patient has had less than three doses of the vaccine;

2. the patient has had three or more doses of the vaccine, but it has been more than 10 years since the last dose; or

3. the patient has had three or more doses of the vaccine but the last dose was more than 5 years ago *and* the wound is dirty or severe.

Tetanus immune globulin (TIG) is given only if the patient had fewer than three doses of the tetanus vaccine *and* it is a dirty or severe wound.

Contacts of a case of pertussis (whether by direct or indirect contact) are usually treated with erythromycin or trimethoprim-sulfamethoxazole (Bactrim or Septra) for 14 days. If they have not completed their series of DTP or the last dose was more than 3 years ago, a booster is administered.

EVALUATION It is recommended that the patient stay ▲▲▲▲▲▲▲▲▲▲ in the clinic area for at least 15 minutes to be sure there is no reaction to the vaccine. Assess the patient for any shortness of breath, wheezing, or drop in blood pressure. These may indicate an anaphylactic reaction to the vaccine.

Often, the nurse will not hear about other reactions to vaccinations until the next appointment. Those reactions now considered to be contraindications to the DTP vaccine are anaphylaxis and encephalopathy. Other reactions are now only precautions, which indicates that the vaccine may still be given but requires close observation. These reactions include a fever above 105°F, collapse, persistent crying (for more than 3 hours or any that is high pitched), and seizures. Any neurological disorder not related to DTP administration is also considered a precaution.

MEASLES, MUMPS, AND RUBELLA VACCINE

The measles, mumps, and rubella (MMR) vaccine is a live virus vaccine that produces artificially acquired active immunity. Ask about allergies, because persons allergic to neomycin or eggs, which produce anaphylactic reactions, should not receive this vaccine. The patient should also not be pregnant, be breast-feeding, or have an active case of tuberculosis.

MMR vaccination is recommended at age 12 to 15 months or older and then once more in 10 years (or possibly at the time of entering school). Children younger than 12 months may be vaccinated with MMR if they are at high risk for development of the disease, but they must then be revaccinated later. The injection is given subcutaneously into the upper outer arm. The dose of 0.5 mL must be reconstituted with the specific diluent provided by the manufacturer. Administer the solution immediately after reconstitution because light begins to destroy the vaccine in minutes. You may wish to caution the patient or parents about possible side effects, including a local irritation such as burning or stinging, a rash that may appear in about 7 to 10 days, or even mild symptoms of the diseases. Warn female patients not to get pregnant within 3 months of receiving the vaccination because of the possible fetal defects that may result.

Precautions should be taken not to give the MMR vaccine within 3 months of a patient's receiving human immune globulin.

A rubella titer can be used to evaluate effectiveness of this vaccine. This blood test counts the number of antibodies found for rubella.

ORAL POLIOVIRUS VACCINE

The oral poliovirus vaccine (OPV) is a live virus vaccine. Because it contains three strains of poliovirus, it is often termed trivalent oral poliovirus vaccine (TOPV). Assess the patient for fever, vomiting, or diarrhea and delay administration if these are present. Patients with immunosuppression, or who live with family members with immunosuppression, should not receive OPV.

OPV is given orally at a dose of 0.5 mL. The solution should be kept frozen until immediately before administration. Vaccination is recommended at ages 2, 4, and 6 months and between the ages of 4 and 7 years. Side effects are unusual, but parents or patients should be made aware of the possibility of a rare paralysis.

Persons with immunosuppression or a family member with immunosuppression should receive inactivated poliovirus vaccine (IPV) because OPV permits the excretion of the poliovirus and may pose a threat to these people.

HAEMOPHILUS INFLUENZAE TYPE B (HIB) VACCINE

HibTITER is used to produce artificially acquired active immunity against *Haemophilus influenzae* type b. This bacterium is a common cause of meningitis in young children. Question whether the child is allergic to the diphtheria toxoid or is immunosuppressed; both prohibit the administration of this vaccine.

This vaccination is now currently recommended at ages 2, 4, 6, and 18 months. The vaccine is given intramuscularly into the vastus lateralis or the deltoid muscle at a dose of 0.5 mL. You may wish to warn the parents of the possibility of a fever, gastrointestinal upset, or local reaction after the vaccination.

VARICELLA VIRUS VACCINE LIVE

Varicella virus vaccine live (Varivax) has recently been approved and become available to the general public. Varivax contains a live, attenuated varicella virus. Administration of the vaccine results in the production of antibodies. The duration of protection by Varivax is as yet unknown, but clinical trials continue. Studies to date indicate that the immunity will persist for at least 6 years after administration of the vaccine.

The most common adverse effects observed during clinical trials are complaints of pain or redness at the injection site. Some patients also experienced swelling, a rash with itching, a hematoma, induration, and stiffness. Patients receiving the injection may also develop a rash. A generalized chickenpox-like rash is

most likely to occur 5 to 26 days after administration. A rash localized at the injection site may occur 8 to 19 days after the injection.

Other adverse effects recorded include a fever, upper respiratory illness, cough, irritability, diarrhea, joint pain, and rare febrile seizures. The adverse effects appear to be similar regardless of the age of the recipient.

Varivax should be given to children at 12 months of age in a single dose of 0.5 mL. It is administered subcutaneously. If the child does not receive the vaccine at 12 months of age, vaccine can be administered at the same dosage up to age 12 years. For clients 13 years old or more, the vaccine should be given in two 0.5-mL doses. Approximately 4 to 8 weeks should separate the two doses for the best development of immunity. It is as yet unknown if a booster dose will be necessary.

The use of Varivax vaccine is contraindicated in patients with hypersensitivity to gelatin, neomycin, or components of the vaccine. It should also not be given to those with immunodeficiency, active untreated tuberculosis, current febrile infection, blood dyscrasias, leukemia, lymphomas, or other malignant neoplasms of the bone marrow or lymphatic system. Varivax should not be given to pregnant women, and female clients of childbearing age should be cautioned to avoid pregnancy for 3 months following the vaccination.

One exception to these contraindications is children or adolescents with acute lymphoblastic leukemia who are in remission. These can receive the vaccine under an investigational protocol that is approved by the FDA. Be sure to caution the client or parents that this is an experimental procedure.

Any cases of children developing varicella infection after administration of this vaccine should be reported to the FDA for investigational purposes. And as always, any adverse effects your patients experience should also be reported.

INFLUENZA VIRUS VACCINES

The influenza virus vaccine produces artificially acquired active immunity only against those strains of influenza virus it contains. These strains are generally those expected to cross the continental United States. Vaccination is recommended for persons who fall into any of the following groups:

• Persons older than 65 years
• Residents of long-term care facilities who have chronic medical conditions
• Persons with chronic pulmonary or cardiovascular conditions, including asthma

- Persons with chronic metabolic, renal, hematopoietic, or immunosuppressive diseases
- Children ages 6 months to 18 years receiving long-term aspirin therapy (to decrease their risk of Reye's syndrome)
- Physicians, nurses, and other health care workers and household members of persons in the other high-risk groups

Ask patients whether they are allergic to eggs, chickens, feathers, chicken dander, or neomycin because each may indicate an allergy to the vaccine. Assess the patient's reaction to any previous doses; if seizures or other neurological disorders occurred, the vaccine is contraindicated. Delay the influenza injection if the patient has a fever or has received the pertussis vaccine within the last 3 days.

The influenza virus vaccine must be given yearly. It is usually given in October or November so that antibodies will be at a peak during the peak influenza season. This season starts in December. Children younger than 9 years should receive two doses if they have never had the vaccine before. The second dose should be given no later than November 1.

Administer the influenza virus vaccine intramuscularly. If the patient is older than 3 years, the usual dose is 0.5 mL. Between the ages of 6 months and 3 years, the dose is only 0.25 mL. An acellular form of the vaccine is recommended for use with young children. Advise the patient that a local reaction is common. Fever, malaise, or myalgia may also occur.

Some potential patients may be afraid of the influenza virus vaccine because of its previous association with Guillain-Barré syndrome, a disorder causing temporary paralysis. Recent influenza virus vaccines have not produced this syndrome, however.

True influenza is a reportable disease, meaning that cases of it should be reported to the health department. The state Department of Health keeps statistics of immunizations given and cases reported.

PNEUMOCOCCAL VACCINE

The pneumococcal vaccine (Pneumovax) produces artificially acquired active immunity against the strains of pneumococcus it contains. It is recommended for persons in the following categories:

- Persons older than 50 years
- Persons with chronic illnesses, such as cardiac, respiratory, hepatic, renal, and hematopoietic diseases or diabetes
- Persons with alcohol abuse
- Persons with Hodgkin's disease
- Persons in residential schools, nursing homes, or other institutions

Assess for allergies or any previous pneumococcal vaccination. Pneumovax is given only once. No repetition of the vaccine should be administered. It is given intramuscularly or subcutaneously at a dose of 0.5 mL. Caution the recipient of the vaccine about possible side effects, including local inflammation, rash, arthritis, arthralgia, myalgia, hives, swollen lymph glands, and malaise. Pneumovax is not given to children younger than 2 years.

Closely observe the recipient of the pneumococcal vaccine who has severe cardiac or respiratory disease or who presents with a fever. The patient with a fever may wish to delay the vaccination.

BCG VACCINE

BCG vaccine is a live vaccine containing bacille Calmette-Guérin, a strain of *Mycobacterium bovis*. It is used for immunizing against tuberculosis, but generally only if the patient is at high risk. People at high risk for tuberculosis include persons living in or traveling to an area of high incidence of the disease, persons who have a family member with active tuberculosis, and health care workers who are routinely exposed to the disease.

Determine whether the patient is immunosuppressed or receiving steroids. Immunosuppression and steroid therapy could cause the vaccine to produce the disease.

BCG vaccine is given percutaneously by rubbing it on the skin and then causing a small puncture to the skin. The area should be kept dry for 24 hours but not dressed. Approximately 0.2 to 0.3 mL of vaccine is used. The most common side effect is swollen lymph glands.

The patient who has received BCG vaccine should be made aware that any subsequent tuberculin skin tests will show positive results. A chest x-ray is required if screening is necessary.

HEPATITIS B VACCINE

Hepatitis B vaccine (Heptavax-B) is an attenuated virus vaccine that produces artificially acquired active immunity. It gives immunity to hepatitis type B, but not to other types of hepatitis.

It is recommended that the hepatitis B vaccine be given to persons in the following categories:

- Health care workers
- Patients on hemodialysis or who receive blood frequently
- Persons at high risk for sexually transmitted disease (STD)

• Drug users
• Household, work, or classroom contacts of persons with persistent hepatitis B

It is also now being administered to infants as a routine immunization.

The hepatitis B vaccine is given intramuscularly into the deltoid muscle, usually at a dose of 1.0 mL; 0.25 mL is given into the vastus lateralis muscle for infants. The patient will need to receive three injections, the second a month after the first, and the third 6 months after the first (but at least 2 months after the second dose). The infant schedule is usually begun at birth or at 1 month of age. Warn the patient of possible local inflammation, headache, gastrointestinal upset, or upper respiratory illness.

If the patient has been exposed to hepatitis B virus, the patient should receive hepatitis B immune globulin at the time of administration of the first vaccine for faster protection.

Closely observe the patient who has a cardiopulmonary disease or infection after the administration of the vaccine. The person with an infection may wish to delay the vaccination.

RH$_O$(D) IMMUNE GLOBULIN

Rh$_o$(D) immune globulin (RhoGAM) is used for an Rh-negative mother if her fetus is Rh-positive. This is to prevent the mother from forming antibodies against the Rh factor in the event of maternal-child blood exchange. It is necessary to prohibit formation of these antibodies to protect subsequent fetuses from being attacked in the event that their blood is also Rh-positive. RhoGAM or MICRhoGAM should be given in case of spontaneous or therapeutic abortion, amniocentesis, pregnancy, or delivery.

RhoGAM is given intramuscularly at a dose of 300 µg. The patient may experience some local discomfort and possibly a slight fever or, rarely, anaphylaxis. The injection must be given within 72 hours of an abortion, amniocentesis, or birth. A half-dose injection is now given prophylactically to Rh-negative mothers at 28 weeks' gestation. Teach all Rh-negative mothers that they must have another injection each time they have an abortion or Rh-positive infant.

Before administration of the drug, be sure to ask about religious objections to receiving serum.

Serum is drawn from the mother to determine her Rh factor. Cord blood is used to determine the infant's Rh factor. RhoGAM should be given if the infant's Rh factor is unknown. Check the injection site for signs of abscess formation.

MISCELLANEOUS IMMUNIZATIONS

Rabies

A vaccine and a serum are available, and both are from human sources. The serum, rabies immune globulin, may be given in combination with the vaccine, but not after the eighth day following the vaccine. Often, half of the serum is applied to the wound itself, and half is given intramuscularly.

Immune Globulin

Immune globulin (Gamastan) is given intramuscularly and can protect against hepatitis A, rubeola (measles), varicella (chickenpox), rubella, and immunoglobulin deficiencies (except immunoglobulin A deficiency). Allergies are rare to this serum, and skin test is not recommended. The dose varies by the disease.

Immune Globulin Intravenous

Immune globulin intravenous (Gamimune N IV) is given in cases of immunodeficiencies (except deficiency of immunoglobulin A). To increase platelet production, it is given to patients with idiopathic thrombocytopenic purpura, a disease that causes seriously low platelet levels.

E X E R C I S E S

CASE STUDIES

1. S.E. is brought to the immunization clinic for her "shots." S.E. is 20 months old and has received only one DTP and one polio vaccine. Her mother states that she forgot to bring the child back after her first visit. What vaccines should S.E. receive today? Would it be necessary to start her series of vaccines over? Would you recommend that S.E. receive all possible vaccines today or be scheduled to return later?

2. S.E.'s mother calls the clinic later in the day and states that the child is running a fever of 100.6°F. She wants to give S.E. acetaminophen syrup as she was instructed but is unsure of the amount. You have standing orders that read to give 120 mg. The mother's bottle reads 80 mg/5 mL. How much should S.E. receive?

3. D.B. is brought to the physician's office to receive a scheduled DTP. D.B. is 2 months old and suffered a seizure at birth. Although D.B. is receiving medication, he still has occasional seizures. What immunization should D.B. receive today?

MENTAL AEROBICS

Visit an immunization clinic. Pay special attention to immunization schedules, conditions that contraindicate immunizations, and techniques used to improve compliance.

ANTISEPTICS AND GERMICIDES

LEARNING OBJECTIVES

After studying this chapter, you should be able to:

1. Discuss the action of and adverse reactions to antiseptics and germicides and nursing responsibilities appropriate for patients using them.

2. List the conditions under which antiseptics and germicides are used.

3. Name examples of antiseptics and germicides.

4. Prepare an appropriate teaching plan for patients using antiseptics or germicides.

DRUGS YOU WILL LEARN ABOUT IN THIS CHAPTER

Antiseptics

hexachlorophene (pHisoDerm, pHisoHex)

boric acid

gentian violet

Germicides

alcohol, isopropyl

alcohol, ethyl 70%

iodine

iodine tincture

povidone-iodine (Betadine)

chlorhexidene (Hibiclens, Hibistat)

benzalkonium (Zephiran)

hydrogen peroxide

potassium permanganate

Louis Pasteur (1822–1895) is credited with founding microbiology. Antisepsis, the practice of reducing microorganisms on the patient and in the environment, is fairly new to medical science. Since Pasteur's time, researchers have identified numerous agents that are effective against microbes.

ACTIONS AND USES An *antiseptic* is an agent that can slow or stop the growth of microorganisms. These agents do not kill the microbes themselves. Antiseptics make the environment less than ideal for the microbe. A *disinfectant* is an agent that can kill microbes. Disinfectants work in many different ways. One possible mode of action is to denature the cell material of the microbe. Disinfectants are not generally used on skin because they can injure the skin cells also. A *germicide* is an agent that kills microbes, but a germicide can be used on the skin and possibly on mucous membranes.

Other terms sometimes used interchangeably with antiseptic and germicide are bactericidal and bacteriostatic. *Bactericidal* means the agent kills bacteria. The word does not expressly include other microorganisms in the definition. *Bacteriostatic* means the agent slows or stops the growth of bacteria. It, too, does not include other microbes.

All of the agents explained in this chapter are topical antiseptics or topical germicides. An in depth analysis of major disinfectants used in infection control is beyond the scope of this text.

Topical antiseptics or germicides are used to decrease the presence of bacteria on the skin, on mucous membranes, and sometimes even in wounds. The most common adverse reactions from these agents are skin irritation, a rash, pruritus, or an allergic response.

ASSESSMENT Before use of an antiseptic or germicide, ▲▲▲▲▲▲▲▲▲▲ be sure to check the patient for a history of allergies to any of the ingredients in the specific agent. Check the order for specific directions for the use of the agent and where the agent is to be applied. Assess the patient's skin or mucous membranes for any open areas.

PLANNING AND IMPLEMENTATION Store any antiseptic ▲▲▲▲▲▲▲▲▲▲▲▲▲▲▲▲▲▲▲▲▲▲▲▲▲▲▲▲ or germicide in a safe place away from children or confused patients. Never transfer the agent into any other container from the original labeled one provided by the pharmacy. For example, if the agent is poured into a medicine cup and stored until use near the patient's bed, it may be mistaken for oral medication. Most of these agents cause toxic effects if the patient were to mistakenly drink them.

If the agent is liquid, remember to pour from the bottle away from the label. The label must remain legible to prevent accidents.

If the patient is to go home before use of the agent is discontinued, or if the patient is to be involved in the use of the agent while in a care facility, teach the patient how to use it. Show the patient the exact procedure for administration of the agent. Allow time for questions. Then arrange for the patient to give a return demonstration. Correct any misunderstandings the patient may exhibit during the demonstration. If necessary, arrange for a repeated demonstration, additional teaching, or another practice session.

Be sure the patient understands where to use the agent and that the agent is *not* to be used elsewhere.

N U R S I N G   A L E R T
▼▼▼▼▼▼▼▼▼▼▼▼▼▼▼▼▼▼▼▼▼▼▼▼▼▼▼▼▼▼

Emphasize the treatment if accidental contact with mucous membranes or the eyes occurs (if these are not the areas ordered for administration). Flushing of the mucous membranes or the eyes with normal saline must be done immediately. Contact the physician for further evaluation.

▲▲▲▲▲▲▲▲▲▲▲▲▲▲▲▲▲▲▲▲▲▲▲▲▲▲▲▲▲▲

EVALUATION In addition to evaluating the patient's ▲▲▲▲▲▲▲▲▲ ability to perform administration of the agent, also evaluate for any adverse reactions. If any occur, do not perform the next procedure and contact the physician.

Evaluation of the effectiveness of the agent is determined by improved signs or symptoms of infection in the area or by the prevention of such signs and symptoms.

ANTISEPTICS

Hexachlorophene

Hexachlorophene (pHisoHex, pHisoDerm) is a bacteriostatic agent. It is used to cleanse a surgical site or as a hand scrub. It is not to be used on any open skin, on mucous membranes, on burns, or on infants.

Repeated use of hexachlorophene has been shown to produce increased effectiveness. The agent leaves a residue on the skin that is difficult to remove with simple handwashing. As a result, the effects may last for several days. Additional use during this time, therefore, increases the amount of residue left behind.

Use of hexachlorophene has been associated with adverse reactions, such as a rash, photosensitivity, and dermatitis.

N U R S I N G   A L E R T
▼▼▼▼▼▼▼▼▼▼▼▼▼▼▼▼▼▼▼▼▼▼▼▼▼▼▼▼▼▼

It has also been demonstrated that hexachlorophene can be absorbed through the skin with repeated use. This may lead to toxicity. Signs or symptoms of toxicity include cerebral irritation, central nervous system stimulation, and even seizures. For this reason, always rinse any area on which hexachlorophene has been applied. Alcohol removes the residue left behind, if desired.

▲▲▲▲▲▲▲▲▲▲▲▲▲▲▲▲▲▲▲▲▲▲▲▲▲▲▲▲▲▲

Boric Acid

Although boric acid is considered only mild bacteriostatic, it is also fungicidal. As a liquid, boric acid may be used as a mild eyewash, a gargle, or an irrigant. An ointment is also available for minor first-aid treatment of such problems as dry or chapped skin, minor rashes, minor burns or abrasions, and insect bites.

Boric acid is generally considered to be nontoxic.

N U R S I N G   A L E R T
▼▼▼▼▼▼▼▼▼▼▼▼▼▼▼▼▼▼▼▼▼▼▼▼▼▼▼▼▼▼

The patient may exhibit adverse reactions related to toxicity in three specific cases: if the liquid is used full strength, if boric acid is applied to large areas of the body, or if the agent is taken internally.

▲▲▲▲▲▲▲▲▲▲▲▲▲▲▲▲▲▲▲▲▲▲▲▲▲▲▲▲▲▲

Gentian Violet

Gentian violet is a dye with bacteriostatic properties. It can be used as a "swish and spit" mouth rinse for thrush or as an irrigant for vaginal yeast infections.

GERMICIDES

Alcohol

Alcohol is one of the most commonly used germicidal agents in the hospital, nursing home, physician's office, or patient's home. Isopropyl alcohol is the most germicidal form. It is not diluted. Ethyl alcohol, at 70% strength, is also used.

Both types of alcohol are used to cleanse the skin before injections and may at times be used to cleanse wounds. The major disadvantage is the stinging the patient may experience on open skin.

Alcohol may also be used to cleanse instruments. Isopropyl alcohol is preferred for any instrument that has rubber or metal because it is less corrosive to these materials.

Iodine, Iodine Tincture, and Iodophors

Iodine or iodine-containing preparations are bactericidal, fungicidal, and virucidal. Iodine or a tincture of iodine can stain both the skin and clothing, however. If this form is used, be sure to protect the patient's clothing during administration. If leakage of the agent is possible after administration, protect the clothing by applying padding. Do not use an occlusive dressing; prolonged exposure to iodine causes an increased risk of skin irritation.

An iodophor is an agent produced by combining iodine and a water-soluble agent. Povidone-iodine (Betadine) is an example of an iodophor. Povidone-iodine does not stain either skin or clothing. It has the added benefit of less irritation to the skin and less discomfort or stinging on open wounds. Povidone-iodine may be used as a skin cleanser, wound cleanser, surgical scrub, douche, or vaginal suppository.

N U R S I N G   A L E R T

▼▼▼▼▼▼▼▼▼▼▼▼▼▼▼▼▼▼▼▼▼▼▼▼▼▼▼▼▼▼▼▼▼▼▼

Before administering any iodine preparation, check the patient for a history of allergic response to iodine. An allergy to seafood may also indicate an increased chance of allergy.

▲▲▲▲▲▲▲▲▲▲▲▲▲▲▲▲▲▲▲▲▲▲▲▲▲▲▲▲▲▲▲▲▲▲▲

Chlorhexidene

Chlorhexidene (Hibiclens, Hibistat) is commonly used as a bactericidal scrub for hands or surgical sites. The physician may order a whole body scrub before surgery. This can best be accomplished in the shower with two separate applications of chlorhexidene separated by thorough rinsing. Chlorhexidene may also be used as a wound cleanser. The most common adverse reactions include a rash, photosensitivity, and dermatitis. It has not been demonstrated to be absorbed through the skin. Chlorhexidene should not be administered on mucous membranes.

Chlorhexidene can stain clothing and linens. If accidental spillage occurs, rinse the area immediately with lukewarm water; if the agent is allowed to dry, it will be set. Next wash with a mild soap. Never wash the item with chlorine bleach because this will cause an ugly brown stain. If additional whitening is necessary, use hydrogen peroxide after washing.

Benzalkonium

Benzalkonium (Zephiran) can be a bactericidal agent if it is used at a strong enough strength. Weaker solutions are bacteriostatic. Strengths can range from 1:10,000 to 1:750. Be sure the physician orders the strength to be used. Do not apply an occlusive dressing if benzalkonium is used on the skin because irritation is then more likely.

Benzalkonium is often used on the skin or mucous membranes as a cleanser. It may be ordered as a wound cleanser or as an irrigant for body cavities, such as the bladder or vagina. At weak strengths, it is used as an eye irrigant.

Oxidizing Agents

Oxidizing agents are solutions that release a free oxygen molecule on coming in contact with protein. The protein may be blood, microorganisms, mucus, or other substances. The excess oxygen then kills the microorganisms that are present. A change in the agent occurs when the oxygen is released.

Hydrogen peroxide (H_2O_2) is one example of an oxidizing agent. When hydrogen peroxide contacts protein, it foams. It is used to cleanse wounds, the mouth, and inanimate objects.

Potassium permanganate ($KMNO_4$) is also an oxidizing agent. When potassium permanganate contacts protein, it turns from purple to brown. Be sure the solution is purple before using it. Permanganate may also stain clothing or other objects. Therefore, protect the patient's possessions during administration. If the agent is used as a vaginal irrigant, pad the underclothing in case of leakage.

E X E R C I S E S

CASE STUDIES

1. A new nurse on your shift is concerned about possible allergic reactions to the cleansing agents used to scrub hands. What allergies prohibit the use of some agents? What symptoms of allergic reaction should the nurse watch for?

2. Your patient is to have surgery in the morning. The physician ordered a whole body scrub with chlorhexidene for tonight. What is the best method for application? What would you do if the patient splashed some of the chlorhexidene onto personal clothing?

3. A patient with an open wound is to perform dressing changes, eventually without supervision. The procedure is to include a wound irrigation with povidone-iodine. How would you teach the patient the procedure?

4. Another nurse on the unit has heard that hexachlorophene leaves a residue on the skin that helps protect against bacteria with increasing effectiveness on each use. This nurse believes that the unit should switch to use of hexachlorophene for all routine handwashing. Based on your knowledge, what would be your best response to this nurse?

5. The physician has ordered potassium permanganate as a vaginal irrigant for your patient. What precautions should you use? How does permanganate work? Name another agent in this category that works in a similar way.

MENTAL AEROBICS

1. Take a tour of the central supply department of a hospital or other health care facility. Focus on products used by the facility for the purposes of antisepsis or disinfection. Ask the personnel why this particular product is used and under what circumstances.

2. Talk with the infection control nurse of your facility. What antiseptics or germicides are routinely used at the facility? Why does this nurse recommend these products? What precautions are necessary with these products?

DRUGS THAT AFFECT NEOPLASMS

Patients who have a diagnosis of cancer may be treated with three main types of therapy:

1. surgical removal of the cancer or neoplasm;
2. chemotherapy, or drug therapy, which attempts to kill the abnormal cells; and
3. radiation therapy, which attempts to shrink or destroy the abnormal cells.

The various types of cancer respond differently to each therapy. The location of the cancer also influences the mode of treatment recommended to the patient.

Because of the many variables in disease and treatment, patients are often referred to an oncology department. Here, physicians and others who special-ize in the treatment of tumors recommend the best mode of therapy for the patient. Many patients receive treatment with a combination of therapies.

Cancer treatment always involves the question of quality of life versus quantity of life. With therapeutic treatment, the goal is to help the patient live as long as possible and as comfortably as possible. The therapies themselves may cause considerable pain or discomfort, so there is sometimes difficulty in achieving both longevity and comfort. When this becomes an issue, the goal of treatment often changes to palliation, which seeks to offer comfort to the patient even if life is indirectly shortened.

ANTINEOPLASTIC DRUGS

LEARNING OBJECTIVES

After studying this chapter, you should be able to:

1. Discuss the actions and uses of the various classes of antineoplastic drugs.

2. Briefly explain the various methods of administration to patients and family.

3. Explain the difference between therapeutic and palliative treatments.

4. List common adverse effects of chemotherapeutic agents.

5. Discuss nursing interventions that are appropriate for prevention or control of adverse effects or that provide comfort to those experiencing adverse effects.

DRUGS YOU WILL LEARN ABOUT IN THIS CHAPTER

Alkylating Agents

mechlorethamine HCl (Mustargen, nitrogen mustard)

cyclophosphamide (Cytoxan)

cisplatin (Platinol)

busulfan (Myleran)

chlorambucil (Leukeran)

Antimetabolites

methotrexate (Mexate, Folex)

6-mercaptopurine (6-MP, Purinethol)

fluorouracil (5-FU)

Antibiotics

dactinomycin (Cosmegen)

doxorubicin (Adriamycin)

bleomycin (Blenoxane)

Miscellaneous Mitotic Inhibitors

vinblastine sulfate (Velban)

vincristine sulfate (Oncovin)

Hormonal Therapy

Androgens

testosterone suspension

testolactone (Teslac)

fluoxymesterone (Halotestin)

Estrogens

chlorotrianisene (Tace)

estrone (Ogen, Theelin)

Antiestrogens

tamoxifen citrate (Nolvadex)

Progestogens

hydroxyprogesterone caproate (Delalutin, Duralutin)

medroxyprogesterone acetate (DepoProvera, Provera)

Adrenocorticosteroids

prednisone (Deltasone, Meticorten)

Drugs That Modify Biological Responses

161

erythropoietin, epoetin alfa (Epogen, Procrit)

filgrastim (granulocyte colony–stimulating factor, G-CSF, Neupogen)

Chemotherapy involves the use of antineoplastic medications that inhibit the growth of neoplasms.

ACTIONS AND USES Antineoplastics act in various ways; therefore, the use of each varies with the type of medication. The types of antineoplastics are alkylating agents, antimetabolites, antibiotics, mitotic inhibitors, and hormones.

ASSESSMENT Because of expected side effects, certain laboratory assessments must be completed before the first administration of chemotherapy. This is to establish baseline values for comparison with the results of tests performed before each subsequent treatment. Complete blood count (CBC) and determination of blood urea nitrogen (BUN) and creatinine levels are often included in these tests. Treatments may be omitted if the laboratory values are seriously altered.

Weigh patients accurately because dosage is calibrated for each kilogram of body weight. Perform a thorough cephalocaudal assessment, and document the findings as baseline data.

PLANNING AND IMPLEMENTATION Antineoplastic medications may be given by the oral, intramuscular, or intravenous routes. Sometimes they are injected into an artery or injected or instilled into a body cavity.

Special catheters and reservoirs are often used to administer chemotherapy. Right atrial catheters, such as Hickman or Broviac catheters, are inserted surgically into the right upper chest. There, they are threaded into the right subclavian vein, with the distal end at the superior vena cava or entrance to the right atrium. These catheters may be used for intravenous (IV) hydration, for medication administration, or to obtain venous blood samples. They provide access for long-term intermittent use of chemotherapeutics, blood products, and hyperalimentation. Care of these catheters includes special dressing procedures, with cleansing of the skin and application of an occlusive dressing according to institutional policy.

Other subclavian lines (e.g., triple-lumen catheters) are inserted while the patients remain in their own rooms. These are frequently used for total parenteral nutrition (TPN) and IV infusion or to obtain laboratory samples when veins are difficult to access.

Some patients have reservoirs, such as the Infusaid or Infuse-a-Port, which are surgically implanted. These devices have a well or reservoir that is closed with a self-sealing rubber material. This area is called a port. Medications can be injected through the port and stored inside, then gradually released. The port can be palpated through the skin. The port reseals after each injection. At the base of the port, a catheter is inserted into an artery or a vein for direct infusion to an area (Fig. 25–1). Blood may be withdrawn from the device, but the first 5 cc must be discarded because it has been heparinized to prevent clots from forming in the catheter. Injections and blood draws are performed with special needles.

There is no care for the device after the skin incision is healed. The patient may participate in normal activities, such as swimming, bathing, and exercising. The patient should carry a special identification card. Teach the patient the purpose and function of the device.

The Ommaya reservoir is a similar device. The reservoir is inserted under the scalp; silicone tubing leads into a ventricle of the brain, on the patient's nondominant side. The reservoir is used to distribute chemotherapeutic medications into the cerebrospinal fluid. It is also used to measure the pressure of the cerebrospinal fluid and to remove a sample of fluid for laboratory testing.

These ports or reservoirs are permanent unless complications occur. Some of the complications that may occur are infection and blockage or displacement of the catheter.

Chemotherapeutic drugs can also be instilled into the pleural, pericardial, and peritoneal cavities for treatment of effusions and ascites that result from metastases. The excessive fluid is first removed from these cavities through thoracentesis or paracentesis procedures, then the medication is instilled. The patient may experience considerable pain. The physi-

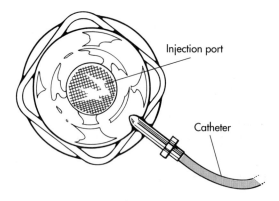

Figure 25–1. Surgically implantable infusion devices are made up of an injection port, which stores medication, and a catheter, which carries the released drug to a direct area.

cian may order various position changes for the patient to distribute the medication throughout the cavity. Nausea and vomiting may persist for 2 to 3 days.

Bladder instillations are sometimes done through a Foley catheter for treatment of bladder tumors. The bladder is drained, the medication is instilled, and the catheter is clamped for the time ordered by the physician. If the patient complains of distress before the ordered time for unclamping, the clamp must be released early. Adverse effects include irritation, burning, and hematuria.

Much of the detail of the administration technique has been omitted from this chapter because oncology is a highly specialized field. Chemotherapeutic agents should be administered only by people who have special training in this field.

The medications are often highly toxic, and special precautions may be required during their preparation. Special gloves, gowns, and protective eyewear should be worn to prepare many of the injectable medications. Mixing and aspiration of drugs into syringes should be done in a special area with a laminar airflow hood, which minimizes the inhalation of droplets that become airborne during the procedure. Materials used in the administration of the medication must be disposed of properly according to institutional policy.

There are often specific recommendations for administration, and some require "rescue" procedures to be initiated at a specific time. Rescue is the administration of an antidote that is specific for the chemotherapeutic agent being used. Timing of the administration of the antidote is critical.

One to 2 liters of IV fluid may be given immediately before treatment to ensure hydration and adequate renal function. Many drugs cause nausea and vomiting, so specific antiemetic medications are sometimes given immediately before treatment.

If the drug is nephrotoxic, a Foley catheter may be inserted to accurately monitor hourly outputs. Some drugs are neurotoxic and may cause lethargy and diminished level of consciousness. Safety measures must be maintained at all times.

Keep patients and family as informed as possible. Give physical and emotional support. An attitude of hopefulness should be maintained. Suggest realistic expectations.

Anaphylaxis may occur with administration of any medication. The caregivers should anticipate and be prepared to perform resuscitative measures unless the patient has an advanced directive or "do not resuscitate order" documented on the current chart.

If alopecia is expected, inform the patient that it is usually temporary. Many people wish to choose a wig before hair loss, so color and texture can be matched. Hats and scarves may be used as alternatives.

Special rubber gloves are used to administer these medications. If the skin comes in contact with the medication, irrigate the area as soon as possible to prevent irritation and sloughing. "Spill kits" are available for this purpose and must be nearby when these medications are infused. IV and intra-arterial sites must be monitored carefully for infiltration. If infiltration occurs, infusions are discontinued immediately to prevent or minimize sloughing of tissue.

Monitor carefully for signs and symptoms of blood vessel inflammation and thromboses. Handle the patient gently to prevent the occurrence of bruising or petechiae. Document and report their presence.

Give oral hygiene three or four times a day and assess the mouth every day for the appearance of irritation or lesions. If they occur, use "toothettes" or some other type of soft toothbrush for care. Monitor food intake; diminished appetite may be the first clue that chewing is difficult or that the throat is sore. Teach the patient to avoid foods that are acidic. Provide a variety of soft foods from which to choose.

Because the platelets are lowered, monitor stools and urine for blood. Many physicians request that all stools be tested for occult blood. Also be alert for bleeding gums and epistaxis. Monitor vital signs frequently. Avoid safety razors.

Skin is very fragile. Pad side rails if patients are restless. Avoid use of tape on the skin if at all possible, because skin tears occur easily. If tape must be used, be extremely careful in removing it.

Because of bone marrow depression, the patient is more susceptible to infection. Monitor vital signs and observe for signs and symptoms of infection anywhere in the body. Yeast or fungal infections commonly occur in body orifices and cavities. Encourage good oral hygiene, pericare, and handwashing as preventive measures. Caregivers must be conscientious with handwashing and aseptic technique, as they should be with all of their patients. No one with an infection should care for the patient. Provide a private room if possible. If this is not possible, be certain the roommate is free of infection. Encourage good nutrition with intake of foods from all the food groups and intake of at least 1500 mL per day.

It is always important to understand the reason a medication is ordered for a particular patient to provide accurate teaching about the medication. The advantages of a therapeutic regimen must always be weighed against the disadvantages of the adverse effects of the medication. When hormones are ordered for treatment of a malignant neoplasm, the intended effect is to prolong life. The adverse effect of masculinization of the female appearance (and vice versa for males) may lose its importance in this situation. See related chapters for additional information.

Understand the goal of the treatment and document

assessments. Compare assessment findings with the baseline documentation.

EVALUATION Observe for signs that drugs are effective, ▲▲▲▲▲▲▲▲▲▲ such as decrease in pain, increase in appetite, increase in weight or strength, and increased participation in activities of daily living.

Compare vital signs and other daily assessment findings with those documented as the baseline values. Monitor blood counts and other laboratory test results and compare with normal values. Report abnormalities.

ALKYLATING AGENTS

Alklylating agents interfere with cell division in rapidly growing tissues. Some examples are mechlorethamine hydrochloride (Mustargen, nitrogen mustard), cyclophosphamide (Cytoxan), cisplatin (Platinol), busulfan (Myleran), and chlorambucil (Leukeran).

All cell growth is dependent on certain "building blocks," such as amino acids, purines, and intact DNA. The alkylating agents interfere with the supply and use of these substances so the cells cannot divide and reproduce.

Alkylating agents are used to treat gestational choriocarcinoma, Hodgkin's disease, childhood acute lymphocytic leukemia, Wilms' tumor and retinoblastoma, and others.

Adverse actions include bone marrow depression, alopecia, nausea and vomiting, and ulceration of the gastrointestinal mucosa. There may be thromboses and irritation and sloughing of skin if there is contact through a spill or infiltration from a needle or catheter. Amenorrhea and aspermatogenesis may occur. Patients may experience drowsiness, fever, or tinnitus. Aphasia may occur.

Because of the high frequency of toxicity associated with alkylating agents, they are generally used in cases of inoperable or widely metastasized cancer.

ANTIMETABOLITES

Antimetabolites interfere with cell metabolism, function, or growth. Examples include methotrexate (Mexate, Folex), 6-mercaptopurine (6-MP, Purinethol), and fluorouracil (5-FU).

Antimetabolites are especially effective in the treatment of leukemia. The most common adverse actions are bone marrow depression, ulceration of the gastrointestinal tract, nausea and vomiting, jaundice, fever, anorexia, and malaise.

ANTIBIOTICS

Some antibiotics bind with DNA and interfere with DNA or RNA synthesis (production). This delays or inhibits cell division or reproduction. These antibiotics are not used for anti-infective properties because they are extremely toxic. Examples of this classification are dactinomycin (Cosmegen), doxorubicin (Adriamycin), and bleomycin (Blenoxane).

These chemotherapeutic agents are especially toxic to rapidly dividing cells, such as cancer cells, but also to the bone marrow and the cells of the gastrointestinal tract. Signs and symptoms of this toxicity may not be apparent until days or even weeks after therapy is completed. Maximal effects and adverse effects may not be reached for 1 or 2 additional weeks.

Infiltration of the intravenous site may cause severe localized tissue reactions. Doxorubicin produces red urine, which is *not* hematuria.

MISCELLANEOUS MITOTIC INHIBITORS

Mitotic inhibitors have different or unknown modes of action that interfere with cell division. Examples include plant alkaloids such as vinblastine sulfate (Velban) and vincristine (Oncovin).

These chemotherapeutic agents may be used to treat Hodgkin's disease and choriocarcinomas that are resistant to other therapy. They sometimes relieve pain and other symptoms. Adverse reactions include cellulitis and severe localized reactions if infiltration occurs at the intravenous site. Toxic symptoms may occur as described previously with other classifications.

HORMONAL THERAPY

Several classifications of hormones are used as chemotherapeutic agents or as an adjunct to chemotherapy. This type of therapy is based on the finding that tumors of the reproductive organs and the accessory organs are dependent on the sex hormones for their normal growth and development. For example, breast and ovarian tumors grow best in an estrogen environment, and testicular and prostate tumors grow best in the presence of testosterone. If possible, surgical removal of the ovaries or testes is done to eliminate the primary source of sex hormones.

The specific action of the hormones is unknown, but they are believed to alter the growth pattern of hormone-dependent tumors by making the cellular environment less favorable. Decreasing or antagonizing the specific hormone seems to decrease the growth of the malignant neoplasm.

Androgens

Androgens, such as testosterone, testolactone (Teslac), and fluoxymesterone (Halotestin), may be used to treat mammary cancers in women during childbearing years. Adverse effects include masculinization of the appearance and fluid retention. (For more details, see Chapter 61.)

Estrogens

Estrogens, such as chlorotrianisene (Tace) and estrone (Ogen, Theelin), may be ordered for treatment of prostate tumors. Adverse effects include feminization of the appearance and fluid retention (see Chapter 62).

Antiestrogens

Antiestrogens, such as tamoxifen citrate (Nolvadex), block the actions of estrogen on breast tumors. Adverse effects include menopausal symptoms and fluid retention (see Chapter 62).

Progestogens

Progestogens, such as hydroxyprogesterone caproate (Delalutin, Duralutin) or medroxyprogesterone acetate (Depo-Provera, Provera), may be ordered for treatment of uterine and endometrial cancers. Adverse effects include fluid retention, nausea and vomiting, breast tenderness, and pain at the injection site (see Chapter 63).

Adrenocorticosteroids

Adrenocorticosteroids, such as prednisone (Deltasone, Meticorten), are often used to produce remissions of susceptible leukemias and lymphomas in children. They are of little benefit in adult leukemias. They are also used to treat Hodgkin's disease, lymphosarcoma, multiple myeloma, and chronic lymphatic leukemia. Adverse effects depend on the dose used, but all systems may be affected (see Chapter 58).

BIOLOGICAL RESPONSE MODIFIERS

Recent advances in technology have permitted the development of new drugs that are used to counteract the adverse effect of bone marrow suppression caused by chemotherapeutic agents.

Erythropoietin and Epoetin Alfa

Erythropoietin is a hormone manufactured and released by the kidney. It stimulates the bone marrow to increase production of erythrocytes (red blood cells), which transport oxygen and carbon dioxide. Release of this hormone is triggered by decreased oxygen levels in the blood, which would be seen in anemia.

Epoetin alfa (Epogen, Procrit) is produced by recombinant DNA techniques. It acts to stimulate the production of erythrocytes just as erythropoietin does. It is used to treat anemia in patients with malignant neoplasms when the anemia is due to the adverse effects of chemotherapeutic drugs. (It is *not used* to treat other types of anemias in cancer patients, such as those caused by deficiencies or hemorrhage, because there are other more appropriate treatments for these.) It is also used to treat anemia due to reduced production of erythropoietin in end-stage renal disease and anemia due to zidovudine therapy in patients infected with human immunodeficiency virus (HIV).

Adverse actions are sometimes difficult to differentiate from those typical in advanced stages of cancer. Nausea, vomiting, diarrhea, rash, headache, and elevated platelet count may be seen. Hypertension, pulmonary embolism, or cerebrovascular accident may be related to the increase in hematocrit. Seizures may occur and are considered to be a life-threatening reaction. Because this drug acts as a growth factor, there is the possibility that the tumor cells may also be stimulated to grow. It has not yet been determined whether use of this drug is safe for treatment of children or pregnant or lactating women.

Assess the patient and the chart for evidence of uncontrolled hypertension or for other conditions that may be contraindications to use of epoetin, such as known hypersensitivity to mammalian cell–derived products or to human albumin, sickle cell anemia, porphyria, coagulation disorders, pregnancy, or lactation. Also assess for history of cardiovascular disorders or seizures; these patients must be monitored carefully for adverse effects.

Serum erythrocyte counts, hematocrit, and erythropoietin levels are obtained and recorded as baseline data. Treatment is not recommended for patients with erythropoietin levels above 200 mU/mL. Vital signs are assessed and documented as baseline data.

Vials contain doses of 2000, 3000, 4000, or 10,000 units per milliliter. The solution does not contain preservatives and must be discarded after one dose. *Read labels carefully* to avoid dosage errors and wasting. Store vials at 36° to 46°F (2° to 8°C). Do not freeze or shake vials because this may inactivate the medication. Discard the vial if the solution is discolored or contains particles. There has been no documentation of interactions with other drugs.

The recommended starting dose is 150 units per kilogram subcutaneously (SC) three times a week. Serum hematocrit levels should be monitored weekly. If the serum hematocrit level exceeds 40%, the dose should be held until the level falls to 36%. Dosages are reduced by 25% when they are resumed and are titrated to maintain the desired hematocrit levels. If hematocrit levels do not increase above baseline levels within 8 weeks, dosage may be increased to 300 units per kilogram SC three times a week.

Advise patients that pain or discomfort in the bones, coldness, and sweating sometimes occur within 2 hours of receiving an injection and may persist for as long as 12 hours.

Monitor vital signs daily (or more frequently, if necessary) and teach patients to continue this monitoring at home. Physicians should establish acceptable parameters. Inform patients to notify the physician if these are not maintained.

Careful handwashing and other techniques of asepsis must be maintained to prevent infection. Monitor the patient for signs and symptoms of infection and teach the patient and caregivers to report their occurrence.

Advise women of the potential risk to a fetus and provide contraceptive information as desired. Also advise nonmenstruating women that menses have sometimes resumed after epoetin therapy.

Teach that driving and other hazardous activities should be avoided until response to the drug has been determined.

Monitor serum erythrocyte and hematocrit levels for improvement. Monitor vital signs and compare with parameters established by the physician.

Filgrastim

White blood cells (WBC, leukocytes) are part of the defense system of the body. Neutrophils and monocytes are types of WBC. They defend the body from infection by destroying microorganisms that have invaded the tissues or bloodstream. They do this by a process called phagocytosis, by which the invaders are ingested into the cell and digested. If the number of WBC is significantly reduced, a condition called leukopenia develops, and the person is at increased risk for development of infections.

Filgrastim (Neupogen) is a granulocyte colony–stimulating factor (G-CSF) or glycoprotein that is genetically engineered from *Escherichia coli* bacteria. It binds to specific receptors on the surface of bone marrow cells.

Filgrastim stimulates the growth and maturation of neutrophils. It is used to decrease the risk of infection in patients with neutropenia due to treatment with chemotherapeutic agents.

Adverse actions include skeletal pain, fever, hematuria and proteinuria, alopecia, osteoporosis, and enlargement of the spleen (splenomegaly). The number of thrombocytes may decrease (thrombocytopenia) and predispose the patient to clotting difficulty or inability to clot blood normally when injury occurs. Because this drug acts as a growth factor, there is the possibility that the tumor cells may also be stimulated to grow. It has not yet been determined whether use of this drug is safe for treatment of pregnant or lactating women.

A complete blood count (CBC) and platelet count must be obtained before initiation of therapy. Assess for signs and symptoms of infection and document. Assess vital signs and document results as baseline data. Assess for hypersensitivity to proteins derived from *E. coli* and report this to the physician immediately.

Dosage for adults and children is 5 mcg per kilogram per day. It is given as a single dose by SC or IV route. Therapy is usually initiated when the WBC count drops below 1000/mm^3. Doses may be increased in increments of 5 mcg per kilogram for each chemotherapy cycle as determined by the WBC count. CBC and platelet counts should be monitored at least twice weekly. Dosage is given daily for up to 2 weeks or until the WBC count has returned to 10,000/mm^3. Do not administer filgrastim within 24 hours of chemotherapy because these drugs may destroy the new WBC.

Vials contain doses of 300 mcg per milliliter. The solution does not contain preservatives and must be discarded after one dose. Do not freeze or shake vials because this may inactivate the medication. Store vials at 36° to 46°F (2° to 8°C). Vials that have been at room temperature for more than 6 hours must be discarded. Also discard the vial if the solution is discolored or contains particles.

Bone pain may be relieved through use of comfort measures, such as position changes and relaxation therapies, along with non-narcotic analgesics except aspirin.

Careful handwashing and other techniques of asepsis must be maintained to prevent infection. Monitor the patient for signs and symptoms of infection and teach the patient and caregivers to report their occurrence.

Monitor CBC and platelet counts. Monitor vital signs and signs and symptoms of infection.

E X E R C I S E S

CASE STUDY

Ms. F.K. is receiving chemotherapy with IV antineoplastic medications. She has refused most of her meals for the past 2 days, and her liquid intake has diminished. This morning, when the nurse was assisting Ms. F.K. with her oral hygiene, the toothbrush was tinged pink. Prepare a care plan for Ms. F.K. that addresses actual and potential problems associated with IV chemotherapy.

LEARNING ACTIVITIES

1. Accompany one of your patients to the oncology department for chemotherapy. List the medications the patient receives. For each drug, list the classification, actions and uses, planning and implementation, and evaluation. Note the patient teaching that was done by the oncology nurse and whether the patient was knowledgeable about the treatments. Note whether the purpose of the treatment is therapeutic or palliative. Note the mood of the patient and the "tone" of the discussions during treatment. Discuss whether the patient and caregivers seemed depressed, hopeful, angry, or accepting.

2. Interview a nurse who specializes in oncology. Ask which chemotherapeutic drugs are commonly administered at that facility. Ask the nurse which side effects are commonly seen. Ask what interventions (if any) are initiated to prevent the occurrence of side effects and what interventions are initiated after side effects occur. Note the classifications of the drugs discussed. Present your report to the class.

RADIATION THERAPY

LEARNING OBJECTIVES

After studying this chapter, you should be able to:

1. Provide a basic explanation of the purpose of radiation therapy in the treatment of patients with cancer.

2. Explain the difference between external and internal sources of radiation.

3. List three methods of protecting caregivers from the adverse effects of radiation therapy.

4. List the adverse effects of external and internal radiation.

5. Provide appropriate interventions to prevent adverse effects or to provide comfort to those experiencing the adverse effects of radiation.

6. Prepare an appropriate plan of care for a patient receiving treatment with radiation therapy.

RADIOACTIVE SOURCES YOU WILL LEARN ABOUT IN THIS CHAPTER

External Sources

X-ray machines

Cobalt machines

Linear accelerators

Internal Sources

Gold Au 198

Sodium iodide I 131

Sodium iodide I 125

Sodium phosphate P 32

Radium implants

Cesium implants

Radiation is used in medicine both as a tool for diagnosis and as a mode of treatment. Radioactivity is based on the ability of certain atoms to decompose spontaneously into other atoms. The energy released as the atom decomposes is called radioactivity. Some radioactive elements occur naturally; others are produced mechanically and are referred to as isotopes.

The two methods of administering radiation are externally and internally. External sources of radiation are the x-ray machines, cobalt machines, and linear accelerators. Internal sources are isotopes or elements that are injected or ingested into the body or implanted into a body cavity. Examples are gold Au 198, sodium iodide I 131 or I 125, sodium phosphate P 32, and radium and cesium implants.

Special applicators are used to insert implants into the vaginal vault. The implants may be shaped as rods or pellets. Special needles are used to insert the implants into other areas, such as the cheek and tongue.

Nurses are not responsible for administration of radioactive substances or for the insertion of the implants or devices, but they are often present at or assist with these procedures. They are also responsible for the care of patients during their treatment with the radioactive elements and are responsible for the safety of all who may be exposed to the radiation. For these reasons, we have chosen to include this information in this text.

ACTIONS AND USES The radioactive rays act to disrupt ▲▲▲▲▲▲▲▲▲▲▲▲▲▲▲▲ the function of cells. Rapidly growing cells are particularly vulnerable. External sources are used to shrink or destroy tumors. Pain may be decreased when the pressure from a tumor on another organ or a nerve is relieved.

Internal sources are used in low doses to diagnose and treat various conditions. ^{131}I and ^{125}I are used to tag other substances to determine their absorption, distribution, or excretion. They are particularly helpful in diagnosis of thyroid disease because of the ability of the thyroid gland to capture and concentrate iodine from the blood. Higher concentrations may be used to treat tumors of the thyroid gland. Further information on radioactive iodine is available in Chapter 59.

^{32}P is used to treat leukemia and polycythemia vera. ^{198}Au is not used often because of its cost. It is injected into a cavity, where its particles are confined because they are not absorbed into the blood to any great extent.

Adverse effects of internal radiation include nausea, vomiting, and blood dyscrasias (such as leukopenia, anemia, and thrombocytopenia). In addition, radioactive implants may cause irritation and sloughing of tissues surrounding the implant.

External radiation may cause redness and drying of the skin at the site being irradiated.

All forms of radiation may cause teratogenic effects on the ova, sperm, embryo, or fetus.

ASSESSMENT Perform a cephalocaudal assessment, including vital signs and weight; document findings as baseline data. Assess the patient's chart for the complete blood count (CBC) and results of any other laboratory tests, x-ray studies, or special diagnostic procedures that may have been ordered. To anticipate and prevent complications, caregivers should be aware of laboratory results. If the patient is of childbearing age, inquire about the possibility of pregnancy.

PLANNING AND IMPLEMENTATION Alpha, beta, and gamma rays are major types of charged particles that cause chemical reactions in the matter through which they pass. These reactions can occur in the patient and caregiver alike, so there are vital facts that the caregiver needs to know about the element or isotope to protect self and others from the harmful effects of the radiation. The three main factors to consider in thinking of protection are *time, distance, and shielding.*

The radiologist and others in the nuclear medicine department determine the amount of time the patient needs to be exposed to the material. This varies with diagnostic and treatment procedures. Members of that department also determine the maximal amount of time a caregiver may be exposed and still avoid potential injury. Caregivers need to use their organizational skills to provide required care in a minimal amount of time. Cooperation and teamwork are required of personnel to limit the amount of time any one person is exposed to the source.

The nuclear medicine department issues special badges to be worn whenever a caregiver is in the vicinity of radioactive material. These badges are used to monitor the amount of radiation exposure incurred by the person wearing the badge. By monitoring the badges, the nuclear medicine department can notify a caregiver if radiation exposure is approaching a caution level. Specific instructions are given at that time. To maintain accurate monitoring of exposure levels, badges must never be borrowed from another.

Protocols determined by the nuclear medicine department indicate the distance the patient is to be placed from an external source of radiation to receive adequate exposure for treatment. Caregivers should always minimize the dose they receive by staying as far away from the source as possible.

Lead is the best shield for radioactive rays. Machines that contain radioactive sources have lead enclosures around the source. When external radiation is to be used, special marks or tattoos are placed on the skin to designate the exact area to be treated. These are to remain on the skin until treatment is completed to ensure irradiation of the same area with each treatment. Healthy tissue surrounding a tumor is often protected from radiation by the use of lead blocks that have been melted and molded into a specific shape for each patient. Treatment rooms in the x-ray and nuclear medicine departments have lead linings in the walls and doors. Technicians and therapists wear lead-lined aprons to protect themselves. Special procedures may be performed behind lead shields.

Women of childbearing age who require diagnostic x-ray testing should have the gonads protected with lead shielding. Men of childbearing age should also protect the gonads by lead shielding. Women who are pregnant should avoid exposure to therapeutic doses of radiation at all times.

The first day that the patient receives external radiation treatment is time-consuming because of the examinations, marking of the area, and measuring for blockers. Anticipate that the patient may need to rest after treatment. Offer liquids and a light snack with a meal after the rest period.

Patients receiving external radiation are permitted to shower or bathe but should avoid soaps, lotions, powders, and colognes on the area being irradiated because these may irritate the skin. Those products that have a metallic base may alter the direction of the radioactive rays. Do not expose treated areas to direct sunlight because the skin may burn easily. Even after treatments are completed, irradiated areas of skin need to be protected from sunlight.

Irradiated areas will have a temporary hair loss.

Other areas of the body will not lose hair. If the head is to be treated, a wig, hat, or scarf may be desired by the patient.

Anemia and leukopenia are common for all patients receiving radiation. Encourage nutrition from the basic food groups. Encourage small, frequent meals and protein supplements if the patient has a poor appetite. Encourage or provide basic hygiene measures for the patient to prevent infection. Caregivers must use appropriate handwashing and aseptic technique. Those with infections should not be in the patient's room.

When radioactive isotopes have been ingested, any excreta may be radioactive. In addition to the blood and body fluid precautions used with all patients, the nuclear medicine department should provide specific instructions for disposal of emesis, urine, and other excrement and any items that may have been soiled with them.

When radioactive implants are used, specific instructions should be provided about position of the patient.

Women with vaginal implants will have a Foley catheter in place to minimize the irradiation of the bladder and to prevent a distended bladder. Considerable discomfort may be experienced from the weight of the implant, the applicator holding it in place, and the packing that secures it in place. Analgesics should be offered as ordered by the physician.

Pregnant women and young children are not permitted to visit patients with implants or those who have ingested isotopes. Caregivers should use lead shielding appropriate for their activities and should follow guidelines from the nuclear medicine department about the time of exposure and the distance to remain from the patient. These patients are cared for in private rooms with lead doors and walls to prevent exposure of other patients.

Offer emotional support for patients. They may be depressed because of the diagnosis, the isolation and limited visitors, or the lack of energy accompanying the adverse effects of treatment.

EVALUATION Assess patients and compare findings ▲▲▲▲▲▲▲▲▲▲ with baseline documentations. Monitor laboratory values and report abnormalities. External radiation treatments may be suspended for several days or discontinued if the blood counts drop too low. Monitor the results of x-rays, scans, and other tests to be aware of the patient's progress.

E X E R C I S E S

CASE STUDY

Ms. J.G. had surgery last month to remove a malignant ovarian tumor. Currently, she is receiving daily radiation treatments in the nuclear medicine department. She seems anxious and withdrawn. She has asked her family not to visit, telling them it is better if they just phone to comfort her. When you approach her today to assist with her bath, she asks whether you are worried about being in the room with her for such an extended time. Discuss your impressions of her actions and your methods of attempting to verify your impressions. Prepare a teaching plan for Ms. J.G. that will correct her misconceptions and offer emotional support for her.

LEARNING ACTIVITIES

Accompany one of your patients to the nuclear medicine department for radiation treatment. Observe as the patient is positioned. Note the use of markings or tattoos to identify the area. Note the use of blockers. Indicate the length of time the patient is treated. Discuss the treatment with the patient. Indicate the patient's version of what is being done. How many treatments will be done for this patient's therapy? Is the patient experiencing any side effects? Are any anticipated? Share your report with the class.

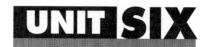
DRUGS THAT AFFECT THE MUSCULOSKELETAL SYSTEM

The musculoskeletal system is actually two separate systems that work together intricately: the muscles, including tendons and ligaments, and the bones, including joints.

There are three different types of muscle tissue: cardiac, smooth, and skeletal. Drugs addressed in Chapter 29 primarily affect skeletal muscles. The cells of a muscle are also referred to as muscle fibers. Movement of the muscle on the whole depends on the contraction of muscle fibers. Contraction of muscle fibers depends on the brain, primarily the cerebrum and cerebellum.

For the human body to remain in an upright position with proper posture, the muscles must be slightly contracted at all times. This slight contraction is called muscle tone. For a muscle to have tone, it must be capable of polarization and depolarization. This is the process by which an electrical impulse is generated and produces movement. For this electrical impulse to be generated within the muscle, a nerve impulse must stimulate the muscle. The origin of the nerve impulse is the brain. From the brain, the nerve impulse passes along neurons, or nerve fibers. It passes from one neuron to another by crossing a synapse. The synapse is a small space between the end processes (axons) of one neuron and the beginning processes (dendrites) of another. A special chemical, called a neurotransmitter, carries the nerve impulse across this space (Fig. VI–1). The main chemicals involved in this process are acetylcholine, acetylcholinesterase, epinephrine, and norepinephrine. See Unit VII for more information on these neurotransmitters.

The drugs we focus on in Chapters 27 and 28 deal with diseases of the joints. A joint may be referred to as an articulation; the ends of the bones involved in the joint are the articular surfaces. Covering the articular surfaces is articular cartilage. The space between the two bones is the joint cavity. The joint cavity is encapsulated by the joint capsule. The capsule is lined with synovial membrane and filled with synovial fluid, both of which promote the smooth movement of the joint by decreasing friction (Fig. VI–2).

The diseases of the joints are forms of arthritis. There are many different types of arthritis. The most common type found in the aging population is osteoarthritis, a degenerative disease that causes destruction of the bone and joint from constant wear and tear. It does not involve any inflammation, but it does involve pain, stiffness, and limitation of movement.

Another common type of arthritis is rheumatoid arthritis. There are actually numerous forms of rheumatoid arthritis. Rheumatoid arthritis may be found in patients of any age, although a peak occurrence is found between the ages of 20 and 50 years. All the types of rheumatoid arthritis involve inflammation. Often the joints are swollen, red, tender, and warm. There is considerable pain and limitation of movement. The patient may experience fatigue, muscle stiffness (especially in the morning), muscle atrophy, and eventual ankylosis (permanent fusion of the joint). In the progression of the disease within the joint, rheumatoid arthritis begins with synovitis, an inflammatory process of the synovium (synovial membrane) and the synovial fluid. The synovitis allows the formation of overgrowth tissue called pannus. The pannus invades the entire joint space and surrounding bone. The pannus eventually converts to scar tissue, and the joint becomes stiff. When the scar tissue is replaced with bony tissue, this is called ankylosis (Fig. VI–3).

Another type of arthritis is gouty arthritis, often simply referred to as gout. This type of arthritis is brought on by an increase in the amount of circulating serum uric acid. Uric acid is a by-product of the metabolism of purine, which is contained in certain foods, such as oatmeal, red meats, glandular meats, tomatoes, alcohol, shellfish, mushrooms, peas, spinach, and fatty foods. As you can see, it would be difficult for a patient to simply look at a food and know it has purines in it. The patient must be taught which foods are high in this element.

When uric acid is elevated in the bloodstream, it accumulates and deposits as crystals in tissues, including joints. An exacerbation of gouty arthritis

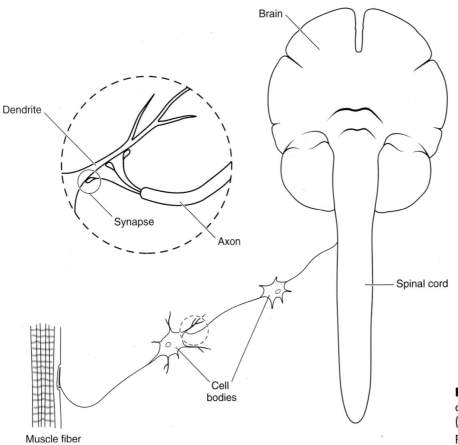

Figure VI–1. A neurotransmitter carries a nerve impulse from the end processes (axons) of one neuron to the beginning processes (dendrites) of another.

Figure VI–2. A normal joint or articulation.

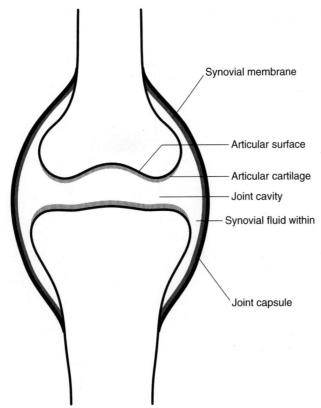

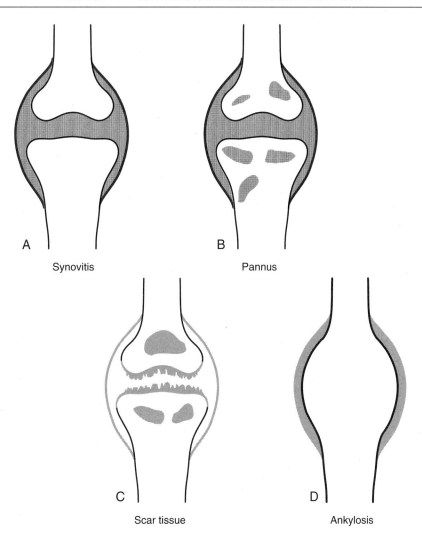

Figure VI–3. The four stages of rheumatoid arthritis. *A.* Synovitis is an inflammatory process of the synovium (synovial membrane) and the synovial fluid. *B.* Pannus is the formation of overgrowth tissue resulting from synovitis. *C.* The pannus eventually converts to scar tissue, and the joint becomes stiff. *D.* Ankylosis occurs when the scar tissue is replaced by bony tissue.

includes severe pain of one or more joints, swelling, redness, and warmth. The patient often has a systemic temperature of 101° to 103°F and may have albumin in the urine. Tophi, the accumulation of the crystals under the surface of the skin, may also be present.

Another problem for which the physician may prescribe these drugs is bursitis. Bursitis is inflammation of the bursa, a small enclosed space found in some joints. This space is lined with synovium and contains a small amount of synovial fluid, which helps promote joint movement by decreasing friction. Bursitis can arise when the bursa is infected, traumatized, or overused or when calcium or lime deposits accumulate. The patient experiences pain aggravated by movement. This pain is also aggravated by warmth as the synovium and synovial fluid swell. The shoulder and knee are the most common sites for bursitis.

With this overview of these common disorders, we are now ready to look at the medications that may be prescribed for each problem.

ANTIRHEUMATIC DRUGS

LEARNING OBJECTIVES

After studying this chapter, you should be able to:

1. Define antirheumatic, analgesic, anti-inflammatory, and antipyretic.

2. Identify the uses of salicylates as an antirheumatic.

3. Identify symptoms of salicylism and other adverse reactions to salicylates.

4. State appropriate patient teaching for patients receiving a salicylate.

5. Demonstrate how to administer salicylates by use of the nursing process.

6. Identify uses of pyrazolone derivatives.

7. Identify adverse reactions to pyrazolone derivatives.

8. State appropriate patient teaching for patients receiving a pyrazolone derivative.

9. Demonstrate how to administer pyrazolone derivatives by use of the nursing process.

10. Define NSAIDs and steroids.

11. Identify uses of and adverse reactions to the NSAIDs and steroids.

12. State types and common examples of NSAIDs and steroids.

13. State appropriate patient teaching for patients receiving NSAIDs and steroids.

14. Demonstrate how to administer NSAIDs and steroids by use of the nursing process.

15. Define immunosuppressives.

16. State uses of penicillamine, Plaquenil, and the gold salts.

17. Identify nursing implications of the miscellaneous drugs and the immunosuppressives.

DRUGS YOU WILL LEARN ABOUT IN THIS CHAPTER

Salicylates

aspirin or acetylsalicylic acid (ASA, ZORprin, Ecotrin, Bufferin)

salsalate (Disalcid, Mono-Gesic, Salflex)

choline magnesium trisalicylate (Trilisate)

Pyrazolone Derivatives

phenylbutazone

Nonsteroidal Anti-inflammatory Drugs (NSAIDs)

Propionic acid derivatives

ibuprofen (Advil, Motrin, Nuprin, Rufen)

flurbiprofen (Ansaid)

ketoprofen (Orudis)

fenoprofen calcium (Nalfon)

naproxen (Anaprox, Naprosyn, Aleve)

Other NSAIDs

indomethacin (Indocin)

sulindac (Clinoril)

diflunisal (Dolobid)

piroxicam (Feldene)

meclofenamate sodium (Meclomen)

diclofenac sodium (Voltaren)

tolmetin sodium (Tolectin)

ketorolac tromethamine (Toradol)

Steroids

cortisone (Cortone)

hydrocortisone (Cortef, Solu-Cortef)

prednisone (Deltasone)

prednisolone (Hydeltrasol)

methylprednisolone (Depo-Medrol, Medrol, Solu-Medrol)

triamcinolone (Aristocort, Kenalog)

betamethasone (Celestone, Valisone)

dexamethasone (Decadron)

Immunosuppressives

methotrexate (Rheumatrex)

cyclophosphamide (Cytoxan)

azathioprine (Imuran)

Gold Salts

gold sodium thiomalate (Myochrysine)

aurothioglucose (Solganal)

auranofin (Ridaura)

Miscellaneous Drugs

penicillamine (Cuprimine)

hydroxychloroquine sulfate (Plaquenil)

Antirheumatic drugs are used to treat rheumatoid conditions. Many are also used for osteoarthritis and other joint diseases. They are divided into several subclasses: salicylates, pyrazolone derivatives, non-steroidal anti-inflammatory drugs (NSAIDs), steroids, immunosuppressives, gold salts, and miscellaneous drugs.

SALICYLATES

ACTIONS AND USES Salicylates are used to treat joint ▲▲▲▲▲▲▲▲▲▲▲▲▲▲ diseases because of their three main properties: anti-inflammation, antipyresis, and analgesia. The salicylates relieve the pain of the joint diseases temporarily, decrease the warmth around a joint, decrease a systemic temperature, and reduce inflammation. They may delay the crippling effects of these diseases, but they are *not* a cure.

Salicylates may also be used for other conditions, such as headache, muscle aches, menstrual pain, and toothaches. They reduce the risk of a transient ischemic attack (TIA) or stroke.

Salicylates can cause gastrointestinal (GI) reactions, including nausea and vomiting, epigastric burning (or heartburn), and GI bleeding. They may also lead to easy bruising and bleeding.

N U R S I N G   A L E R T
▼▼▼▼▼▼▼▼▼▼▼▼▼▼▼▼▼▼▼▼▼▼▼▼▼▼▼▼▼▼▼▼

Salicylates have been known to cause asthmatic attacks in susceptible persons.

Be alert to the symptoms of salicylism, which is an overdose of salicylate. The most common symptom and often the first to appear is tinnitus. If ringing in the ears or dizziness does develop, discontinue the drug and notify the physician.

▲▲▲▲▲▲▲▲▲▲▲▲▲▲▲▲▲▲▲▲▲▲▲▲▲▲▲▲▲▲▲▲

The patient may also experience tachycardia, hyperventilation, headache, fever, dehydration, sweating, drowsiness, vertigo, confusion, electrolyte imbalances, and an altered blood pH.

You may often hear patients tell you that they use acetaminophen because it is less irritating to the stomach. Because acetaminophen does not have any anti-inflammatory properties, it is best to advise the patient to seek medical advice if the patient is taking the drug for an arthritic condition.

ASSESSMENT Before initiation of a salicylate, be famil-
▲▲▲▲▲▲▲▲▲▲ iar with the patient's condition, including location of pain, severity of pain, and presence of inflammation. Also check for any history of renal insufficiency, liver dysfunction, gastritis, or peptic ulcers; these conditions call for extra caution when a salicylate is administered.

N U R S I N G   A L E R T
▼▼▼▼▼▼▼▼▼▼▼▼▼▼▼▼▼▼▼▼▼▼▼▼▼▼▼▼▼▼▼▼

Use caution if the patient is younger than 12 years. Children or teens who have a viral infection, especially chickenpox or the flu, are at special risk for the development of Reye's syndrome.

▲▲▲▲▲▲▲▲▲▲▲▲▲▲▲▲▲▲▲▲▲▲▲▲▲▲▲▲▲▲▲▲

If the patient has a toothache, advise the patient to seek the attention of a dentist. If the patient experiences pain or inflammation that lasts more than 10 days, a physician should be consulted.

PLANNING AND IMPLEMENTATION Because of the high ▲▲▲▲▲▲▲▲▲▲▲▲▲▲▲▲▲▲▲▲▲▲▲▲▲▲▲▲▲▲▲ risk of GI disturbance, the patient may wish to take this drug with meals. Instruct the patient to report any symptoms of GI bleeding, such as dyspepsia or black tarry stools.

Teach your patient the signs and symptoms of salicylism. Caution that the drug must be stopped immediately and the physician informed. Other symptoms that should be reported to the physician include easy bruising, flare-ups of the arthritic symptoms, or anything unusual. It is possible that the dose may need to be adjusted or a different drug prescribed.

EVALUATION Evaluation of the effectiveness of these ▲▲▲▲▲▲▲▲▲▲ drugs is accomplished by comparing the level of symptoms with the baseline report. Note level of pain, ability to perform range of motion, and amount of inflammation. Use the patient's report of these as your guide.

Salicylates interact with numerous drugs. When salicylates are used together, the effects of both drugs are increased. The effects of the salicylate are decreased when it is used with corticosteroids. The effects of the other drug are increased, sometimes to the point of toxicity, if salicylates are used with anticoagulants, oral hypoglycemics, penicillin, thyroxine, thiopental, phenytoin, valproic acid, carbonic anhydrase inhibitor diuretics, sulfapyrazole, naproxen, warfarin, steroids, or methotrexate (Box 27–1).

Aspirin or Acetylsalicylic Acid

Aspirin (ASA, ZORprin, Ecotrin, Bufferin) is one of the most commonly used over-the-counter drugs, yet medical science is only now beginning to realize the vast uses possible for this drug. It is not a miracle drug, but research has shown it to be possibly effective in many different conditions.

There are numerous brand name and generic aspirin products on the market. Encourage the patient to read the label carefully to determine the presence of other products. Bufferin, for example, is aspirin with calcium carbonate, magnesium oxide, and magnesium carbonate. These additives buffer the effects of the aspirin on the GI system, thus decreasing the risk of GI distress.

Ecotrin is an enteric coated aspirin. This prevents the aspirin from being absorbed by the lining of the

---

Box 27–1. Drug Interactions with Salicylates

Increased effects of both drugs
Other salicylates

Decreased effects of salicylates
Corticosteroids

Possible drug toxicity of other drug
Anticoagulants
Penicillin
Thiopental
Valproic acid
Naproxen
Steroids
Carbonic anhydrase inhibitor diuretics
Oral hypoglycemics
Thyroxine
Phenytoin
Sulfapyrazole
Warfarin
Methotrexate

---

stomach and therefore decreases the risk of GI distress.

ZORprin is aspirin, but it is a slightly larger dose than most other aspirin products. Most commonly, aspirin comes in 300- to 325-mg tablets or occasionally as 650-mg tablets. ZORprin tablets are 800 mg.

The average dose recommended for this salicylate is 600 to 650 mg every 4 hours. No more than 3600 to 3900 mg should be taken in a 24-hour period.

Salsalate

ACTIONS AND USES Salsalate (Mono-Gesic, Salflex, ▲▲▲▲▲▲▲▲▲▲▲▲▲▲▲▲ Disalcid) is used for many of the same conditions as aspirin is. It does not cause bleeding tendencies or asthmatic attacks as other salicylates can. However, it is associated with Reye's syndrome in children.

ASSESSMENT If a patient is allergic to aspirin, the ▲▲▲▲▲▲▲▲▲▲ patient will be allergic to salsalate. The use of this product is contraindicated in such patients. It is also contraindicated in pregnant women or nursing mothers. Specifically ask about these conditions.

PLANNING AND IMPLEMENTATION The dose of salsalate ▲▲▲▲▲▲▲▲▲▲▲▲▲▲▲▲▲▲▲▲▲▲▲▲▲▲▲▲▲▲▲ is individualized but, in general, is 3000 mg per day in divided doses. Monitor serum levels of salicylic acid. The therapeutic range is 10 to 30 mg per 100 mL.

N U R S I N G   A L E R T

Salsalate toxicity is increased if the patient eats or drinks large amounts of acidifying foods or medications. Alkalinizing foods or medications decrease the effectiveness of salsalate.

EVALUATION The effectiveness of the drug is determined by noting presence or absence of symptoms.

Choline Magnesium Trisalicylate

Choline magnesium trisalicylate (Trilisate) is absorbed by the body as salicylate; therefore, all information about the salicylates also applies to this drug. However, it is not associated with bleeding tendencies. There is less risk of interaction with anticoagulants.

The usual dose of choline magnesium trisalicylate is 1500 mg twice a day or 3000 mg once a day. The therapeutic blood levels are 15 to 30 mg per 100 mL.

Acidifying and alkalinizing agents of foods affect trisalicylate the same as they do salsalate.

PYRAZOLONE DERIVATIVES

Pyrazolone derivatives are toxic to the body. The main example still in use is phenylbutazone.

Phenylbutazone

ACTIONS AND USES Phenylbutazone shares the three properties of the salicylates: anti-inflammation, antipyresis, and analgesia. It is also a mild uricosuric (see Chapter 28). Phenylbutazone is used to treat the symptoms of all types of arthritis and acute gout. It is recommended for use only after other medications have been tried but failed because of its high risk of agranulocytosis and aplastic anemia.

N U R S I N G   A L E R T

Blood dyscrasias, a fairly common side effect of phenylbutazone, are more likely to occur in the elderly and in women. These dyscrasias can be fatal.

Other side effects can be serious also. Hepatitis, renal necrosis, gastrointestinal (GI) bleeding, and ulceration have been reported from this drug. Some of the milder reactions include edema, rash, nausea and vomiting, increased value of liver function tests, and asthma attacks in asthmatic patients.

ASSESSMENT Because of the wide variety of adverse reactions possible to phenylbutazone, be aware of the patient's condition and history. Know what condition the drug is prescribed for and what drugs were used previously. What symptoms is the patient experiencing?

N U R S I N G   A L E R T

Check the chart and ask the patient whether there is any history of bronchospasms, especially those brought on by taking aspirin or other antirheumatic drugs.

Check laboratory values for any blood dyscrasias, kidney disease, or liver disease. Ask the patient whether there is a history of cardiac failure, pancreatitis, parotitis, stomatitis, GI ulcerations, or inflammatory conditions.

PLANNING AND IMPLEMENTATION Phenylbutazone is available as tablets or capsules and is taken orally. The usual dose is 100 to 200 mg daily after a "loading dose" of a larger amount has been administered. Caution the patient to take this drug with milk or meals.

Teach the patient to discontinue the drug immediately and inform the physician if symptoms of a blood dyscrasia develop. These include fever, sore throat, or lesions in the mouth. The same action is called for in the event of symptoms of GI ulceration, such as dyspepsia, anemia, GI bleeding, or black tarry stools. The patient should also inform the physician right away in the event of a skin rash, weight gain, or other signs of edema.

EVALUATION Effectiveness of this drug is determined by decreased symptoms.

N U R S I N G   A L E R T

Also check frequently, however, for any symptoms of toxic effects. These include any GI upset or bleeding or a change in level of consciousness, including restlessness, dizziness, hallucinations, seizures, or coma. Vital signs may be altered and electrolyte levels impaired. The patient may become cyanotic and experience respiratory arrest. Kidney failure, liver failure, and blood dyscrasias are also considered signs of toxic effects.

If the patient does not experience significant reduction in the baseline symptoms, the physician should discontinue the drug.

Phenylbutazone interacts with many drugs. Evaluate for changes in the effectiveness of the drug. The effects of the other drug may be enhanced to the point of toxicity if phenylbutazone is used with nonsteroidal anti-inflammatory drugs, anticoagulants, oral hypoglycemics or insulin, sulfonamides, lithium, valproate, phenytoin, or methotrexate. The effects of the other drug are decreased if phenylbutazone is used with digitoxin or cortisone products. The effects of phenylbutazone are decreased if it is used with barbiturates, promethazine, chlorpheniramine, rifampin, or corticosteroids (Box 27–2).

Box 27–2. Drug Interactions with Phenylbutazone

Toxicity of other drug
Nonsteroidal anti-inflammatory drugs (NSAIDs)
Oral hypoglycemics
Insulin
Valproate
Methotrexate
Anticoagulants
Sulfonamides
Lithium
Phenytoin

Decreased effects of other drug
Digitoxin
Cortisone products

Effects of phenylbutazone decreased
Barbiturates
Chlorpheniramine
Corticosteroids
Promethazine
Rifampin

NONSTEROIDAL ANTI-INFLAMMATORY DRUGS

ACTIONS AND USES Nonsteroidal anti-inflammatory drugs (NSAIDs) are anti-inflammatory, antipyretic, and analgesic, just as the salicylates are. The NSAIDs are also used for osteoarthritis, rheumatoid conditions, and other joint conditions.

NSAIDs can produce side effects. Gastrointestinal (GI) disturbances, such as nausea, vomiting, constipation, abdominal pain, and even GI bleeding, are common events. Other side effects often seen are central nervous system effects, like nervousness, dizziness, tinnitus, and changes in vision (such as blurriness or dimness). Some patients may complain of headache, rhinitis, rash, edema, or even urinary tract infections.

ASSESSMENT Be familiar with the patient and the condition for which the drug is prescribed. What symptoms does this patient have and to what degree? Ask about pain, especially pain on movement, and ability to perform range of motion before the first dose of the medication. If the drug is being used for its antipyretic property, take a baseline temperature.

Ask the patient and check the file for history of conditions that would put the patient at a higher risk for complications. These include liver and kidney dysfunction; cardiac dysfunction; hypertension; anemia; and GI bleeding, ulceration, and perforation.

N U R S I N G   A L E R T

If bronchospasms have ever been precipitated in the patient by taking aspirin or some other NSAID, the patient is at risk for development of bronchospasms from this drug as well.

Assess the patient for any signs or symptoms of infection. The actions of this drug may mask symptoms of an infection after the drug is started.

Monitor laboratory work reports for clotting times because NSAIDs can affect these adversely.

PLANNING AND IMPLEMENTATION NSAIDs should be given 30 to 60 minutes before or 2 hours after meals to promote the best absorption. Encourage the patient to take the drug with at least 8 ounces of water to decrease GI upset. Even with this precaution, it may be necessary to give the drug with food or milk, or the physician may order it to be given with an antacid. Advise the patient to remain sitting or standing upright for at least 30 minutes after the medication is taken. Lying down may increase GI disturbances.

Institute appropriate safety precautions to protect the patient in case of dizziness or drowsiness. These include walking with the patient, having the patient dangle before getting up, and cautioning the patient not to drive or operate hazardous machinery after returning home. It may be possible to lift these precautions after it is noted how an individual patient responds to the drug. Remember, adverse reactions can occur at any time.

Teach your patient not to mix this drug with any other substance without asking the physician. Of particular importance are alcohol, aspirin, and acetaminophen. Each of these can increase the frequency of side effects. Prolonged use of an NSAID with acetaminophen, for example, may cause renal dysfunction.

If the physician prescribes an NSAID to be given with a narcotic analgesic, monitor the patient's response to this combination carefully. It may be possible for the physician to lower the dosage of the narcotic because of the additive effect.

Advise the patient to tell a surgeon or dentist about therapy with this type of drug before any invasive treatment is done, such as surgery, root canal surgery, or tooth extraction.

EVALUATION Effectiveness of this drug is determined ▲▲▲▲▲▲▲▲▲▲ by improvement of the symptoms with which the patient presented. Once again, ask the patient about pain and assess the ability to perform range of motion. Take the temperature.

N U R S I N G   A L E R T
▼▼▼▼▼▼▼▼▼▼▼▼▼▼▼▼▼▼▼▼▼▼▼▼▼▼▼▼▼▼▼▼

Be especially alert to any signs of infection, even minor or subtle ones. Remember, NSAIDs can mask these symptoms.

▲▲▲▲▲▲▲▲▲▲▲▲▲▲▲▲▲▲▲▲▲▲▲▲▲▲▲▲▲▲▲▲

Check for any interactions with other drugs. It is to be expected that NSAIDs will interact with anticoagulants. The result is usually an increased tendency to bleed. The concomitant use of NSAIDs with aspirin decreases the effects of the NSAID and therefore is discouraged. The effects of certain diuretics are also decreased. The effects of propranolol are increased.

Propionic Acid Derivatives

Ibuprofen

Ibuprofen (Motrin, Advil, Nuprin, Rufen) is one of the most commonly prescribed NSAIDs. It may also be used for mild to moderate pain or primary dysmenorrhea.

Caution is used if visual disturbances develop.

N U R S I N G   A L E R T
▼▼▼▼▼▼▼▼▼▼▼▼▼▼▼▼▼▼▼▼▼▼▼▼▼▼▼▼▼▼▼▼

Ibuprofen should be discontinued if the patient experiences blurred or diminished vision, changes in color vision, or a decrease in the central portion of the vision.

▲▲▲▲▲▲▲▲▲▲▲▲▲▲▲▲▲▲▲▲▲▲▲▲▲▲▲▲▲▲▲▲

Ibuprofen is given orally. The usual dose is 1200 to 3200 mg per day in divided doses.

In addition to interactions common to NSAIDs in general, be alert for increased chances of toxic effects of methotrexate or lithium.

Flurbiprofen

Flurbiprofen (Ansaid) is available as tablets. The usual dose is 200 to 300 mg per day in divided doses. Information listed under NSAIDs pertains to flurbiprofen.

Ketoprofen

Ketoprofen (Orudis) is also used for mild to moderate pain and for primary dysmenorrhea. It is given in capsule form orally, 150 to 300 mg per day in three or four divided doses. Encourage the patient to take the medication with food or milk, or the physician may order it to be given with an antacid.

In addition to interactions common to NSAIDs in general, note possible electrolyte imbalances and increased risk of renal dysfunction when ketoprofen is used with hydrochlorothiazide, a diuretic. The effects of ketoprofen are decreased when it is used with probenecid, an antigout agent. Ketoprofen may cause toxic effects when it is used with methotrexate or lithium.

Fenoprofen Calcium

Fenoprofen calcium (Nalfon) is given 200 to 600 mg four times a day average. Full therapeutic benefits may not be seen until the drug has been taken regularly for 2 or 3 weeks, however. Be sure the patient understands the need for patience.

Fenoprofen interacts with phenobarbital, hydantoin, and sulfonamides.

Naproxen

Besides being ordered for joint disorders, like all the NSAIDs, naproxen (Naprosyn, Anaprox, Aleve) is effective against mild to moderate pain and primary dysmenorrhea. It is also useful against acute stages of gouty arthritis. Naproxen is given orally as either tablets or a suspension. The usual dose is 250 to 500 mg twice a day. Once again, you will need to caution the patient that improvement of signs or symptoms of the disorder is not expected for 2 to 4 weeks.

In addition to the interactions common to all NSAIDs, naproxen interacts with propranolol and other beta-blockers, methotrexate, and probenecid.

Other NSAIDs

Indomethacin

Indomethacin (Indocin) is useful for treatment of joint diseases, including gout. However, it is associated with numerous adverse reactions, in addition to those already mentioned for NSAIDs in general. The frequency of these adverse reactions tends to increase with the patient's age.

If the patient experiences blurred vision, report this immediately. It may indicate the development of retinal or corneal changes.

N U R S I N G A L E R T
▼▼▼▼▼▼▼▼▼▼▼▼▼▼▼▼▼▼▼▼▼▼▼▼▼▼▼▼▼▼▼

Indomethacin can cause drowsiness, headache, blood dyscrasias, jaundice, and even fatal hepatitis.

▲▲▲▲▲▲▲▲▲▲▲▲▲▲▲▲▲▲▲▲▲▲▲▲▲▲▲▲▲▲▲

Ask the patient information about his or her medical history. The suppository form of this drug is contraindicated if there is a history of proctitis or rectal bleeding. Depression, epilepsy, and parkinsonism may be aggravated by use of this drug.

Institute safety precautions until the individual patient's reaction to this drug can be determined. Report any of the side effects or symptoms of them because the drug may need to be discontinued.

Indomethacin is available in capsules, suspension, or suppository form. The usual dose is 25 to 50 mg two or three times a day.

In addition to other interactions possible with NSAIDs, indomethacin interacts with probenecid, methotrexate, lithium, some diuretics, and antihypertensives.

Sulindac

Sulindac (Clinoril) is useful in treatment of joint diseases, including gout. Given orally, sulindac is generally kept at levels below 400 mg per day.

Sulindac does not have the same interactions as other NSAIDs do. In fact, it has only a few in common. The effects of sulindac are decreased if the patient takes it with aspirin. The effects of sulindac are increased if it is taken with probenecid. The effects of methotrexate may become toxic if it is taken with sulindac.

Diflunisal

Much of the information presented under the general classification of NSAIDs applies to diflunisal (Dolobid). It is given orally, usually at a dose of 500 mg every 8 to 12 hours. Often, a "loading" dose, or a dose larger than subsequent doses, is given.

In addition to those interactions listed previously, diflunisal also affects the actions of antacids, acetaminophen, methotrexate, and indomethacin.

Piroxicam

Piroxicam (Feldene) acts and reacts in much the same way as other NSAIDs do, but it is also capable of producing other adverse reactions.

N U R S I N G A L E R T
▼▼▼▼▼▼▼▼▼▼▼▼▼▼▼▼▼▼▼▼▼▼▼▼▼▼▼▼▼▼▼

Piroxicam has been associated with jaundice and even fatal hepatitis.

▲▲▲▲▲▲▲▲▲▲▲▲▲▲▲▲▲▲▲▲▲▲▲▲▲▲▲▲▲▲▲

Bleeding tendencies and GI bleeding are also known to occur with some frequency.

Piroxicam is given in capsule form, generally 20 mg every day.

Meclofenamate Sodium

Meclofenamate sodium (Meclomen) is also associated with additional adverse reactions: GI disturbances (such as nausea, vomiting, and diarrhea), fever, and rash. The drug is given orally, 50 to 100 mg every 4 to 6 hours.

Meclofenamate is not associated with the same interactions of the other NSAIDs. It is known to react with warfarin by increasing bleeding tendencies. The effectiveness of this drug is decreased if it is given with aspirin.

Diclofenac Sodium

Diclofenac sodium (Voltaren) causes less risk of GI bleeding than salicylates or other NSAIDs do, but the possibility still exists. It is an enteric coated tablet, which may account for this fact.

N U R S I N G   A L E R T
▼▼▼▼▼▼▼▼▼▼▼▼▼▼▼▼▼▼▼▼▼▼▼▼▼▼▼▼▼▼▼▼

The nurse cannot encourage the use of diclofenac with food or milk, without special instruction from the physician, because this greatly delays the absorption of this drug.

▲▲▲▲▲▲▲▲▲▲▲▲▲▲▲▲▲▲▲▲▲▲▲▲▲▲▲▲▲▲▲▲

The usual dosage is 50 to 75 mg two or three times a day.

Diclofenac may cause hyperkalemia if it is given with potassium-sparing diuretics. Toxicity is more likely to develop with use of digitoxin, methotrexate, cyclosporine, and lithium. Aspirin decreases the effects of diclofenac.

Tolmetin Sodium

N U R S I N G   A L E R T
▼▼▼▼▼▼▼▼▼▼▼▼▼▼▼▼▼▼▼▼▼▼▼▼▼▼▼▼▼▼▼▼

Tolmetin sodium (Tolectin) may cause jaundice and fatal hepatitis. Carefully monitor liver function test reports. Tolmetin can also cause visual disturbances. Report these immediately. Caution the patient to

have frequent eye examinations throughout tolmetin therapy.

▲▲

Inform the patient that therapeutic response of signs or symptoms of the disorder is not expected for a few days to a week.

The usual dose for this oral drug is 200 to 600 mg three times a day. If the patient experiences gastric upset, ask the physician if it may be given with food or milk. This will decrease the absorption to some degree. It is preferable that the physician order it to be given with an antacid, because antacids do not decrease the absorption or effectiveness of this drug.

In addition to interactions listed for all NSAIDs, tolmetin can also increase the chances of toxic reaction to methotrexate.

Ketorolac Tromethamine

Although ketorolac tromethamine (Toradol) shares the same properties of the other NSAIDs, its analgesic property is of special interest. Compared with meperidine and morphine, 30 or 90 mg of ketorolac produces the equivalent pain relief of 100 mg of meperidine or 12 mg of morphine; 10 mg of ketorolac is equivalent to 50 mg of meperidine or 6 mg of morphine. The duration of pain relief from ketorolac is longer than that from either of these narcotic analgesics. Ketorolac also causes less drowsiness and less nausea or vomiting than the two narcotics do.

Ketorolac is prescribed by the physician for short-term pain relief only. It is given intramuscularly. It should not be given with other NSAIDs, however, because adverse reactions are more likely. The effects of ketorolac are diminished if the patient also takes aspirin.

STEROIDS

ACTIONS AND USES Steroidal drugs suppress inflam-
▲▲▲▲▲▲▲▲▲▲▲▲▲▲▲▲▲ mation and therefore are useful in the treatment of joint diseases, but steroids affect the body as a whole. The endocrine and immune systems are dramatically affected by any steroidal drug.

Because of the many effects, steroids can be used for many other diseases or conditions besides joint disorders. Steroids may be used for

• Endocrine disorders, such as adrenocortical insufficiency

- Collagen diseases, such as systemic lupus erythematosus
- Dermatological diseases, such as dermatitis or psoriasis
  - Allergic states like asthma or drug allergies
  - Ophthalmic diseases, such as optic neuritis

Steroids may be ordered for treatment of gastrointestinal (GI) diseases, such as ulcerative colitis, but extreme caution is warranted because there is an increased risk of GI perforation. These drugs are useful in the treatment of several disorders (Box 27–3):

- Respiratory diseases, such as sarcoidosis or pneumonitis
- Hematological diseases, such as hemolytic anemia or leukemias
  - Nephrotic syndrome
  - Multiple sclerosis

When a patient is receiving a steroid, it is possible that adrenal suppression will occur, especially with long-term therapy.

N U R S I N G   A L E R T

If the patient is a child, adrenal suppression may even lead to growth declines or cessation.

Cushingoid syndrome or signs and symptoms of diabetes can occur (Box 27–4). The skin may become

---

Box 27–3. Possible Uses of Steroids

Joint disorders
Systemic lupus erythematosus
Psoriasis
Allergies
Ulcerative colitis
Pneumonitis
Hemolytic anemia
Multiple sclerosis
Adrenocortical insufficiency
Dermatitis
Asthma
Optic neuritis
Sarcoidosis
Nephrotic syndrome
Leukemia
Others

Box 27–4. Symptoms of Cushing's Syndrome

Increased fatty tissue deposits
Fatigue
Weakness
Osteoporosis
Loss of protein tissues
Amenorrhea/impotence
Edema
Skin discolorations and plethora
Abnormal hair growth
Development of diabetes mellitus

---

hyperpigmented or hypopigmented. Menstrual irregularities are common.

N U R S I N G   A L E R T

Effects on the immune system include masking signs and symptoms of infection and decreased resistance to infection.

Reaction to skin testing may also be diminished or absent. Impaired or delayed wound healing occurs. This may also be due to the fragility of the skin and easy bruising from steroid use.

Long-term use of steroids can lead to cataracts, glaucoma, hypertension, and psychic derangement. Hypocalcemia may result from increased serum calcium excretion. Bones become brittle because of osteoporosis, and pathological fractures, such as vertebral compression, may occur. Other fluid and electrolyte imbalances are also possible. Muscle weakness and loss of muscle mass may be related to endocrine or electrolyte effects.

N U R S I N G   A L E R T

Gastrointestinal effects can be mild, such as nausea and vomiting; severe and even fatal effects include peptic ulcer with perforation, pancreatitis, and ulcerative esophagitis.

Central nervous system effects can include headache, vertigo, increased intracranial pressure, or seizures. If signs of these occur, notify the physician, but do *not* discontinue the medication. Steroids must be withdrawn slowly.

N U R S I N G   A L E R T
▼▼▼▼▼▼▼▼▼▼▼▼▼▼▼▼▼▼▼▼▼▼▼▼▼▼▼▼▼▼▼▼▼▼▼▼

Abrupt withdrawal of steroids may lead to adrenal crisis.

▲▲▲

To better compare the relative effectiveness of different cortisone and cortisone-like drugs, a relative potency number is assigned to the drug on the basis of its actions compared with hydrocortisone. Therefore, the relative potency of hydrocortisone is 1. The strength (in milligrams) of the tablet of the different drugs is multiplied by the relative potency. This gives us the equivalent value of the drug. For example, prednisolone has a relative potency of 4 compared with hydrocortisone. The usual tablet strength given is 5 mg. $4 \times 5 = 20$. The equivalent value of prednisolone is 20. If you look at Table 27–1, you will note that most of the steroidal drugs have an equivalent value of 20 or near 20. This means the actions expected from each of these drugs at the given tablet strength are approximately the same. Hydrocortisone 20 mg is approximately equal to prednisolone 5 mg, which is approximately equal to triamcinolone 4 mg.

Dexamethasone 0.75 mg is only slightly less effective than these other drugs. Prednisolone and prednisone are equal in value to one another with equal tablet strengths. Methylprednisolone and triamcinolone are equal in value to one another with equal tablet strengths. Cortisone requires a tablet strength of 25 mg to equal the value of these other drugs.

ASSESSMENT Baseline assessments necessary before
▲▲▲▲▲▲▲▲▲▲▲ establishment of steroid therapy include signs and symptoms of the condition for which the drug is prescribed. Check the height and weight of children. Assess for any symptoms of adrenal insufficiency, such as hypotension, weight loss, nausea or vomiting, lethargy, or confusion.

Look for any signs of a serious infection, especially fungal infections. These conditions contraindicate the use of steroids. One important exception to this is some types of meningitis.

Ask the patient whether there is a history of hypothyroidism or cirrhosis. The effects of steroids are enhanced in such patients.

PLANNING AND IMPLEMENTATION When planning the
▲▲▲▲▲▲▲▲▲▲▲▲▲▲▲▲▲▲▲▲▲▲▲▲▲▲▲▲▲▲▲ best time of day to give a steroid, consider the body's natural cycles. It is best to give steroids in the morning; this is when the body normally secretes glucocorticoids.

Table 27–1. Steroidal Comparisons

DRUG	TABLET STRENGTH		RELATIVE POTENCY		EQUIVALENT VALUE
Cortisone	25　mg	×	0.8	=	20
Hydrocortisone	20　mg	×	1	=	20
Prednisone	5　mg	×	4	=	20
Prednisolone	5　mg	×	4	=	20
Methylprednisolone	4　mg	×	5	=	20
Triamcinolone	4　mg	×	5	=	20
Dexamethasone	0.75 mg	×	25	=	18.75

Data from *Physicians' Desk Reference,* 1991.

Because of the effects of steroids on the GI system, encourage the patient to take them with meals. This decreases the frequency of GI distress. The physician may order the drug to be given with antacids to prevent the formation of GI ulceration.

Teach the patient the signs and symptoms of adrenal insufficiency and caution that these symptoms must be reported to the physician immediately. Also caution the patient not to stop taking the medication abruptly. Steroids must be gradually withdrawn to prevent adrenocortical insufficiency.

During steroid therapy, encourage the patient to eat a diet high in protein, calcium, and potassium but do not encourage high amounts of sodium or carbohydrates.

Teach the patient to report any increased level of stress because this may necessitate an increase of the steroid dosage.

Because of the effect on the immune system, teach the patient to avoid people with contagious diseases, even the common cold. Teach other measures that will promote an adequate immune response, such as staying out of drafts and adequate intake of vitamins and minerals. Caution the patient that live vaccines cannot be received with steroid therapy because the immune response is so altered that the patient may contract the disease.

You will see many diagnostic tests performed periodically while the patient is receiving steroid therapy. Monitor the results of these tests and report abnormalities at once. Common tests ordered can include urinalysis, blood sugar, chest x-ray, daily weight, and daily blood pressure. An upper GI x-ray series may also be ordered if the physician suspects that the patient has an ulceration or is experiencing dyspepsia.

EVALUATION To evaluate the effectiveness of steroid ▲▲▲▲▲▲▲▲▲▲ therapy, continue to monitor signs and symptoms of the patient's condition. Look for evidence of improvement or worsening.

Evaluate for the many side effects of the drug. Include in your observations any signs or symptoms of infection anywhere in the body, signs or symptoms of adrenal insufficiency, and height and weight in children below normal ranges.

Be aware of the possibility of interactions with many drugs. It is known that steroids can increase the frequency of hypokalemia if they are given with amphotericin B, diuretics, or several of the antibiotics from the penicillin group. The dose of either insulin or oral hypoglycemics may need to be increased by the physician as a result of interaction with steroids. The effects of steroids are lessened if they are given with phenytoin (Dilantin, an anticonvulsant), phenobarbital (anticonvulsant, sedative-hypnotic), rifampin (antitubercular), or oral contraceptives.

Cortisone

Cortisone (Cortone) is the drug with which all other steroids are compared. This is not to indicate that it is the best.

Cortisone may be given orally or intramuscularly. The oral dose is generally 25 to 300 mg per day; 20 to 300 mg per day is given intramuscularly. The dose within this range depends on the disease to be treated.

Hydrocortisone

Hydrocortisone (Cortef, Solu-Cortef) is usually used as an emergency drug when it is given intramuscularly or intravenously. The form given by these routes is Solu-Cortef. The initial dose of 100 to 500 mg can be repeated every 2 to 6 hours.

The oral form of hydrocortisone is Cortef. The dose is 10 to 320 mg per day in divided doses.

Prednisone

Prednisone (Deltasone) is available in tablet form and given initially at 5 to 60 mg per day. The level is determined by the disease to be treated. Maintenance doses are individualized.

Prednisolone

Prednisolone (Hydeltrasol) can be given either orally, intramuscularly, or intravenously. The dose is 5 to 60 mg daily in divided doses. Maintenance doses are individualized.

Methylprednisolone

Methylprednisolone is given as Medrol tablets orally at a dose of 4 to 48 mg per day. It is also possible to see doses ordered in excess of 200 mg per day for multiple sclerosis.

Methylprednisolone can be given intramuscularly or intra-articularly as Solu-Medrol or Depo-Medrol. These products should *not* be diluted. The dose for these routes is 4 to 120 mg per day.

The dose of methylprednisolone depends on the disease being treated or the size of the joint affected.

Triamcinolone

Triamcinolone (Aristocort, Kenalog) is available as a suspension for administration by intramuscular, intra-articular, or intrasynovial injection. It is also available as tablets for oral administration. The injectable forms are generally used when oral therapy is not feasible.

Use a 24-gauge needle or larger for this suspension. It is possible for the patient to experience "post-injection flare" after intra-articular administration. This causes arthropathy with pain.

N U R S I N G   A L E R T
▼▼▼▼▼▼▼▼▼▼▼▼▼▼▼▼▼▼▼▼▼▼▼▼▼▼▼▼▼▼

If triamcinolone suspension is accidentally given subcutaneously, the tissue may atrophy.

▲▲▲▲▲▲▲▲▲▲▲▲▲▲▲▲▲▲▲▲▲▲▲▲▲▲▲▲▲▲

Triamcinolone may be diluted with normal saline or sterile water. It may also be diluted by adding equal parts of saline and 1% procaine or another local anesthetic. It may be given full strength. Be sure the order clearly specifies how the physician wants the drug administered. A dilution of triamcinolone may be made up ahead of time and kept for as long as 1 week.

The usual dose of triamcinolone is 3 to 48 mg per day initially. The maintenance dose is then individualized. Average maintenance doses are oral, 40 mg; intramuscular, 40 mg; intra-articular, 25 mg.

Betamethasone

Betamethasone (Celestone, Valisone) is given orally or intramuscularly. Orally, the dose is 0.6 to 7.2 mg a day. Intramuscularly, up to 9 mg may be administered. Betamethasone can also be given intravenously or intra-articularly.

Dexamethasone

Dexamethasone (Decadron) is a synthetic glucocorticoid. It produces almost no sodium retention. It is available as an elixir, tablets, or injectable solution for intravenous, intramuscular, or intra-articular administration. It can also be used ophthalmically, by inhalation, as a topical cream, or as a nasal spray.

The initial oral dose is 0.75 to 9 mg per day. Intramuscular or intravenous doses are 0.5 to 9 mg per day. Each is then individualized to the disease and patient.

IMMUNOSUPPRESSIVES

Immunosuppressives may be used to treat rheumatoid conditions. The theory of their use for this purpose is to reduce the body's autoimmune response to its own tissue. See Chapter 25 for a full discussion of these drugs.

Methotrexate

Methotrexate (Rheumatrex) is an antimetabolite. It is available as tablets or for injection by the intramuscular, intravenous, intra-articular, or intrathecal route.

Cyclophosphamide

Cyclophosphamide (Cytoxan) appears to be related to nitrogen mustard. See Chapter 25 for a full discussion of this drug.

Azathioprine

Azathioprine (Imuran) is an antimetabolite.

N U R S I N G   A L E R T
▼▼▼▼▼▼▼▼▼▼▼▼▼▼▼▼▼▼▼▼▼▼▼▼▼▼▼▼▼▼

Azathioprine is associated with an increased risk of neoplasms and hematological toxic effects.

▲▲▲▲▲▲▲▲▲▲▲▲▲▲▲▲▲▲▲▲▲▲▲▲▲▲▲▲▲▲

Azathioprine is given orally or intravenously.

GOLD SALTS

ACTIONS AND USES The gold salts are expensive, but
▲▲▲▲▲▲▲▲▲▲▲▲▲▲▲▲▲ these drugs appear to suppress the synovitis associated with rheumatoid diseases.

Gold salt drugs are associated with numerous potential adverse reactions. Some of these can be fatal. Adverse reactions most likely to occur include dermatitis, itching, alopecia, loss of the nails, inflammation of the mouth, inflammation of the tongue or gums, metallic taste in the mouth, serious blood dyscrasias, nephrotic syndrome or glomerulitis, gastrointestinal distress, ulcerative enterocolitis (potentially fatal), confusion, hallucinations, and seizures.

ASSESSMENT Before initiating gold salt therapy, the ▲▲▲▲▲▲▲▲▲▲ patient must be thoroughly evaluated for the presence of many diseases. Those that necessitate extreme caution with gold salts include a history of blood dyscrasias, drug allergies, a current skin rash, any kidney or liver disease, marked hypertension, poor circulation of cerebrum or cardiovascular bed, diabetes, or congestive heart failure. Those that preclude the use of gold salts (contraindications) include systemic lupus erythematosus (SLE) and severe debilitation.

PLANNING AND IMPLEMENTATION Before the first dose, ▲▲▲▲▲▲▲▲▲▲▲▲▲▲▲▲▲▲▲▲▲▲▲▲▲ be sure a baseline complete blood count and urinalysis have been obtained. These are necessary for comparison after therapy has begun.

Different gold salt preparations are available for either intramuscular injection or oral administration. These drugs should be given under the careful direction of a physician who is familiar with their use.

EVALUATION Evaluate for the effectiveness of the drug ▲▲▲▲▲▲▲▲▲▲ by evaluating the level of pain, range of motion, and other symptoms of the patient's condition. If gold salt therapy does not prove effective in a given time, the drug is discontinued.

N U R S I N G   A L E R T
▼▼▼▼▼▼▼▼▼▼▼▼▼▼▼▼▼▼▼▼▼▼▼▼▼▼▼▼▼▼▼

Throughout gold salt therapy, be attuned to the possibility of toxic effects. If any of the following symptoms should appear, the drug is stopped immediately and the physician notified: low hemoglobin level, leukopenia, eosinophilia, low platelet count, albuminuria, hematuria, pruritus, rash, stomatitis, or persistent diarrhea.

▲▲▲▲▲▲▲▲▲▲▲▲▲▲▲▲▲▲▲▲▲▲▲▲▲▲▲▲▲▲▲

Gold Sodium Thiomalate

Gold sodium thiomalate (Myochrysine) is an injectable gold salt medication. The first weekly injection is usually 10 mg. The second weekly injection is 25 mg. The third and all subsequent weekly injections are 25 to 50 mg until clinical improvement occurs. If there is no clinical improvement, the drug is discontinued. If clinical improvement occurs, the drug is then given every other week for up to 20 weeks. Injections can then be further decreased to every third or fourth week.

Aurothioglucose

Aurothioglucose (Solganal) is given intramuscularly only. The dose and schedule are like those of gold sodium thiomalate.

Auranofin

Auranofin (Ridaura) is an oral form of gold salt. Adverse reactions are less likely with this form of the drug. Auranofin is available as capsules and is given 6 mg per day.

MISCELLANEOUS DRUGS

Penicillamine

ACTIONS AND USES Penicillamine (Cuprimine) may be ▲▲▲▲▲▲▲▲▲▲▲▲▲▲▲▲ given for severe rheumatoid arthritis and also for Wilson's disease, but it is associated with potentially fatal adverse reactions, such as blood dyscrasias. The most common reactions include a rash and itching, gastrointestinal upset, peptic ulcer, blunted sense of taste and mouth ulcerations, renal dysfunction, myasthenia gravis, and serious blood dyscrasias.

ASSESSMENT Be aware of the patient's condition, in- ▲▲▲▲▲▲▲▲▲▲ cluding the condition that is to be treated with penicillamine, and any historical conditions. The use of penicillamine is contraindicated in patients with a history of blood dyscrasias or kidney disease. Patients who are currently pregnant cannot receive penicillamine.

PLANNING AND IMPLEMENTATION Penicillamine should ▲▲▲▲▲▲▲▲▲▲▲▲▲▲▲▲▲▲▲▲▲▲▲▲▲▲▲ be given on an empty stomach. Direct the patient to take the drug 1 hour before or 2 hours after any meal and at least 1 hour apart from any other drug. Be sure the physician is aware of any and all drugs the patient is taking, including over-the-counter drugs.

The initial dose of penicillamine is 125 to 250 mg in a single dose per day. This will be increased approximately every 1 to 3 months by doubling the dose until a therapeutic response is achieved or intolerance occurs. If no response is seen after 3 or 4 months at the level of 1000 to 1500 mg per day, it is presumed that the drug will not work for this patient, and the physician discontinues the drug.

N U R S I N G   A L E R T

▼▼▼▼▼▼▼▼▼▼▼▼▼▼▼▼▼▼▼▼▼▼▼▼▼▼▼▼▼▼▼▼▼

Teach the patient to report any signs or symptoms of blood dyscrasias, such as fever, sore throat, chills, bruising, or bleeding from any site.

If the patient complains of itching or a rash appears on the skin or mucous membranes, do not give the next dose of the drug and notify the physician at once. A rash on the skin or mucous membranes may indicate the beginning of drug fever, and the drug will need to be discontinued.

▲▲▲▲▲▲▲▲▲▲▲▲▲▲▲▲▲▲▲▲▲▲▲▲▲▲▲▲▲▲▲▲▲

This rash is not to be confused with a lupus-like syndrome that can result from the use of penicillamine. There is no need to discontinue the drug if this syndrome occurs.

Because penicillamine can decrease the sense of taste and cause ulcerations in the mouth, the patient may need encouragement to eat nutritionally balanced meals. Report ulcerations to the physician. A topical anesthetic may be prescribed.

Penicillamine may cause deficiencies of iron or pyridoxine regardless of the patient's intake. It may be necessary for the physician to order supplements. Be sure to assess for symptoms of deficiencies and encourage foods that are high in these nutrients.

The use of penicillamine may cause fragile skin. Be sure to take extra precautions when moving or turning the patient or when removing tape. Skin tears occur more easily. Skin breakdown occurs faster. An immobilized patient must be cared for with great caution.

EVALUATION Because of the many potential adverse
▲▲▲▲▲▲▲▲▲▲ reactions, many tests are performed frequently throughout the therapy. These include urinalysis and complete blood counts every 2 weeks. A yearly kidney x-ray will be ordered to look for the formation of a cystine kidney stone, which can occur when penicillamine is used for more than 6 months. Liver function tests should be performed frequently to look for liver damage. Evaluate the patient for hematuria or proteinuria as warning signs of renal damage.

Caution the patient that it may take 2 to 3 months for any clinical improvement. Continue to evaluate for changes in the patient's condition.

Hydroxychloroquine Sulfate

Hydroxychloroquine sulfate (Plaquenil) is an antimalarial drug also used for systemic lupus erythematosus and for rheumatoid conditions such as arthritis. See Chapter 22 for additional information on this drug.

E X E R C I S E S

CASE STUDIES

1. Mr. C.G. has osteoarthritis. His physician has prescribed large doses of a salicylate each day. What are your responsibilities for Mr. C.G.? What teaching does he require? What drug interactions should you evaluate for?

2. Mr. N.R. was diagnosed with rheumatoid arthritis and has been prescribed various drugs over the years. Presently, he has been prescribed penicillamine. He is also taking an oral drug for hypertension. What drug regimen should Mr. N.R. be on if the antihypertensive drug is given every 8 hours?

What assessments and evaluations should you do for Mr. N.R.?

3. Ms. E.D., age 56, has been prescribed a steroidal anti-inflammatory for her rheumatoid arthritis. What adverse reactions should you look for when you are evaluating Ms. E.D.? What would be the important points to place on her plan of care?

MENTAL AEROBICS

1. Visit the offices of an orthopedic specialist. How commonly does this physician see patients with some form of arthritis? What medications are these patients prescribed? What teaching is done?

2. Take a survey of patients on a medical-surgical floor in the hospital. How many patients are receiving a form of steroid? What conditions are the steroids prescribed for? Which form is most common? Do any of these patients take other prescribed drugs that can potentially cause a drug interaction? Is the potential interaction noted in the plan of care? (If not, please inform the patient's nurse.)

ANTIGOUT DRUGS

LEARNING OBJECTIVES

After studying this chapter, you should be able to:

1. Define antigout, enzyme inhibitor, and uricosuric agent.

2. Identify types of antigout drugs.

3. State the actions, uses, and common examples of each type of antigout drug.

4. Identify adverse reactions to antigout drugs and appropriate nursing interventions for patients receiving them.

5. Demonstrate how to administer antigout drugs by use of the nursing process.

6. State drugs with which uricosuric agents interact.

DRUGS YOU WILL LEARN ABOUT IN THIS CHAPTER

Colchicine

Uricosuric Agents

sulfinpyrazone (Anturane)

probenecid (Benemid)

colchicine and probenecid (ColBenemid)

Enzyme inhibitors

allopurinol (Zyloprim)

Drugs given to treat patients who have gouty arthritis focus on different aspects of uric acid formation, distribution, or excretion. The three main types are colchicine, uricosuric agents, and enzyme inhibitors.

COLCHICINE

ACTIONS AND USES Colchicine is a medication in a ▲▲▲▲▲▲▲▲▲▲▲▲▲▲▲▲ class by itself. The true mechanism of its action is not fully understood. However, it appears to decrease the inflammatory reaction of uric acid crystals and to decrease phagocytosis at the site of a gout attack. It is not useful for anti-inflammation of other disorders.

Colchicine is associated with several adverse reactions. It can cause severe gastrointestinal (GI) upset, especially diarrhea. These GI symptoms may occur even if the medication is given intravenously, although the frequency is decreased. Colchicine may also cause serious blood dyscrasias, peripheral neuritis, and myopathy.

ASSESSMENT Before the initial dose of colchicine, thor- ▲▲▲▲▲▲▲▲▲▲ oughly assess the patient for signs and symptoms of gout. These usually include signs of inflammation (warmth, redness, swelling) as well as the presence of tophi, which are large deposits of uric acid crystals in joints or under the skin. Be sure to include in your assessment the patient's systemic temperature, ability to perform range of motion, and level of pain (Fig. 28–1).

Colchicine should not be given to patients with certain disorders. Ask the patient and consult the chart for any serious GI, renal, hepatic, or cardiac diseases currently present or in the medical history.

Extra caution is warranted when colchicine is given to patients with other conditions. This includes the elderly or debilitated. The physician may need to decrease the dose if severe GI upset occurs. Also check the patient's history for any tendency to the development of thrombophlebitis, because this can be precipitated by colchicine.

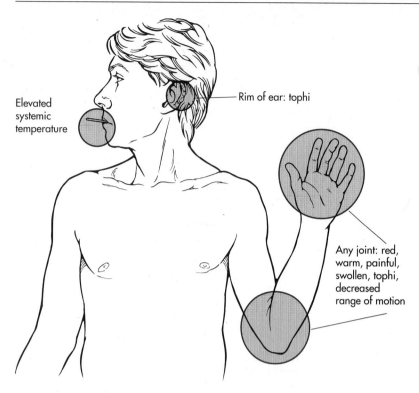

Elevated
systemic
temperature

Rim of ear: tophi

Any joint: red,
warm, painful,
swollen, tophi,
decreased
range of motion

Figure 28–1 Symptoms of gout include signs of inflammation (warmth, redness, swelling), tophi (large deposits of uric acid crystals in joints or under the skin), elevated systemic temperature, and decreased range of motion.

PLANNING AND IMPLEMENTATION Colchicine may be given orally or intravenously (IV).

N U R S I N G   A L E R T

If the medication is accidentally given subcutaneously or intramuscularly, this may result in severe tissue irritation. Watch the IV site carefully for any signs of infiltration because tissue damage may develop. If infiltration does occur, treat the site with heat or cold applications. The physician may order analgesics.

When colchicine is given IV, it is preferred that the nurse inject the medication into a previously established IV line that is in a large vein. The drug should be diluted with normal saline, and the IV line should be infusing with normal saline. Do not give with dextrose 5% in water. The registered nurse should administer the drug in a 2- to 5-minute period.

The initial dose is approximately the same whether it is given orally or intravenously. The usual dose is 0.5 mg every 6 hours until relief occurs (or severe adverse reactions occur). This cannot exceed 4 mg in a 24-hour period. Doses above this amount have resulted in death. Do not give colchicine again for at least 7 days after a patient has received a full 4 mg of

the drug. After relief has occurred, colchicine may be used as a maintenance drug. Usually, it is prescribed orally at dosages of 0.5 to 1.0 mg once or twice a day.

EVALUATION To establish whether colchicine is effective for the patient, reassess the patient for signs and symptoms of gout and compare these findings with the baseline assessments. Ask the patient whether improvement has been noted.

Be aware of the possibility of drug interactions with colchicine. This drug is known to cause malabsorption of vitamin B_{12}. It also increases the effects of central nervous system (CNS) depressants and sympathomimetics.

N U R S I N G   A L E R T

Be alert to symptoms of colchicine overdose. These include severe GI upset and possibly hemorrhage. The patient may also complain of burning pain in the throat, in the stomach, or on the skin. Muscle weakness and even paralysis may occur. In its most severe stage, this paralysis may produce respiratory failure. Myocardial injury and resultant shock can occur. Colchicine may also damage the liver, kidneys, and lungs. Blood dyscrasias, alopecia, and stomatitis can also be associated with colchicine overdose.

Overdose with this drug can be fatal. It is a medical emergency, and the physician or nurse should consult the poison control center in the area to determine the best treatment.

▲▲▲▲▲▲▲▲▲▲▲▲▲▲▲▲▲▲▲▲▲▲▲▲▲▲▲▲▲▲▲▲▲▲▲▲

URICOSURIC AGENTS

ACTIONS AND USES Uricosuric agents cause the body
▲▲▲▲▲▲▲▲▲▲▲▲▲▲▲▲▲ to excrete more uric acid. It is drawn from both the bloodstream and the tissues. Therefore, the symptoms of gouty arthritis eventually abate, and attacks do not recur while the patient is receiving the medication. However, this therapeutic response may take a lengthy time, and during this time, while the uric acid is being mobilized out of the bloodstream, acute attacks of gout can actually be precipitated by the medication. These attacks gradually shorten, and the length of time between each attack becomes longer.

The uricosurics also cause the resorption of tophi. They do not decrease the signs and symptoms of an acute attack; they only prevent further exacerbation.

ASSESSMENT In addition to knowing the patient's
▲▲▲▲▲▲▲▲▲▲ current symptoms, also check for a history of peptic ulcer disease. Uricosurics in such patients must be used with caution because a peptic ulcer can be aggravated or reopened.

Use of uricosurics is contraindicated in patients with a history of blood dyscrasias or kidney stone formation.

PLANNING AND IMPLEMENTATION Because uric acid is
▲▲▲▲▲▲▲▲▲▲▲▲▲▲▲▲▲▲▲▲▲▲▲▲▲▲▲▲▲▲ mobilized by the uricosurics, uric acid kidney stones may form. Encourage the patient to drink an increased amount of fluid throughout the day, unless a coexisting disorder prohibits this. Also discourage foods that acidify the urine. This may be referred to as an alkaline-ash diet (Box 28–1). Alkaline urine decreases the chance of the formation of this type of kidney stone.

Because of the effects on the gastrointestinal (GI) system, you may need to encourage the patient to take the medication with food or milk. The physician may order uricosurics to be given with antacids.

EVALUATION Evaluate the patient for decreased pain
▲▲▲▲▲▲▲▲▲▲ and decreased symptoms of inflammation around the site of the current exacerbation. Also check for any additional sites of inflammation. Compare the ability to perform range of motion with the baseline information.

N U R S I N G   A L E R T
▼▼▼▼▼▼▼▼▼▼▼▼▼▼▼▼▼▼▼▼▼▼▼▼▼▼▼▼▼▼▼▼▼▼▼

Be sure to evaluate for drug interactions. Be especially alert to any mention of the use of salicylates. The uricosurics and salicylates are antagonistic. Because aspirin and other salicylates are readily available over-the-counter, ask the patient frequently about their use.

▲▲▲▲▲▲▲▲▲▲▲▲▲▲▲▲▲▲▲▲▲▲▲▲▲▲▲▲▲▲▲▲▲▲▲▲

Sulfinpyrazone

Sulfinpyrazone (Anturane) is a pyrazolone derivative. Therefore, it is chemically related to phenylbutazone (Butazolidin). You may wish to review information about this drug. If a patient is sensitive to phenylbutazone, sensitivity to sulfinpyrazone is likely.

In addition to the adverse reactions common to all uricosurics, sulfinpyrazone may also cause a rash. It is not normally necessary to discontinue the drug if this occurs. Overdose with sulfinpyrazone may cause GI upset and pain, ataxia, dyspnea, seizures, and coma.

The usual dose is 200 to 400 mg orally in two divided doses each day. This may then be gradually increased to as much as 800 mg every day. Once serum levels of uric acid are controlled, the dose may once again be reduced to 200 mg.

In addition to interaction with salicylates, sulfinpyrazone may also potentiate some sulfonamides, oral hypoglycemics, insulin, and anticoagulants. Be aware of the toxic effects of these drugs.

Probenecid

Along with its use as a uricosuric, probenecid (Benemid) may also be used to prolong the effectiveness of penicillin and other antibiotics. The antibiotic remains in the body longer because probenecid inhibits its excretion.

Probenecid is associated with numerous adverse reactions, including mild discomforts such as head-

---

Box 28–1. The Alkaline-Ash Diet

Avoid each of the following as much as possible:

Cranberries	Cereal	Meats
Prunes	Nuts	Fish
Plums	Legumes	Cheese
Corn	Eggs	

ache, dizziness, GI upset, sore gums, urinary frequency, and flushing. More serious reactions can include dermatitis, alopecia, nephrotic syndrome, and liver dysfunction.

Probenecid should not be initiated during an acute attack of gout. After the attack subsides, the usual dose is 0.25 g twice a day for the first week; the dose is then increased to 0.5 g twice a day. If an acute attack of gout occurs during therapy, the drug should *not* be discontinued.

In addition to the drug interactions common to uricosurics, probenecid also inhibits the excretion of several drugs. These drugs are then effective in the body for a longer time, possibly overlapping with the next dose. This increases the frequency of toxic effects. Longer effectiveness is likely with aminosalicylic acid, indomethacin and other nonsteroidal anti-inflammatory drugs (NSAIDs), some steroids, pantothenic acid (a vitamin), lorazepam (a sedative-hypnotic), rifampin, acetaminophen, phenolsulfonphthalein, and methotrexate. Use of probenecid may cause falsely high results of serum theophylline determinations. The anesthesiologist should be notified that the patient is taking probenecid if the patient goes to surgery. The dose of anesthesia may need to be reduced.

Colchicine and Probenecid (ColBenemid)

The actions and uses of and the nursing implications for this drug are the same as for the ingredients it contains.

ENZYME INHIBITORS

Allopurinol

ACTIONS AND USES As an enzyme inhibitor, allopurinol (Zyloprim) decreases the production of uric acid by inhibiting the enzyme that causes uric acid to form. It is therefore used for prophylactic treatment of those with recurrent gout. It may also be used for patients with diseases receiving medications that may elevate serum uric acid levels.

Allopurinol may cause severe rash. This rash may indicate an allergy to the drug and may lead to Stevens-Johnson syndrome, vasculitis, toxic liver effects, and possibly even death. Other adverse reactions may include gastrointestinal upset, blood dyscrasias, pruritus, fever, chills, arthralgia, and jaundice.

ASSESSMENT Be familiar with the patient's history. What is the drug being used for? If the drug is used to prevent acute attacks of gout, assess the patient for signs or symptoms of gout before the first dose.

Check for a history of kidney stones. These may be precipitated by allopurinol.

PLANNING AND IMPLEMENTATION Allopurinol is given orally. The usual dose is 200 to 800 mg every day. The dose is started at the lower end of the scale and increased by 100 mg each week until a therapeutic level is found for the individual patient. Caution the patient that a therapeutic response may take between 2 and 6 weeks.

Teach the patient to take the medication with meals if gastric upset occurs.

N U R S I N G   A L E R T

Allopurinol should be discontinued immediately, and the physician notified, if a rash, dysuria, hematuria, conjunctivitis, or swollen lips or mouth is noted.

Inform the patient not to "double-up" on doses if a dose is forgotten. Encourage the patient to drink increased fluids unless this is contraindicated by another condition. This is to prevent uric acid kidney stone formation. An alkaline-ash diet also decreases this risk. The physician may prescribe alkalinizing agents.

Because allopurinol can cause drowsiness, caution patients not to drive or operate hazardous machinery until the individual patient's response is known.

EVALUATION Compare signs and symptoms, including frequency of gout attacks, with baseline information to establish therapeutic response to the drug.

Look for signs of allopurinol toxicity, including liver dysfunction, rash, and vasculitis, if the drug is given with thiazide diuretics.

The doses of mercaptopurine (an antineoplastic) and azathioprine (an immunosuppressive) may need to be decreased if they are given with allopurinol. The effects of anticoagulants are enhanced by allopurinol. The effects of both allopurinol and a uricosuric are decreased if they are used together.

Evaluate the patient for anorexia, weight loss, or pruritus frequently. These may indicate impending liver dysfunction. The physician should order liver function tests if these signs are noted.

Evaluate for signs and symptoms of kidney stones, including renal colic.

E X E R C I S E S

CASE STUDIES

1. Mr. J.R. has been diagnosed with acute gout. Colchicine has been ordered. As his nurse, what major adverse reactions should you watch for?

In addition to the colchicine, Mr. J.R. is prescribed probenecid. By what action does probenecid treat gout? What medication should Mr. J.R. be warned to avoid when he returns home?

A few weeks after Mr. J.R. returns home, his order is changed to allopurinol. By what action does allopurinol treat gout? What should Mr. J.R. do if he begins having symptoms of gout while taking allopurinol? What should he do if a rash develops?

What type of diet will Mr. J.R. most likely be ordered?

2. Mr. R.S. is admitted to the hospital for bronchial pneumonia. The following orders are given:

amoxicillin 500 mg bid

probenecid 0.25 mg bid

For what reason has Mr. R.S. been prescribed probenecid? What should he do if a rash develops?

MENTAL AEROBICS

Write a care plan for a patient with gout who has been prescribed probenecid. Include important points of care and teaching for the patient.

MUSCLE RELAXANTS

LEARNING OBJECTIVES

After studying this chapter, you should be able to:

1. Define skeletal muscle relaxant, centrally acting, and peripherally acting.

2. State actions and uses of and adverse reactions to the centrally acting skeletal muscle relaxants.

3. Classify common examples of centrally acting skeletal muscle relaxants.

4. State actions and uses of and adverse reactions to the peripherally acting skeletal muscle relaxants.

5. Identify nursing responsibilities for the patient receiving either a centrally acting or peripherally acting skeletal muscle relaxant.

6. Demonstrate how to administer skeletal muscle relaxants by use of the nursing process.

DRUGS YOU WILL LEARN ABOUT IN THIS CHAPTER

Centrally Acting Muscle Relaxants

methocarbamol (Robaxin)

cyclobenzaprine (Flexeril)

chlorzoxazone (Paraflex, Parafon Forte)

metaxalone (Skelaxin)

orphenadrine (Norflex)

carisoprodol (Soma)

baclofen (Lioresal)

Peripherally Acting Muscle Relaxants

dantrolene (Dantrium)

Neuromuscular Blockers

succinylcholine (Anectine)

vecuronium bromide (Norcuron)

pancuronium bromide (Pavulon)

Several types of drugs may be used clinically to produce muscle relaxation. The muscle relaxants are divided as follows:

• Centrally acting drugs—the main site of action is in the central nervous system (CNS)
• Peripherally acting drugs—the main site of action is outside the CNS, possibly in the muscle itself or the nerve endings

CENTRALLY ACTING MUSCLE RELAXANTS

ACTIONS AND USES The centrally acting muscle relaxants, also called skeletal muscle relaxants, are used for two major purposes:

1. to treat spasticity associated with spinal cord diseases or lesions; and
2. as an adjunct in the treatment of acute musculoskeletal conditions that cause pain.

These drugs do not work directly on either muscle or nerve fibers. Instead, they cause generalized CNS depression and block neuronal activity at the spinal cord. This produces relief of the symptoms but does not treat the cause of these symptoms.

As a result of these actions, the centrally acting muscle relaxants are associated with adverse reactions. The most common is drowsiness. The patient may also complain of a dry mouth, dizziness, fatigue, nausea and vomiting, constipation, headache, and nervousness. You may note signs of confusion, tachycardia, and other cardiac arrhythmias.

ASSESSMENT Before the first dose of the medication, be ▲▲▲▲▲▲▲▲▲▲ fully aware of your patient's symptoms, condition, and medical history. To help determine the effectiveness of the drug later, be sure to assess the patient for level of pain, degree of muscle stiffness, and ability to perform range of motion in affected extremities. If spasms are part of the condition, determine whether anything makes the spasms worse or better, when they are most likely to appear, and what other symptoms are associated with them.

Be sure to check the patient's medical history. The use of centrally acting muscle relaxants is contraindicated in persons with a history of cardiac arrhythmias, hyperthyroidism, congestive heart failure, or heart block and in the acute recovery phase of myocardial infarction.

N U R S I N G   A L E R T
▼▼▼▼▼▼▼▼▼▼▼▼▼▼▼▼▼▼▼▼▼▼▼▼▼▼▼▼▼▼▼▼

Centrally acting muscle relaxants should also not be used if the patient is receiving monoamine oxidase (MAO) inhibitors.

▲▲▲▲▲▲▲▲▲▲▲▲▲▲▲▲▲▲▲▲▲▲▲▲▲▲▲▲▲▲▲▲

Other conditions to check for in the medical history include urinary retention, liver or kidney disease, closed-angle glaucoma, and increased intraocular pressure. Caution must be exercised if the drug must be used in this patient because each of these conditions may be worsened by the drug.

PLANNING AND IMPLEMENTATION Because drowsiness ▲▲▲▲▲▲▲▲▲▲▲▲▲▲▲▲▲▲▲▲▲▲▲▲▲▲ is such a prevalent adverse reaction with this class of drugs, be especially cautious of safety hazards. The patient may not be able to ambulate or transfer as easily as normal. Be sure the pathway is clear of any clutter, and be sure the pathway is well lit at night. Do not allow the patient to perform dangerous actions without direct supervision, for example, smoking, self-administering medications, or getting out of bed alone.

Teach the patient to avoid driving or operating hazardous machinery if the drug causes drowsiness. Also teach the patient to avoid alcohol and other CNS depressants while taking this drug because the depressant actions will be potentiated.

EVALUATION To evaluate the effectiveness of the drug, ▲▲▲▲▲▲▲▲▲▲ reassess the patient's level of pain, fre-

quency of spasms, and ability to perform range of motion or other activities. The patient may be your best source of information, because small or subtle changes may be apparent only to the person.

Evaluate the patient's posture and balance. In some cases, spasticity helps the patient maintain an upright posture or perform certain movements. It is not appropriate to lose function from medication.

Also evaluate for signs of drug interaction. Additive effects can be expected if the patient is given both muscle relaxants and another CNS depressant, such as alcohol, antihistamines, antidepressants, narcotic analgesics, or sedative-hypnotics.

N U R S I N G   A L E R T
▼▼▼▼▼▼▼▼▼▼▼▼▼▼▼▼▼▼▼▼▼▼▼▼▼▼▼▼▼▼▼▼▼

Some muscle relaxants interact with MAO inhibitors to produce hyperpyretic crisis. The patient may experience severe convulsions and even death.

▲▲▲▲▲▲▲▲▲▲▲▲▲▲▲▲▲▲▲▲▲▲▲▲▲▲▲▲▲▲▲▲▲

Anticholinergics and antihypertensives given with relaxants may cause hypertension.

Methocarbamol

Methocarbamol (Robaxin), a common muscle relaxant, can be given orally, intramuscularly (IM), or intravenously (IV).

In addition to the adverse reactions common to all muscle relaxants, methocarbamol can also produce a rash or urticaria with pruritus, conjunctivitis, nasal congestion, fever, flushing, blurred vision, diplopia, nystagmus, metallic taste in the mouth, and bradycardia.

N U R S I N G   A L E R T
▼▼▼▼▼▼▼▼▼▼▼▼▼▼▼▼▼▼▼▼▼▼▼▼▼▼▼▼▼▼▼▼▼

When methocarbamol is given IV, carefully watch the site. Accidental infiltration may result in thrombophlebitis or sloughing of tissue.

▲▲▲▲▲▲▲▲▲▲▲▲▲▲▲▲▲▲▲▲▲▲▲▲▲▲▲▲▲▲▲▲▲

The patient should be lying down during and immediately after an IV administration of the drug. IV solutions of this drug should be administered no faster than 3 mL per minute by IV push.

With IM administration, no more than 5 mL of solution (a total of 1000 mg) should be given into each gluteus medius muscle. This can be repeated every 8 hours until symptoms are relieved. The physician will most likely change the route to oral at that point.

The usual dose given orally is 750 to 1500 mg four times a day.

Cyclobenzaprine

Cyclobenzaprine (Flexeril) is related to the tricyclic antidepressants. It is not effective against muscle spasms from CNS diseases, such as cerebral palsy.

In addition to the adverse reactions common to all muscle relaxants, cyclobenzaprine can also cause paresthesia, an unpleasant taste in the mouth, and blurred vision.

The usual dose for this oral drug is 10 mg three times a day. It is recommended that the drug not be used for periods longer than 2 to 3 weeks. Withdrawal after prolonged use may cause nausea, headache, and malaise, but this does not indicate that an addiction to the drug has occurred.

Be alert for signs of overdose of this drug, which may include confusion, hallucinations, agitation, hyperactive reflexes, muscle rigidity, hyperpyrexia, and nausea and vomiting.

Chlorzoxazone

Chlorzoxazone (Paraflex, Parafon Forte) seldom causes adverse reactions. When it does, it is most likely to be gastrointestinal upset or, occasionally, drowsiness, dizziness, or overstimulation.

The usual dose for this oral drug is 250 to 750 mg three or four times a day. As improvement occurs in the clinical picture, the physician may reduce the dosage.

Be alert for signs of overdose. These are normally an exaggeration of the adverse reactions but may also include headache, malaise, lack of muscle tone, inability to produce movement (but the patient retains the ability to feel), and, in severe overdose, respiratory depression and low blood pressure. Shock is not associated with overdose from this drug.

Metaxalone

Although most information that relates to the muscle relaxants can be applied to metaxalone (Skelaxin), also be aware that this drug can produce serious blood dyscrasias as an adverse reaction. For this reason, its use is contraindicated in persons with a tendency to anemia, especially hemolytic anemia.

If glucose testing must be done, remember that metaxalone can cause false-positive results if Benedict's solution is used.

The usual dose for this oral drug is 800 mg three or four times a day.

Orphenadrine

The actions of orphenadrine appear to be slightly different from those of most muscle relaxants. It is thought that orphenadrine (Norflex) owes its therapeutic effects to analgesic properties. It may also be an anticholinergic.

N U R S I N G   A L E R T

▼▼▼▼▼▼▼▼▼▼▼▼▼▼▼▼▼▼▼▼▼▼▼▼▼▼▼▼▼▼▼▼▼▼▼▼▼

Orphenadrine in its injectable form contains sulfite. Ask patients about allergies to sulfites before administration. Sulfite allergy is more common in asthmatics.

▲▲▲▲▲▲▲▲▲▲▲▲▲▲▲▲▲▲▲▲▲▲▲▲▲▲▲▲▲▲▲▲▲▲▲▲▲

In addition to common side effects, orphenadrine can also cause urinary retention, dilated pupils, agitation, and tremors. These adverse reactions can be attributed to its anticholinergic qualities. Also because of its anticholinergic actions, this drug is contraindicated in patients with glaucoma, pyloric or duodenal obstruction, peptic ulcers, prostatic hypertrophy, cardiospasm, or myasthenia gravis.

The usual oral dose of this drug is 100 mg twice a day. The IM or IV dose is 60 mg every 12 hours.

Evaluate the patient for any interaction if it is given with propoxyphene. The effects may be additive, producing tachycardia, cardiac decompensation, coronary insufficiency, or cardiac arrhythmias.

Carisoprodol

Carisoprodol (Soma) is related to meprobamate (Equanil). Persons with allergies to meprobamate may also be allergic to carisoprodol. Another contraindication to the use of this drug is porphyria. Adverse reactions may include irritability, insomnia, or hiccups.

This oral drug is given four times a day at a dose of 350 mg. Overdose may produce stupor, coma, respiratory depression, shock, and even death.

Baclofen

Baclofen (Lioresal) is classified as both a muscle relaxant and an antispasmodic. It works at the spinal cord level to inhibit reflexive spasms. Therefore, it is useful in the treatment of spasms from multiple sclerosis or other spinal cord diseases or injuries. It helps relieve the pain and rigidity associated with these spasms.

In addition to the adverse reactions common to other muscle relaxants, baclofen is associated with several other serious reactions. The patient may complain of insomnia or urinary frequency. The blood pressure may be unstable or low. Ovarian cysts or an enlarged adrenal gland can develop. Use of baclofen in patients susceptible to seizures may cause an increase in the frequency of these seizures. This may occur even in previously well controlled epileptics.

N U R S I N G   A L E R T
▼▼▼▼▼▼▼▼▼▼▼▼▼▼▼▼▼▼▼▼▼▼▼▼▼▼▼▼▼▼▼▼▼

Baclofen should not be withdrawn abruptly. Caution the patient not to stop taking the medication without consulting the physician. Sudden withdrawal can lead to hallucinations and seizures.

▲▲▲▲▲▲▲▲▲▲▲▲▲▲▲▲▲▲▲▲▲▲▲▲▲▲▲▲▲▲▲▲▲

Check your patient's history for kidney disease or past stroke. Both of these conditions require extra precaution in the use of baclofen.

The dose of baclofen is individualized. The patient normally receives between 40 and 80 mg a day in three divided doses. Be alert for signs of an overdose. The patient may experience vomiting, muscle hypotonia, drowsiness, coma, respiratory depression, and seizures.

PERIPHERALLY ACTING MUSCLE RELAXANTS

Dantrolene

ACTIONS AND USES Dantrolene (Dantrium) works di-
▲▲▲▲▲▲▲▲▲▲▲▲▲▲▲▲▲ rectly on the muscle fiber, not on the nerves. It is used to treat spasms from spinal cord injuries or diseases, such as multiple sclerosis or cerebral palsy, and from stroke. The amount of control of the spasms achieved from dantrolene varies with the person. It can range from an increased ability to perform the activities of daily living to just minor changes that are apparent only to the patient. These minor changes may still be significant to the patient.

Dantrolene may also be used to help treat malignant hyperthermia, a serious adverse reaction experienced by some patients from anesthesia. Since the advent of this drug, the death rate from malignant hyperthermia has declined to such a point that it is now considered rare if treatment is instituted promptly. At one time, the death rate was approximately 50%.

The adverse reactions associated with dantrolene are similar to those of other muscle relaxants. These include drowsiness, dizziness, weakness, malaise, fatigue, and diarrhea. Most of these reactions usually decrease as therapy continues. The diarrhea, however, may be so severe that the drug must be discontinued for a short time and then restarted slowly. If the diarrhea occurs again, the drug is generally discontinued permanently.

Patients may also experience photosensitivity reactions of the skin, hepatitis or hepatotoxic effects, seizures, or pleural effusion.

ASSESSMENT Be familiar with the patient's current
▲▲▲▲▲▲▲▲▲▲ status and the rationale for the drug's use. Determine the frequency and severity of spasms, ability to perform activities or range of motion, and pain level. The use of dantrolene is contraindicated when spasticity produces improved posture or helps the patient maintain balance.

Check the patient's medical chart for evidence of any active liver disease. This contraindicates the use of this drug. Report your findings to the physician. Those with previous liver disease, pulmonary disease, or cardiac disease require extra precautions when being given this drug.

PLANNING AND IMPLEMENTATION The dose of dan-
▲▲▲▲▲▲▲▲▲▲▲▲▲▲▲▲▲▲▲▲▲▲▲▲▲▲▲▲▲ trolene is individualized. The practitioner generally begins at 25 mg every day and then slowly increases the dose each week. The therapeutic range is usually achieved at doses below 400 mg a day. If no therapeutic effects are achieved at doses below this level, it is presumed that the drug is not effective for this patient.

Dantrolene can be given orally or by intravenous solution. Intravenous administration is normally used for malignant hyperthermia because the effects must be achieved quickly.

N U R S I N G   A L E R T
▼▼▼▼▼▼▼▼▼▼▼▼▼▼▼▼▼▼▼▼▼▼▼▼▼▼▼▼▼▼▼▼▼

Watch the site carefully. Accidental infiltration (extravasation) may cause sloughing of the tissue.

▲▲▲▲▲▲▲▲▲▲▲▲▲▲▲▲▲▲▲▲▲▲▲▲▲▲▲▲▲▲▲▲▲

Because of the potential for hepatotoxic effects, the physician should order frequent liver function testing. You should monitor the results of these tests and report any abnormalities to the physician immediately.

Because of the risk of photosensitivity, caution the patient to stay out of sunlight and protect exposed skin areas when this is not possible.

Safety is a priority concern for this patient. The patient will probably already be experiencing spasms that interfere with ambulation or transfers. The drug may cause drowsiness, weakness, or dizziness, all of which may further affect the patient's mobility.

EVALUATION To evaluate the effectiveness of the drug, look for improvement in pain level, frequency or severity of spasms, ability to perform activities, posture, and balance. The patient may be able to notice improvement that you cannot see. If no improvement is noted after 45 days of treatment, the physician discontinues the drug.

Evaluate the patient for any signs of impending liver dysfunction. Be familiar with the signs and symptoms of hepatitis. This adverse reaction can be fatal.

Evaluate for signs of drug interactions. Patients receiving dantrolene and estrogen at the same time are at higher risk for hepatotoxic effects. If given with verapamil (Calan), dantrolene may produce circulatory collapse.

NEUROMUSCULAR BLOCKERS

ACTIONS AND USES Neuromuscular blockers can also be called curariform drugs. They work directly on the nerve endings to inhibit neuromuscular transmission. This produces a flaccid paralysis. Although all skeletal muscles can be affected, the effects generally start in the face, progress downward to the muscles of the throat (especially the glottis) and then the respiratory muscles, and finally reach all other skeletal muscles. The neuromuscular blockers do not affect consciousness or the ability to feel sensations.

Because of the actions, neuromuscular blockers are used as adjunct drugs to general anesthesia. They are also used to facilitate endotracheal intubation or mechanical ventilation, because they inhibit the patient's normal reaction to fight these procedures.

Adverse reactions to the neuromuscular blockers are normally exaggerations of the actions. The patients may experience profound muscle relaxation with apnea. Other reactions include cardiac arrhythmia or even arrest, malignant hyperthermia, hypertension or hypotension, increased intraocular pres-

sure, acute renal failure, excessive salivation, or rash. The patient should also be warned that there may be postoperative muscle pain.

ASSESSMENT Before surgery, check the patient's history for malignant hyperthermia and determine whether there is a family history of this reaction. If either is present, use of a neuromuscular blocker is contraindicated. Other contraindications include myopathies, closed-angle glaucoma, and open eye injuries.

PLANNING AND IMPLEMENTATION The neuromuscular blockers should be administered by an anesthetist or anesthesiologist. The dose is individualized to the patient.

EVALUATION After surgery in which a neuromuscular blocker was used, evaluate the patient's respiratory status carefully.

N U R S I N G   A L E R T

Neuromuscular blockers can result in prolonged respiratory depression.

Drug interactions may also become apparent after surgery (Box 29–1). The drugs are often discontinued before surgery, or if this is not possible, the anesthesiologist may choose not to use neuromuscular blockers. At other times, the drugs may be used together.

Box 29–1. Drug Interactions with Neuromuscular Blockers

Increased effects of neuromuscular blocker with
Nonpenicillin antibiotics
Promazine
Beta-blockers
Lidocaine
Magnesium salts
Chloroquine
Other muscle relaxants
Oxytocin
Quinidine
Procainamide
Lithium
Quinine
Some anesthetics

Increased and longer effects of the neuromuscular blocker may be anticipated if the patient is receiving any of the following drugs: certain antibiotics (usually nonpenicillin), oxytocin, promazine, quinidine, beta-blockers, procainamide, lidocaine, lithium, magnesium salts, quinine, chloroquine, and some anesthetics, especially inhaled anesthetics. Other muscle relaxants produce synergistic effects with neuromuscular blockers.

Succinylcholine, Vecuronium Bromide, and Pancuronium Bromide

All three of these drugs are neuromuscular blockers with similar effects. Pancuronium bromide (Pavulon) is the longest acting, followed by vecuronium bromide (Norcuron); succinylcholine (Anectine) is the shortest acting. Vecuronium is the most potent. Often, vecuronium and succinylcholine are used during the same surgery. Succinylcholine is used first because its actions occur faster. Vecuronium is then started for its more prolonged effects.

All of these drugs are much more potent in the patient with myasthenia gravis. For this reason, these patients may be given much smaller doses.

All three drugs are given intravenously, but succinylcholine may also be given intramuscularly. The drugs should be given only by an anesthesiologist or anesthetist.

E X E R C I S E S

CASE STUDIES

1. Ms. M.L. has been prescribed a muscle relaxant by her physician. The drug is to relieve muscle spasms she experiences in her back after an automobile accident. As her nurse, what assessments should you perform?

What precautions should you take while Ms. M.L. is in the hospital?

After discharge, Ms. M.L. forgot your instructions to avoid alcohol while taking the drug and had a glass of wine at a social gathering. What effects would you expect her to experience?

2. Your patient, Mr. J.E., is to go to surgery. He is expected to receive vecuronium while under anesthesia. For what effects is this drug used during surgery? Why must anesthesia also be used?

Mr. J.E. is also a manic-depressive and is receiving lithium. What effect does this have on the plan to use a neuromuscular blocker?

During surgery, Mr. J.E. experiences symptoms indicating malignant hyperthermia. The anesthesiologist immediately begins treatment with a medication. What medication is this likely to be?

MENTAL AEROBICS

1. Observe the anesthesiologist or anesthetist during surgery. Make an inventory of the drugs used. Which are neuromuscular blockers? What precautions did the anesthesiologist take because these drugs were used?

2. Tour an intensive care unit where patients are maintained with mechanical ventilation or have an endotracheal tube in place. Determine which of the drugs are used to facilitate these procedures.

3. Visit an orthopedic clinic, an office of an orthopedic practitioner, or a hospital ward that specializes in orthopedic conditions. Take an inventory of the patients receiving muscle relaxants. What is the relaxant being used for in each case? What teaching is done at the facility about these drugs?

UNIT SEVEN

DRUGS THAT AFFECT THE NERVOUS SYSTEM

Neurons are the basic cells of the nervous system. They are composed of a cell body, axons, and dendrites. Neurons are responsible for carrying a nerve impulse from one part of the body to another. Axons carry the message away from the cell body, and dendrites carry it to the cell body. The message is passed from the end of one neuron to the beginning of another through the use of neurohormones.

Sometimes, the neurons can become too active, or hyperexcited. This means that they are putting out messages at a rapid and irregular rate. The messages are often distorted and sent in wrong directions. The person then has a seizure. There are many different types of seizures. The neurons react in different ways, and the behavior of the person is different. For the purposes of this discussion, we use the following terminology for the different seizure types.

A tonic-clonic seizure, sometimes called a grand mal or generalized seizure, is what most people think of when we say seizure or convulsion. The patient experiences a preictal (or preseizure) stage, which may include an aura (a warning that a seizure is about to occur), followed by an epileptic cry; the patient then loses consciousness. This signals the end of the preictal stage. Next comes the tonic stage, during which the patient's muscles clench. The clonic stage follows. During this phase, the patient experiences the convulsive portion of the seizure. The muscles alternately contract and relax. The patient is often incontinent or involuntary of stool. After the clonic stage, the patient enters the postictal stage. The patient may awaken with a headache, confusion, and the desire to sleep.

Another common type of seizure is the partial seizure, also called an absence attack or sometimes petit mal. During this seizure, there is no convulsive activity. Instead, the patient loses consciousness for a few seconds during which he appears to simply stare. After the seizure, he typically does not realize the seizure occurred unless something in his line of vision moved.

Myoclonic seizures, often referred to now as minor motor seizures, are also a type of partial seizure. During this seizure, a limb or even the entire trunk of the body will jerk. This is no cause for alarm if it happens occasionally during your twilight sleep, for this is a normal part of the sleep cycle. It becomes abnormal if it happens when you are awake or occurs excessively at night and disturbs sleep significantly.

Psychomotor seizures, another partial seizure, may also be called temporal lobe seizures. During this seizure, the patient repetitively performs an inappropriate act, perhaps certain hand movements, walking motions, or swimming motions. Because the patient is acting oddly, this type of seizure is often confused with psychosis until diagnostic tests are done.

Jacksonian seizures, or focal seizures, are convulsions of just one part of the body. Therefore, they are also partial seizures. Convulsive movement may occur in just an arm, a leg, or even an entire half of the body. This type of seizure may include sensory problems, such as transient numbness or tingling in an area.

The term status refers to a series of seizures. If the patient is experiencing a series of petit mal seizures, we call this petit mal status. A series of psychomotor seizures is called psychomotor status. A series of grand mal seizures, however, is called status epilepticus. This constitutes a medical emergency because the patient does not regain consciousness between seizures and suffers oxygen deprivation if left untreated. If it continues, the patient could die.

The autonomic nervous system controls many body functions. It is composed of two parts, the sympathetic and the parasympathetic nerves.

The sympathetic nerves can also be called adrenergic. Functions controlled by these nerves constitute the fight-or-flight mechanism—those functions vital to survival when the body must either fight (react) or run away. When presented with such a situation (meeting an enemy, nearly having an accident), the body shunts blood and nerve stimulation past parts and organs not vital to survival in this immediate situation. It is not necessary to digest or eliminate food, so these smooth muscles relax. Peripheral blood vessels constrict because blood is more vitally needed elsewhere. Extra blood and nerve stimulation are sent to areas needed in a fight or in running. The bronchi relax and dilate to improve intake of oxygen. Coronary arteries dilate to improve myocardial oxygenation. The brain is stimulated, and the patient is alert with quickened reflexes. Muscle strength increases. Persons have been known to perform feats of great strength during moments of crisis. The heart beats faster, respirations increase, and pupils dilate. Fats are liberated, and blood glucose is used more easily for a "quick burst of energy."

The sympathetic nerves use two neurohormones: epinephrine (adrenaline), produced by the adrenal gland, and norepinephrine (noradrenaline), produced at the nerve endings.

The parasympathetic nervous system may also be referred to as cholinergic. This system of nerves works to conserve your energy, slow your heart, digest your food and eliminate waste, and produce sexual hormones. Just as the sympathetic division is said to control the fight-or-flight mechanism, the parasympathetic division controls "feed or breed" functions.

The parasympathetic nerves use two neurohormones. Acetylcholine acts by transmitting nerve impulses. Acetylcholinesterase inactivates acetylcholine and therefore stops the nerve impulse.

In this unit, we discuss drugs that decrease the ability of the neurons and brain to detect sensation or react to it. Some have effects that alter the functioning of the mind. These are sometimes called psychotropic drugs and include some of the analgesics, anesthetics, sedative-hypnotics, alcohol, hallucinogens, and psychotherapeutic drugs.

Psychotherapeutic drugs are those used to treat specific disorders of the mind. The main classifications are the tranquilizers, antidepressants, and antipsychotic drugs.

Many of the psychotropic and psychotherapeutic drugs are controlled substances and are subject to restrictions imposed by the Comprehensive Drug Abuse Prevention and Control Act, which is also called the Controlled Substances Act.

In Chapter 34, we address the drugs used to stop or decrease seizures. Chapter 35 looks at drugs that stimulate various parts of the nervous system. Chapter 36 focuses on the drugs used to treat a specific neurological disease, parkinsonism.

Chapters 37 to 40 discuss drugs that affect the autonomic nervous system. Although these drugs are used to produce different actions, their mode of action is through the stimulation or blocking of the autonomic nervous system.

ANALGESICS

LEARNING OBJECTIVES

After studying this chapter, you should be able to:

1. Identify examples of the various subclasses of analgesics.

2. List the general adverse effects of drugs in each subclass.

3. Assess the effectiveness of analgesic medications.

4. State nursing interventions that are appropriate for patients receiving these drugs.

5. Prepare an appropriate plan of care for a patient receiving one of these drugs.

DRUGS YOU WILL LEARN ABOUT IN THIS CHAPTER

Narcotics

  Opiates

    morphine sulfate

    codeine sulfate

    heroin

  Synthetics

    meperidine HCl (Demerol)

    methadone HCl (Dolophine)

    hydromorphone HCl (Dilaudid)

    levorphanol tartrate (Levo-Dromoran)

Narcotic Antagonists

    levallorphan tartrate (Lorfan)

    naloxone HCl (Narcan)

Non-narcotics

  Synthetics

    pentazocine (Talwin)

    nalbuphine HCl (Nubain)

    butorphanol tartrate (Stadol)

  Salicylates

    acetylsalicylic acid or aspirin (Ecotrin, Aspergum, ASA)

  Salicylate combination drugs

    Equagesic

    Excedrin

    Darvon Compound-65

    Vanquish

  Nonsalicylates

    acetaminophen (Tylenol, Datril, Liquiprin, Tempra)

  Other non-narcotics

    NSAIDs

    carbamazepine (Tegretol)

Pain is an unpleasant stimulus that is perceived differently by each person. Some people appear to feel pain at a less intense level than others do. In addition, there are varying degrees of painful stimuli and varying kinds or types of pain. Pain may be acute (lasting less than 6 months) or chronic (lasting longer than 6 months). Some other words commonly used to explain or describe pain include sharp, dull, aching, mild, moderate, or severe.

In addition to the physical discomfort of the pain itself, other symptoms are caused by the painful stimuli. These are associated with autonomic nervous system responses and include hypertension, tachycardia, diaphoresis, pallor, restlessness and anxiety, dilated pupils, grimacing, tensed muscles, and inability to concentrate.

The physiological mechanism of pain and the perception of pain are two concepts that are difficult to distinguish. Pain receptors are located throughout the body, in the skin and surrounding the body organs. When an injury occurs, pain-producing substances are released in the area. These substances include histamine, kinins, serotonin, and prostaglandins, which cause inflammation and increase the irritability of the pain receptors.

Pain impulses are transmitted by afferent (sensory) nerve fibers across nerve synapses to the spinal cord and then to the brain, where the perception of pain occurs. The brain releases chemicals called enkephalins and endorphins, which act in several ways to control or moderate the pain. Enkephalins and endorphins may occupy specific receptors, called opiate receptors, in the brain, brain stem, and spinal cord. When the opiate receptors are occupied, the release of neurotransmitters is prevented at the synapse. This blocks or stops the transmission of the pain impulse to the brain.

There are many ways to control pain that do not involve the use of medications. The use of analgesics is but one approach that modifies the patient's perception of the pain. Just as there are many different kinds of pain, there are also many different kinds of pain relievers. The two main groups of analgesics are narcotics and non-narcotics. These drugs and their dosages are listed in Table 30–1.

Analgesics may be administered by many routes. In addition to the usual oral (PO), subcutaneous (SC), intramuscular (IM), and intravenous (IV) routes, they are sometimes administered sublingually, rectally, and through special infusion systems. Surgically implanted devices such as the Infusaid implantable pump, the Cormed implantable pump, and epidural catheters offer unique methods of control for those with terminal illnesses. Patient-controlled analgesia (PCA) systems allow the patient to release premeasured IV doses of analgesic at intervals chosen by the patient. Each system is designed to provide better pain control than the usual intermittent administration schedules.

Some aspects of the nursing process are applicable to all patients receiving analgesics.

Table 30–1. Analgesics

DRUG	DOSAGE
Narcotics	
Morphine sulfate	Adults: 5–15 mg SC or IM q4h; 30–60 mg PO or per rectum q4h
MS Contin *oxycontin*	Adults: 30- or 60-mg tablets PO q12h
Hydromorphone hydrochloride (Dilaudid)	Adults: 1–6 mg PO q4–6h prn; 2–4 mg IM, SC, or IV q4–6h prn; 3 mg rectal suppository hs
Codeine phosphate (codeine)	Adults: 15–60 mg SC or IM q4h prn
Codeine sulfate (codeine)	Adults: 15–60 mg PO q4h prn Children: 3 mg/kg qd PO in divided doses q4h prn
Levorphanol tartrate (Levo-Dromoran)	2–3 mg PO or SC q6–8h prn
Meperidine hydrochloride (Demerol)	Adults: 50–150 mg PO, IM, or SC q3–4h prn Children: 1 mg/kg PO, IM, or SC q4–6h prn (maximum, 100 mg q4h prn)
Methadone hydrochloride (Dolophine)	2.5–10 mg PO, IM, or SC q4–12h prn or around the clock (also used in narcotic withdrawal programs and given in dosages of 15–40 mg PO qd, with maintenance doses individually titrated at 20–120 mg PO qd according to federal and state regulations)

Table 30–1. Analgesics Continued

DRUG	DOSAGE
Oxycodone hydrochloride (Roxicodone)	1–3 rectal suppositories qd prn
Propoxyphene hydrochloride (Darvon, Doraphen, Pargesic 65)	65 mg PO q4h prn
Combination Drugs	
Propoxyphene napsylate (Darvocet-N, Darvon-N)	100 mg PO q4h prn
Darvon Compound-65	propoxyphene HCl 65 mg, aspirin 389 mg, with caffeine 32.4 mg PO q4h prn
Empirin with Codeine #2, 3, or 4	aspirin 325 mg with codeine phosphate 15–60 mg PO q4h prn
Fiorinal with Codeine #1, 2, or 3	butalbital 50 mg, caffeine 40 mg, aspirin 200 mg, acetaminophen 325 mg, with codeine phosphate 7.5–30 mg PO q4h prn
Tylenol with Codeine #1, 2, 3, or 4	acetaminophen 300 mg with codeine phosphate 7.5–60 mg PO q4h prn
Percocet-5	acetaminophen 325 mg with oxycodone HCl 5 mg PO q6h prn
Percodan	oxycodone HCl 45 mg, oxycodone terephthalate 0.38 mg, with aspirin 325 mg PO q6h prn

Table 30–1. Analgesics Continued

DRUG	DOSAGE
Narcotic Antagonists	
Levallorphan tartrate (Lorfan)	Adults: 1 mg IV, followed by 1 to 2 doses of 0.5 mg at 10- to 15-min intervals prn (maximum total dose, 3 mg) Children: 0.02 mg/kg IV followed by 0.01–0.02 mg/kg in 10–15 min Neonates: 0.05–0.1 mg IV into umbilical vein immediately after delivery; may repeat in 10–15 min
Naloxone hydrochloride (Narcan)	Adult concentration (0.4 mg/mL): 0.4–2 mg IV, SC, or IM; may repeat q 2–3 min prn to a total of 10 mg; if there is no response after 10 mg, another diagnosis should be considered Child/neonate concentration (0.02 mg/mL): Child: 0.01 mg/kg IV, IM, or SC; may repeat q 2–3 min Neonate: 0.01 mg/kg IV into umbilical vein, IM, or SC; may repeat q 2–3 min for 3 doses
Non-Narcotics	
Pentazocine hydrochloride, pentazocine lactate (Talwin)	50–100 mg PO q3–4h prn (maximum, 600 mg qd), or 30 mg IV, IM, or SC q3–4h prn (maximum, 360 mg qd)

Table continued on following page

Table 30–1. Analgesics *Continued*

DRUG	DOSAGE
Nalbuphine hydro-chloride (Nubain)	10–20 mg q3–6h prn (maximum, 160 mg qd)
Butorphanol tartrate (Stadol)	0.5–2 mg IV q3–4h prn or 1–4 mg IM q3–4h prn
Salicylates	
Acetylsalicylic acid or aspirin (Ecotrin, Aspergum, ASA)	Dosage depends on use Adults: **arthritis:** 26–52 g PO qd in divided doses; **pain/fever:** 325–650 mg PO or rectal suppository q4h prn; **thrombotic disorders:** 325–650 mg PO qd–bid Children: **arthritis:** 90–130 mg/kg PO qd in divided doses q4–6h; **fever:** 40–80 mg/kg PO or rectal suppository qd in divided doses q6h; **pain:** 65–100 mg/kg in divided doses PO or rectal suppository q4–6h prn
Aspirin (combined products)	
Anacin	aspirin 400 mg with caffeine 32 mg PO q4h

Table 30–1. Analgesics *Continued*

DRUG	DOSAGE
Equagesic	aspirin 250 mg, ethohepta-zine citrate 75 mg, with meprobamate 150 mg PO q4–6h prn
Excedrin	aspirin 250 mg, acetamino-phen 250 mg, with caffeine 65 mg PO q4–6h prn
Nonsalicylates	
Acetaminophen (Tylenol, Datril, Liquiprin, Tempra)	Adults and children older than 10 y: 325–650 mg PO or rectal suppository q4h prn (maximum, 26 g qd) Infants 0–2 y: 15–60 mg PO or rectal suppository q4h prn; maximum 12 g qd; dosage may be increased by 60 mg for each year to age 5 (240 mg) Children 5–10 y: 325 mg q4h prn

ASSESSMENT Assess and document the patient's complaints about the pain. Include descriptions of the type of pain, location, onset, and influencing factors. Assess and document the vital signs as baseline information for comparisons and also before each dose of analgesic. Also document objective signs of pain that the patient displays. Assess the physician's order for frequency and route of administration.

PLANNING AND IMPLEMENTATION Assess the pain before administration of the analgesic and 30 to 60 minutes after administration. Document the response. It is often helpful to ask the patient to qualify the degree of pain being experienced by assigning a number value to the pain, for example, 1 to indicate mild pain and 10 to indicate severe pain. Document the system being used so that others may interpret the patient's complaint in the same manner.

Teach the patient to report the need for analgesic before the pain becomes severe. If the patient is nonverbal, monitor for signs and symptoms that might indicate the presence of pain. When you keep pain under control, rather than allowing the roller-coaster effect of severe pain followed by sedation, the patient perceives analgesics as being more effective.

Some types of pain are better controlled when analgesics are administered throughout a 24-hour schedule rather than on an as-needed (prn) basis. In these cases, it may be necessary for caregivers to awaken the patient at night to give a dose on schedule.

If the analgesic is expected to cause sedation, monitor the vital signs before each dose and 30 to 60 minutes after administration. If vital signs are not within the ranges documented on the assessment, withhold administration of the medication, notify the physician, and request parameters for the vital signs. A narcotic antagonist may be ordered if severe respiratory depression occurs. (In some cases of severe, chronic pain of the type that may occur in terminally ill persons, there may be physician orders to the contrary.)

If painful nursing procedures are to be performed, they are best done when the analgesic effect is at its peak, usually 1 to 2 hours after administration.

Provide safety factors as needed for patients, such as raising side rails, placing signal cords in reach, and assisting with ambulation. Teach patients to rise slowly and dangle before ambulating. Teach patients who take these medications at home to avoid driving and other hazardous activities.

Supplement the medication regimen with physical comfort measures, such as therapeutic touch, position changes, heat or ice application (if permitted by the physician), relaxation techniques or other distractions such as music or TV, and emotional support.

Teach patients to control constipation by increasing fluid intake, ingesting more roughage and fruit juices, and increasing physical activity, if possible.

Observe federal and institutional regulations for documentation of the use of controlled substances.

EVALUATION Document the patient's response to the analgesic. Describe appearance, muscle tenseness, or grimacing. Request that the patient qualify the pain by use of the number system. Report to the physician if the patient requests analgesic more frequently than it is ordered or if the patient complains that the medication does not relieve the pain. Remember that some analgesics are not effective for some people, or there may be a more serious problem causing increased or continued pain.

NARCOTICS

There are two main types of narcotics, the opiates and the synthetics. Opiates, such as morphine, codeine, and heroin, are derived from the unripe pod of a certain type of white poppy plant that is grown in Turkey and the Far East. These drugs are sold to the United States for legal and illegal use.

The synthetic narcotics, which are manufactured from chemicals other than the plant sources, include such products as meperidine hydrochloride (Demerol) and methadone hydrochloride (Dolophine).

Most drugs in this classification belong to Schedule II of the Controlled Substances Act, which means they may lead to severe psychological and physical dependence. Some combination products that contain small amounts of these narcotics are classed in Schedule IV of the Controlled Substances Act. This means they have limited potential for psychological and physical dependence and therefore are not abused as frequently as are those of higher classifications. Antitussive syrups that contain narcotics (usually codeine) are classed in Schedule V of the Controlled Substances Act because they have limited potential for abuse.

Narcotics are used to treat acute pain that is of moderate to severe intensity. They act to alter the perception of pain, and the emotional response to pain, by binding with opiate receptors in the central nervous system to block the transmission of the painful impulse. The term narcotic agonist is used to describe a narcotic that mimics this activity.

Some narcotics, especially codeine, also produce antitussive effects by suppressing the cough reflex in the medulla. Narcotics are often used as preanesthetic agents to relax the patient and potentiate the effects of the anesthesia. Some anesthetics are also narcotics.

Adverse effects include respiratory depression, depressed level of consciousness, constricted pupils, nausea, vomiting, constipation, anorexia, urgency or difficulty in voiding, hypotension, and others. In addition, if narcotics are used for a long time, physical dependence and addiction may result. Tolerance to the drug with decreased analgesic effect may also occur with long-term use.

Caregivers must remember the difference between addiction and tolerance and their implications for care. Addiction does not occur in a few days of use during acute pain. Do not withhold the drug on the basis of your own perception of the patient's pain. Remember that not all people perceive pain in the same manner or demonstrate the same response to pain.

The physician titrates analgesic dosages on the basis of the patient's statement of the severity of pain, the age and size of the patient, the patient's tolerance to the medication, and sometimes the cause of the pain.

Some patients develop tolerance to a medication after a time and may require increased dosage or increased frequency of dosage to obtain relief. If there is a question about the need for analgesic, discuss the situation with the physician.

Narcotics are generally contraindicated in patients with head injuries, those with increased intracranial pressure, those with decreased respiratory reserve, and those who are comatose. They should be used with caution in patients with seizure disorders, acute alcoholism, hypothyroidism, and bronchial asthma.

Alcohol, phenothiazines, and tricyclic antidepressants potentiate the depressant effects of narcotics on the central nervous system and should be used with caution. Use of narcotics with cholinergic blockers may cause urinary retention or severe constipation.

The physician may order a narcotic antagonist if the patient becomes overly sedated with a narcotic. The following additional information relates to specific narcotics.

Morphine

Morphine sulfate is capable of relieving severe pain, and it has long been considered the prototype or standard with which all other narcotics are compared. It primarily affects the central nervous system and the bowel. Extremely large doses can cause convulsions and severe respiratory depression. It is effective by many routes of administration, including oral (PO), intravenous (IV), intramuscular (IM), subcutaneous (SC), rectal, sublingual, epidural, and intrathecal routes. Adult dose ranges are 5 to 15 mg SC or IM, 30 to 60 mg PO or per rectum. Doses are usually ordered to be given every 4 hours on a prn basis or on a 24-hour schedule. MS Contin, a long-acting oral form, has recently become available in the United States and is available in 30- or 60-mg tablets administered every 12 hours.

Hydromorphone

Hydromorphone hydrochloride (Dilaudid) is a potent narcotic with a rapid onset but short action that is particularly useful in the elderly or those with unstable metabolism. Adult dose ranges are 1 to 6 mg PO every 4 to 6 hours prn; 2 to 4 mg IM, SC, or IV every 4 to 6 hours prn; 3 mg rectal suppository at bedtime prn.

IV administration may cause respiratory depression or severe hypotension. Administer the drug slowly with the patient in the recumbent position and monitor vital signs frequently.

Other Narcotics

Codeine, oxycodone, and propoxyphene are often combined with other drugs, such as aspirin, caffeine, or acetaminophen. These combination products are weaker and are used for mild to moderate pain. A number is sometimes used after the codeine products to indicate the amount of narcotic contained. A product labeled #1 contains 1/8 grain, #2 contains 1/4 grain, #3 contains 1/2 grain, and #4 contains 1 grain of codeine. Examples include Empirin with Codeine #2, 3, or 4; Fiorinal with Codeine #1, 2, or 3; Tylenol with Codeine #1, 2, 3, or 4; and Percocet-5 and Percodan.

NARCOTIC ANTAGONISTS

ACTIONS AND USES Narcotic antagonists displace narcotic analgesics at their receptors. These drugs act to block the activity of a previously administered narcotic. They are used to treat a narcotic overdose. Expected actions are an increase in respiratory and pulse rates, an increase in level of consciousness, and increased activity. Adverse effects may include a sudden return of pain (if the narcotic was administered to a patient in pain), excitement, hypertension, hypotension, ventricular tachycardia or fibrillation, and pulmonary edema.

Examples of narcotic antagonists include levallorphan tartrate (Lorfan) and naloxone hydrochloride (Narcan).

ASSESSMENT Assess for history of narcotic intake. Assess and document vital signs and level of consciousness.

PLANNING AND IMPLEMENTATION Nursing actions are based on the situation. Maintain an airway and cardiopulmonary circulation, prevent aspiration, and provide safety factors. Monitor vital signs and level of consciousness frequently.

EVALUATION Compare the vital signs and level of consciousness with the baseline documentation.

NON-NARCOTICS

There is a group of newer drugs that are not narcotics, but they are potent, even several times more potent than morphine. For this reason, many institutions lock them up and use security measures, just as they do with narcotics. Principles of nursing care are the same as those listed for narcotics. Examples of non-narcotics include pentazocine hydrochloride, pentazocine lactate (Talwin), nalbuphine hydrochloride (Nubain), and butorphanol tartrate (Stadol).

Each of these may also act as a narcotic antagonist and should not be used in combination with narcotics. These products may produce withdrawal symptoms in persons addicted to narcotics.

Other non-narcotic analgesics are used for mild to moderate pain. These include the salicylates and nonsalicylates.

Salicylates

Salicylates include acetylsalicylic acid or aspirin (Ecotrin, Aspergum, ASA). Aspirin may be combined with another agent such as caffeine, which potentiates its analgesic effect. Examples include Anacin, Equagesic, and Excedrin.

Aspirin may also be combined with antacid products, such as aluminum hydroxide or magnesium hydroxide, to decrease the possibility of gastrointestinal distress. An example of this is Vanquish.

ACTIONS AND USES The actions of the salicylates are not clearly understood. It is believed that the salicylates produce analgesia by affecting the thalamus to suppress pain perception. The anti-inflammatory effects result from blocking of prostaglandin production in the peripheral areas. Antipyretic effects are due to the effect on the hypothalamus. Vasodilation and increased activity of the sweat glands result in cooling of the skin by evaporation.

Adverse effects include nausea, vomiting, burning sensation, and other gastrointestinal distress or bleeding. Anemia may occur. Bruising may be noted, and the bleeding time is prolonged because of factors that inhibit the clumping of platelets. (This may be a desired effect in patients with a tendency to thromboembolic problems.)

The adverse effect of salicylism may occur after repeated large doses. Symptoms include tinnitus, headache, confusion, drowsiness, nausea, and vomiting; the temperature, pulse, and respirations are elevated. In addition to these symptoms and signs, toxic doses also cause restlessness, excitement, incoherent speech, tremors, delirium, hallucinations, euphoria, or convulsions. Allergic reactions include swelling of the lips, tongue, and throat. Dyspnea and hypotension are also signs of an allergic response. Even death is possible.

ASSESSMENT Assess the patient and the medical record for history of allergy to aspirin or aspirin products. Assess also for history of bleeding disorders, increased bruising, or low platelet counts.

PLANNING AND IMPLEMENTATION Do not administer salicylates to children younger than 8 years because of the possibility of Reye's syndrome. Give with food, milk, or a large glass of water to minimize gastrointestinal irritation. Teach patients to report increases in bruising, petechiae, epistaxis, bleeding gums, hematuria, or black stools.

Urine acidifiers and carbonic anhydrase inhibitors may increase blood levels and predispose the patient to toxicity. Monitor closely. Teach the patient to avoid aspirin if an anticoagulant is being taken because bleeding tendencies will increase.

Antacids in large doses, urine alkalinizers, and corticosteroids decrease salicylate levels, so physicians may order increased doses.

EVALUATION Monitor for the desired effect and the presence of adverse effects. Physicians may order periodic prothrombin times and platelet counts.

Nonsalicylates

The nonsalicylates, such as acetaminophen (Tylenol, Datril, Liquiprin and Tempra), are coal tar derivatives. These products are often preferred for adults who should not take aspirin and for children younger than 8 years because of the risk of Reye's syndrome.

ACTIONS AND USES Nonsalicylates produce analgesia by blocking pain impulses. Antipyretic action occurs in the hypothalamus. Acetaminophen does *not* possess anti-inflammatory properties. Adverse actions include gastrointestinal upset, allergic reactions, hemolytic anemia, and hepatic necrosis; a link to hepatic cancer is possible.

ASSESSMENT Assess for a history of allergy. The physician may wish to order baseline liver function tests if therapy is to be prolonged.

PLANNING AND IMPLEMENTATION Teach patients to avoid alcohol ingestion. Effects of anticoagulants may be increased if acetaminophen is taken, so teach patients to report bruising and petechiae.

EVALUATION The physician may wish to order laboratory tests to monitor liver function at intervals. Monitor for signs of increased bruising.

Other Non-narcotics

Nonsteroidal anti-inflammatory drugs (NSAIDs) are often used to prevent chronic pain associated with the menstrual cycle or headaches and for chronic muscle, bone, or joint pain. They act to prevent the release of prostaglandins. More information on this classification is available in Chapter 27.

Carbamazepine (Tegretol) is an anticonvulsant drug that is structurally related to the tricyclic antidepressants. It is also used to control the pain of trigeminal neuralgia (tic douloureux). More information is available on this drug in Chapter 34.

E X E R C I S E S

LEARNING ACTIVITIES

Mr. C.Q. is terminally ill with cancer. His physician is discharging him with a prescription for liquid morphine sulfate to control his pain. Prepare a written plan to teach the patient and his spouse about his medication.

ANESTHETICS

LEARNING OBJECTIVES

After studying this chapter, you should be able to:

1. Name classifications of, rationales for, and examples of drugs commonly used in preoperative medications.

2. Define anesthesia, local, general, and balanced anesthesia.

3. List routes of administration for local and general anesthetics.

4. Differentiate between the rationales for local and general anesthesia.

5. Describe the physiological changes that occur in the four stages of anesthesia.

6. Relate at least two factors that affect the stages of anesthesia.

7. Outline nursing care related to anesthesia by use of the nursing process.

DRUGS YOU WILL LEARN ABOUT IN THIS CHAPTER

Local Anesthetics

  ethyl chloride

  lidocaine (Xylocaine)

  procaine (Novocaine)

  tetracaine (Pontocaine)

  dibucaine (Nupercainal)

General Anesthetics

  thiopental sodium (Pentothal)

  methohexital sodium (Brevital)

  succinylcholine chloride (Anectine)

  pancuronium bromide (Pavulon)

  tubocurarine chloride

  droperidol and fentanyl (Innovar)

  fentanyl (Sublimaze)

  ketamine (Ketalar)

  cyclopropane

  nitrous oxide ("laughing gas")

  halothane

  ether

In 1850, Dr. Richard Long discovered anesthesia. Until then, surgery went on without anesthesia. Long discovered the anesthetic use of ether by observing its anesthetic effects in guests at illicit parties he gave. Ether was used at these parties to lower inhibitions. The guests and the party got a bit wild, but the guests also felt no pain if they happened to hurt themselves.[1]

---

[1] *What the Doctor Ordered*, by James Burke, PBS Special.

ACTIONS AND USES The word anesthesia means a state
▲▲▲▲▲▲▲▲▲▲▲▲▲▲▲▲ of painlessness. Today, anesthesia is used in many different ways, including for surgical procedures, to stitch a wound, and in the dentist's office.

In actuality, when a patient is given anesthesia, the physician is aiming for a state of "balanced anesthesia." This means giving other drugs to counteract the potent side effects of the anesthetics. For example, some anesthetics can cause an increase of respiratory and gastrointestinal secretions, nausea or vomiting, and an emergence reaction. Generally, these other drugs are given as part of a preoperative medication regimen.

PREOPERATIVE ASSESSMENT

Thoroughly assess the patient before giving a preoperative medication. The normal reaction to surgery is fear or anxiety. Some patients may not admit it. Some patients may have heard stories from well-meaning but misguided friends and relatives, or the patient may have even known someone who died in surgery. The patient may also be afraid of a future diagnosis; of the anesthesia, pain, disfigurement, or disability; or of becoming a burden to others. Assess for undue depression or acute anxiety because these increase the patient's surgical risk.

Also assess for other factors that place the patient at high risk. Those with other physical impairments, such as patients with poor respiratory exchange or cardiac patients, are more likely to have problems during surgery or after. Those with poor nutrition or who are dehydrated are less resistant to infection, and their wounds tend to heal more slowly.

PLANNING AND IMPLEMENTATION

The purpose of preoperative care is to prepare the patient both physically and psychologically. This takes a cooperative effort between the physician and the nursing team.

Be sure to give thorough explanations and teach the patient how to perform actions that will be expected postoperatively. Items taught preoperatively, such as deep-breathing or coughing exercises, have a better cooperation rate than those that are taught postoperatively. Teach these exercises to any patient with lung problems. The physician may also order blow bottles, incentive spirometry, or nebulization. The patient can become familiar with these before surgery.

Teach the patient to change position in bed frequently. Let the patient know that early ambulation will be required. Listing the benefits of this helps ensure cooperation. Teach any special measures that are specific to the type of surgery, such as crutch walking.

Explain the procedures that will be performed and what the schedule of events will be preoperatively. The physician performs a physical examination if it was not done in the office. X-rays, laboratory tests, and other diagnostic studies may be ordered. Some physicians order preoperative enemas or laxatives for the night before surgery. Some require a shave prep of the skin. Insertion of an indwelling catheter may be ordered. The patient will usually not be allowed anything to eat or drink for a certain length of time before surgery. If a sedative is ordered before bedtime, let the patient know. If preoperative medication is ordered, inform the patient of the time it is ordered and its purpose. Let the patient know what time the surgery is scheduled for and what time she can expect to leave her room. Inform the patient's family of what time they should be at the hospital and where they can wait, get coffee, and the like.

Spiritual care is also important. If the patient requests a spiritual advisor, provide one. You may wish to be subtle in suggesting this. We do not want to add to the patient's fears, but listen carefully for any cues from the patient.

NURSING ALERT

Be sure the operative permit is signed by the patient before any sedation is given, after the patient has received a thorough explanation from the physician and with a witness to the signature.

It may be the nurse's responsibility in your facility to see that the permit is signed. Such a permit protects the hospital, physician, and nurse from any lawsuit for unsanctioned surgery. It does not protect against lawsuits based on errors made. A minor must have a parent or legal guardian sign the permit.

Try to ensure that the patient has a bath and oral care before surgery. Caution the patient not to swallow while brushing the teeth. The patient is then dressed in a clean hospital gown without underwear. No make-up, nail polish, hairpins, wigs, contacts, glasses, dentures, or jewelry should remain on the patient. Some exceptions may be made. Be sure the patient has an identification band on. Check that all ordered laboratory test results as well as the history and physical examination findings are on the chart. Mark any allergies clearly. Assess the patient's vital signs.

Often, facilities have a surgical check list that is on or in the chart. See an example in Table 31–1.

EVALUATION

After the patient returns from surgery, much of the nurse's responsibilities are due to the effects of anesthesia. Immediately ensure that the patient has a clear airway. Check for respirations, respiratory effort, the patient's color, and the rate of respirations. Check the pulse and blood pressure also. Check all dressings for placement and any drainage. Check intravenous lines for any swelling, redness, or warmth at the site. Check also the drip rate (formula: cubic centimeters per hour ordered divided by minutes to be delivered multiplied by the drop factor) and solution, and compare with the order. Check all drainage tubes for placement and drainage. Determine the patient's level of consciousness. Position the patient properly according to the type of anesthesia used.

Table 31-1 Surgical Check List

Patient's Name _____ Room _____	
ID band on	
Surgical permit signed	
History and physical	
Allergies	
Operative area prepped	
Preop enema (if ordered)	
NPO after _____	
Blood work done	
Urinalysis	
Vital signs taken	
Voided or catheterized	
Consultation	
Jewelry removed or secured	
Hairpins, make-up, and nail polish off	
Contact lenses and glasses removed	
Dentures removed	
Surgical cap and gown	
Preop medication of _____	
Time given _____	
Side rails up	
Date _____ Nurse_____	

Most often, after general anesthesia, the patient will not be allowed to eat or drink anything for a certain length of time. Then the patient is placed on a progressive diet. After nausea subsides, the patient can attempt to take ice chips, then sips of water, then clear liquids and full liquids, then a soft diet, and finally a regular diet.

Vital signs are assessed frequently after surgery. A common schedule is immediately, then every half-hour for two checks, then every hour for four checks, and then every 4 hours for at least the next 24 hours.

Activity levels are ordered by the physician. In general, ambulation is encouraged as early as possible. The patient will dangle first at the side of the bed, then sit up in a chair. A walk in the hall with assistance is the next step. This is often accomplished within 24 hours of the surgery.

Deep-breathing or coughing exercises, frequent turning in bed, and possibly nebulization may be ordered to ensure the removal of respiratory secretions.

Be aware of orders for any medications. It is common for physicians to order medications for pain and nausea for their postoperative patients. The patient should also be on intake and output monitoring. Also check for any orders for diagnostic testing that may be continued postoperatively.

Always be alert for any complications arising from surgery or the anesthesia. Look for signs and symptoms of hemorrhage or shock, thrombophlebitis or embolism, airway obstruction, hypostatic pneumonia, singultus (hiccups), wound infection, evisceration or dehiscence, urinary retention or infection, nausea or vomiting, paralytic ileus, tympanites, pain, or insomnia.

COMMON CLASSIFICATIONS OF PREOPERATIVE MEDICATIONS

Some of the most common medications given preoperatively are the narcotic analgesics. The narcotic analgesic is given to help relax the patient and also to lower the basal metabolic rate. Examples include meperidine hydrochloride (Demerol) and morphine sulfate.

NURSING ALERT

Before giving a preoperative medication with a narcotic analgesic in it, always check the respirations first. Remember that narcotics can lower the respirations.

Have the patient void before you give the drug so that a fall due to dizziness or drowsiness can be avoided. Make sure all side rails are in the up and locked position. Caution the patient not to get up now without help. Also avoid excess noise because this may tend to confuse the patient.

Sedative-hypnotics are also commonly given to the preoperative patient. Most often, these are ordered at bedtime, again to relax the patient and to lower the metabolic rate. Examples include the barbiturates, such as pentobarbital (Nembutal) or secobarbital (Seconal). The nursing responsibilities are the same as for the narcotic analgesics.

Anticholinergics are often included in the medication given immediately before surgery. This is to reduce the secretions of the respiratory and gastrointestinal tracts, to minimize spasms of both of these tracts, to maintain a clear airway, and to reduce nausea and vomiting. Examples are atropine and glycopyrrolate (Robinul). Caution the patient that the mouth may become dry, but liquids are still not permitted preoperatively.

Tranquilizers may also be included in a preoperative medication. The rationales for use of these drugs are to reduce apprehension and to reduce nausea and vomiting. Examples include promethazine (Phenergan), hydroxyzine (Vistaril), chlorpromazine (Thorazine), and prochlorperazine (Compazine). Be sure the patient's side rails are in the up and locked position. Instruct the patient to ask for help before getting up. Have the patient void before giving the medication. Avoid excess noise.

Examples of common preoperative medications are given Table 31–2.

LOCAL ANESTHESIA

There are two major classes of anesthesia: local and general. Local anesthesia may be administered topically, by infiltration or injection, or by regional blocks.

Topical Applications

Topical anesthesia is applied to the nerve endings in the mucous membranes or to broken skin. These drugs interfere with the conduction of the nerve impulses at the site. Examples of uses for this type of anesthetic include eye drops, throat sprays, burn ointments, and rectal and vaginal ointments. Examples of medications used topically include ethyl chloride, which is sprayed onto skin before a small incision is made, such

Table 31–2. Common Preoperative Medications

Narcotic analgesics	meperidine hydrochloride (Demorol) morphine sulfate
Sedative-hypnotics	pentobarbital (Nembutal) secobarbital (Seconal)
Anticholinergics	atropine glycopyrrolate (Robinul)
Tranquilizers	promethazine (Phenergan) hydroxyzine (Vistaril) chlorpromazine (Thorazine) prochloperazine (Compazine)
Common Local Anesthetics	
Ethanes or vapocoolants	ethyl chloride
Caine family	lidocaine (Xylocaine) procaine (Novocaine) tetracaine (Pontocaine) dibucaine (Nupercainal)
Common General Anesthetics	
Short-acting barbiturates	thiopental sodium (Pentothal) methohexital sodium (Brevital)
Muscle relaxants	succinylcholine chloride (Anectine) pancuronium bromide (Pavulon) tubocurarine chloride
Neuroleptics	droperidol and fentanyl (Innovar) droperidol (Inapsine) fentanyl (Sublimaze)

Table 31–2. Common Preoperative Medications *Continued*	
Common General Anesthetics	
Dissociative gases	ketamine (Ketalar) cyclopropane nitrous oxide
Volatile vapors	halothane ether

as to drain an area of infection; lidocaine (Xylocaine); and dibucaine (Nupercainal), an over-the-counter medication for hemorrhoids.

Anesthesia by Infiltration or Injection

Anesthesia given by infiltration is injected along the line of a wound. These drugs affect the local nerve endings but not the nerve trunks. Vasoconstrictive drugs are also sometimes given with these local anesthetics to decrease the systemic absorption of the drug and to decrease bleeding in local wounds. Examples of uses for this type of anesthetic are for sewing up lacerations and doing minor surgical procedures. Medications that may be used in this manner are lidocaine (Xylocaine), tetracaine (Pontocaine), and procaine (Novocaine).

Regional Blocks

Regional blocks can be subdivided into categories. A peripheral block is a type of regional block. A peripheral block drug is injected into a nerve or group of nerves that supply feeling to the area to be incised. Examples of nerves that may be blocked in this manner are the sciatic, femoral, ulnar, intercostals, trigeminal, and pudendal.

Central blocks are also a type of regional block. Central block medications are injected into or just outside of the dura mater of the spinal cord. Central blocks are often referred to by different names, depending on the area of the spinal cord blocked. For example, for the spinal block, the drug is injected into the subarachnoid space between L-3 and L-4 or L-4 and L-5. For the saddle block, the drug is injected near

the dura mater between S-1 and S-2 or sometimes a little higher. For the epidural and caudal blocks, the drug is injected near the dura mater near the base of the spinal column (Fig. 31–1).

N U R S I N G   A L E R T

▼▼▼▼▼▼▼▼▼▼▼▼▼▼▼▼▼▼▼▼▼▼▼▼▼▼▼▼▼▼▼▼▼▼▼▼▼

Complications with central blocks can occur if too much medication is injected or if the anesthetic rises in the spinal fluid.

▲▲▲▲▲▲▲▲▲▲▲▲▲▲▲▲▲▲▲▲▲▲▲▲▲▲▲▲▲▲▲▲▲▲▲▲▲

This can lead to nervousness, fear, disorientation, confusion, vertigo, nausea and vomiting, convulsions, depressed respirations or even respiratory failure due to the paralysis of respiratory muscles, coma, slow pulse, arrhythmias, cardiac arrest, hives, and bronchospasms.

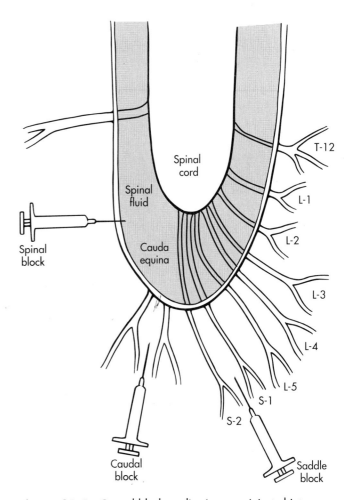

Figure 31–1. Central block medications are injected into or just outside of the dura mater of the spinal cord.

N U R S I N G   A L E R T

▼▼▼▼▼▼▼▼▼▼▼▼▼▼▼▼▼▼▼▼▼▼▼▼▼▼▼▼

After the central block wears off, the patient may have headaches (may be called "spinal headaches"), numbness, palsy, and paraplegia of the area supplied by that portion of the spinal cord.

▲▲▲▲▲▲▲▲▲▲▲▲▲▲▲▲▲▲▲▲▲▲▲▲▲▲▲▲

GENERAL ANESTHESIA

General anesthesia may be administered in several different ways. One of the most common is by the intravenous route. This delivers the medication through the bloodstream directly to the brain centers and depresses the nerve cells at their origin. Examples of drugs that may be used for this type of anesthesia include the following:

Short-acting barbiturates: thiopental sodium (Pentothal), methohexital sodium (Brevital)

Muscle relaxants: succinylcholine chloride (Anectine)

Neuroleptics: droperidol and fentanyl (Innovar), droperidol (Inapsine), fentanyl (Sublimaze)

Dissociative anesthetics: ketamine (Ketalar), also a narcotic analgesic

General anesthesia may also be delivered by inhalation. This route may be referred to as topical. The patient breathes in the vapors or gases. The drug is then exchanged in the lungs to the circulatory system and then travels to the brain to depress the central nervous system. Anesthetics delivered by inhalation must always be given with oxygen.

Examples of gases that may be used for anesthesia are cyclopropane and nitrous oxide. The student may recognize the layman's term for this last example: laughing gas.

Examples of liquids that are given as a vapor are halothane and ether. Although ether was the first anesthetic to be discovered, it is not often used today because of the danger of fire and explosion and the frequency of nausea experienced by the patient.

Stages of General Anesthesia

As the level of anesthesia in the bloodstream increases, different groups of nerve cells become depressed. The part of the brain most sensitive is the reticular activating system (RAS). This is in the midbrain and functions to keep a person conscious. Table 31–3 shows the stages of anesthesia.

Table 31–3. Stages of Anesthesia	
Stage I (early induction)	Decreased awareness of sensory stimuli, loss of consciousness
Stage II (delirium or excitement)	Psychomotor excitement, depressed inhibition of movement, hyperreflexes, dilated pupils
Stage III (surgical anesthesia)	Complete relaxation, flushed skin, constricted pupils, decreased eyelid reflexes, regular respirations and pulse
Stage IV (medullary paralysis)	Respiratory arrest, cardiac arrest, cardiovascular collapse, artificial ventilation needed

In stage I of anesthesia, or early induction, consciousness becomes progressively cloudy. The patient's awareness of sensory stimuli, such as hearing and vision, becomes disrupted. The patient may state that she is feeling "floaty" or even numb. Loss of consciousness ends stage I.

Stage II is also called delirium or excitement. The patient is unconscious but may experience psychomotor excitement from depression of the inhibitory area of the central nervous system. Signs of this stage include increased respirations, increased pulse, hyperactive reflexes, muscle contractions, reaction to painful stimuli, and dilated pupils.

N U R S I N G   A L E R T

▼▼▼▼▼▼▼▼▼▼▼▼▼▼▼▼▼▼▼▼▼▼▼▼▼▼▼▼

Protect the patient from injury during this stage.

▲▲▲▲▲▲▲▲▲▲▲▲▲▲▲▲▲▲▲▲▲▲▲▲▲▲▲▲

Stage III is called surgical anesthesia because this is the stage during which surgery is performed. The patient's respirations and pulse become regular again and at a more normal rate for the patient. The pupils constrict, and the patient loses the eyelid reflexes. The skin is flushed. The patient is in a state of complete relaxation.

Stage IV of anesthesia is called medullary paralysis.

It is not a stage the anesthesiologist is trying for. The anesthesia must be reversed before this stage occurs. At this stage, the patient will experience respiratory arrest and complete cardiovascular collapse. The patient must be artificially ventilated if this stage is reached.

The stages of anesthesia are affected by many things. The type of anesthetic (gas, vapor, intravenous) and the drug and dose used are important factors. The physical condition of the patient also affects the stages of anesthesia. Factors that may affect the stages include respiratory disease, circulatory conditions, and liver disease. The preoperative medications used can also affect the stages of anesthesia.

After the patient's anesthesia has been reversed, the vital signs decrease.

N U R S I N G   A L E R T

The patient should be in an area of quiet. Excessive noise during the waking period may cause the patient to have an emergence reaction.

Signs of an emergence reaction include confusion, restlessness, and hallucinations.

The patient may also require lowered doses of analgesia postoperatively after the use of certain anesthetics, especially droperidol and fentanyl (Innovar), fentanyl (Sublimaze), and ketamine (Ketalar).

E X E R C I S E S

CASE STUDIES

1. Your patient is ordered to be given a preoperative medication containing meperidine (Demerol), hydroxyzine (Vistaril), and glycopyrrolate (Robinul). What nursing responsibilities do you have for your patient?

The physician orders the following:

Demerol 20 mg IM 1 h preop

Vistaril 15 mg IM 1 h preop

Robinul 0.05 mg IM 1 h preop

Check a reliable drug information source to determine which, if any, of these drugs can be administered in the same syringe.

How much of each drug, in milliliters, would you include in the preoperative medication if the vials read as follows:

meperidine HCl (Demerol) 50 mg/mL

hydroxyzine (Vistaril) 50 mg/mL

glycopyrrolate (Robinul) 0.2 mg/mL

2. You have a patient with a cardiac condition who is going to surgery. The physician orders the following:

Penicillin G 100,000 U IM 12 h preop

The vial reads:

Penicillin G 2,000,000 U. Inject 23 mL of sterile water to yield 25 mL of solution.

How many milliliters of solution will you give the patient?

MENTAL AEROBICS

Observe the administration of general anesthesia to a patient. What drugs are used? What drugs were used preoperatively? What was the purpose of these drugs? How was the anesthesia reversed? What care did nurses give to the patient after anesthesia? What care was given to the patient for the next 24 hours? What was the purpose of each intervention?

SEDATIVES AND HYPNOTICS

LEARNING OBJECTIVES

After studying this chapter, you should be able to:

1. Describe the action of sedatives and hypnotics.

2. Discuss the normal sleep cycle.

3. Explain the adverse effects of having interrupted sleep cycles.

4. List three classifications of drugs used for their sedative-hypnotic effects.

5. Discuss adverse effects of each of these classifications.

6. Prepare an appropriate teaching plan for a patient taking one of these drugs.

7. List several nursing interventions appropriate for a patient receiving one of these drugs.

DRUGS YOU WILL LEARN ABOUT IN THIS CHAPTER

Barbiturates

amobarbital (Amytal)

amobarbital sodium (Amytal Sodium)

pentobarbital (Nembutal)

pentobarbital sodium (Nembutal Sodium)

secobarbital (Seconal)

secobarbital sodium (Seconal Sodium)

phenobarbital (Barbita, Luminal)

phenobarbital sodium (Luminal Sodium)

Miscellaneous Sedative-Hypnotics

chloral hydrate (Noctec)

glutethimide HCl

Benzodiazepines

flurazepam HCl (Dalmane)

temazepam (Restoril)

triazolam (Halcion)

Psychotropic drugs affect the functioning of the mind. Drugs that have a sedative or hypnotic action are included in this group of drugs because they depress the central nervous system. The sedative-hypnotics are barbiturates, benzodiazepines, and miscellaneous types. These drugs are metabolized by the liver and excreted by the kidneys. They accumulate in the body, so repeated use may lead to toxicity. These drugs and their dosages are summarized in Table 32–1.

ACTIONS AND USES Hypnotic drugs are sometimes referred to as soporifics. The difference between a sedative and a hypnotic is a matter of degree because the effects are dose related. Small doses of these drugs relieve anxiety and cause sedation by decreasing excitability and activity and increasing relaxation. They are sometimes prescribed to assist in control of stress-related hypertension. Moderate doses cause drowsiness and sleep. They are usually administered at bedtime or are used preoperatively to potentiate other medications. Large doses produce generalized anesthetic effects.

Rapid eye movement (REM) sleep may decrease as an adverse effect of hypnotics, which could result in personality changes. Use of hypnotics lowers inhibitions, slows thought processes, and increases reaction time. Rashes, dizziness, nausea, vomiting, weakness, vertigo, confusion, and "hangover" symptoms some-

Table 32–1. Sedative-Hypnotics

DRUG	DOSAGE
Barbiturates	
amobarbital (Amytal) amobarbital sodium (Amytal Sodium)	**Sedation** Adults: 30–50 mg PO bid or tid (possible 15–120 mg bid–qid) Children: 3–6 mg/kg qd PO, divided into 4 equal doses **Insomnia** Adults: 65–200 mg PO or deep IM at hs Children: 3–5 mg/kg deep IM at hs **Preanesthesia Sedation** Adults and children: 200 mg PO or IM 1–2 h preoperatively
pentobarbital (Nembutal) pentobarbital sodium (Nembutal Sodium)	**Sedation** Adults: 20–40 mg PO bid–qid Children: 6 mg/kg PO in divided doses **Insomnia** Adults: 100–200 mg PO at hs; 150–200 mg deep IM; 100 mg initially IV, then additional doses up to 500 mg; 120–200 mg rectally Children: 3–5 mg/kg IM (maximum dose, 100 mg); rectal doses: 2 mo–1 y; 30mg; 1–4 y; 30–60 mg; 5–12 y; 60 mg; 12–14 y; 60–120 mg
secobarbital (Seconal) secobarbital sodium (Seconal Sodium)	**Sedation** Adults: 200–300 mg PO 1–2 h preoperatively Children: 50–100 mg PO or 4–5 mg rectally 1–2 h preoperatively **Insomnia** Adults: 100–200 mg PO or IM Children: 3–5 mg/kg IM not to exceed 100 mg; 4–5 mg rectally

Table 32–1. Sedative-Hypnotics *Continued*

DRUG	DOSAGE
phenobarbital (Barbita, Luminal) phenobarbital sodium (Luminal Sodium)	**Sedation** Adults: 30–120 mg PO qd in 2 or 3 divided doses Children: 6 mg/kg PO divided into 3 doses **Insominia** Adults: 100–320 mg PO or IM Children: 3–6 mg/kg PO **Preoperative** Adults: 100–200 mg 60–90 min before procedure Children: 16–100 mg 60–90 min before procedure
Miscellaneous Sedative-Hypnotics	
chloral hydrate (Noctec)	Adults: 500 mg–1 gm 15–30 min before retiring Children: 50 mg/kg (maximum dose, 1 gm); available in oral capsules, solution, and rectal suppositories
glutethimide hydrochloride	250–500 mg PO at hs
Benzodiazepines	
flurazepam hydrochloride (Dalmane)	15–30 mg PO at hs
temazepam (Restoril)	15–30 mg PO at hs
triazolam (Halcion)	0.125–0.5 mg PO at hs

times occur. Additive effects occur with use of multiple drugs. These drugs belong to Schedule II, III, and IV of the Controlled Substances Act, so adverse effects include psychological and physical dependence. If dependence occurs, physical symptoms of withdrawal include wakefulness, depression, anxiety, nightmares, agitation, delirium, psychoses, seizures, coma, or death.

Sleep is a temporary state of altered consciousness. It is characterized by amnesia and a decreased perception of and response to the environment, although sleep can be interrupted if the stimuli are strong enough. Sensory and motor activities are suspended during sleep, and body processes and metabolism are slowed. Sleep is a time for the body and mind to repair themselves and prepare for the next activity cycle that will accompany the awake state.

Stages of sleep are not steady but consist of rest and activity cycles that last 60 to 120 minutes each. These cycles have been determined by monitoring of motor activity, vital signs, and brain wave patterns during sleep. The cycles are believed to be related to the fluctuating cycles of productivity and efficiency that occur during awake hours.

There are two main periods of sleep, REM (rapid eye movement) and NREM (non–rapid eye movement). The NREM period has been divided into four stages that occur in sequence of I to IV, which then reverse IV to I and are followed by a period of REM sleep. People are easy to awaken in stage I and progress to hard to awaken and slow to arouse in stage IV. REM sleep is when most dreams occur. This period lasts 5 to 20 minutes of each 90 to 120 minutes of sleep. The length of this period increases with each sleep cycle. The person is difficult to arouse during REM sleep.

If sleep is interrupted for any reason, the person returns to stage I NREM sleep. If these disruptions recur frequently, the person is deprived of REM sleep; an abnormal sleep cycle eventually develops, and the cycle begins with the REM phase.

Disruptions of the sleep-wake cycle (dyssomnia) or absence of sleep (insomnia) will cause problems with the maintenance of body temperature, hormone secretion, mental alertness, and psychomotor function. Therefore, caregivers should be concerned that they and their patients attain and maintain normal sleep cycles to maintain health and promote healing.

It takes approximately 2 weeks to readjust a sleep cycle to a normal pattern. This is of particular concern to people who work other shifts and must be awake at night and sleep during the day. Complications occur for people who must rotate shifts frequently because they do not have time to readjust and regain a normal sleep cycle.

ASSESSMENT Assess the vital signs and level of consciousness of the patient, and document these findings as baseline data. Assess the patient and review the chart for history of allergy. Also assess for renal or hepatic disease because it may impede detoxification and excretion of drugs. Review the entire drug regimen for medications that may interact in an adverse manner.

PLANNING AND IMPLEMENTATION Sedative-hypnotics potentiate analgesics and anesthetics. Do not administer these drugs at the same time or shortly after one another unless the physician orders this (for example, as a preoperative medication or to control some types of pain).

Most of these medications are classed as Schedule IV drugs by the Controlled Substances Act, with the exception of many of the barbiturates, which are Schedule II drugs. Either group must be kept locked and signed out to the patient receiving them.

Monitor the vital signs of the patient. Be alert for respiratory depression and hypotension. Monitor the level of consciousness and maintain safety precautions because sedation is an expected effect. If these medications are prescribed for outpatient use, teach the patient to avoid driving or operation of hazardous equipment.

Caregivers must be aware of the reason for use to anticipate and evaluate the effect.

NURSING ALERT

Sudden discontinuation of sedative-hypnotics in a patient accustomed to their use may produce withdrawal symptoms.

Teach the patient to avoid alcohol and to use caution with analgesics and other central nervous system (CNS) depressants. These substances potentiate the CNS and respiratory depression. Nonprescription medications should not be taken without consulting the physician.

Caution patients that these medications are teratogenic. Offer contraceptive information if it is desired.

If the patient will be taking a sedative-hypnotic on a regular basis, encourage and teach the use of mental and physical relaxation techniques, such as music therapy, backrubs, and warm baths. Teach the avoidance of naps; if a nap is necessary or desirable, teach the advantages of scheduling it early in the afternoon.

EVALUATION Monitor the vital signs and level of consciousness; compare findings with the baseline data. Compare symptoms of the diagnosis to determine whether the intended effect is being achieved.

BARBITURATES

ACTIONS AND USES Barbiturates produce a general-
▲▲▲▲▲▲▲▲▲▲▲▲▲▲▲▲▲ ized depressant effect on all organs, not just the central nervous system (CNS). The
main action is on the CNS and the respiratory and
gastrointestinal systems. Barbiturates produce mood
alteration in the forms of mild excitation, mild
sedation, hypnosis, and deep coma. Some barbiturates
are detoxified by the liver, but others are excreted
unchanged by the kidneys.

An additional adverse effect is the occurrence of the
Stevens-Johnson syndrome, which is characterized by
fever, cough, muscle aches and pains, headache, and
the appearance of wheals or blisters on the skin and
mucous membranes or other organs. This syndrome
can be fatal.

Toxicity is indicated by coma, constricted pupils,
cyanosis, clammy skin, and hypotension. Death may
result.

ASSESSMENT Basic Assessments are the same for all
▲▲▲▲▲▲▲▲▲▲ sedative-hypnotics.

PLANNING AND IMPLEMENTATION Oral forms are eas-
▲▲▲▲▲▲▲▲▲▲▲▲▲▲▲▲▲▲▲▲▲▲▲▲▲▲▲▲ ily absorbed by the
gastrointestinal system. Do not mix injectable forms
with other drugs because they may precipitate in
the container. Barbiturates may be given intravenously. Do not administer intramuscularly unless
it is absolutely necessary because they cause pain
and possible necrosis at the injection site. Administer intramuscular doses into a large muscle mass,
rotate injection sites, and monitor the sites for irritation.

Use of barbiturates is contraindicated for women in
labor. They may cause respiratory depression in the
infant at birth and shortly after.

Monoamine oxidase (MAO) inhibitors block the
metabolism of barbiturates and may cause prolonged
CNS depression. Rifampin may cause decreased blood
levels of barbiturates.

Barbiturates should not be used as hypnotics for
longer than 2 weeks because of the potential for
dependence and abuse. The following examples are
Schedule II drugs unless indicated otherwise.

EVALUATION Monitor the vital signs and level of
▲▲▲▲▲▲▲▲▲▲ consciousness; compare findings with the
baseline data. Compare symptoms of the diagnosis to
determine whether the intended effect is being
achieved.

MISCELLANEOUS SEDATIVE-HYPNOTICS

The miscellaneous sedative-hypnotics have the same
general side effects and precautions as the barbiturates do. Assessments and evaluations are generally
the same.

Chloral Hydrate

Chloral hydrate (Noctec) is a Schedule IV drug. It is
contraindicated in patients with renal or hepatic
impairment. Gastric disorders also contraindicate
use. Dilute liquid preparations and administer capsules with a large glass of liquid to prevent gastric
irritation and mask unpleasant taste. Effects of
anticoagulants are increased, so use caution when
administering these drugs together. Monitor prothrombin times frequently.

Glutethimide Hydrochloride

Glutethimide hydrochloride is a Schedule III drug.
Be aware of additional adverse effects that include
excitation, ataxia and dizziness, dry mouth, blurred
vision, and bladder atony.

Assess the history of male patients for evidence of
prostatic hypertrophy. Monitor for urinary urgency,
hesitancy, and retention.

Assess also for a history of glaucoma. Monitor
complaints of headache and visual disturbances; note
whether pupils are dilated.

Gastrointestinal irritation or ulcer may occur.
Document and report complaints of gastrointestinal
distress.

Withdraw the drug gradually. Abrupt withdrawal
may cause nervousness, tremors, tachycardia, hallucinations, and convulsions.

BENZODIAZEPINES

The following examples are on Schedule IV of the
Controlled Substances Act.

Flurazepam, temazepam, and triazolam act on the
limbic system (the part of the brain that has to do with
feelings, emotions, and survival behaviors), the thalamus, and the hypothalamus of the central nervous
system to produce hypnotic effects.

Flurazepam hydrochloride (Dalmane) may produce
the additional adverse effects of leukopenia and
granulocytopenia. Assess the chart for results of the
white blood cell count. Assess the patient for signs of

infection. Document these and report them to the physician.

E X E R C I S E S

LEARNING ACTIVITIES

Role play the following situations with a classmate.

1. Your patient, Ms. M.H., recently had a major bowel surgery. She has been in the hospital for 2 1/2 weeks. During that time, she has often had difficulty sleeping at night and was given a sedative-hypnotic. Now that she is being discharged, she has requested a prescription for this medication to use at home. When her physician omitted writing a prescription for this drug, she became upset. What teaching will you do to help her understand that this was not an oversight? Why does insomnia often occur during a hospitalization? What alternatives will you suggest to her so that she can obtain her needed rest?

2. Mr. S.P. is scheduled for surgery in 2 hours. When you arrive with his ordered dose of Nembutal and explain that the physician ordered a preoperative sedative, he replies that he is not anxious about the surgery and would rather not take any sedation. How will you explain and encourage him to accept this medication?

3. Your classmate complained that her baby has chickenpox and is restless and fussy. She states that she was awakened every 1 1/2 to 2 hours last night to soothe the baby. While she says that each time she was able to return to sleep immediately after, she complains of feeling tired and is having difficulty thinking today. Explain what is happening to her because of the interruption in her sleep cycles.

PSYCHOTHERAPEUTIC DRUGS

LEARNING OBJECTIVES

After studying this chapter, you should be able to:

1. List the three major classifications of psychotherapeutic drugs.

2. List the subclasses or groups of each of the three major classes.

3. List examples of each classification.

4. List the conditions for which each of these is used.

5. Discuss the adverse effects common to drugs of each class.

6. State nursing interventions appropriate for patients receiving each of these drugs.

7. Prepare an appropriate plan of care for a patient receiving one of these medications.

DRUGS YOU WILL LEARN ABOUT IN THIS CHAPTER

Antianxiety Medications

Benzodiazepine compounds

diazepam (Valium)

chlordiazepoxide HCl (Librium)

oxazepam (Serax)

alprazolam (Xanax)

lorazepam (Ativan)

Miscellaneous minor tranquilizers

hydroxyzine pamoate (oral Vistaril)

hydroxyzine HCl (injectable Vistaril, Atarax)

buspirone (BuSpar)

meprobamate (Equanil, Miltown)

Antidepressant Medications

Tricyclic antidepressants

amitriptyline HCl (Elavil, Metavil)

doxepin (Adapin, Sinequan)

imipramine (Tofranil)

nortriptyline (Aventyl)

protriptyline (Vivactil)

Monoamine oxidase (MAO) inhibitors

phenelzine sulfate (Nardil)

tranylcypromine sulfate (Parnate)

isocarboxazid (Marplan)

Miscellaneous antidepressants

maprotiline HCl (Ludiomil)

amoxapine (Asendin)

trazodone HCl (Desyrel)

bupropion HCl (Wellbutrin)

fluoxetine (Prozac)

Antipsychotic Agents/Neuroleptics

reserpine (Serpasil)

rauwolfia (Raudixin)

Phenothiazines

223

chlorpromazine HCl (Thorazine, Chlorzine, Ormazine)

promazine HCl (Sparine)

Miscellaneous antipsychotics

droperidol (Inapsine)

haloperidol (Haldol)

lithium carbonate (Lithane, Lithizine)

lithium citrate (Cibalith-S)

Psychotherapeutic drugs (also called psychoactive drugs) are used to treat disorders of the mind. They were first introduced in the 1950s and have radically changed psychiatric care. Patients who were once residing in institutions are now back in their communities. Many are once again productive members of society. The degree of mind change produced by the medication depends on the particular drug being taken, the dosage, and the response of the patient.

Included in the classification of psychotherapeutics are the subclassifications of antianxiety drugs, antidepressant drugs, and antipsychotic drugs, each of which is discussed separately. Patients may be taking one type of medication or a regimen of medications from each of the subclassifications, depending on the particular symptoms being experienced. Table 33–1 lists common psychotherapeutic drugs and their dosages.

The actions of the psychotherapeutics vary with the specific type of drug and are discussed individually. Uses are for disorders of thought, agitation, and psychoses.

Adverse actions include food and alcohol interactions, hypotension, restlessness, tachycardia, dry mouth, decreased motor and cognitive abilities, alterations in sleep patterns with decrease in rapid eye movement (REM) sleep, and hangover effects. Sexual activity may be affected by an increase or decrease in libido (conscious or unconscious sex drive), impotence (inability to achieve or maintain an erection), or achievement of an erection but inability to ejaculate.

With all types of therapeutics, caregivers must assess the patient's vital signs and current mental status. Assess the chart for a history of depression and alcohol or drug dependence or abuse because these may be contraindications to use. Document findings as baseline data.

Some general points are especially important to remember in administering medications to patients with mental disturbances.

Table 33-1. Psychotherapeutic Drugs

DRUG	DOSAGE
Benzodiazepine Compounds	
diazepam (Valium)	Adults: 2–10 mg PO tid or qid Children older than 6 mo: 1–2.5 mg PO tid or qid Parenteral doses may be used to stop seizures, to treat anxiety, or as preoperative medications: Adults: 5–10 mg IV initially; may use up to 30 mg in 1 h depending on the response Children older than 5 y: 1 mg IV or IM slowly q 2–5 min to a maximum of 10 mg; may be repeated q2–4h
chlordiazepoxide hydrochloride (Librium)	Adults: 5–25 mg PO tid–qid Children older than 6 y: 5–10 mg PO bid–tid For alcohol withdrawal: Adults: 50–100 mg PO, IM, or IV (maximum, 300 mg qd) For preoperative sedation Adults: 50–100 mg IM 1 h before procedure
oxazepam (Serax)	For alcohol withdrawal or severe anxiety: 15–30 mg PO tid or qid
Alprazolam (Xanax)	For anxiety: 0.25–0.5 PO tid to a maximum of 4 mg in divided dosages; elderly start at 0.25 mg bid or tid

Always check to be sure that patients swallow oral preparations. Be certain they drink sufficient liquid to prevent their holding the tablet or capsule in the mouth. To assess this, ask the patient to open the

Table 33-1. Psychotherapeutic Drugs *Continued*

DRUG	DOSAGE
lorazepam (Ativan)	For anxiety or organic disorders (adults): 2–6 mg PO qd in divided doses (maximum 10 mg qd) For preoperative sedation in adults: 2–4 mg IM or IV
Miscellaneous Minor Tranquilizers	
hydroxyzine pamoate (oral Vistaril) hydroxyzine hydrochloride (injectable Vistaril, Atarax)	200–400 mg PO or IM qd
buspirone (BuSpar)	5–10 mg PO tid
meprobamate (Equanil, Bamate, Miltown)	Adults: 1.2–1.6 g PO in 3–4 divided doses (maximum 2.4 g qd) Children 6–12 y: 100–200 mg PO bid or tid
Tricyclic Antidepressants	
amitriptyline hydrochloride (Elavil, Meravil)	50–100 mg PO hs, increasing to 200 mg qd (maximum, 300 mg qd) 20–30 mg IM qid or 80–120 mg IM qd at hs
doxepin (Adapin, Sinequan)	50–75 mg PO qd in divided doses (maximum, 300 mg qd); entire dose may be given at hs
imipramine (Tofranil)	75–100 mg PO or IM qd in divided doses; may increase by 25 to 50-mg increments up to 200 mg qd (maximum, 300 mg qd)

Table 33-1. Psychotherapeutic Drugs *Continued*

DRUG	DOSAGE
nortriptyline (Aventyl)	25 mg PO tid or qid; may gradually increase to a maximum of 150 mg qd; entire dose may be given at hs
protriptyline (Vivactil)	15–40 mg PO qd in divided doses; may gradually increase to a maximum of 60 mg
Monoamine Oxidase (MAO) Inhibitors	
phenelzine sulfate (Nardil)	45 mg PO qd in divided doses, increasing to 60 mg qd (maximum, 90 mg qd)
tranylcypromine sulfate (Parnate)	10 mg PO bid; may increase to a maximum of 30 mg qd after 2 wks
isocarboxazid (Marplan)	30 mg PO qd in divided doses; reduce to 10–20 mg qd when symptoms improve
Miscellaneous Antidepressants	
maprotiline hydrochloride (Ludiomil)	75 mg PO qd; dose may be increased to 150 mg qd; maximum dose of 225 mg in patients who are not hospitalized; maximum dose of 300 mg qd in severely depressed, hospitalized patients

Table continued on following page

Table 33-1. Psychotherapeutic Drugs *Continued*

DRUG	DOSAGE
amoxapine (Asendin)	50 mg PO tid × 3 days; then may increase to 100 mg tid × 2 wk, then evaluate; hospitalized patients: maximum dose of 600 mg PO qd
trazodone hydrochloride (Desyrel)	150 mg PO qd in divided doses; may increase by 50 mg qd q 3–4 days; average dose: 150–400 mg qd (maximum, 600 mg qd)
fluoxetine (Prozac)	20 mg PO every morning, may increase after several weeks to 20 mg bid with doses given morning and noon; may progressively increase if needed to a maximum of 80 mg qd in divided doses
Phenothiazines	
chlorpromazine hydrochloride (Chlorzine, Ormazine, Thorazine)	Intractable hiccups, alcohol withdrawal: 25–50 mg PO or IM tid–qid Nausea, vomiting: 10–25 mg PO or IM q4–6h, prn; 50–100 mg rectally q6–8h prn Psychosis: 500 mg PO qd in divided doses, increasing gradually to 2 g; 25–50 mg IM q1–4h prn
promazine hydrochloride (Sparine)	Psychoses: 25–200 mg. PO or IM q4–6h Acute agitation: up to 1 gm qd. IV in concentrations up to 25 mg/mL; initial concentrations 50–150 mg; repeat in 5–10 min prn

Table 33-1. Psychotherapeutic Drugs *Continued*

DRUG	DOSAGE
Miscellaneous Antipsychotics	
droperidol (Inapsine)	2.5–10 mg IM 30–60 min preoperatively Induction of general anesthesia: 2.5 mg IV per 20–25 lb weight Maintenance in general anesthesia: 1.25–2.5 mg IV
haloperidol (Haldol)	Adult psychotic disorders: 0.5–5 mg PO bid or tid; 2–5 mg IM q4–8h (maximum, 100 mg PO qd Control of tics in tourette's syndrome: 0.5–5 mg PO bid or tid, increasing prn
lithium carbonate (Lithane, Lithizine) lithium citrate (Cibalith-S)	300–600 mg PO up to qid, increasing on the basis of serum drug levels to achieve optimum dose Lithium citrate (liquid) contains 8 mEq lithium, which is equal to 300 mg lithium carbonate

mouth and lift the tongue. Patients with suicidal tendencies may save medications until they have enough to produce a lethal dose.

Observe the patient after medication administration to prevent self-induced vomiting. Many patients are suspicious and may vomit the medication because they fear some harm will be produced by the medication.

Assessment for therapeutic effects and adverse effects is a 24-hour-a-day responsibility. Many patients may be unable to express themselves to describe signs and symptoms of adverse effects. Caregivers may have to rely on nonverbal clues to subjective symptoms.

Teach patients who will be self-administering medications not to alter their medication regimen without consulting the physician. Many people decrease dosage or abruptly discontinue medications when they feel better or when they experience adverse effects. This may result in subtherapeutic blood levels of the drug or withdrawal symptoms. Encourage patients to report all unusual symptoms because they may indicate the onset of adverse effects.

Encourage patients to keep all appointments with the physician and counselor. Some patients rely on the medication to "make them well" and may tend to cancel appointments when they decide they are better. Remind them that the medications are intended to assist them in controlling some aspect of their behavior but that it is imperative to continue with counseling. Counseling is intended to assist them in gaining insights into their behaviors and in learning positive coping skills that will help them attain stable behaviors.

Teach patients not to take over-the-counter medications without consulting their physician. Patients should also provide a list of all of their medications to all of the physicians who are prescribing treatments for them.

Caution patients to avoid driving and operation of hazardous machinery. Make them aware of any specific safety risks. Postural hypotension is common with many of these medications, so caution patients to change position slowly and to dangle before rising. Monitor blood pressure while the patient changes from lying to sitting and to standing positions.

Some medications require that certain foods be omitted because they may precipitate the onset of side effects. Teach patients about foods that may cause problems and provide them with a written list of these foods. Alcohol is contraindicated with all of these classifications of medications.

Psychotherapeutic drugs cause sedation when therapy is first initiated. Patients frequently show decreased response to the environment, drowsiness, and inability to focus on a task or conversation. Tolerance to the sedative effects develops rapidly, and symptoms of sedation diminish.

Caregivers should not permit patients to draw them into detailed discussions of their sexual difficulties because this may also be a symptom of their illness. Instead, recognize and acknowledge the distress that may be caused by difficulties with sexual function in patients who may already be experiencing difficulty with relationships of all types. Offer counseling *by appropriate professionals* to patients who indicate a need or concern for it.

Caregivers must know the expected actions of the drug to evaluate its effectiveness. Note particularly whether behavior changes occur after medication is received or before the next assigned dose.

ANTIANXIETY MEDICATIONS

ACTIONS AND USES Antianxiety medications are also called tranquilizers, ataractic agents, or anxiolytics. They act on subcortical areas of the brain (below the cortex) to produce a calm feeling and to reduce nausea. They are sometimes divided into groups called minor tranquilizers.

Antianxiety medications are used to treat neuroses, psychosomatic conditions (conditions in which mental stressors cause physical symptoms), mild anxiety, and panic disorders. Minor tranquilizers are sometimes used as skeletal muscle relaxants for chronic pain, such as back pain, when muscle spasm is a part of the pain. They are sometimes used in patients undergoing alcohol withdrawal and also as anti-convulsant agents. Many of these drugs have additive actions when they are combined with other central nervous system (CNS) depressants.

Adverse actions include drowsiness and dizziness. Drug dependence is possible, as are serious episodes of depression.

The main type of antianxiety agent is the benzodiazepine compound. Miscellaneous minor tranquilizers are also included in this section.

ASSESSMENT Assess vital signs and current mental status. Assess the chart for a history of depression and alcohol or drug dependence or abuse because these may be contraindications to use. Document findings as baseline data.

PLANNING AND IMPLEMENTATION Caution patients to avoid alcohol ingestion. Caution patients about the possibility of dependence or tolerance. Monitor and observe for indications of dependence or tolerance. Encourage patients to participate in self-help programs that teach techniques of management for anxiety or chronic pain.

EVALUATION Evaluate the patient's statements of effectiveness of therapy. Evaluate signs and symptoms of dependence or tolerance. Monitor for improvement in seizure control.

Benzodiazepine Compounds

Examples of benzodiazepine compounds are diazepam (Valium), chlordiazepoxide hydrochloride (Librium), oxazepam (Serax), alprazolam (Xanax), and lorazepam (Ativan). An additional action of the benzodiazepines is amnesia, which is of a patchy quality not usually recognized by the patient. It is usually amnesia for events just after administration, so it has an advantage for preoperative use in that the patient often does not remember the unpleasant events of immediate postoperative pain and recovery room events. This is also true of use in seizure episodes.

Benzodiazepines are metabolized by the liver and excreted by the kidneys. Adverse effects are more common among the elderly and may contraindicate use. Assess the chart for a history of renal or hepatic impairment or laboratory results that may indicate these problems.

Because of the amnesia effects, the patient may not recall preoperative teaching or teaching and explanations given in the immediate postoperative period. Important points usually need to be repeated several times.

Avoid mixing injectable forms of these drugs with others because many are incompatible. Powdered forms contain specific instructions for mixing. Diluent may be included in the package. Read instructions carefully before preparation and administration of the drug. Adminster intramuscular (IM) preparations deep into a large muscle mass.

Assess for history of glaucoma because this may also contraindicate use. Encourage patients to report headache, eye pain or discomfort, and blurred vision that may indicate the occurrence of increased intraocular pressure. Assess for bloodshot appearance to the eyes. Document and report findings to the physician.

These are Schedule IV drugs of the Controlled Substances Act. Long-term use of these medications is contraindicated because of the potential for dependence or tolerance. Patients should have a medical evaluation at least monthly to determine whether continued use is indicated.

Flumazenil (Romazicon) is a benzodiazepine antagonist that may be ordered for intravenous (IV) administration to reverse adverse effects of anesthetics or overdose. The duration of action is 1 to 4 hours, which allows easy adjustment of dosage.

Miscellaneous Minor Tranquilizers

In addition to the uses described for the antianxiety medications, hydroxyzine pamoate (oral Vistaril) and hydroxyzine hydrochloride (injectable Vistaril, Atarax) are used for their antiemetic actions and to treat urticaria and pruritus due to allergic conditions.

The parenteral form is for IM use only, never IV. It is irritating to tissues, so it must be injected deep into a large muscle mass. Aspirate carefully. Rotate injection sites and monitor for irritation at the site.

Buspirone

Buspirone (BuSpar) acts as an agonist of serotonin and dopamine. It effectively relieves anxiety without producing significant sedation, drowsiness, or amnesia.

Adverse effects are insomnia, dizziness, nervousness, nausea, headache, tinnitus, fatigue, and chest pain.

Initial dosages are lower until response is evaluated. Doses are then increased progressively.

Meprobamate

Meprobamate (Equanil, Miltown) has additional adverse actions that include thrombocytopenia, leukopenia, palpitations, tachycardia, and rashes. Monitor for signs and symptoms of infection and for increased bruising and petechiae.

Give oral preparations with meals to reduce gastric distress. Administer IM preparations deep into a large muscle mass.

Because of an increase in street use and abuse of this drug, many physicians do not order meprobamate as frequently as they previously did.

Monitor laboratory values of the complete blood count (CBC) and results of hepatic function tests. Monitor serum drug levels. Therapeutic levels are 0.5 mg to 2 mg per 100 mL of blood. Levels above 20 mg per 100 mL may cause coma and death.

ANTIDEPRESSANT MEDICATIONS

The three main groups of antidepressant drugs are the tricyclic antidepressants, the monoamine oxidase (MAO) inhibitors, and the non-MAO inhibitors (or miscellaneous antidepressants).

Tricyclic Antidepressant Medications

ACTIONS AND USES Included in this group are amitriptyline hydrochloride (Elavil, Meravil), doxepin (Adapin, Sinequan), imipramine (Tofranil), nortriptyline (Aventyl), and protriptyline (Vivactil). Tricyclic and tetracyclic antidepressants have become the most widely used drugs for treatment of depression. It is believed that they act to gradually increase the norepinephrine or serotonin in the central nervous system (CNS). It takes approximately 2 weeks to note significant effects. These medications act to elevate the mood, increase the appetite, and increase alertness in patients with depression. They are used for the depressive phase of bipolar disorder (formerly called manic-depressive disorder) and the depressive reactions due to organic brain syndromes. They have little effect in neurotic depressions and agitated depressions.

All of the tricyclic antidepressants cause anticholinergic effects, such as dry membranes, constipation, blurred vision, and urinary retention. Some sedation is possible. Rash, photosensitivity, and jaundice may appear. Blood dyscrasias, swelling of the testes, gynecomastia, and impotence may also occur. Some patients note a slight tremor of the hands, numbness and tingling of the extremities, and sometimes extrapyramidal effects. Orthostatic hypotension is common. Tachycardia, arrhythmias, and congestive heart failure have been known to occur on occasion. Patients taking large doses may experience seizures.

ASSESSMENT Assess male patients for a history of prostatic hypertrophy because this may predispose them to urinary retention. Assess also for a history of cardiac conditions. Assess vital signs and document findings as baseline data.

PLANNING AND IMPLEMENTATION Chewing gum or sucking hard candy or ice may relieve dry mouth. Monitor intake and output, especially in men with prostatic hypertrophy.

Increased intake of fluids may relieve constipation. Increasing intake of fruits, vegetables, and whole-grain products may also help. If these measures are not adequate, consult the physician about use of a stool-softening agent.

Caution patients and caregivers about the possibility of sedation, especially early in therapy. Initiate appropriate safety measures.

Exercise caution when MAO inhibitors are used and monitor for symptoms of drug interaction, such as severe excitation, high fevers, and convulsions. Barbiturates may decrease blood levels of the antidepressant medications and allow symptoms of the illness to increase.

EVALUATION Monitor laboratory values of the complete blood count (CBC). Monitor for improvement of symptoms.

Monoamine Oxidase Inhibitors

ACTIONS AND USES Monoamine oxidase (MAO) is an enzyme partly responsible for destruction of certain body chemicals, such as epinephrine, norepinephrine, and serotonin. Inhibiting this enzyme results in an increase in CNS stimulation and a decrease in depression. The enzyme takes several weeks to regenerate, resulting in longer term therapeutic effects of the drugs.

Included in this group are phenelzine sulfate (Nardil), tranylcypromine sulfate (Parnate), and isocarboxazid (Marplan). These drugs are limited in use because of their adverse reactions. Mild adverse effects include anticholinergic effects of dry mouth and blurred vision, excessive stimulation, and allergic reactions. The physician can sometimes eliminate the excessive stimulation by decreasing the dosage or by starting with smaller doses and gradually increasing them.

All MAO inhibitors can produce orthostatic *hypotension*. This is contrary to the expected effect.

The most serious adverse effects are due to interactions with other medications. A hypertensive crisis may be precipitated by administering with a tricyclic antidepressant. Depressant effects of opiates are potentiated.

Hypertensive crisis and death may also result when these medications are taken with foods containing tyramine. Examples of tyramine-containing foods are aged cheeses, yogurt, pickled herring, liver, chocolate, bananas, dried fruits, beer, and wine.

ASSESSMENT Assess vital signs and document findings as baseline data. Assess the patient's drug regimen for medications that are contraindicated. Document and report these to the physician. Assess for a history of kidney dysfunction, cardiovascular disease, pregnancy, pheochromocytoma, and epilepsy; these may contraindicate use.

PLANNING AND IMPLEMENTATION Monitor vital signs frequently. Caregivers should be taught to recognize the signs of impending hypertensive crisis. The crisis usually begins with an occipital headache followed by a stiff neck, nausea, and vomiting. Cerebrovascular accident (CVA) or death may result from the hypertension.

N U R S I N G   A L E R T

Teach patients the importance of avoiding tyramine and give them a written list of foods that contain tyramine. Foods that commonly cause interactions include dried, fermented, and pickled foods.

Medications containing phenylethylamine, phenylephrine, and other vasoconstricting agents are contraindicated. Cold remedies and other vasoconstricting products often contain the harmful ingredients. Teach patients not to take over-the-counter drugs without consulting the physician.

Because of the potentially lethal effects that may occur with some drugs, a 2-week interval is recommended when a MAO inhibitor is discontinued and therapy with a tricyclic antidepressant is initiated. If the patient has previously been taking a tricyclic antidepressant, the same 2-week interval is recommended before initiation of therapy with the MAO inhibitor.

EVALUATION Evaluate compliance with the diet and
▲▲▲▲▲▲▲▲▲▲ medication regimen. Evaluate vital signs and compare findings with baseline data.

Miscellaneous Antidepressants

There are multiple drugs in this group. They are sometimes referred to as non-MAO inhibitors, tetracyclics, or second-generation antidepressant drugs. Many have actions similar to the tricyclics and most offer little, if any, advantage over the previously mentioned drugs. Examples include maprotiline hydrochloride (Ludiomil), amoxapine (Asendin), trazodone hydrochloride (Desyrel), and bupropion hydrochloride (Wellbutrin).

Trazodone Hydrochloride

Trazodone hydrochloride (Desyrel) is reported to have fewer anticholinergic and cardiotoxic effects than the other antidepressants. It can cause priapism (prolonged, painful penile erections), and prolonged use can cause impotence.

Bupropion Hydrochloride

Bupropion hydrochloride (Wellbutrin) has the added advantage of achieving therapeutic drug levels within 2 hours of oral administration. This drug has the potential to cause seizures. It also has serious drug interactions with MAO inhibitors, levodopa, and agents that lower the seizure threshold.

Fluoxetine

Fluoxetine (Prozac) has recently become controversial because an increase in the frequency of suicide attempts (in patients not previously recognized as suicidal) has caused concern. Caregivers should maintain suicide precautions for any person receiving this medication.

ANTIPSYCHOTIC AGENTS/NEUROLEPTICS

Antipsychotic agents or neuroleptics include drugs sometimes referred to as the major tranquilizers: the phenothiazines, rauwolfia alkaloids, and a group of miscellaneous drugs. These drugs block dopamine receptors in the brain. They modify psychotic symptoms but do not cure. They are used to treat acute and chronic psychoses, especially in cases involving panic, agitation, hostility, and aggression such as is seen in schizophrenia, organic psychoses, and bipolar disorders.

Examples of the rauwolfia drugs are reserpine (Serpasil) and rauwolfia (Raudixin). They are the oldest of the tranquilizers, but their value is currently more historic than practical. They are not often used because they have unclear actions, require large doses, and produce major adverse effects. They can be used to treat agitated psychoses and severe hypertension.

Phenothiazines

The first of the phenothiazines to be introduced for therapy was chlorpromazine hydrochloride (Chlorzine, Ormazine, Thorazine). Another example is promazine hydrochloride (Sparine).

ACTIONS AND USES The phenothiazines act on the ce-
▲▲▲▲▲▲▲▲▲▲▲▲▲▲▲▲ rebral cortex, the basal ganglia, the hypothalamus, and the medulla. They block peripheral adrenergic and cholinergic impulses. These drugs are used to treat psychoses, bipolar disorder (manic-depressive disorder), agitation, and delirium tremens (DTs). Some are also used for their antiemetic effects.

Adverse actions include hypotension, dizziness, fainting, bradycardia, blood dyscrasias, confusion, restlessness, lethargy, pruritus, urticaria, jaundice, photosensitivity, photophobia, dry mouth, headache, nausea, vomiting, and diarrhea. Men may also experience impotence.

Extrapyramidal effects may also be seen. These include a shuffling gait, pill rolling, agitation, rigidity, and spasms.

Tardive dyskinesia is the most serious of the neurological syndromes that can result from these medications; 60% to 70% of these symptoms are not reversible after the drug is discontinued. Symptoms include involuntary buccofaciomandibular or buccolingual movements, such as sucking, smacking lips, and lateral movements of the jaw and tongue.

ASSESSMENT Assess vital signs and document findings ▲▲▲▲▲▲▲▲▲▲ as baseline data. Assess for a history of cardiac conditions. A complete blood count (CAC) should also be obtained before therapy is initiated.

PLANNING AND IMPLEMENTATION Teach patients to ▲▲▲▲▲▲▲▲▲▲▲▲▲▲▲▲▲▲▲▲▲▲▲▲▲▲▲▲▲ avoid exposure to the sun. Exposed parts of the body should be protected by application of sunblock and by wearing large-brimmed hats. Skin should also be monitored daily for rash or jaundice.

Monitor vital signs, especially early in the course of treatment. To avoid injury from postural hypotension, teach patients to change positions slowly and to dangle before rising. Observe for sudden cardiac arrest and be prepared to perform resuscitative procedures. Anticipate and try to prevent suicide attempts. Administer intramuscular (IM) injections deep into a large muscle mass.

EVALUATION Monitor vital signs and the behavior of ▲▲▲▲▲▲▲▲▲▲ the patient. Hypotension, central nervous system (CNS) depression, and extrapyramidal reactions may indicate overdosage.

Miscellaneous Antipsychotics

Examples of the miscellaneous antipsychotics include droperidol (Inapsine), haloperidol (Haldol), lithium carbonate (Lithane, Lithizine, Lithobid), and lithium citrate (Cibalith-S).

Droperidol

Droperidol (Inapsine) is an antipsychotic medication, but the Food and Drug Administration (FDA) has approved use *only* for induction and maintenance of anesthesia. This drug is more likely to cause extrapyramidal reactions than are other antipsychotic agents. Other adverse actions include respiratory depression, apnea, and muscle rigidity, which could lead to respiratory arrest.

Monitor vital signs preoperatively and document as baseline findings. Assess for a history of hypotension, impaired hepatic or renal function, cardiovascular disease, or Parkinson's disease. Monitor vital signs frequently during treatment and compare findings with baseline data. Do not place patients in Trende-

lenburg position because it promotes respiratory arrest. A narcotic antagonist and resuscitative equipment must be on hand.

Haloperidol

Haloperidol (Haldol) has additional adverse actions that include transient leukopenia and leukocytosis. Assess the chart for baseline results of the complete blood count (CBC). Monitor the patient for signs and symptoms of infection and compare results of repeated CBC tests with baseline data.

There is a high frequency of severe extrapyramidal reactions. Monitor for these symptoms, document them, and report their occurrence.

Drug interactions include lethargy and confusion with large doses of lithium and symptoms of dementia with methyldopa. Monitor patients for symptoms.

Haloperidol is contraindicated in Parkinson's disease, coma, or CNS depression. Use with caution in the elderly, those with allergies, and those with severe cardiovascular disorders.

Oral and IM preparations are available. Protect solutions from light. There is a slight yellowish appearance to the liquid. Discard the solution if it is markedly discolored.

Do not suddenly withdraw this medication from the patient. Notify the physician if adverse effects are noted or changes are desired.

Lithium Carbonate

Lithium carbonate (Lithane, Lithizine) is an oral preparation; lithium citrate (Cibalith-S) is a liquid.

ACTIONS AND USES Lithium was first used in the ▲▲▲▲▲▲▲▲▲▲▲▲▲▲▲▲ 1800s for treatment of gout. It has been used since that time as a hypnotic and as a salt substitute. There were many negative effects from these uses until the 1960s, when lithium was used to treat manic behaviors of those with bipolar disorder. It may be also ordered to supplement counseling and behavior modification therapies for some behavioral disorders in children, such as attention deficit hyperactivity disorder (ADHD).

Lithium calms the patient by controlling symptoms, such as flight of ideas, elation, talkativeness, restlessness, poor judgment, hostility, aggressiveness, and decreased sleep time. It does not produce sedative or euphoric effects.

Many patients fail to continue the ordered regimen when they feel better. This is sometimes believed to be due to fear of side effects or a desire to return to the euphoric phase of the illness.

Peak serum levels are achieved within 1 to 4 hours of ingestion, but therapeutic effects are not seen for 7 to 10 days. Excretion is by the kidneys. A lowered sodium intake slows the excretion of lithium and results in accumulation and toxicity. Use of diuretics also predisposes to toxicity. Symptoms of thirst and polyuria resembling diabetes insipidus may continue throughout therapy.

Severity of the adverse reactions depends on the serum levels of the drug. Dry mouth and metallic taste are fairly common. Early toxic symptoms include nausea, vomiting, diarrhea, drowsiness, and weakness. Later, ataxia, giddiness, blurred vision, tinnitus, and polyuria may be seen. Some people experience transient hyperglycemia, goiter, and hypothyroidism. Toxic reactions also include tremors, blackouts, seizures, stupor, arrhythmias, hypotension, albuminuria, and circulatory collapse.

ASSESSMENT Assess for a history of thyroid disease, ▲▲▲▲▲▲▲▲▲▲ epilepsy, renal or cardiovascular disease, and brain damage. Assess the chart for baseline electrocardiographic (ECG) recordings, thyroid test results, serum glucose determinations, renal studies, and electrolyte levels.

PLANNING AND IMPLEMENTATION Monitor   lithium ▲▲▲▲▲▲▲▲▲▲▲▲▲▲▲▲▲▲▲▲▲▲▲▲▲▲▲▲▲ concentrations frequently. Adverse effects are generally mild if blood levels are maintained below 1.5 mEq/liter.

Minor toxic effects usually subside after the first few weeks of therapy. Monitor for signs of toxicity and report these to the physician. Depending on the serum level at that time, the dose may be decreased or stopped for 24 hours. It is usually resumed at a decreased dosage.

Monitor intake and output. Unless it is contraindicated, fluid intake of 2500 to 3000 cc should be maintained each day. Diet should be low calorie if weight gain is a problem and include approximately 2 g of salt each day. Teach patients to weigh themselves daily to monitor for edema and weight gain.

Teach patients not to discontinue the drug abruptly and to avoid over-the-counter preparations unless the physician is consulted before use. Patients should carry an identification card that lists toxic symptoms and emergency measures.

This drug should be used with caution with many other medications. The physician should monitor the medication regimen and consult pharmaceutical references if new medications are added.

Monitor the patient for signs and symptoms of hyperglycemia.

This drug is known to be teratogenic. Female patients should be aware of this and offered counseling about birth control practices.

EVALUATION Periodic assessments of serum lithium ▲▲▲▲▲▲▲▲▲▲ levels are imperative. An ECG may be ordered if symptoms of cardiovascular symptoms arise. (Reversible ECG changes are not unusual.) Other laboratory tests that may be ordered at intervals include specific gravity and other tests of renal function, thyroid tests, and blood glucose determinations.

E X E R C I S E S

CASE STUDIES

1. Mr. D.K. is taking the phenothiazine Thorazine for treatment of his mental disorder. After taking this medication without difficulty for 2 years, he is now displaying the following symptoms: pill rolling, shuffling gait, spasms, and unusual movements of his tongue and lips. Discuss the implications of these symptoms.

2. Ms. S.F. is scheduled for surgical removal of a neuroma from her foot. Her preoperative medication order includes meperidine and diazepam. Explain the role of diazepam as a preoperative medication.

ANTICONVULSANTS

L E A R N I N G   O B J E C T I V E S

After studying this chapter, you should be able to:

1. Define anticonvulsant, hydantoin, benzodiazepine, succinimide, oxazolidinedione, and barbiturate.

2. Identify actions and uses of and adverse reactions to each type of anticonvulsant.

3. State appropriate nursing interventions for a patient receiving each type of anticonvulsant.

4. State common examples of each type of anticonvulsant.

5. Identify symptoms of the toxic effects of dilantin.

6. Relate laboratory tests necessary with dilantin therapy.

7. Prepare an appropriate teaching plan for a patient receiving an anticonvulsant.

8. Demonstrate how to administer anticonvulsants by use of the nursing process.

DRUGS YOU WILL LEARN ABOUT IN THIS CHAPTER

Barbiturates

phenobarbital (Luminal)

primidone (Mysoline)

Hydantoins

phenytoin (Dilantin)

mephenytoin (Mesantoin)

Benzodiazepines

diazepam (Valium)

clonazepam (Klonopin) (formerly Clonopin)

clorazepate dipotassium (Tranxene)

Oxazolidinediones

trimethadione (Tridione)

paramethadione (Paradione)

Succinimides

ethosuximide (Zarontin)

methsuximide (Celontin)

Valproic Acid and Derivatives

valproic acid (Depakene)

divalproex sodium (Depakote)

Tricyclics

carbamazepine (Tegretol)

Other Anticonvulsants

gabapentin (Neurontin)

ACTIONS AND USES The anticonvulsants work on the ▲▲▲▲▲▲▲▲▲▲▲▲▲▲▲▲ central nervous system. They often work directly on the neurons. A person who suffers from seizures may be prescribed an anticonvulsant. Just as there are many different types of seizures, there are also many different types of anticonvulsants. Some of these drugs work for different types of seizures; not all of them work for all people. In some cases, people simply cannot tolerate every type of anticonvulsant.

Several of the different types of anticonvulsants can cause liver damage. Others in this classification can cause serious blood dyscrasias because they interfere with hematopoiesis (the process of making blood). Some of the anticonvulsants can lead to kidney disease.

Many anticonvulsants cause drowsiness, nystagmus, confusion, ataxia, dizziness, and gastrointestinal upset.

ASSESSMENT Be aware of your patient's history. Often, the physician does not give certain types of anticonvulsants or lowers the dosage if the patient has a history of liver disease. Even an otherwise healthy person should have a baseline liver function profile (tests that show how well the liver functions before the first dose of the drug).

If patients have a history of a blood dyscrasia, they will probably not be given certain drugs. Check the chart and ask the patient for his or her medical history. The physician will order a baseline complete blood count with white cell differential.

Patients are unlikely to receive such a drug if there is a history of kidney disease, or a reduced dose may be used. A baseline urinalysis is obtained.

PLANNING AND IMPLEMENTATION When patients are prescribed any type of anticonvulsant, they should receive some information about the general classification of the drug. Warn them to inform the physician of any seizures they may experience because their medication may need to be changed or the dosage adjusted.

Teach patients to carry or wear an identification tag or card that states they are subject to seizures. This is for their protection. Should they suffer a seizure, this information is vital to an emergency department physician faced with a patient who is unconscious or confused.

Inform patients that this type of drug is for control only. Anticonvulsants do not cure seizures. Should they stop taking their medication, the seizures will recur, and they run the risk of entering status epilepticus.

The patients need to be aware of the possibility of drowsiness. Warn patients not to operate any hazardous machinery, such as an automobile, or perform any hazardous acts that require their full attention and alertness until stabilized on their drug regimen.

Apprise the patient of the effect of drinking alcohol while taking an anticonvulsant. The sedative effects of both the anticonvulsant and the alcohol are increased, leading to severe drowsiness or even stupor. Driving during this period would be deadly, for the patient and for others.

Gastrointestinal upset may be dealt with by lowering the dosage and then slowly increasing it as the patient can tolerate it. This must be ordered by the physician. Some of the drugs can be taken with food to decrease this side effect.

The serum concentration level of a drug needed by the patient for seizure control is highly individualized. Generic drugs can be 10% above or below the efficacy of the trade name drug. If a patient gets a different brand name of drug each time the prescription is filled, a different serum level will be achieved. Because the blood level range required is so narrow for each person, many physicians order a prescription to be filled with a trade name drug only. You may be required to explain this to the patient.

EVALUATION During therapy with an anticonvulsant, the patient is required to have periodic blood tests. These are drug blood levels that tell us how much of the drug is available in the bloodstream. There are three main reasons for these blood tests: (1) to check whether the drug has reached the therapeutic level; (2) to check that the drug has *not* reached the toxic level; and (3) to check for compliance of the patient to the dosage schedule. The blood levels of phenytoin (Dilantin) are especially difficult to regulate. The serum levels of this drug rise quickly with only small increases of dosage. The serum levels of all the other anticonvulsants tend to rise linearly, that is, if the blood level is currently 5 and the physician wants to raise it to 10, the dose is doubled also. Even with these drugs, the serum levels confirm how the drug reacted for the individual patient.

The physician orders frequent repeats of the liver profile during drug therapy. If the tests become abnormal, the physician may change the dose or the drug or discontinue the drug altogether. Evaluate your patient during drug therapy for jaundice or edema.

Blood tests are repeated frequently during drug therapy, and the physician will probably stop the drug if a dyscrasia develops. Warn the patient to inform the physician or nurse of any signs or symptoms of infection, any bleeding or bruising, or any rash.

Urinalysis is periodically repeated throughout drug therapy. The physician will stop the medication if albuminuria develops; this is a symptom of nephrosis.

BARBITURATES

Phenobarbital

ACTIONS AND USES Phenobarbital (Luminal) is a central nervous system (CNS) depressant. It can be used as a sedative-hypnotic, with anesthesia, or as an anticonvulsant. Phenobarbital decreases both sensation and motion, causing the patient to feel drowsy and sedated. The patient will have less rapid eye movement (REM) sleep, and therefore withdrawal from the drug may cause an increase in dreams, nightmares, and insomnia; the physician will withdraw the drug slowly.

In addition to the other side effects listed for anticonvulsants, phenobarbital can lead to nervousness, anxiety, and headache. It can also cause anemia, which can be treated with folic acid and does not necessarily indicate a need to discontinue the drug.

ASSESSMENT Assess the patient's history. A history of porphyria is a contraindication to phenobarbital. Porphyria is a metabolic disorder.

Because phenobarbital is a CNS depressant, it depresses respirations. It may also mask pain, so be alert to safety hazards and signs of complications. Also ask the patient if she is pregnant because phenobarbital is known to cause fetal abnormalities.

PLANNING AND IMPLEMENTATION Phenobarbital may be prescribed orally, intramuscularly, or intravenously. For anticonvulsant use, the oral dose is 100 to 300 mg per day. Up to 600 mg can be given intravenously. The intravenous dose for status epilepticus is based on the patient's weight.

When phenobarbital is given intramuscularly, choose a large muscle and inject deeply.

N U R S I N G   A L E R T

Intravenous phenobarbital should be given slowly. If it is given too quickly, intravenous phenobarbital can cause laryngospasms, apnea, and hypotension.

Regardless of the route, monitor the vital signs carefully because phenobarbital can cause bradycardia, hypotension, and slowed pulse.

EVALUATION Be aware that phenobarbital is habit forming. It can produce both physical and psychological dependencies. Therefore, be aware of an increased need for the drug and possible withdrawal effects if the patient is removed from the drug.

Caution the patient to alert the physician or nurse about any seizure activity that may be experienced. This may indicate a need to increase the dosage or change medications altogether.

Last, because phenobarbital can precipitate otherwise unknown cases of porphyria, look for symptoms of this disease, including abdominal pain, neurological disorders, and photosensitivity.

Phenobarbital interacts with several other medications. Box 34–1 describes drug interactions with phenobarbital.

Primidone

Primidone (Mysoline) is an oral anticonvulsant given for tonic-clonic, psychomotor, and focal seizures. As this drug is metabolized in the body, it is broken down into its main ingredient—phenobarbital. For this reason, it shares the information listed for phenobarbital. The usual maintenance dose for primidone is 250 mg

---

Box 34–1. Drug Interactions with Phenobarbital

Increased effects of phenobarbital
Steroids
Central nervous system depressants
Monoamine oxidase inhibitors

Decreased effects of phenobarbital
Griseofulvin
Other anticonvulsants
Hormones

Increased effects of concurrent drug
Dilantin
Steroids

Decreased effects of concurrent drug
Anticoagulants
Doxycycline
Oral contraceptives
Estrogens

three or four times a day. The dosage must be reached gradually, starting at around 125 mg once a day.

HYDANTOINS

Phenytoin

ACTIONS AND USES Phenytoin (Dilantin) works by decreasing the hyperexcitability of the neurons. It is one of the drugs of choice for partial seizures and is still used to treat tonic-clonic or generalized seizures. It may also be prescribed for the prevention and treatment of seizures during and after neurological surgeries.

During phenytoin therapy, note side effects. In addition to those listed for anticonvulsants, phenytoin may cause a rash, slurred speech, confusion, insomnia, nervousness, twitching, hyperglycemia, gingival hyperplasia, respiratory depression, lymphadenopathy, and headache.

N U R S I N G   A L E R T

It is especially important to note that blood dyscrasias are possible from phenytoin.

Other serious complications of phenytoin therapy may include lupus and immunoglobulin abnormalities.

ASSESSMENT Be aware of the type of seizure activity the patient has been experiencing. Because phenytoin can cause hyperglycemia, assess the patient's chart for any history of diabetes. In addition, this drug should not be given to someone with altered liver function.

PLANNING AND IMPLEMENTATION Phenytoin may be given orally, intramuscularly (IM), or intravenously (IV). The dose is individualized and should be established in a 7- to 10-day period. The IM route gives a sustained-release action to phenytoin. IV phenytoin must be given slowly and directly into a large vein. It must never be added to IV solutions because it will precipitate. After the slow IV injection, inject sterile saline into the portal to decrease the chance of vein irritation. Regardless of the route, monitor the patient's respirations for any signs of depression.

Because of possible blood dyscrasias, inform the patient that periodic blood work is needed. Not only

are phenytoin therapeutic levels checked, but also a complete blood count with differential is obtained.

Phenytoin can cause unusual overgrowth of some tissues, including enlarged lips and gingival hyperplasia. Teach the patient the importance of good oral hygiene and dental care. Patients should inform their dentist that they are taking this drug.

Lymphadenopathy from phenytoin therapy can be confused with other more serious disorders. The nurse's role is careful observation of the placement of the enlargement.

Also be careful in your description of a patient's rash. In this case, the type of rash determines whether the drug can be restarted or must be changed to another anticonvulsant.

EVALUATION Evaluate the patient for absence of seizure activity. This includes all portions of a seizure. Include in the evaluation the number of seizures experienced, what type of seizure, and the severity of each.

If a patient takes an overdose, signs of the toxic effects of phenytoin include nystagmus, ataxia, slurred speech, lethargy, nausea and vomiting, joint pains, and tremors.

Evaluate growth patterns in younger patients and symptoms of osteomalacia in older patients because phenytoin interferes with the metabolism of vitamin D. There are numerous other drugs with which phenytoin interacts (Box 34–2).

Box 34–2. Drug Interactions with Phenytoin

Increased effects of phenytoin

Alcohol	Phenothiazines
Chloramphenicol	Salicylates
Chlordiazepoxide	Succinimides
Diazepam	Sulfonamides
Anticoagulants	Phenobarbital
Hormones	Valproic acid
Isoniazid	

Decreased effects of phenytoin

Carbamazepine	Calcium
Reserpine	Antidepressants
Sucralfate	Phenobarbital
Antacids	Valproic acid

Decreased effects of concurrent drug

Steroids	Hormones
Anticoagulants	Furosemide
Digitoxin	Rifampin
Quinidine	Theophylline
Doxycycline	Vitamin D

Mephenytoin

Mephenytoin (Mesantoin) is used to treat both generalized and partial seizures. It is usually given only after safer drugs have failed to control the patient's seizures.

Mephenytoin is given orally. The dose is initially low, and the physician increases the dose slowly until a therapeutic level is reached for the patient.

Mephenytoin produces the same side effects as phenytoin. In addition, there may be diplopia. Teach the patient to report any signs of infection, bleeding, bruising, rash, or swollen glands; any of these may indicate a need to change to a different anticonvulsant.

BENZODIAZEPINES

Diazepam

ACTIONS AND USES Diazepam (Valium) is used as an ▲▲▲▲▲▲▲▲▲▲▲▲▲▲▲ anticonvulsant because it decreases the hyperexcitability of the neurons. It can also be used for other disorders, including anxiety, alcohol withdrawal, and skeletal muscle spasms or strains.

Diazepam is known to cause drowsiness, fatigue, ataxia, and possibly blood dyscrasias.

ASSESSMENT Assess the patient's history. Be aware of ▲▲▲▲▲▲▲▲▲▲ the type of seizures that have been experienced as well as accompanying symptoms. Also be aware of any history of glaucoma because diazepam is contraindicated with closed-angle glaucoma.

PLANNING AND IMPLEMENTATION Diazepam may be ▲▲▲▲▲▲▲▲▲▲▲▲▲▲▲▲▲▲▲▲▲▲▲▲▲▲▲▲▲▲ given orally, intramuscularly, or intravenously. The dose is 2 to 10 mg up to four times a day. An extended-release tablet is available; the dose for this form is 15 to 30 mg once a day.

For intramuscular administration, choose a large muscle and inject the drug deeply. It should not be mixed with any other solutions. When given intravenously, it is given slowly into a large vein. Once again, it may not be mixed with other solutions.

Because diazepam is known to cause drowsiness and ataxia, warn the patient against hazardous tasks, such as driving or operating dangerous machinery.

The physician will order periodic blood studies to check for blood dyscrasias. Teach the patient about these blood tests and the importance of complying with these orders.

Box 34–3. Drugs that Potentiate Diazepam

Potentiate diazepam effects
Phenothiazine
Narcotics
Barbiturates
Monoamine oxidase inhibitors
Antidepressants

Potentiates diazepam blood levels
Cimetidine

Mutual potentiation
Alcohol
Other central nervous system depressants

Because diazepam can cause physical or psychological dependency, a patient may have withdrawal symptoms if the drug is stopped. These may include convulsions, tremors, nausea and vomiting, sweating, and cramping. As with any anticonvulsant, diazepam should not be withdrawn abruptly because it may lead to status epilepticus.

EVALUATION Effectiveness is determined by the same ▲▲▲▲▲▲▲▲▲▲ measures as for other anticonvulsants. Monitor the reports of blood cell studies and inform the physician of any abnormalities.

Be aware that diazepam may interact with some drugs. Box 34–3 lists drugs that can potentiate the effects or blood levels of diazepam.

Clonazepam

As another benzodiazepine, clonazepam (Klonopin, formerly Clonopin) shares many of the properties of diazepam. This drug is most often given for absence attacks and myoclonic seizures.

Clonazepam is given orally in three equally divided doses per day. It may be necessary to increase the dose every 3 days to reach a maintenance dose for the patient. Tolerance may occur after 3 months, and the dose may need to be increased again. The daily dose should not exceed 20 mg per day.

Clonazepam can increase salivation and the frequency of tonic-clonic seizures or worsen chronic respiratory disease.

Clonazepam shares all of the drug interactions of diazepam. Also, if used with the valproic acid drugs, clonazepam may cause absence attacks.

Clorazepate Dipotassium

Clorazepate dipotassium (Tranxene) is an oral anti-convulsant that may be used for anxiety, partial seizures, and alcohol withdrawal. It is contraindicated with closed-angle glaucoma and also with depressive psychosis or neurosis. In addition to evaluating for the effectiveness of the drug, be aware of possible interactions with other drugs (Box 34–4).

OXAZOLIDINEDIONE DERIVATIVES

Trimethadione

ACTIONS AND USES Trimethadione (Tridione) is used for absence attacks, but only if other less toxic drugs have failed to control the patient's seizures. In addition to the side effects that are common to all anticonvulsants, trimethadione may also cause eye damage, systemic lupus erythematosus, lymphadenopathy, a myasthenia gravis–like syndrome, grand mal seizures, personality changes, bleeding gums, epistaxis, and paresthesia.

ASSESSMENT Be careful to assess for seizure activity. Absence attacks can easily be missed or misinterpreted.

PLANNING AND IMPLEMENTATION Trimethadione is an oral drug given at a dose of 300 to 600 mg three or four times a day. The dosage is started low and gradually increased in a period of several weeks until a therapeutic maintenance dose is found for the patient.

Box 34–4. Drug Interactions with Clorazepate

Increased effects of clorazepate
Barbiturates
Narcotics
Phenothiazines
Monoamine oxidase inhibitors
Antidepressants

Increased effects of concurrent drug
Barbiturates
Alcohol
Other central nervous system depressants
Chlorpromazine
Hypnotics

N U R S I N G   A L E R T

Teach the patient to have frequent eye examinations because of the possible damage that can be done from this drug.

If a rash develops during the course of drug therapy, trimethadione should be stopped. Inform the physician immediately if you see a rash on your patient's skin.

EVALUATION Effectiveness of the drug is based on the absence or decrease of seizure activity. Neurological deficits may be determined by a neurological examination, including pupil assessment, hand grasps, and level of consciousness with orientation.

Paramethadione

Paramethadione (Paradione) is closely related to trimethadione and therefore shares its properties.

SUCCINIMIDES

Ethosuximide

ACTIONS AND USES Ethosuximide (Zarontin) is a succinimide anticonvulsant used for absence attacks. Many physicians now consider it to be one of the drugs of choice for generalized seizures.

Ethosuximide has many possible side effects.

N U R S I N G   A L E R T

Ethosuximide may lead to blood dyscrasias, liver or kidney disease, or even lupus.

Advise the patient of the possibility of other side effects, including gingival hyperplasia, drowsiness, dizziness, ataxia, gastrointestinal upset, headache, euphoria, hiccups, irritability, lethargy, hyperactivity, nightmares, urticaria, and myopia. Some of these side effects may appear contradictory to the student. This is because the drug reacts differently in different people. The importance of accurate nursing observation becomes obvious.

ASSESSMENT Be aware of the patient's history and what type of seizures have been experienced. Ethosuximide can increase the frequency of tonic-clonic seizures or precipitate them. Perform the same baseline assessments as for patients receiving other anticonvulsants.

PLANNING AND IMPLEMENTATION Ethosuximide is an oral drug. The patient is not immediately prescribed a maintenance dose. The physician will start low and slowly increase the dose until the patient's seizures are well controlled. The maintenance dose generally does not exceed 750 mg given twice a day.

Because ethosuximide may also cause gingival hyperplasia, emphasize to the patient the need to maintain good dental and oral hygiene.

Because of possible drowsiness or dizziness, take safety precautions in the hospital setting, such as having the patient dangle before arising, instructing the patient to call for help before getting up, keeping the call light close at hand, and answering the call promptly. Further instruct the patient to refrain from operating hazardous machinery, such as automobiles or factory equipment, until stabilized on the drug regimen.

EVALUATION The effectiveness of this drug is determined by the decreased frequency of seizure activity. Make accurate observations and record and report them.

Laboratory work-ups specific to each of the adverse reactions are ordered periodically throughout drug therapy. Monitor the results and report abnormalities to the physician.

Ethosuximide interacts with some other drugs. If the patient is taking either phenytoin or phenobarbital concurrently with ethosuximide, the effects of these two drugs may be increased. In addition, concurrent use with valproic acid may either increase or decrease the effects of ethosuximide.

Methsuximide

Methsuximide (Celontin) is an oral succinimide anticonvulsant closely related to ethosuximide. As such, information on ethosuximide applies to methsuximide. In addition, caution the patient not to leave this drug in high temperatures, such as in an automobile, because the drug can be altered in this manner.

VALPROIC ACID AND DERIVATIVES

Valproic Acid

ACTIONS AND USES Valproic acid (Depakene) is used to treat absence attacks and multiple seizures that include absence attacks as part of their make-up. Be aware of the type of seizure being treated.

N U R S I N G   A L E R T

Valproic acid has been known to cause fatal hepatotoxic effects, most often in the age group younger than 2 years.

Other adverse reactions include gastrointestinal (GI) upset, blood dyscrasias, sedation, dizziness, ataxia, tremors, headache, nystagmus, alopecia, rash, photosensitivity, depression, psychosis, hyperactivity, amenorrhea, breast enlargement, and edema.

ASSESSMENT Be aware of other aspects of the patient's history, including liver disease. Valproic acid is contraindicated in liver disease. The physician will most often order liver function tests before prescribing this drug.

Baseline laboratory tests are ordered before the first dose to check for blood dyscrasias. Most often, a complete blood count with white cell differential is obtained.

PLANNING AND IMPLEMENTATION Valproic acid is an oral drug that is given in increasing doses until the therapeutic dose for the patient is reached. This should not be higher than 60 mg per kilogram of body weight per day.

The increase of dosage must be done slowly, especially if GI irritation arises. If the patient continues to have GI irritation, the physician may opt to switch to divalproex sodium (see later). Caution the patient not to chew the drug, or the mouth and throat may become irritated.

Valproic acid can cause a false-positive urine ketoacidosis test result. The diabetic patient may need to switch to blood evaluations while taking this drug.

Changes in thyroid function tests have also been noted. Patients who have abnormal thyroid function may be better treated with another anticonvulsant.

Teach the patient to avoid hazardous tasks, such as driving or operating hazardous machinery, because of possible sedation and dizziness. Advise the patient of the possibility of adverse reactions.

Teach the patient to refrain from using alcohol while taking this drug. The effects of both the alcohol and valproic acid are potentiated.

EVALUATION In addition to evaluating for the effectiveness of this drug, monitor the results of all laboratory work, such as complete blood count, white cell differential, and liver function studies.

Also be aware of possible drug interactions. Valproic acid may interact with aspirin, carbamazepine, dicumarol and other anticoagulants, phenytoin, phenobarbital, and alcohol.

In the case of an overdose of valproic acid, the patient should receive a counteractive dose of naloxone, which is given subcutaneously, intramuscularly, or intravenously.

Divalproex Sodium

Divalproex (Depakote) is closely related to, and indeed derived from, valproic acid. Its main advantage is the decreased chance of GI irritation. Once again, however, this drug should be slowly increased to the therapeutic level to lessen this side effect. If GI irritation does occur even with divalproex, the drug can be sprinkled on a small amount of food. Caution the patient not to chew the pellets.

Divalproex shares the information listed for valproic acid. Many physicians now consider divalproex to be one of the drugs of choice for generalized seizures.

TRICYCLICS

Carbamazepine

ACTIONS AND USES Carbamazepine (Tegretol) is used to treat psychomotor, tonic-clonic, and mixed seizures. In fact, it is the first drug of choice for partial seizures. It is also the specific analgesic for the treatment of trigeminal neuralgia.

Adverse reactions can include dizziness, drowsiness, immune system dysfunction, gastrointestinal upset, congestive heart failure, coronary artery disease, thrombophlebitis, dyspnea, pneumonia, kidney dysfunction, blurred vision, muscle and joint aches, and impotence.

ASSESSMENT Be aware of the patient's presenting history, including type of seizure, neurological status, and any pre-existing conditions.

N U R S I N G   A L E R T

Carbamazepine is contraindicated if the patient has a history of blood dyscrasias.

The physician will most often order baseline blood work, including a complete blood count (CBC) with white cell differential.

N U R S I N G   A L E R T

Carbamazepine is also contraindicated in liver disease, so liver function tests are routinely ordered for baseline purposes.

Because this drug can adversely affect the immune system, a urinalysis is also commonly ordered before the first dose.

Carbamazepine should not be given to persons who have demonstrated an intolerance to any tricyclic compound, including the antidepressants.

Be aware that carbamazepine can activate psychosis, confusion, or agitation. It can also worsen increased intraocular pressure and cardiac or kidney disease. Therefore, continually monitor these patients for any increase in their symptoms.

PLANNING AND IMPLEMENTATION Carbamazepine is an oral drug that can be given as chewable tablets or as a liquid. This eases the use of this drug by children. The dose is slowly increased over time until the therapeutic dose is achieved for the patient. The usual maintenance dose range is 800 to 1200 mg per day given in divided doses.

Because carbamazepine can cause dizziness, drowsiness, and ataxia, caution the patient to avoid hazardous tasks. Take safety precautions in the hospital setting.

Instruct the patient to report any signs or symptoms of infection, bruising, bleeding, or ulcers in the mouth. Any of these may indicate serious side effects.

Box 34–5. Drug Interactions with Carbamazepine

Decreased effects of carbamazepine
Phenobarbital
Phenytoin
Oral contraceptives

Decreased effects of concurrent drug
Phenytoin
Doxycycline
Theophylline
Warfarin
Haloperidol
Valproic acid

Increased effects of carbamazepine
Erythromycin
Cimetidine
Isoniazid
Calcium channel blockers

Increased neurotoxic effects
Lithium

EVALUATION Effectiveness of the drug is determined ▲▲▲▲▲▲▲▲▲▲ by the absence or decreased frequency of seizure activity.

Carbamazepine can change results of some diagnostic tests. Thyroid function test results may be decreased; blood levels of sodium may be decreased, indicating hyponatremia. The patient should continue to have periodic CBCs with white cell differentials, urinalysis, and liver function tests. Blood level determinations of carbamazepine concentration are also recommended.

Be aware of possible drug interactions (Box 34–5). Also, carbamazepine should not be used with monoamine oxidase (MAO) inhibitors.

OTHER ANTICONVULSANTS

Gabapentin

Gabapentin (Neurontin) is a new drug that has been introduced for use in partial seizures. It is recommended for adjunctive therapy (used with another drug) rather than for use alone. Gabapentin has not been fully tested in children. Its mode of action is unknown, but it does closely resemble the neurotransmitter gamma-aminobutyric acid. The most common adverse reactions are central nervous system effects,

such as sleepiness, dizziness, ataxia, fatigue, and nystagmus.

Gabapentin is given in three doses per day to a total of 900 to 1800 mg. The patient must be brought up slowly to this dosage level.

No drug interactions have as yet been found. This is no doubt because the drug is not metabolized by the body. Persons with kidney dysfunction should be monitored closely and the dose lowered. Gabapentin does cause false-positive responses for urinary protein with use of the Ames N-Multistix SG dipstick test.

NEW DRUGS

Watch for these drugs that are new on the market or in late clinical trials. Vigabatrin and tigabine are new drugs that work on the neurotransmitter gamma-aminobutyric acid. Vigabatrin has already been approved for use in Europe, as has another new drug, lamotrigine. Two others to watch for are topiramate and dezinamide.

Felbamate was approved for use in the United States but then voluntarily taken off the market when new serious adverse reactions appeared.

E X E R C I S E S

CASE STUDIES

1. Mr. B.T. has been diagnosed with seizures. His physician has prescribed phenytoin. What patient teaching should Mr. B.T. receive specific to his drug? What laboratory work will most likely be ordered for him? What symptoms would you watch for that may indicate toxic drug effects?

2. Anticonvulsant drugs often have an adverse effect on the hematopoietic system. What symptoms would you need to be observant for because of this effect?

3. A 3-year-old girl has been diagnosed with partial seizures and is prescribed carbamazepine. What diagnostic tests may be altered by this drug? What diagnostic tests should be ordered periodically throughout drug therapy? Why is it important for you to be aware of the need for these tests and their results? What body systems might be affected by this drug?

4. D.S., age 15 months, is taking valproic acid for absence attacks. What adverse effect is D.S. more susceptible to because of her age? The child's mother reports that D.S. vomits after each dose of the drug. What might be useful in this case? What precaution needs to be emphasized for administration of this drug?

MENTAL AEROBICS

Memory games are often useful when groups of information must be learned. In the case of the subgroups of anticonvulsants, the student may notice that many of them contain a person's name, for example, Barb for barbiturates, Dan for hydantoins, Ben for benzodiazepines, and Sue for succinimides. A story may be concocted to help the student remember these names. The more humor used in the story, the easier it will be to remember the subgroups. The authors believe that if you make up your own story, you will be better able to recall the information. Think how much better you would remember if you and your fellow students then acted out the story you invented. Have fun!

STIMULANTS

LEARNING OBJECTIVES

After studying this chapter, you should be able to:

1. Define CNS stimulant, psychomotor stimulant, analeptic, amphetamine, and anorexiant.

2. Identify actions and uses of and adverse reactions to the CNS and psychomotor stimulants.

3. Discuss potential overuse of the amphetamines and anorexiants.

4. State common examples of each type of the CNS stimulants and psychomotor stimulants.

5. Demonstrate how to administer the CNS stimulants or psychomotor stimulants by use of the nursing process.

DRUGS YOU WILL LEARN ABOUT IN THIS CHAPTER

Central Nervous System (CNS) Stimulants

Analeptics

  caffeine

  doxapram HCl (Dopram)

Amphetamines

  methamphetamine HCl (Desoxyn)

  amphetamine (Biphetamine)

  dextroamphetamine (Dexedrine)

Anorexiants

  phenmetrazine HCl (Preludin)

Psychomotor Stimulants

  methylphenidate HCl (Ritalin)

  pemoline (Cylert)

CENTRAL NERVOUS SYSTEM STIMULANTS

Do you drink coffee? How about tea? Do you reach for a chocolate candy bar for a quick "pick-me-up"? Maybe cola or Mountain Dew soft drink is more your style. All harmless food items, right? Wrong! They are all central nervous system (CNS) stimulants.

CNS stimulants can be classified into three groups: analeptics, amphetamines, and anorexiants.

Analeptics

ACTIONS AND USES Analeptics are used to fight fatigue, to alleviate mild pain, to counteract the effects of other drugs such as narcotics, and to relieve respiratory distress. Most of us are familiar with the most common member of this family: caffeine. Users of analeptics in any form (including "harmless" food items) may experience a wide range of adverse reactions including sneezing, nausea, vomiting, flushing, restlessness, irritability, and insomnia. Some users of analeptics abuse the drug and can become addicted. Withdrawal causes symptoms just like those the addict experiences on withdrawal from illicit drugs.

ASSESSMENT Before beginning the use of an analeptic drug, assess the patient's mental status for any agitation or difficulty sleeping. Use of this type of drug will only aggravate these problems.

PLANNING AND IMPLEMENTATION Teach all of your patients the hidden sources of caffeine. Caffeine can interfere with normal activities of daily living as well as with sleep. Caution the patient against using caffeine sources routinely to counteract fatigue or sleepiness. This can lead to a never-ending cycle wherein the patient stimulates the body to stay awake by using caffeine, experiences difficulty sleeping that night, and then must use caffeine to stay awake again the next day. Teach the patient other methods for inducing sleep, such as doing relaxation exercises before bedtime, maintaining the bed always as a place of sleep rather than as a place to watch television or read, using white sound devices, and eating or drinking a source of protein (especially one high in tryptophan).

EVALUATION Evaluate your patient for the appearance of any of the adverse reactions. Take note of the patient's ability to sleep. Ask the patient if sleep was restful. Do not assume the person is rested just because the person was asleep.

If the caffeine is given as a component of a pain reliever, evaluate for effectiveness of pain relief. If the analeptic is used to relieve respiratory distress, do a thorough respiratory evaluation, including breath sounds, respiratory rate and rhythm, respiratory effort, and the patient's complaints.

Caffeine

Caffeine is a common ingredient or component of many foods, drinks, and drugs. It is found in coffee, tea, colas and other soft drinks, chocolate or cocoa, NōDōz over-the-counter stimulant, Anacin pain reliever, Excedrin Extra-Strength pain reliever, and Aspirin Free Excedrin. It is used to enhance the effectiveness of the pain relievers or to fight fatigue.

Doxapram Hydrochloride

ACTIONS AND USES Doxapram hydrochloride (Dopram) is a respiratory stimulant that increases tidal volume and slightly increases the rate of respiration. It is most often used for patients with respiratory depression after anesthesia, for patients with chronic obstructive pulmonary disease with acute hypercapnia, and in drug-induced CNS depression.

The patient receiving doxapram may experience many adverse reactions. These can include pyrexia or a feeling of warmth throughout the body, anxiety, disorientation, dizziness, seizures, pruritus, paresthesia, headache, dyspnea or tachypnea, cough, increased blood pressure, increased or decreased pulse, arrhythmias, phlebitis, nausea, vomiting, diarrhea, spontaneous voiding, or urinary retention. Doxapram can also cause an elevated hemoglobin level, hematocrit, or red blood cell count while decreasing the white blood cell count under certain circumstances. The patient can experience an elevated blood urea nitrogen concentration or albuminuria.

ASSESSMENT Perform a thorough respiratory assessment before initiating doxapram. Also check the patient's history for previous convulsive disorders, cardiovascular disorders, or mechanical respiratory disorders. All of these contraindicate the use of doxapram. Other contraindications include head injuries and mechanical ventilation. Doxapram should not be used in newborns because it contains benzyl alcohol as a preservative.

PLANNING AND IMPLEMENTATION Doxapram is an injectable drug given intravenously. It may be mixed with 5% to 10% dextrose in water or in normal saline. It should never be added to or hung "piggyback" with intravenous solutions containing thiopental sodium, bicarbonate, or aminophylline. Each of these causes a precipitate or a gas to form.

EVALUATION Evaluate for effectiveness by repeating the respiratory assessment you performed. Compare your results with these baseline data. Watch the patient carefully for any signs of increasing distress or adverse reactions. Monitor laboratory values for any of the drug's effects here.

Amphetamines

ACTIONS AND USES Amphetamines are sympathomimetic amines (see Chapter 37 for more information). As a CNS stimulant, amphetamines may be prescribed by the physician for treatment of obesity. However, because amphetamines have a high potential for abuse, they are reserved for the patient in whom other treatments did not work. Amphetamines may also be used for narcolepsy or treatment of attention deficit disorder (ADD) with hyperactivity (previously known as minimal brain dysfunction).

Amphetamines commonly cause restlessness, nervousness, and insomnia. The patient may complain of a headache or a dry mouth. The blood pressure and pulse may increase. The patient can experience dizziness, tremors, diarrhea or constipation, or impotence. Amphetamines are known to aggravate tics or Tourette's syndrome. With overuse, symptoms of Parkinson's disease or amphetamine psychosis can develop.

Some examples of amphetamines are methamphetamine hydrochloride (Desoxyn), amphetamine (Biphetamine), and dextroamphetamine (Dexedrine).

ASSESSMENT Before initiating this drug, assess the patient for mental status. Also note the patient's weight, blood pressure, and pulse. Because amphetamines should not be given to patients with a history of certain disorders, check the patient's history for any mention of glaucoma, cardiovascular disease, hyperthyroidism, drug abuse, agitation, tics, or Tourette's syndrome.

In children, take baseline height and weight measurements and plot the expected growth on a growth chart curve.

With your female patients of childbearing age, do a pregnancy test.

Also check your patient's medication orders. Most amphetamines should not be given with monoamine oxidase (MAO) inhibitors because this will lead to hypertensive crisis.

PLANNING AND IMPLEMENTATION Most amphetamines are tablets or other oral forms. Because tolerance develops in only a few weeks, the patient should be removed from the drug when this occurs. A larger dose should not be administered because this increases the likelihood of addiction.

Caution your female patients to let the physician know immediately if pregnancy is suspected; if the woman is nursing a child, she should stop. Teach all patients about safety concerns, such as not driving or operating hazardous machinery while under the influence of this drug.

If the drug is being used for obesity, encourage your patient by setting reachable goals. Weigh the patient once a week and keep a chart of the patient's progress. Give praise not only for results but for effort as well. Be sure to emphasize the patient's worth as a person, not as a successful dieter.

EVALUATION Continue to monitor the patient's weight and, in children, the height as well. In children with ADD, monitor reports of the child's ability to stay on task, distractibility, and activity level. Continue to monitor the vital signs and for any adverse reactions.

N U R S I N G   A L E R T

If the patient has taken an overdose, the person may experience panic, hallucinations, combativeness, fever, circulatory collapse, seizures, and coma.

You may wish to initiate a pill count periodically if you have any doubts about the patient's use of the drug.

Anorexiants

Anorexiants are also sympathomimetic amines. As such, they have many of the same actions as amphetamines and the same high potential for abuse. Anorexiants are used primarily for obesity. Phenmetrazine hydrochloride (Preludin) is available as a tablet.

PSYCHOMOTOR STIMULANTS

ACTIONS AND USES Psychomotor stimulants have uses similar to those of central nervous system (CNS) stimulants, but the mechanism of action is poorly understood. It is theorized that the medications activate the brain stem and cortex. Although it would not at first seem that children with attention deficit disorder (ADD) need further stimulation, it is believed that the drug activates the portions of the CNS that inhibit impulsive behaviors. Therefore, it allows the child to be more attentive and sit more quietly in a learning situation.

The most common use of the psychomotor stimulants is for ADD with hyperactivity. They can also be used to treat narcolepsy and senility. However, drug treatment is not considered appropriate for all children with ADD. Methylphenidate hydrochloride (Ritalin) has been the focus of much controversy; some groups of researchers claim that it is the most overused drug in history, and other groups claim that it is not prescribed quickly enough to help the child experiencing ADD problems.

The child who is taking methylphenidate may experience nervousness and insomnia. Some children contrarily experience drowsiness. The patient may have an increased or decreased blood pressure and pulse, arrhythmias, a headache, or gastrointestinal distress. Allergic reactions are also fairly common.

Pemoline (Cylert) is not used as often for children with ADD because of additional serious adverse reactions, including liver dysfunction. It does cause less dystonic movements that can be seen with other psychomotor stimulants.

ASSESSMENT Before the initiation of a psychomotor ▲▲▲▲▲▲▲▲▲▲ stimulant, the nurse and a multidisciplinary team evaluate the behavior of the child. Diagnostic testing is used to rule out other disorders. These tests may include an electroencephalogram, psychological testing, vision and hearing screening, and evaluation for learning disability. The child should be assessed in an environment that is familiar to the child. This does not include the physician's office.

Take a baseline reading of the patient's blood pressure and pulse. Psychomotor stimulants are given only with caution if the blood pressure is elevated. These medications are contraindicated in patients with anxiety, agitation, a history of seizures, glaucoma, tics or Tourette's syndrome, and depression.

Weigh and measure the height of the child who is prescribed a psychomotor stimulant. Plot the expected growth curve for the child.

PLANNING AND IMPLEMENTATION Psychomotor stimu-
▲▲▲▲▲▲▲▲▲▲▲▲▲▲▲▲▲▲▲▲▲▲▲▲▲▲▲▲▲▲▲▲ lants are oral medications, most often tablets. Methylphenidate is also available as a sustained-release tablet, so the actions of the drug last longer through the school day. The dose of medication is timed so that effectiveness is at a peak during school hours. It may be necessary for the child to receive an additional dose midway through the day. The medication should not be administered after noon so that the child will not experience sleep difficulties.

EVALUATION Evaluation of the effectiveness of the ▲▲▲▲▲▲▲▲▲▲ drug is best accomplished with the input of the multidisciplinary team. The parents, teachers, psychologist, counselors, school nurse, and physician should each be involved. Evaluate the child's behavior for increased attention span, decreased distractibility, and decreased activity. The child's grades are only one indicator of the effectiveness of the drug.

Be alert to any new drugs initiated during psychomotor stimulant therapy. These drugs will decrease the effectiveness of guanethidine (an antihypertensive). They also increase the effects of monoamine oxidase (MAO) inhibitors, anticonvulsants, coumarin, and tricyclic antidepressants. Dosages of these drugs may need readjustment during psychomotor stimulant therapy.

Continue to monitor the child's growth patterns and the blood pressure and pulse. Look also for other adverse reactions and report them to the physician immediately.

E X E R C I S E S

CASE STUDIES

1. Your patient is admitted with palpitations. During the course of your nursing care, you note that the patient has had three cups of coffee and it is only 10:30 AM. How is this information related? What other effects might you expect? What teaching should you do for the patient?

2. Mrs. K.R., age 42 years, is 5 feet 3 inches tall and weighs 230 pounds. She has tried many different diet and exercise programs but has never been able to successfully lose the weight she desires. She has been prescribed methamphetamine HCl. What disorders should you check her chart for before initiating the medication? What assessments are necessary?

Mrs. K.R. is discharged on methamphetamine. What safety teaching should you do? How can you determine whether Mrs. K.R. is taking the drug appropriately when she returns to her weekly clinic appointments? What symptoms would you expect Mrs. K.R. to exhibit if she took too many of the tablets?

3. J.T., 7 years old, is having difficulty in school. He is highly distractible and has a short attention span; the teacher states that he never sits still. If you were the school nurse, who would you involve in J.T.'s assessment?

J.T. is later diagnosed with ADD with hyperactivity. He is prescribed methylphenidate HCl. His mother thinks that giving J.T. the medication before bedtime would fit into their family schedule best. What should your response be to this? What assessments should you perform before the initiation of the drug?

MENTAL AEROBICS

1. Visit a weight loss clinic that is supervised by a physician. What teaching is done? What medications are used? Are they used routinely for all patients? What psychosocial interventions are used by the staff?

2. Ask to observe a school nurse. Does the nurse deal with children with ADD? What medications are they receiving? What assessments does the nurse make?

3. Attend a support group for parents of children with ADD. What problems do they encounter? What needs do they all have? What do they wish their children would receive from health care workers?

ANTIPARKINSONIAN DRUGS

LEARNING OBJECTIVES

After studying this chapter, you should be able to:

1. Define dopamine.

2. Identify the actions and uses of and adverse reactions to antiparkinsonian drugs.

3. State common examples of antiparkinsonian drugs.

4. State nursing implications for patients receiving antiparkinsonian drugs.

5. Demonstrate how to administer antiparkinsonian drugs by use of the nursing process.

DRUGS YOU WILL LEARN ABOUT IN THIS CHAPTER

Dopamines

 levodopa (Larodopa)

 carbidopa and levodopa (Sinemet)

Dopamine Receptor Agonists

 bromocriptine mesylate (Parlodel)

 pergolide mesylate (Permax)

Anticholinergics

 trihexyphenidyl HCl (Artane)

Other Antiparkinsonian Drugs

 amantadine HCl (Symmetrel)

Parkinsonism, or Parkinson's disease, is caused by a lack of available dopamine at the synapses. Most drugs for the treatment of parkinsonism are forms of levodopa—the precursor of dopamine—or an anticholinergic used as an adjunct to levodopa.

DOPAMINES

ACTIONS AND USES As a precursor of dopamine, levodopa crosses the blood-brain barrier; dopamine itself does not. Therefore, levodopa can be administered to increase the availability of dopamine in the brain and decrease the occurrence of parkinsonism symptoms.

The patient who is taking a dopamine should be watched for any adverse reactions, the most common of which are choreiform or dystonic movements. The patient could also experience arrhythmias, orthostatic hypotension, ataxia, depression, suicidal tendencies, psychosis, aggression, hypersexuality, urinary retention, gastrointestinal bleeding, nausea, vomiting, diarrhea, dry mouth, hemolytic anemia, agranulocytosis, and seizures.

ASSESSMENT Thoroughly assess all body systems of the patient who is to receive a dopamine. Be especially alert for any signs of liver or kidney dysfunction, hematopoietic dysfunction, cardiovascular disease, or pulmonary disease. Closely monitor the patient with a history of either peptic ulcer disease or psychosis for any onset of reactions. The use of dopamines is contraindicated in combination with monoamine oxidase (MAO) inhibitors or in patients with closed-angle glaucoma or a history of melanoma.

PLANNING AND IMPLEMENTATION The dose of dopamines is highly individualized. The physician generally starts with a low initial dosage and gradually increases the level by small increments.

Because the patient is at an increased risk for nausea from the dopamines if he is ingesting caffeine, the diet should be low in sources of this drug-like ingredient. Be aware of coffee, tea, chocolate, colas and some other soft drinks, and even many medications that contain caffeine.

N U R S I N G   A L E R T
▼▼▼▼▼▼▼▼▼▼▼▼▼▼▼▼▼▼▼▼▼▼▼▼▼▼▼▼▼▼▼▼▼

Pyridoxine (vitamin B$_6$) interferes with the metabolism of the dopamines, decreasing their effectiveness. For this reason, the patient should be on a diet that is low in vitamin B$_6$ foods.

▲▲▲▲▲▲▲▲▲▲▲▲▲▲▲▲▲▲▲▲▲▲▲▲▲▲▲▲▲▲▲▲▲

Implement safety precautions appropriate for dizziness, depression or suicide, and aggression.

EVALUATION The effectiveness of this type of drug is
▲▲▲▲▲▲▲▲▲▲ determined by the decrease of parkinsonism symptoms with the absence of major adverse reactions. Continue to monitor liver and kidney function test results, complete blood counts (CBCs), and vital signs. Continue to monitor the patient's mental status throughout drug therapy.

N U R S I N G   A L E R T
▼▼▼▼▼▼▼▼▼▼▼▼▼▼▼▼▼▼▼▼▼▼▼▼▼▼▼▼▼▼▼▼▼

An early sign of overdose of dopamines is blepharospasm. Evaluate the patient often for this phenomenon and ask the patient about "tics" in the eye.

▲▲▲▲▲▲▲▲▲▲▲▲▲▲▲▲▲▲▲▲▲▲▲▲▲▲▲▲▲▲▲▲▲

Be aware that some people never tolerate the dopamines because of adverse reactions. The physician may try different dosages and preparations or may add anticholinergic drugs to decrease the reactions.

Levodopa

Available as tablets and capsules, levodopa (Larodopa) is the precursor of dopamine without additives. The usual dose is 0.5 to 1.0 g daily. The dose is gradually increased to a level that benefits the patient most, but this amount is not to exceed 8 g a day.

Carbidopa and Levodopa

Carbidopa is added to levodopa (Sinemet) to decrease the destruction of levodopa by the body before it crosses the blood-brain barrier. This causes more levodopa to be available for activity in the brain, but less is present in other tissues. Thus, the necessary dose is less, and adverse reactions of peripheral tissues and organs, especially cardiac arrhythmias, are lessened. The usual dose is 75 to 150 mg of carbidopa and 300 to 1500 mg of levodopa in three to four divided doses. Other adverse reactions of the central nervous system (CNS) may occur sooner. This is especially true of choreiform and dystonic movements.

Before initiation of carbidopa and levodopa, any other form of plain levodopa must be stopped for at least 8 hours. This helps prevent additional adverse reactions.

DOPAMINE RECEPTOR AGONISTS

ACTIONS AND USES Those drugs classified as dopa-
▲▲▲▲▲▲▲▲▲▲▲▲▲▲▲▲▲ mine receptor agonists help activate receptors of dopamine and increase the action of all available dopamine in the body. These drugs are therefore often used as adjuncts to levodopa.

In addition to increasing levodopa activity, the dopamine receptor agonists help decrease the CNS adverse reactions associated with levodopa, especially choreiform and dystonic movements. The dopamine receptor agonists are also used to treat hyperprolactinemia, to prevent lactation, and to treat acromegaly.

The most common adverse reactions with this class are CNS reactions, such as confusion, hallucinations, depression, and ataxia. The patient may also experience nausea and vomiting, shortness of breath, dry mouth, and blepharospasms.

These drugs can also cause some much more serious adverse reactions. The dopamine receptor agonists can precipitate orthostatic hypotension or severe hypertension. They can also lead to seizures or strokes.

ASSESSMENT Be especially alert to any factors that
▲▲▲▲▲▲▲▲▲▲ increase the patient's risk of complications from these drugs. Be sure a baseline test result is available on the chart for liver and kidney function tests. If dysfunction of either of these systems were to develop, the available drug in the body would build up, leading to more adverse reactions.

Have a baseline CBC available for comparison and take baseline vital sign readings, especially blood pressure.

The use of dopamine receptor agonists is contraindicated in patients with uncontrolled hypertension, toxemia in pregnancy, or allergy to ergot derivatives for certain preparations.

PLANNING AND IMPLEMENTATION The dose of this ▲▲▲▲▲▲▲▲▲▲▲▲▲▲▲▲▲▲▲▲▲▲▲▲▲ group of drugs is individualized. Just as with the dopamines, the initial dose is relatively small and increased in gradual increments.

Because of the potential for orthostatic hypotension or seizures, institute appropriate safety precautions. No activities requiring alertness should be attempted, such as driving or operating hazardous machinery.

EVALUATION Continue to monitor the patient's status ▲▲▲▲▲▲▲▲▲▲ throughout drug therapy. Monitor liver and kidney function test results, CBC, and blood pressure readings carefully.

N U R S I N G   A L E R T
▼▼▼▼▼▼▼▼▼▼▼▼▼▼▼▼▼▼▼▼▼▼▼▼▼▼▼▼▼▼▼▼▼▼

Be especially alert to any complaint of headache or visual disturbances. Those patients who suffer seizures or strokes often complain or a progressively severe headache or visual disturbances before the event.

▲▲▲▲▲▲▲▲▲▲▲▲▲▲▲▲▲▲▲▲▲▲▲▲▲▲▲▲▲▲▲▲▲▲▲

Bromocriptine Mesylate

As an ergot derivative, bromocriptine mesylate (Parlodel) is capable of causing allergic reactions in those sensitive to ergot derivatives. The usual dose is 1.25 mg twice a day initially, which is gradually increased. The patient should not receive more than 100 mg a day. Those receiving phenothiazines may experience a decreased effectiveness of this drug.

Pergolide Mesylate

Pergolide mesylate (Permax) is similar to bromocriptine and is also used as an adjunct to levodopa.

Box 36–1. Anticholinergics Used in the Treatment of Parkinsonism

benztropine mesylate (Cogentin)
diphenhydramine hydrochloride (Benadryl)
biperiden hydrochloride and biperiden lactate (Akineton)
procyclidine hydrochloride (Kemadrin)
hyoscyamine sulfate (Levsin; Levsinex, a timed-release form)

ANTICHOLINERGICS

ACTIONS AND USES The anticholinergics are covered in ▲▲▲▲▲▲▲▲▲▲▲▲▲▲▲▲ more detail in Chapter 40. As therapy for parkinsonism, the anticholinergics act by inhibiting the parasympathetic nervous system. This blocks the nerve impulses, thus decreasing symptoms and also adverse reactions from levodopa. The therapeutic properties are similar to those of atropine. The anticholinergics are used primarily as an adjunct rather than as a first-line drug.

The adverse reactions are those of anticholinergics (see Chapter 40). The patient using an anticholinergic for symptoms of parkinsonism is most likely to experience confusion and gastrointestinal distress.

Box 36–1 lists anticholinergics used in the treatment of parkinsonism.

ASSESSMENT See Chapter 40 for assessment of the ▲▲▲▲▲▲▲▲▲▲ patient receiving anticholinergics.

PLANNING AND IMPLEMENTATION The physician usu-▲▲▲▲▲▲▲▲▲▲▲▲▲▲▲▲▲▲▲▲▲▲▲▲▲▲▲▲▲▲ ally begins with a small dose of an anticholinergic for parkinsonism and gradually increases the amount until maximal benefits are achieved.

If the patient experiences gastrointestinal distress, these drugs can be given with food to decrease this reaction.

EVALUATION See Chapter 40 for evaluation of the ▲▲▲▲▲▲▲▲▲▲ patient receiving anticholinergics.

Trihexyphenidyl Hydrochloride

The usual dose of trihexyphenidyl hydrochloride (Artane) is 1 mg a day initially, increased by 2-mg increments every 3 to 5 days. The patient attains maximal benefit in the range of 6 to 15 mg a day. Trihexyphenidyl is available as tablets, an elixir, and sustained-release capsules.

OTHER ANTIPARKINSONIAN DRUGS

Amantadine Hydrochloride

ACTIONS AND USES The mechanism of
▲▲▲▲▲▲▲▲▲▲▲▲▲▲▲▲
action of amantadine hydrochloride (Symmetrel) in relation to parkinsonism is largely unknown. It is known to increase the release of dopamine in the brain. It is less effective than levodopa. Amantadine is also an antiviral agent active against influenza type A virus.

The patient may experience gastrointestinal upset, headache and insomnia, dizziness and orthostatic hypotension, a dry mouth, and depression and hallucinations.

ASSESSMENT Check the patient's history for any sei-
▲▲▲▲▲▲▲▲▲▲ zures. Seizures can be precipitated by amantadine in those with a history. Also check the history for congestive heart failure, which can also be aggravated.

The patient should have baseline kidney and liver function studies performed before initiation of this drug. Take baseline readings of the vital signs, especially the blood pressure.

PLANNING AND IMPLEMENTATION The usual dose of
▲▲▲▲▲▲▲▲▲▲▲▲▲▲▲▲▲▲▲▲▲▲▲▲▲▲▲ amantadine is 100 mg twice a day if it is used alone. However, if it is used with other antiparkinsonian agents, the same dose is given only once a day.

Institute safety precautions because of the risk of blurred vision and drowsiness. Teach the patient to avoid activities that require alertness, such as driving.

EVALUATION The effectiveness of this drug is deter-
▲▲▲▲▲▲▲▲▲▲ mined by the decrease of parkinsonism symptoms and absence of drug reactions. Continue to monitor kidney and liver function test results and vital signs.

E X E R C I S E S

CASE STUDIES

1. Mr. N.D., age 45 years, has been diagnosed with parkinsonism. He is prescribed a dopamine drug. What foods should Mr. N.J. avoid while taking this drug? Name three drugs that cause an interaction with the dopamine group. What safety precautions would you institute for Mr. N.J.?

2. Mr. N.J.'s physician decided to change his medication to carbidopa and levodopa. Before initiation of this drug, what must be done?

3. Ms. S.A., age 57 years, has been taking levodopa for a considerable time. Her physician has decided to add bromocriptine to her drug regimen. What is the rationale for this? If Ms. S.A. begins to complain of a headache, what should you do?

4. Mr. J.M., age 62 years, is taking levodopa and trihexyphenidyl. What is the rationale for the trihexyphenidyl? What could you as the nurse do if Mr. J.M. experiences nausea during drug therapy?

MENTAL AEROBICS

DIRECTED RESEARCH Research the major anticholinergics used for parkinsonism. What are the major differences between them? Why would a physician choose one over the other for particular patients?

ADRENERGIC AGONISTS

LEARNING OBJECTIVES

After studying this chapter, you should be able to:

1. Identify general actions of and name the sympathetic neurohormones.

2. Identify actions and uses of and adverse reactions to the adrenergic drugs.

3. Differentiate between catecholamines and noncatecholamines.

4. State appropriate patient teaching for a patient receiving an adrenergic.

5. Define sympathetic nervous system.

6. State common examples of both types of adrenergics.

7. Demonstrate how to administer adrenergics by use of the nursing process.

DRUGS YOU WILL LEARN ABOUT IN THIS CHAPTER

Catecholamines

   epinephrine (Adrenalin, Primatene)

   norepinephrine (Levophed)

   isoproterenol (Isuprel)

   dopamine (Intropin)

Noncatecholamines

   ephedrine (Efedron)

   phenylephrine (Neo-Synephrine)

   mephentermine (Wyamine)

   metaraminol (Aramine)

ACTIONS AND USES The adrenergic nerves lend their name to a classification of drugs that act similarly. These are the adrenergic agonists. Just as the nerves have two names, so does this classification of drugs—adrenergic agonists or sympathomimetics (*sympatho,* sympathetic; *mimetic,* to mimic).

In general, adrenergic agonists are used for hypotension, surface bleeding, bronchospasms, and nasal congestion.

The sympathomimetics (adrenergic agonists) can be further divided into two subgroups, the catecholamines and the noncatecholamines. Both have similar actions, but whereas catecholamines have a more intense effect, noncatecholamines have a longer lasting effect. Therefore, the catecholamines are more likely to be used as an emergency treatment; noncatecholamines are more likely to be used as a maintenance drug. This is a generalized statement, however, and as with all generalized statements, it has its exceptions, as the student will find as we look at the individual drugs.

Side effects tend to be more intense actions than were intended, that is, hypertension, anxiety, headache, tachycardia that may progress to arrhythmias, and bradycardia.

ASSESSMENT Be familiar with both the patient and the medical history of the patient. Look for conditions that would warrant extra precautions during the administration of adrenergic agonist drugs. Use caution if the patient is elderly, pregnant, psychotic, or neurotic or if the patient has cardiovascular disease, hypertension, diabetes mellitus, or hyperthyroidism.

Baseline information is essential to use of these drugs. Assess vital signs and record them before the first dose of the drug is administered. Determine also the rationale for the use of the drug and any presenting symptoms.

PLANNING AND IMPLEMENTATION Many of these drugs ▲▲▲▲▲▲▲▲▲▲▲▲▲▲▲▲▲▲▲▲▲▲▲▲▲▲▲ can be administered in a variety of ways. Be sure the physician has ordered which route to use. Carefully note this portion of the order.

Because of the emergency nature of some of these drugs, they should be administered by a nurse who is experienced with the actions of this classification. Often, the physician prefers to administer the drug.

EVALUATION Effectiveness of the individual drug is ▲▲▲▲▲▲▲▲▲▲ determined in different ways. Monitor the presenting symptoms as well as the patient's vital signs.

CATECHOLAMINES

Epinephrine

ACTIONS AND USES As a catecholamine, epinephrine ▲▲▲▲▲▲▲▲▲▲▲▲▲▲▲ (Adrenalin, Primatene) has short-lived effects. It is more often useful in emergency situations rather than as a maintenance drug.

Epinephrine may be used in the following ways:

• To treat respiratory distress, bronchospasms, status asthmaticus, and nasal congestion
• To relieve allergic reactions, heart block, cardiac arrhythmias, and open-angle glaucoma
• To relax uterine contractions
• To prolong anesthesia

ASSESSMENT See assessment for adrenergic agonists ▲▲▲▲▲▲▲▲▲▲ in general.

PLANNING AND IMPLEMENTATION Epinephrine can be ▲▲▲▲▲▲▲▲▲▲▲▲▲▲▲▲▲▲▲▲▲▲▲▲▲▲▲▲▲ administered in a variety of ways: by inhalation; by the subcutaneous, intramuscular, intravenous, and intracardiac routes; and ophthalmically. Of the parenteral routes, subcutaneous injection is preferred. Intramuscular injection should not be given in the gluteus muscle. Table 37–1 lists dosages of epinephrine.

EVALUATION Monitor the patient's vital signs, listen to ▲▲▲▲▲▲▲▲▲▲ breath sounds, and always investigate any complaints the patient voices.

Table 37–1. Dosages of Epinephrine

ROUTE	DOSAGE
Inhalation	1–2 puffs (1–2 mg delivered per puff)
Subcutaneous	0.2–1.0 mg; may be repeated as soon as 15 min Maintenance: up to 1.5 mg q6h
Intramuscular	0.2–1.0 mg; may be repeated as soon as 15 min Maintenance: usually achieved with intravenous infusion
Intravenous	Bolus: 0.1–1.0 mg; may be repeated in 5 min Infusion: 1–4 µg/min
Intracardiac	0.1–10. mg, administered by physician; may be repeated in 5 min
Ophthalmic	1 drop once or twice a day

N U R S I N G   A L E R T
▼▼▼▼▼▼▼▼▼▼▼▼▼▼▼▼▼▼▼▼▼▼▼▼▼▼▼▼▼▼▼▼▼▼

Always assess all parenteral sites for possible local necrosis. Also be aware of the possibility of an overdose. An overdose may lead to death from cerebrovascular accident (CVA), pulmonary edema, or ventricular fibrillation.

▲▲▲▲▲▲▲▲▲▲▲▲▲▲▲▲▲▲▲▲▲▲▲▲▲▲▲▲▲▲▲▲▲

Norepinephrine

ACTIONS AND USES Norepinephrine (Levophed) is of-▲▲▲▲▲▲▲▲▲▲▲▲▲▲▲▲▲ ten used to raise the blood pressure in emergency situations, such as in shock or with myocardial infarction. The successful action of this drug is due to its ability to constrict peripheral blood vessels and yet dilate coronary arteries.

ASSESSMENT Check the chart for the medical history ▲▲▲▲▲▲▲▲▲▲ and condition of the patient and for all laboratory reports of blood gas analysis.

N U R S I N G   A L E R T

Norepinephrine should not be used if the patient has a thrombosis, very low partial pressure of oxygen (Po_2), or very high partial pressure of carbon dioxide (Pco_2).

PLANNING AND IMPLEMENTATION The intravenous dose of norepinephrine is titrated by the patient's blood pressure. This is normally 2 to 4 µg per minute. A larger initial or loading dose of up to 12 µg per minute may be used.

Take the blood pressure frequently (as often as every 2 minutes) and assess the patient for a headache. This may indicate that the blood pressure has risen too high.

The nurse is also responsible to check for infiltration of the intravenous site frequently because this will lead to tissue necrosis. For preventive purposes, a large vein must be chosen. Phentolamine mesylate (Regitine), an adrenergic blocker, is used to treat the infiltrated tissue.

N U R S I N G   A L E R T

Norepinephrine should not be stopped suddenly because this may lead to myocardial infarction.

EVALUATION Norepinephrine interacts with other drugs to produce effects on the blood pressure. When norepinephrine is given in conjunction with adrenergic blockers, monoamine oxidase (MAO) inhibitors, tricyclic antidepressants, or any ergot alkaloids, the blood pressure will increase, possibly to dangerous heights. When norepinephrine is given with phenytoin (Dilantin), an anticonvulsant, the blood pressure and pulse will decrease. Norepinephrine should also not be given with haloperidol (Haldol) because they are antagonistic.

Isoproterenol

Isoproterenol (Isuprel) may be used to treat shock, cardiac arrhythmias or arrest, bronchospasms (such as from asthma, emphysema), and status asthmaticus. It may be administered sublingually, by inhalation, rectally, subcutaneously, intramuscularly, intra-

venously, or even by intracardiac injection. Table 37–2 lists dosages of isoproterenol.

Isoproterenol should not be given with epinephrine because this leads to arrhythmias. It is also contraindicated if a cardiac arrhythmia is due to digitalis toxicity.

Caution patients not to overuse isoproterenol as an inhalant because the drug will lose its effectiveness.

Dopamine

Dopamine (Intropin) is the precursor of norepinephrine. It causes increased blood flow to the kidneys, myocardium, and cerebrum. It increases blood pressure and cardiac output. Therefore, dopamine is useful in the treatment of shock due to myocardial infarction, congestive heart failure, septicemia, and trauma. The usual dose range is 2 to 50 µg per kilogram of body weight per minute. The solution must be diluted before administration.

Dopamine is not used in the presence of cardiac arrhythmias or pheochromocytoma. It is used only

Table 37–2. Dosages of Isoproterenol

ROUTE	DOSAGE
Sublingual	10–60 mg/day
Inhalation	Inhaler: 1–2 puffs up to 6 times a day Nebulizer: 2.5 mL of 1% solution up to 5 times a day
Rectal	1–15 mg
Subcutaneous	0.15–0.2 mg
Intramuscular	0.02–1.0 mg
Intravenous	Bolus: 0.01–0.2 mg Infusion: 2–20 µg/min, normally 5 µg/min
Intracardiac	0.02 mg, administered by physician

with caution if the patient has peripheral vascular disease.

See norepinephrine for other information.

NONCATECHOLAMINES

Ephedrine

ACTIONS AND USES Ephedrine (Efedron) has both cat-
▲▲▲▲▲▲▲▲▲▲▲▲▲▲▲ echolamine and noncatecholamine actions. Because this drug can stimulate the myocardium, resulting in an increased pulse and blood pressure, it can be used to treat heart block. Because it stimulates respirations, it is useful in treating overdoses of central nervous system (CNS) depressants, bronchial asthma, and myasthenia gravis. Ephedrine is also useful against enuresis and nasal congestion.

ASSESSMENT Ephedrine should not be administered to
▲▲▲▲▲▲▲▲▲▲ patients with closed-angle glaucoma. Check the patient's medical history.

PLANNING AND IMPLEMENTATION Ephedrine may be
▲▲▲▲▲▲▲▲▲▲▲▲▲▲▲▲▲▲▲▲▲▲▲▲▲▲ given by a variety of routes, including orally, nasally, subcutaneously, in-

Table 37–3. Dosages of Ephedrine	
ROUTE	**DOSAGE**
Oral	25–50 mg every 3–4 h 15–60 mg extended-release forms 2 or 3 times a day
Nasal	1–2 drops every 4 h; also comes as nasal jelly
Subcutaneous	12.5–50 mg; may be repeated up to 150 mg/day
Intramuscular	12.5–50 mg; may be repeated up to 150 mg/day
Intravenous	10–25 mg as a bolus, given slowly; may be repeated in 5 min, up to 150 mg/day

tramuscularly, and intravenously. The dosages of ephedrine are given in Table 37–3.

Check the blood pressure and output frequently. If the patient will be taking ephedrine as a maintenance drug at home, teach the patient not to overuse ephedrine because it will lose its effectiveness. Caution the patient not to take over-the-counter drugs (because many contain antagonists) without checking with the physician. Advise the patient not to take the drug late in the evening because this may cause insomnia.

EVALUATION Evaluation for effectiveness is the same
▲▲▲▲▲▲▲▲▲▲ as for other noncatecholamines.

Phenylephrine

ACTIONS AND USES Phenylephrine (Neo-Synephrine)
▲▲▲▲▲▲▲▲▲▲▲▲▲▲▲▲▲ acts as a noncatecholamine. It is used to treat hypotension, nasal congestion, and bronchial asthma.

ASSESSMENT Phenylephrine should not be given to
▲▲▲▲▲▲▲▲▲▲ patients with closed-angle glaucoma, coronary disease, or arrhythmias.

PLANNING AND IMPLEMENTATION Phenylephrine may
▲▲▲▲▲▲▲▲▲▲▲▲▲▲▲▲▲▲▲▲▲▲▲▲▲▲▲▲ be administered nasally or by subcutaneous, intramuscular, or intravenous injection.

N U R S I N G   A L E R T
▼▼▼▼▼▼▼▼▼▼▼▼▼▼▼▼▼▼▼▼▼▼▼▼▼▼▼▼▼▼▼▼▼▼▼▼

If your patient has been prescribed a nasal spray or drops, teach the patient about rebound phenomenon. This reaction occurs as the nasal mucosa becomes adjusted to or tolerant of the drug and eventually needs larger and more frequent applications of the drug. Severe nasal congestion will result if the patient then tries to stop the drug. To avoid the major effects of rebound phenomenon, the use of nasal decongestants is usually limited to 3 days.

▲▲▲▲▲▲▲▲▲▲▲▲▲▲▲▲▲▲▲▲▲▲▲▲▲▲▲▲▲▲▲▲▲▲▲▲▲▲

The patient may also experience nasal stinging and burning during initial therapy. Generally, patients report that this lasts only for the first few doses.

Overdrying of the nasal mucosa may develop during therapy, possibly leading to cracking and epistaxis. Teach the patient to report this to the physician.

Also teach patients the procedure for nasal spray or drop application. If the medication is intended to reach the sinuses, drops require the patient to lay with the head far back and shoulders up on pillows. The usual order is for 2 to 3 drops or sprays, and application should not be repeated for 4 hours.

Caution your patients about the risks involved with using old nasal spray bottles of the squeeze-type variety, which actually draw nasal drainage and microbes into the bottle when it is released inside the nares. For this same reason, patients should never share bottles with others and should rinse the tip of any nasal application system with warm water after each use. The winged-tip spray bottles do not share this disadvantage.

Doses for the subcutaneous and intramuscular routes are 2 to 5 mg. This injection can be repeated as early as 1 hour.

Ophthalmic solutions are given every 4 hours, 1 to 2 drops each dose.

EVALUATION Effectiveness of this drug is determined ▲▲▲▲▲▲▲▲▲▲ by careful monitoring of the presenting symptoms. Be aware of the purpose for administering the drug to correctly evaluate the effectiveness.

Mephentermine

Mephentermine (Wyamine) has both catecholamine and noncatecholamine actions. It raises cardiac output and is used as a peripheral vasoconstrictor. It has less CNS stimulation than ephedrine.

Mephentermine may be given intramuscularly or intravenously. Evaluate the blood pressure and pulse often, even well into the drug therapy, because tolerance to the drug may develop. Do not give mephentermine if the patient is pregnant because it can bring on uterine contractions.

Metaraminol

Metaraminol (Aramine) is also an effective vasopressor (produces vasoconstriction). This raises the blood pressure and improves blood flow to the myocardium, cerebrum, and kidneys, which makes metaraminol useful in the treatment of shock and hypotension, for example, from trauma, myocardial infarction, or surgery.

Metaraminol may be given intramuscularly, intravenously, and subcutaneously, although subcutaneous administration is rare because it can cause tissue necrosis. Watch the intravenous site for signs of infiltration because this, too, can lead to tissue necrosis.

E X E R C I S E S

CASE STUDIES

1. Mr. A.L. experienced difficulty breathing while at the company picnic and was brought to the emergency department. Because he had a history of asthma, the physician ordered ephedrine IM. After three consecutive doses of epinephrine, Mr. A.L. continued to have moderate respiratory distress. His physician diagnosed status asthmaticus.

As a nurse, you know that epinephrine is an adrenergic catecholamine. What side effects might you expect Mr. A.L. to experience? How long would you expect the effects to last? What site would *not* have been used for injections? What are your responsibilities for the injection sites?

2. Mr. C.B., age 54 years, was brought to the emergency department with a suspected myocardial infarction. His blood pressure is low, the pulse is fast and thready, and the skin is pale and diaphoretic. Dopamine is ordered IV. What are your nursing responsibilities as they relate to the drug? What drug should be near at hand?

If Mr. C.B. has seizures, what drug should not be administered?

3. Your neighbor is using over-the-counter phenylephrine for her seasonal allergies and asks your advice. What teaching should you give your patient? What questions should you ask your neighbor?

MENTAL AEROBICS

The actions of the adrenergic nerves (and therefore drugs) may be difficult to remember because they are diverse. Many learners remember better by using movement.

ROLE PLAYING Act out the actions of the adrenergic drugs on the following body parts: (1) heart; (2) lungs; (3) nose; (4) brain; (5) stomach; (6) muscles; (7) pupils. Pretend you are that body part. (*Author's note:* Although you may feel silly doing this activity, humor reinforces learning. If you do the activity in the group, you will all benefit best if the actions are memorable.)

CHAPTER 38

ADRENERGIC BLOCKERS

LEARNING OBJECTIVES

After studying this chapter, you should be able to:

1. Identify the three types of adrenergic blockers.

2. Evaluate the effectiveness of adrenergic blockers.

3. State common examples of each type of adrenergic blocker.

4. Prepare an appropriate teaching plan for a patient receiving each type of adrenergic blocker.

5. Demonstrate how to administer adrenergic blockers by use of the nursing process.

DRUGS YOU WILL LEARN ABOUT IN THIS CHAPTER

Alpha-Blockers

phenoxybenzamine HCl (Dibenzyline)

phentolamine (Regitine)

ergotamine tartrate (Cafergot, Ergostat, Ergotartrate)

Beta-Blockers

propranolol HCl (Inderal, Inderal LA)

acebutolol HCl (Sectral)

atenolol (Tenormin)

pindolol (Visken)

labetalol HCl (Trandate)

metoprolol tartrate (Lopressor)

nadolol (Corgard)

Neuron Blockers

reserpine (Serpasil)

Adrenergic blockers have opposite effects of the adrenergic agonists because they prohibit the actions of the sympathetic nerves. Therefore, once you are familiar with the fight-or-flight mechanism, the actions of the adrenergic blockers will be easier to learn.

Adrenergic blockers are also called sympathomimetic blockers or sympatholytics. The classification is divided into three subgroups: alpha-blockers, beta-blockers, and neuron blockers.

ALPHA-BLOCKERS

Phenoxybenzamine

ACTIONS AND USES Phenoxybenzamine (Dibenzyline) is a vasodilator that is used to treat peripheral vascular diseases and pheochromocytoma. The patient's blood vessels will dilate, allowing more blood to pass through more freely.

Given orally, phenoxybenzamine may cause gastrointestinal (GI) upset. This drug often causes nasal congestion, dilated pupils, and a drop in the blood pressure. The patient may also complain of drowsiness or weakness.

ASSESSMENT Before initiating the first dose of this drug, take your patient's blood pressure in both the lying and standing positions. This helps provide baseline information for future reference.

Check the patient's chart for any other disorders. Phenoxybenzamine is to be used with caution if other major body systems (such as the cardiovascular, urinary, or respiratory) are impaired. Assess the patient for any history or symptoms of peptic ulcer disease. This disorder also warrants caution.

PLANNING AND IMPLEMENTATION The usual dose of
▲▲▲▲▲▲▲▲▲▲▲▲▲▲▲▲▲▲▲▲▲▲▲▲▲▲▲▲ this oral drug for adults is 10 mg per day in a single dose initially. The physician may increase the dose up to 40 mg per day in small increments.

You may wish to give the drug with food or milk if the patient experiences GI upset. It may also become necessary for the physician to lower the dosage prescribed. Be sure to keep the physician informed of the patient's discomfort.

Safety precautions are important while the patient is ambulating because of possible dizziness or drowsiness. Always have the patient dangle at the side of the bed before standing to lessen the possibility of postural hypotension. If the patient will be taking the drug at home, teach safety precautions for the home. Advise against operating machinery or driving a car. Also caution the patient against standing for long periods because this may produce the same effects.

N U R S I N G   A L E R T

▼▼▼▼▼▼▼▼▼▼▼▼▼▼▼▼▼▼▼▼▼▼▼▼▼▼▼▼▼▼▼▼

Because the patient may experience nasal congestion, caution against the use of over-the-counter decongestants. These drugs contain an antagonist that counteracts the effects of phenoxybenzamine.

▲▲▲▲▲▲▲▲▲▲▲▲▲▲▲▲▲▲▲▲▲▲▲▲▲▲▲▲▲▲▲▲

The patient may have some problems with a dry mouth. This is especially true if nasal congestion is always experienced. List methods the patient may use to lessen the discomfort of a dry mouth. For example, letting ice chips melt in the mouth may feel good; or the patient may suck on hard candy or chew gum. Brushing the teeth and rinsing with mouthwash also help the mouth feel fresh and moist.

EVALUATION Effectiveness of phenoxybenzamine is
▲▲▲▲▲▲▲▲▲▲ determined by evaluating the patient's blood pressure. Also evaluate for any episodes of excessive sweating if the drug is used to treat pheochromocytoma.

Evaluate for orthostatic (postural) hypotension. Check your patient's blood pressure in both the lying and the standing positions. A significant drop on rising may indicate that your patient could become dizzy and fall. Emphasize to the patient the importance of calling for help before arising.

Look for any drug interactions. Phenoxybenzamine is known to decrease the effectiveness of adrenergics, dopamines, ephedrine, and phenylephrine. The effects of antihistamines, antidepressants, and central nervous system (CNS) depressants including alcohol may be enhanced.

Phentolamine

Phentolamine (Regitine) decreases the blood pressure, so it may be used as an antihypertensive. This drug may also be prescribed to treat pheochromocytoma or to treat infiltration of intravenous adrenergics. It may be given by mouth, intramuscularly, or intravenously. When given orally, it too may cause GI distress; therefore, it may be given with food or milk. As with phenoxybenzamine, phentolamine may also cause orthostatic hypotension. See preceding section for appropriate nursing measures.

Ergot Alkaloids

ACTIONS AND USES Ergotamine tartrate is given to
▲▲▲▲▲▲▲▲▲▲▲▲▲▲▲▲ treat vascular headaches, such as migraines. It decreases the cerebral blood supply, thereby decreasing the pain.

ASSESSMENT Assess the patient's condition. Ask the
▲▲▲▲▲▲▲▲▲▲ patient to describe the headaches experienced. How often do they occur? Does anything relieve the pain? Are any other symptoms experienced in conjunction with the pain?

Ergot alkaloids should not be given to pregnant patients or to patients with peripheral vascular disease, infection, or coronary artery disease.

PLANNING AND IMPLEMENTATION Dosage schedules
▲▲▲▲▲▲▲▲▲▲▲▲▲▲▲▲▲▲▲▲▲▲▲▲▲▲▲▲▲▲ lend themselves to easy overdosing by the patient. For example, the schedule for Cafergot, an oral form also containing caffeine, is 2 capsules at the start of the headache, then 1 capsule every 30 minutes until the pain is relieved. However, the patient should not take more than 6 capsules per attack or 10 in a week. The schedule for Ergostat (a sublingual form of ergotamine) is similar.

Because vascular headaches can be precipitated by stress, teach patients stress reduction methods. You may choose visualization, guided imagery, deep breathing, progressive muscle setting and relaxation, or exercise.

Ergot poisoning may develop in patients who overdose on ergot alkaloids. They present with numbness and tingling, weakness, cyanosis, and muscle pain in their extremities. The extremities are also cold. Always withhold further doses of the drug and notify the physician because ergot poisoning can lead to gangrene.

BETA-BLOCKERS

ACTIONS AND USES Beta-adrenergic blockers are commonly given to treat hypertension, angina, and cardiac arrhythmias. Some are also given to prevent the occurrence of migraine headaches. They perform their antagonistic actions by taking up space at a receptor site, effectively blocking sympathomimetic stimulation.

Side effects may include blood dyscrasias, hearing and vision loss, paresthesia, depression, hallucinations, disorientation, nausea, vomiting, and diarrhea.

ASSESSMENT When your patient is prescribed a beta-adrenergic blocker, check the chart and the patient's history carefully for any contraindications or conditions that warrant extra precaution. The use of beta-adrenergic blockers is contraindicated if the patient has bradycardia, second- or third-degree heart block, or cardiac failure or is in cardiogenic shock. They can be used but with caution if the patient has peripheral vascular disease, bronchospasms, diabetes, hyperthyroidism, or any impairment of kidney or liver function.

Assess the patient's blood pressure as well as both the rate and rhythm of the heart beat. These measurements are used as baseline data for comparison with assessment findings after drug therapy has begun.

If the pulse is below 50 beats per minute or irregular, beta-blockers should not be given without consulting the physician.

PLANNING AND IMPLEMENTATION Teach the patient or the home caregiver how to take the pulse and blood pressure. Allow sufficient time for mastery of this procedure. Instruct the patient in pulse and blood pressure norms and reasons to call the physician.

Because the beta-blockers can cause postural hypotension, take safety precautions while the patient is in the care facility. Instruct the patient and family in safety precautions to take at home.

The patient taking a beta-blocker needs to fully understand the importance of continuing the medication and being monitored by the physician on a regular basis. The conditions for which beta-blockers are often prescribed can be "silent" or without symptoms. This may cause the patient to begin thinking that the drug is unnecessary or that regular checkups are uncalled for.

Warn the patient not to stop beta-blockers suddenly because this may lead to cardiac arrest or failure.

EVALUATION To determine the effectiveness of the beta-blocker, continue to monitor the patient's blood pressure and the rate and rhythm of the pulse. If the drug is prescribed to prevent angina or migraines, evaluate for the presence and frequency of pain.

Watch also for any sign of drug interactions. Beta-blockers should not be used in conjunction with over-the-counter cold remedies or nose sprays because many of these contain adrenergics and therefore are antagonistic to the adrenergic blockers. The anesthesiologist must be informed if a patient is taking a beta-blocker before the administration of anesthesia because beta-blockers alter the effectiveness of the anesthesia.

Propranolol Hydrochloride

Propranolol hydrochloride (Inderal) acts on the nerve receptors in the heart muscle and smooth muscles. Therefore, it is useful in treating hypertension, angina, pheochromocytoma, cardiac arrhythmias, and migraines.

Propranolol is given orally or intravenously. The dose depends on the rationale for use. The oral dose ranges from 40 to 240 mg a day. Inderal LA, an oral form of the drug, is a sustained-release capsule given once a day.

Propranolol is used intravenously as an emergency drug to treat tachycardia arrhythmias, such as ventricular tachycardia. The dose is up to 3 mg. It may then be repeated in 2 to 5 minutes. Further doses should not be repeated for another 4 hours.

NURSING ALERT
▼▼▼▼▼▼▼▼▼▼▼▼▼▼▼▼▼▼▼▼▼▼▼▼▼▼▼▼▼▼▼▼▼

Because one of propranolol's main actions is to slow and strengthen the heart, bradycardia is a major side effect. Ascertain that the patient's pulse is at least 60 beats per minute before administering.

▲▲▲▲▲▲▲▲▲▲▲▲▲▲▲▲▲▲▲▲▲▲▲▲▲▲▲▲▲▲▲▲▲▲▲▲

If bradycardia does occur, the physician may order atropine, a cholinergic blocker, to raise the pulse.

NURSING ALERT
▼▼▼▼▼▼▼▼▼▼▼▼▼▼▼▼▼▼▼▼▼▼▼▼▼▼▼▼▼▼▼▼▼

Respiratory distress has also been noted in patients taking propranolol, especially with a history of asthma. Be aware of the patient's history.

▲▲▲▲▲▲▲▲▲▲▲▲▲▲▲▲▲▲▲▲▲▲▲▲▲▲▲▲▲▲▲▲▲▲▲▲

Congestive heart failure has at times been precipitated by the use of propranolol because of fluid retention. Therefore, this drug should be used with caution in the presence of a pre-existing cardiac disorder. Propranolol shares the precautions described for beta-blockers in general.

Acebutolol Hydrochloride

Acebutolol hydrochloride (Sectral) is used to treat cardiac arrhythmias and hypertension. It shares assessments and contraindications with its relatives as described before.

Acebutolol is given orally in capsule form. The normal dose is 400 to 1200 mg a day in a single dose or split and given twice a day. It may lead to fatigue, dizziness, headache, nausea, vomiting, diarrhea, and even dyspnea.

When used in conjunction with nonsteroidal anti-inflammatory drugs (NSAIDs), acebutolol may have a decreased effectiveness.

Atenolol

Atenolol (Tenormin) is given for its antihypertensive and antianginal effects. It may be given orally or intravenously. The normal oral dose range is 50 to 150 mg a day.

Be aware that atenolol may interact with other adrenergic blockers, clonidine (Catapres), and verapamil (Calan).

Pindolol

Pindolol (Visken) is also used for its antihypertensive effects. It is given orally at a dose of 5 mg two or three times a day. Patients may experience distressful sleep disturbances, including insomnia, unusual dreams, and even nightmares. They may also have dizziness, dyspnea, nervousness, pain in the muscles and joints, and gastrointestinal upset.

Labetalol Hydrochloride

Labetalol hydrochloride (Trandate) is another oral antihypertensive. The oral dose ranges from 200 to 400 mg per day. However, it can also be ordered intravenously (IV). The IV dose can be given as a bolus of up to 80 mg at a time, in at least 10- to 15-minute intervals, not to exceed 300 mg in a 24-hour period. Labetalol can also be given by continuous IV drip. Adjust the drip rate to prevent the infusion of more than 2 mg per minute.

In addition to the side effects common to the subgroup beta-blockers, labetalol may cause impotence. Be aware that your patient may not easily report this effect. Therefore, as a nurse, you should routinely ask. Talking about sexuality may not come easily to either you or your patient, but by ignoring this aspect of life, you are ignoring an essential part of patient care. As with most things, the first time you attempt to discuss sexuality with your patient will be the most difficult. Take heart! It does get easier.

Metoprolol Tartrate

Metoprolol tartrate (Lopressor) is antihypertensive and antianginal. It can be administered orally (up to 450 mg per day) or intravenously (5 mg in 2 minutes, repeated up to three times).

In addition to the common side effects, metoprolol may lead to confusion and palpitations.

Nadolol

Nadolol (Corgard) is used for its antihypertensive and antianginal effects. See assessments under labetalol.

This drug has the same side effects as its relatives, including impotence. It is given orally, 40 to 240 mg per day.

NEURON BLOCKERS

ACTIONS AND USES The neuron blockers are also called rauwolfia alkaloids. They are effective in lowering blood pressure, reducing anxiety, and treating psychosis. Unfortunately, the severe side effects associated with them limit their usefulness. They are capable of producing postural hypotension, nasal stuffiness, depression, sedation, and impotence.

N U R S I N G   A L E R T

Neuron blockers can have dangerous effects on the heart, including bradycardia, angina, cardiac arrhythmias, and even cardiac arrest.

ASSESSMENT Before the first dose of the drug, take baseline vital sign readings, especially blood pressure and pulse.

Assess the patient's emotional status and report all findings to the physician.

Check the chart for any history of cardiac disorders. Neuron blockers are used only with extreme caution in the patient with a history of a myocardial infarction.

PLANNING AND IMPLEMENTATION The nurse has responsibilities related to safety for drowsiness and dizziness on arising and after standing for long periods. Walk with the patient and caution the patient to call for help before getting out of bed. Teach the patient to avoid driving or operating hazardous machinery.

Nasal stuffiness often causes the patient to reach for an over-the-counter nasal spray. Caution the patient at the time of drug therapy initiation to avoid these nasal sprays.

Be alert for signs of depression, such as insomnia, change in eating habits, change in sleeping habits, lack of personal hygiene, or statements with morbid themes. The possibility of suicide cannot be ruled out.

The nurse's responsibility to discuss impotence is described earlier (see section on labetalol).

EVALUATION You can help determine the effectiveness of a neuron blocker by frequent monitoring of vital signs. Compare your results with the baseline data you collected.

If the neuron blocker is being used to treat anxiety or psychosis, ask the patient to compare symptoms now with those previously experienced. Note any tremoring, hallucinations, pressured speech, or disorientation.

One of the most commonly experienced drug interactions of this classification is with nasal sprays. Because most are adrenergic agonists, they are therefore antagonistic.

Reserpine

Reserpine (Serpasil) is used to treat hypertension, anxiety, and psychosis. It produces its actions by blocking the bonding of norepinephrine at a receptor site.

In addition to those effects common to all rauwolfia alkaloids, reserpine may lead to gastrointestinal upset, dry mouth, dyspnea, edema, nervousness, headache, dizziness, and muscle aches.

Be aware of the patient's medical history. Reserpine should not be given to patients with depression, to patients receiving electroconvulsive therapy, or to patients with either peptic ulcer disease or ulcerative colitis because it increases gastrointestinal motility and secretions. Reserpine should be used with caution if the patient has any impairment of kidney function because the kidney is the main organ of excretion.

Reserpine is given orally. The usual dose is 0.1 to 0.25 mg per day. This dose may be divided in half and given twice a day.

Warn patients about the possibility of severe side effects. Instruct them to notify the physician of anything unusual.

Be aware of possible drug interactions, including interactions with the monoamine oxidase (MAO) inhibitors. Also, if reserpine is given with digitalis or quinidine, it may lead to cardiac arrhythmias. When reserpine and the tricyclic antidepressants are given in conjunction, the effectiveness of the antidepressant is reduced.

E X E R C I S E S

CASE STUDIES

1. Ms. M.M. has migraine headaches and has been prescribed propranolol (Inderal). The dose she has been ordered is 40 mg. The label on the bottle reads propranolol 80 mg/tablet. How many tablets should you give Ms. M.M.? What needs to appear on the tablet before you will be able to give the correct dose?

2. Mr. J.A. has been prescribed atenolol (Tenormin) for his high blood pressure. What information does Mr. J.A. need before drug therapy can be successful? When would the nurse need to begin his training? What important precaution does the nurse need to stress to Mr. J.A.?

MENTAL AEROBICS

ROLE PLAYING Playing a game may help the student remember the many varied effects this classification can have on the body. In class or in study group or even on your own, act out the effects this class has on (1) the heart, (2) the blood pressure, (3) the blood vessels, and (4) the nose. Remember, humor actually helps you to remember.

DIRECTED RESEARCH Take a tally in the hospital of how many patients are prescribed adrenergic blockers. To limit the workload, you may wish to limit the core group of patients to one floor or one portion of the ward. The student should know the number of patients, the drug each patient is receiving, and the rationale for its use for that patient.

CHOLINERGIC AGONISTS

LEARNING OBJECTIVES

After studying this chapter, you should be able to:

1. Identify general actions of and name the parasympathetic neurohormones.

2. Identify the actions and uses of and adverse reactions to the cholinergics.

3. Differentiate between direct-acting and indirect-acting cholinergics.

4. State appropriate nursing interventions for patients receiving cholinergics.

5. Define parasympathetic nervous system.

6. State common examples of cholinergics.

7. Demonstrate how to administer cholinergics by use of the nursing process.

DRUGS YOU WILL LEARN ABOUT IN THIS CHAPTER

Direct-acting Cholinergic Agonists

　bethanechol (Urecholine)

Indirect-acting Cholinergic Agonists

　demecarium bromide (Humorsol)

　edrophonium chloride (Tensilon)

　neostigmine methylsulfate (Prostigmin)

　pilocarpine (Pilocar)

　pyridostigmine (Mestinon)

ACTIONS AND USES The parasympathetic nervous system lends its name to the classification of drugs called the cholinergic agonists. They may also be called parasympathomimetic, which means "to mimic the parasympathetic."

The cholinergic agonist drugs can be subdivided into two types:

• Direct-acting cholinergic agonists, which mimic acetylcholine (and therefore keep a nerve impulse going)
• Indirect-acting cholinergic agonists, which block acetylcholinesterase (and therefore also keep a nerve impulse going)

Although these drugs are used for a variety of different conditions, many of them produce similar adverse effects. Most can lead to gastrointestinal (GI) upset, increased GI and respiratory secretions, excessive salivation, diaphoresis, flushing, a feeling of warmth, bradycardia, shortness of breath, tremors, rash, and weakness.

Many of these drugs are used to treat myasthenia gravis. Remember that this disease can lead to myasthenia crisis, which is manifested by respiratory weakness and even paralysis.

NURSING ALERT

The overdosage of a cholinergic agonist drug can lead to cholinergic crisis. It is important to differentiate between cholinergic crisis and myasthenia crisis, but it is also difficult to do so. Symptoms of cholinergic crisis include muscle rigidity and spasms, clenched jaw, and excessive salivation. Eventually the muscles weaken, however, and can mimic the effects of myasthenia crisis.

ASSESSMENT Assess the patient's vital signs before the first use of the medication. Other assessments depend on the rationale for the use of the drug.

Be aware of the patient's general health and medical history.

N U R S I N G   A L E R T

The cholinergic agonist drugs should not be used if the patient has a mechanical obstruction of either the GI system or the urinary system. Great caution is exercised if the patient is asthmatic because cholinergic agonists can produce bronchospasms.

PLANNING AND IMPLEMENTATION Many of the cholinergic agonist drugs cause GI upset. If this occurs, the drug may be administered with food or meals.

Instruct the patient to take these drugs exactly as prescribed. The dose has often been individualized to the patient's condition. The patient should not skip a dose. Help the patient devise a plan that will serve as a reminder for each dose. This may include pill boxes with alarms attached.

EVALUATION Effectiveness is determined by the absence or decrease of symptoms for which the drug was prescribed. Compare your evaluations with your baseline assessment findings.

Atropine (a cholinergic blocker) can be used to treat both the GI side effects of cholinergic agonists and cholinergic crisis. However, great care must be taken because atropine can either make the symptoms of myasthenia crisis worse or precipitate cholinergic crisis.

Also evaluate for the appearance of drug interactions. Cholinergic agonists are known to interact with anticholinergics, some types of muscle relaxants, antihistamines, antidepressants, the phenothiazines (certain antiemetics and antipsychotic medications), and some antiarrhythmics.

PYRIDOSTIGMINE

ACTIONS AND USES Pyridostigmine (Mestinon) is an indirect-acting cholinergic agonist given to treat myasthenia gravis. Although it is similar to neostigmine, pyridostigmine lasts longer and has less gastrointestinal upset associated with it.

ASSESSMENT Assess muscle strength, hand grasps, dorsal-plantar flexion, gait and speech, and ability to perform activities of daily living. Record your assessment findings as baseline information.

PLANNING AND IMPLEMENTATION Pyridostigmine can be given orally by tablet, timespan tablet, or syrup at a dose of 60 to 180 mg four times a day. It can also be administered intramuscularly or very slowly intravenously.

EVALUATION Evaluate the effectiveness of this drug through the frequent monitoring of the patient's strength. There should be improvement in hand grasps, dorsal-plantar flexion, ambulation, speech, and activities of daily living.

NEOSTIGMINE METHYLSULFATE

ACTIONS AND USES Neostigmine methylsulfate (Prostigmine) is also an indirect-acting cholinergic agonist used for myasthenia gravis. It can also be used to treat gastrointestinal distention or urinary retention after surgery.

N U R S I N G   A L E R T

Mechanical obstruction is a contraindication to the use of this drug. Neostigmine also should not be used for patients with bowel inflammations, such as peritonitis.

PLANNING AND IMPLEMENTATION Neostigmine can be given orally in tablet form, intramuscularly, intravenously, or subcutaneously. Know that the risk exists for severe adverse reactions, including convulsions, cardiac arrhythmias, dyspnea, bronchospasms, respiratory depression, and even respiratory arrest. Watch the patient's vital signs carefully. Also observe and assess for dizziness, headache, pain in the joints, and tremors.

EVALUATION Evaluate effectiveness with muscle strength. Be aware of the patient's history and be watchful for any symptoms or complaints that indicate an increase of cardiac arrhythmias, peptic ulcer, hyperthyroidism, or asthma.

Also be aware that some antibiotics can increase the effects of neostigmine, including kanamycin, streptomycin, and neomycin. Anesthetics and antiarrhythmics, on the other hand, decrease the effectiveness of neostigmine.

EDROPHONIUM CHLORIDE

Edrophonium chloride (Tensilon) is a very short acting cholinergic agonist. Its action begins in about 60 seconds and lasts only about 10 minutes. It works by inhibiting acetylcholinesterase, which makes it an indirect-acting cholinergic agonist. Most often, edrophonium is used as a diagnostic agent. After administration, if the patient has a brief but dramatic increase of muscle strength, the test result is positive for myasthenia gravis. Because of its brief length of action, edrophonium is not useful as a maintenance drug.

Edrophonium is given either intramuscularly or intravenously. Monitor the patient carefully because this drug can produce dramatic side effects, including respiratory or cardiac arrest. Be especially cautious with patients who have a history of asthma or cardiac arrhythmias.

The patient is evaluated for muscle strength to determine the presence of myasthenia gravis. The nurse may participate in hand grasp and dorsal-plantar flexion evaluation, or the patient may be asked to perform certain exercises before and after drug administration.

BETHANECHOL

ACTIONS AND USES Bethanechol (Urecholine) is a direct-acting cholinergic agonist. It is given to treat neurological urinary retention. When given in tablet form, it produces micturition in about 30 to 60 minutes. When given subcutaneously, bethanechol is even quicker, producing micturition in 5 to 15 minutes.

ASSESSMENT Bethanechol shares many of the same contraindications to use of its relatives. It should not be given to persons with hyperthyroidism, peptic ulcer disease, inflammation of the gastrointestinal (GI) system, weakened wall of the GI tract or genitourinary (GU) tract, mechanical obstruction of either the GI or GU system, parkinsonism, epilepsy, bradycardia, hypotension, coronary artery disease, or bronchial asthma.

PLANNING AND IMPLEMENTATION Bethanechol can be administered either orally or subcutaneously. The initial oral dose of 5 to 10 mg can be repeated hourly if micturition does not occur. The patient may then be prescribed a maintenance dose of 10 to 100 mg up to four times a day. The initial subcutaneous dose is 2.5 mg, which may be repeated every 15 to 30 minutes. The maintenance dose is 2.5 to 10 mg up to four times a day.

N U R S I N G   A L E R T

Keep in mind the purpose of the drug and its expected time of action. Stay nearby or answer the call light immediately. You may even keep the bedpan near the patient if leaving the room is necessary.

However, do not keep the patient on the bedpan or the commode for the entire waiting period. This is uncomfortable and could cause nerve damage in the legs in some instances.

The patient may experience side effects from bethanechol. Warn the patient of this possibility. The patient may have a headache, hypotension, malaise, GI upset, tachycardia, flushing and sweating, bronchospasms, and tearing.

EVALUATION Keep an accurate intake and output record for any patient experiencing urinary retention. Take note of the time the drug was given, the time micturition occurred, and the amount the patient voided. Also evaluate the urine for color, sediment, and odor.

PILOCARPINE

Pilocarpine (Pilocar) is an ophthalmic solution used to treat glaucoma. It works by producing miosis (pupil constriction).

Pilocarpine is administered directly to the conjunctival sac. Wash your hands before and after instillation to prevent transmission of microorganisms and absorption of the drug through your own skin. Compress the tear duct for 5 to 10 seconds after instillation to prevent the drug from entering the nasal passages and being absorbed systemically.

The patient may experience stinging or burning of the eye with tearing and even eyelid twitching. Some patients may have conjunctival redness or inflammation. In addition to the common cholinergic side effects, pilocarpine may produce headache, blurred vision, cyst formation, and even lens opacity.

N U R S I N G   A L E R T

One of the most important evaluations the nurse must make for the patient receiving pilocarpine therapy is for signs or symptoms of pilocarpine poisoning. This may lead to pulmonary edema and even respiratory arrest.

The antidote for pilocarpine poisoning is atropine, a cholinergic blocker. Also evaluate for a decrease of eye pain.

DEMECARIUM BROMIDE

Demecarium bromide (Humorsol) is also an ophthalmic solution. It is an indirect-acting cholinergic agonist. It, too, produces miosis and is therefore useful in the treatment of open-angle glaucoma. It may be ordered after an iridectomy and for cases of strabismus as well. It should not be used if the patient has ophthalmic inflammation.

Demecarium is administered in the same way as pilocarpine is. Use caution when giving it to patients with myasthenia gravis or under anesthesia because it may interfere with drug regimens in place.

Evaluate for a decrease of glaucoma symptoms, including blurring or possibly eye pain.

E X E R C I S E S

CASE STUDIES

1. Ms. P.B. has been experiencing symptoms that the physician believes may be myasthenia gravis. What drug might be used to confirm her diagnosis? What reaction to the drug might the nurse expect if Ms. P.B. does indeed have myasthenia gravis? What evaluations by the nurse might be required for the accurate interpretation of this test?

2. Ms. P.B. is receiving pyridostigmine 2 mg IV. The order reads pyridostigmine 2 mg/500 mL to be given over 4 hours. The IV solution is to run through a pump with a drop factor of 12. How many drops per minute should the IV solution be set for?

3. Mr. J.M. has been diagnosed with glaucoma. He has been prescribed demecarium ophthalmic solution. How should the nurse administer this drug? What side effects might Mr. J.M. experience right away? What systemic effects might demecarium produce?

4. Mr. G.D. has not voided for 7 hours since surgery. His physician has decided to try bethanechol. What is the purpose of this drug? When would the nurse expect the drug actions to begin if Mr. G.D. receives it by mouth? by subcutaneous injection? What actions should the nurse take after the administration of this drug?

MENTAL AEROBICS

ROLE PLAYING Role playing each of the following actions provides the student with a visual concept of the parasympathetic nervous system and the cholinergic drugs.

1. One student will pretend to be acetylcholine and carry a "nerve impulse" from point A to point B (the end of one nerve and the beginning of another).

2. One student will pretend to be acetylcholine, and another student will be acetylcholinesterase. They will need to "fight it out" to perform their jobs.

3. One student will pretend to be a nonfunctioning or weak acetylcholine, one student will be acetylcholinesterase, and one student will be a direct-acting cholinergic drug. Each will perform the assigned job while trying to carry the nerve impulse.

4. One student will be acetylcholine, one student will be acetylcholinesterase, and one student will be an indirect-acting cholinergic drug. Each will perform the assigned job while the nerve impulse is passed.

CHAPTER 40

CHOLINERGIC BLOCKERS

LEARNING OBJECTIVES

After studying this chapter, you should be able to:

1. Identify actions and uses of and adverse reactions to the cholinergic blockers.

2. State common examples of cholinergic blockers.

3. Prepare an appropriate teaching plan for a patient receiving a cholinergic blocker.

4. Demonstrate how to administer cholinergic blockers by use of the nursing process.

DRUGS YOU WILL LEARN ABOUT IN THIS CHAPTER

Cholinergic Blockers

anisotropine methylbromide

atropine sulfate

clidinium bromide (Quarzan)

dicyclomine HCl (Bentyl)

glycopyrrolate (Robinul)

ipratropium bromide (Atrovent)

isopropamide iodide (Darbid)

mepenzolate bromide (Cantil)

propantheline bromide (Pro-Banthine)

scopolamine (Transderm Scōp)

Combination Drugs

Donnagel (kaolin, pectin, atropine sulfate, scopolamine, hyoscyamine sulfate)

Donnagel-PG (kaolin, pectin, atropine sulfate, scopolamine, hyoscyamine sulfate, paregoric)

Donnatal (phenobarbital, atropine sulfate, scopolamine, hyoscyamine sulfate)

Librax (chlordiazepoxide HCl [Librium], clidinium)

ACTIONS AND USES The cholinergic blockers are also ▲▲▲▲▲▲▲▲▲▲▲▲▲▲▲▲ called the parasympathomimetic blockers because they block or are antagonistic to the action of the parasympathetic nervous system. They are at times referred to as parasympatholytics for the same reason; the suffix -lytic means to work against. Last, they may also be referred to as anticholinergics in some sources. They are, however, all the same group of drugs. The difference in names reflects our desire to be exact and concise. Unfortunately, in this case, it has served only to confuse.

The cholinergic blockers work by inhibiting acetylcholine. They therefore cause the nerve impulse to stop, which leads to their many actions. As a group, these drugs can cause drowsiness and a dreamless sleep, dry both respiratory and gastrointestinal (GI) secretions, relax bronchi, and dilate pupils. These many actions can be put to good use. The anticholinergics are often used in preoperative medications to decrease the chance of aspiration. The patient has less risk of vomiting or aspirating when secretions are lessened. They may be useful in the treatment of bronchospasms and in cold or allergy relief. For this reason, we often find cholinergic blockers in over-the-counter preparations. Anticholinergics are often used in the treatment of GI diseases, such as peptic ulcers, colitis, and GI spasms, because of their antispasmodic actions. They may be applied topically to the eye before an examination of the eye so that the examiner may better view the interior.

Most cholinergic blockers cause side effects as well, including dry mouth, photophobia, urinary retention, tachycardia, palpitations, headache, nervousness, insomnia, confusion, dizziness, GI upset, and impotence.

ASSESSMENT Check the patient's medical history carefully. Anticholinergics have many contraindications because of their systemic effects. They should not be used for someone with glaucoma, GI or genitourinary obstruction, ulcerative colitis, GI hemorrhage, or myasthenia gravis.

Be cautious when administering an anticholinergic to a patient with neuropathy, liver or kidney disease, hyperthyroidism, cardiac disease, or hiatal hernia. Any of these diseases may be worsened by the cholinergic blockers.

Other assessments depend on the rationale for use of the drug. If the drug is used for seasonal allergies, assessment of the upper and lower respiratory system is warranted. If the drug is used for colitis, perform a full GI assessment. This highlights the need for you to be knowledgeable of the patient's condition.

PLANNING AND IMPLEMENTATION Warn patients that the drug may cause drowsiness or blurred vision. This can make operating hazardous machinery, such as an automobile, even more dangerous. If the patient will be exposed to high temperatures, whether because of the climate or work conditions, warn the patient that the use of cholinergic blockers in such conditions can precipitate heat stroke. This is due to the drug's ability to decrease sweating.

Assess patients for the occurrence of adverse reactions and formulate appropriate interventions. For example, a dry mouth can be eased by ice chips or when not contraindicated, hard candy. Photophobia can be eased with pulled drapes, dimmed lights, or sunglasses. Other side effects may require the intervention of a physician. Urinary retention that does not respond to conventional nursing measures will require a physician's order, perhaps for medication or for catheterization.

EVALUATION Effectiveness of the drug is determined by the presence, absence, increase, or decrease of the symptoms for which the drug was prescribed. Also look for drug interactions. Cholinergic blockers are known to interact with antihistamines, antacids, quinidine, and any central nervous system (CNS) depressants.

ATROPINE SULFATE

ACTIONS AND USES Atropine sulfate is used for many purposes. It increases respirations and relaxes bronchi. Along with the decrease in respiratory secretions, breathing is eased. This drug also relaxes gastrointestinal smooth muscles and decreases secretions. Therefore, it is useful in treating diseases in which hypermotility predominates, such as spastic colon and spasm of the gallbladder or bile duct. It is used as a preoperative medication. It may be applied before eye examinations to dilate the pupil. It can be given as an antidote when needed for cholinergic overdose.

ASSESSMENT Assessments before use depend on the rationale for use. See assessments for cholinergic blockers in general.

PLANNING AND IMPLEMENTATION Atropine sulfate may be administered orally, subcutaneously, intramuscularly, intravenously, as an inhalant, or ophthalmically. The average oral dose is 0.3 to 1.2 mg given four to six times a day. Subcutaneous and intramuscular doses range from 0.4 to 0.6 mg. This is usually a preoperative dosage given no more than 1 hour before surgery.

Warn patients that they may experience a dry mouth and teach possible interventions to relieve this discomfort. If this is a preoperative medication, warn patients to remain NPO (nothing by mouth) despite the dry mouth. You may observe that the patient becomes restless or talkative. If this seems to distress the patient, explaining that it is a side effect of the drug may help the patient relax. Patients may have a low-grade fever or become flushed after the use of atropine. This should not be confused with signs of an infection. A slight rash may also develop.

EVALUATION Evaluation of the effectiveness of the drug depends on the purpose for administration. You may be noting respirations, level of consciousness, presence of nausea, absence of pain, appetite, or pupil dilatation.

IPRATROPIUM BROMIDE

Ipratropium bromide (Atrovent), a drug similar to atropine, is given by aerosol for its local bronchodilator effects. It is not well absorbed, and therefore the risk of toxic effect is low. It is often given to treat bronchospasms associated with chronic obstructive pulmonary disease. It does not work rapidly and therefore is used only as a maintenance drug, not for acute bronchospasms. Patients take 2 puffs four times a day and as needed between, but not more than 12 puffs in a 24-hour period.

SCOPOLAMINE

ACTIONS AND USES Scopolamine has traditionally ▲▲▲▲▲▲▲▲▲▲▲▲▲▲▲ been used as a preoperative medication and for motion sickness for its anticholinergic effects. In addition to the other cholinergic blocker side effects, the patient may experience dry, itchy, reddened eyes.

ASSESSMENT Assess for the frequency and severity ▲▲▲▲▲▲▲▲▲▲ of motion sickness and precipitating factors.

PLANNING AND IMPLEMENTATION Scopolamine is not ▲▲▲▲▲▲▲▲▲▲▲▲▲▲▲▲▲▲▲▲▲▲▲▲▲▲ used as often as it once was. It may be administered orally, subcutaneously, intramuscularly, or intravenously. The usual parenteral dose is up to 1 mg every 6 to 8 hours as needed.

N U R S I N G   A L E R T

▼▼▼▼▼▼▼▼▼▼▼▼▼▼▼▼▼▼▼▼▼▼▼▼▼▼▼▼▼▼▼▼

Patients should not be given scopolamine for more than 3 days because they may experience withdrawal symptoms.

▲▲▲▲▲▲▲▲▲▲▲▲▲▲▲▲▲▲▲▲▲▲▲▲▲▲▲▲▲▲▲▲

EVALUATION Effectiveness of the drug is determined ▲▲▲▲▲▲▲▲▲▲ by decreased occurrence and severity of motion sickness. When scopolamine is given as a preoperative medication, evaluate for a decrease in respiratory and gastrointestinal secretions, which often presents as dry mouth and thirst.

Transderm Scōp

Transderm Scōp is a trade name form of topical scopolamine. It is used to prevent motion sickness. It should not be used by patients who are allergic to adhesives or who have glaucoma. It is applied by patch in the postauricular area at least 4 hours before the time it is anticipated to be needed. Patients should wash their hands after administration and after removal of the patch to prevent getting the drug in their eyes and to prevent systemic effects. The patch is generally left in place for 3 days. If absolutely needed, another patch may be applied, but the patient will usually experience withdrawal for applications lasting longer than the 3-day period.

DONNAGEL, DONNAGEL-PG

Donnagel (which contains kaolin, pectin, atropine sulfate, hyoscyamine sulfate, and scopolamine) and Donnagel-PG (which contains kaolin, pectin, atropine sulfate, scopolamine, hyoscyamine sulfate, and paregoric) use the combined effects of the ingredients, including the anticholinergics, to treat diarrhea, tenesmus (the urge to defecate without stool in the rectum), and abdominal pain associated with cramping. Because of the anticholinergic components, Donnagel and Donnagel-PG share the contraindications to use of the cholinergic blockers. They also should not be used if the patient has a fever.

Donnagel and Donnagel-PG are both oral drugs. The usual dose is 1 ounce for every loose stool. The patient should allow approximately a half-hour for the drug to begin to work. Neither drug should be used for more than 2 days. This is especially important for Donnagel-PG because the paregoric component is habit forming.

Donnagel and Donnagel-PG should be discontinued if the patient experiences blurred vision or eye pain, tachycardia, or dizziness. Keep an accurate record of intake and output. Record the number, consistency, and quantity of stools or complaints of abdominal pain for any patient with diarrhea.

DONNATAL

Because of the combination of phenobarbital, atropine sulfate, hyoscyamine sulfate, and scopolamine, Donnatal is useful for its antispasmodic action in enterocolitis and irritable bowel syndrome.

Donnatal is an oral drug. The usual dose is 1 to 2 tablets or capsules, or 1 to 2 teaspoons every 3 to 4 hours.

Evaluate the patient for number, consistency, and quantity of stools as well as for pain or cramping.

PROPANTHELINE BROMIDE

ACTIONS AND USES Propantheline bromide (Pro-▲▲▲▲▲▲▲▲▲▲▲▲▲▲▲▲ Banthine) is another cholinergic blocker used to decrease gastrointestinal motility and secretions. It is therefore used to treat peptic ulcer. It shares the contraindications listed for cholinergic blockers.

ASSESSMENT Assess for abdominal pain, frequency of ▲▲▲▲▲▲▲▲▲▲ symptoms, nausea and vomiting, and appetite.

PLANNING AND IMPLEMENTATION Propantheline bro-
▲▲▲▲▲▲▲▲▲▲▲▲▲▲▲▲▲▲▲▲▲▲▲▲▲▲▲ mide is an oral drug. The usual initial dose is 15 mg before every meal and 30 mg before bed. This dose may be adjusted up or down according to the patient's condition.

EVALUATION Effectiveness is determined by the de-
▲▲▲▲▲▲▲▲▲▲ crease in frequency and severity of symptoms. Keep accurate records of food intake, emesis, or complaints of pain. The effects of propantheline may be increased if it is used together with any of the following groups of drugs: central nervous system depressants, narcotic analgesics, antiarrhythmics, antihistamines, phenothiazines, or tricyclic antidepressants. If propantheline is used with the steroid group, the patient is at greater risk for increased intraocular pressure.

CLIDINIUM BROMIDE

Clidinium bromide (Quarzan) also decreases gastrointestinal motility and secretions. It is given orally for treatment of peptic ulcer disease. Evaluate the patient's pain, appetite, and gastric distress. Interestingly, researchers do not list any interactions for clidinium with other drugs.

CHLORDIAZEPOXIDE HYDROCHLORIDE AND CLIDINIUM

Chlordiazepoxide hydrochloride (Librium) combined with clidinium is sold under the trade name Librax. It is often used to treat gastric distress brought on by anxiety. Its properties are those of the two drug components it contains.

ANISOTROPINE METHYLBROMIDE, ISOPROPAMIDE IODIDE, AND MEPENZOLATE BROMIDE

Each of these drugs is used for its anticholinergic effect on the gastrointestinal system. Anisotropine methylbromide, isopropamide iodide (Darbid), and mepenzolate bromide (Cantil) decrease motility and

secretions and consequently are used to treat peptic ulcer disease. They share the general information listed for all cholinergic blockers. Each is an oral agent.

DICYCLOMINE HYDROCHLORIDE

Dicyclomine hydrochloride (Bentyl) is used for its antispasmodic action to treat irritable bowel syndrome and other disorders involving gastrointestinal spasms. Assess for the number, consistency, and quantity of stools; abdominal pain; or nausea and vomiting.

Dicyclomine can be given orally (up to 40 mg every 6 hours) or intramuscularly (up to 20 mg every 6 hours).

N U R S I N G   A L E R T
▼▼▼▼▼▼▼▼▼▼▼▼▼▼▼▼▼▼▼▼▼▼▼▼▼▼▼▼▼▼▼▼▼

Be sure to aspirate when giving dicyclomine intramuscularly because this drug causes thrombosis if it is accidentally given intravenously.

▲▲▲▲▲▲▲▲▲▲▲▲▲▲▲▲▲▲▲▲▲▲▲▲▲▲▲▲▲▲▲▲▲

Dicyclomine has the same properties as the other cholinergic blockers.

Effectiveness of the drug is determined by a relief of symptoms. Therefore, ongoing assessments are required.

GLYCOPYRROLATE

Glycopyrrolate (Robinul) is used for several purposes. It can be used to treat peptic ulcer disease, to dry respiratory secretions, to decrease gastrointestinal secretions, and as a preoperative medication. Appropriate assessments are determined by the purpose of the drug.

You may be administering glycopyrrolate orally, intramuscularly, or intravenously. The usual preoperative dose is 0.1 mg intramuscularly. The usual dose given for a peptic ulcer is 1 to 2 mg every 8 to 12 hours orally.

Evaluation of the effectiveness of this drug depends on the purpose of the prescription. You may be evaluating for pain, appetite, dry mouth and mucous membranes, or gastrointestinal upset. Be aware that glycopyrrolate can lead to ventricular arrhythmias if it is given intravenously in combination with cyclopropane anesthesia. In general, the anesthesiologist will opt for a different combination of drugs.

E X E R C I S E S

CASE STUDIES

1. Ms. J.W. is a nursing student. She is trying to look up the classification cholinergic blockers in a reference book but is unable to find it. What advice could you give her? What other names might she try looking for?

2. Mr. A.J. is to have surgery in an hour. His preoperative medication contains atropine. What teaching would you do for Mr. A.J. to maintain his safety before, during, and after the surgery?

3. After surgery, Mr. A.J. has a low-grade fever and is flushed on his cheeks. The nurse manager states that it is too early for an infection to be occurring. What possible explanation is there for Mr. A.J.'s symptoms?

4. In report, you hear that one of the patients had been given an overdose of medication and was given atropine to counteract it. For what classification of drugs is atropine an antidote?

MENTAL AEROBICS

1. One student will role play the actions of acetylcholine and its effects on a nerve impulse. Another student will role play the actions of a weakened acetylcholinesterase. The students should be able to see the increased nerve impulses passing from one nerve ending to another.

2. The two students in activity 1 continue to role play their parts. A third student is assigned to role play the actions of a cholinergic blocker. Which of the first two students will be aided? What will happen to the nerve impulse?

3. Write one nursing intervention for each possible side effect of the cholinergic blocker classification. This will prepare you for the many times you will see these side effects.

UNIT EIGHT

DRUGS THAT AFFECT THE CARDIOVASCULAR SYSTEM

The cardiovascular system is composed of three major parts:

• The blood and all of its elements, which carry nutrition to all cells and wastes away from cells

• The vascular system, a network of blood vessels through which the blood flows

• The heart muscle with its chambers and valves, which act together to pump the blood throughout the system.

The nervous system provides the electrical stimuli to make the heart contract and relax and the blood vessels dilate and constrict.

There are many classifications of drugs used to alter the function of the heart, the blood vessels, and the blood. Each acts in a specific manner as you will see in Chapters 41 through 45.

DRUGS THAT AFFECT HEART TONE AND RHYTHM

LEARNING OBJECTIVES

After studying this chapter, you should be able to:

1. Identify two major uses of cardiotonics.

2. Explain the difference between a digitalizing dose and a maintenance dose.

3. List the symptoms of digitalis toxicity.

4. Compare the nursing care of a patient being digitalized with that of a patient receiving a maintenance dose of a cardiotonic.

5. List the general adverse effects of drugs in each subclass.

6. State nursing interventions that are appropriate for patients receiving these drugs.

7. Prepare an appropriate plan of care for a patient receiving one of these drugs.

DRUGS YOU WILL LEARN ABOUT IN THIS CHAPTER

Cardiotonics (Cardiac Glycosides)

digitalis leaf

digitoxin (Crystodigin)

digoxin (Lanoxin, Lanoxicaps)

deslanoside (Cedilanid-D)

Cardiac Depressants (Antiarrhythmics)

Group I cardiac depressants

disopyramide (Rhythmodan)

disopyramide phosphate (Norpace, Norpace CR)

lidocaine HCl (Xylocaine)

phenytoin (Dilantin, Infatabs)

phenytoin sodium (Dilantin)

procainamide HCl (Pronestyl, Procan, Procan SR)

quinidine sulfate

quinidine gluconate (Quinaglute)

Group II cardiac depressants

propranolol HCl (Inderal)

Group III cardiac depressants

bretylium tosylate (Bretylol)

Unclassified cardiac depressants

atropine sulfate

The conduction system of the heart is the collection of nervous system stimuli that cause the heart muscle to contract and relax. One of the functions of the medulla oblongata of the brain stem is to control the organs in the chest.

Electrical impulses from the medulla travel by way of the tenth cranial nerve (the vagus nerve) to the sinoatrial (SA) node in the right atrium. The SA node is referred to as the "pacemaker" of the heart because impulses originating from there set the pace for the heart rate. The SA node relays the impulses to all parts of the atria, which causes them to contract.

Next, the impulses travel to the atrioventricular (AV) node located at the septum where the atria and ventricles join. The impulses travel from the AV node down the ventricular septum by way of the bundle of His to the Purkinje fibers. The Purkinje fibers carry the impulse to all parts of the ventricles and cause them to contract.

The *cardiac cycle* refers to the rhythmic contractions of the atria and ventricles. The atria contract together to pump the blood through the valves into the relaxed ventricles. After the ventricles fill, the valves at their entrances close, the valves at their exits open, and the ventricles contract to pump the blood out to the systemic circulation. The atria are now relaxed with their entrance valves open to receive the blood flowing back from the systemic circulation.

The cycle then repeats. When the two atria contract, the two ventricles are relaxed. When the two ventricles contract, the two atria are relaxed. The relaxed chambers are filling while the contracting chambers are emptying.

The ventricles contract more strongly than the atria, so the ventricles can force the blood out through the pulmonary artery to the lungs and through the aorta to the vital organs and the peripheral blood vessels.

Cardiac output refers to the amount of blood leaving the left ventricle with each contraction. If cardiac contractions are uncoordinated, cardiac output decreases. Decreased cardiac output deprives all vital organs of an adequate blood supply. The inadequate blood supply results in a diminished oxygen supply, and cell damage may result.

The body attempts to compensate for the inadequate blood supply by increasing the respiratory rate to take in more oxygen. The body then increases the heart rate to transport that oxygen to all the cells of the body. However, if the heart is beating irregularly at the same time that the rate increases, the irregular beat will worsen. The inadequate oxygen supply to the cells will become worse.

CARDIOTONICS (CARDIAC GLYCOSIDES)

Cardiac glycosides are sometimes called cardiotonics. Glycosides are extracted from plants. Cardiac glycosides are extracts of the digitalis plant.

ACTIONS AND USES Cardiotonics act directly on the ▲▲▲▲▲▲▲▲▲▲▲▲▲▲▲ myocardium to increase the force of the contractions. As a result, the cardiac output increases. Cardiotonics also affect the conduction system of the heart by depressing the sinoatrial node. This slows the conduction of impulses to the atrioven-

tricular node, resulting in a decreased number of beats per minute. Therefore, it is often said that cardiotonics act to slow and strengthen the heart beat.

Examples of cardiotonics include digitalis leaf, digitoxin (Crystodigin), digoxin (Lanoxin, Lanoxicaps), and deslanoside (Cedilanid-D). Cardiotonics differ from one another in their speed and duration of action. These differences allow the physician to individualize the treatment regimens.

Cardiotonics are used to treat congestive heart failure, atrial fibrillation, and paroxysmal tachycardia. Cardiotonics have a narrow margin of safety. This means that there is little difference between a therapeutic dose and a dose that produces adverse effects. Therefore, it is important to monitor for adverse reactions, which can occur at any time.

Digitalis toxicity refers to adverse effects resulting from therapy with *any* of the cardiotonics. Signs and symptoms of toxicity include anorexia, nausea, vomiting, diarrhea, weakness, headache, drowsiness, and blurred vision. Other visual disturbances may occur, such as altered perception of green and yellow or seeing halos around dark objects or lights. Depression, confusion, and delirium sometimes occur. Alterations in the rate and rhythm of the heart can worsen and become life-threatening.

ASSESSMENT Assess vital signs, including apical and ▲▲▲▲▲▲▲▲▲▲ radial pulses (taken simultaneously for a full minute), blood pressure, and respiratory rate. Document findings as baseline data. Make note of any abnormalities, such as cyanosis, plethora (a deep red color due to distention and congestion of blood vessels), dyspnea, or orthopnea. Assess the lung sounds and document findings. Assess for signs of peripheral edema. Weigh the patient. Check for distention of the neck veins. Assess for mucus production and note the color and consistency of the mucus. Note the level of consciousness and state of mental alertness or confusion. Assess the chart for electrocardiogram (ECG) reports and laboratory values, such as electrolyte, blood urea nitrogen, and creatinine levels. Note any history of renal or hepatic impairment.

PLANNING AND IMPLEMENTATION When therapy with ▲▲▲▲▲▲▲▲▲▲▲▲▲▲▲▲▲▲▲▲▲▲▲▲▲▲ a cardiotonic is initiated, the physician often orders the administration of "loading" doses of the drug to be given in divided doses (spread throughout a 24-hour period) until therapeutic effects are achieved. This regimen is referred to as *digitalizing* the patient. The physician then orders the dose decreased to a *maintenance* dose. Table 41–1 contains dosages for cardiac glycosides.

During digitalization, assess the patient every 2 to 4 hours, or as ordered by the physician, or as the

Table 41-1. Typical Dosage Ranges for Cardiotonic Drugs

DRUG	LOADING DOSAGE	MAINTENANCE DOSAGE
digitalis leaf	1.2–1.8 g PO in divided doses in 24-h period	100 mg PO qd
digitoxin (Crystodigin)	Adults: 1.2–1.6 mg IV or PO in divided doses in 24-h period	0.1 mg qd
digoxin (Lanoxin, Lanoxicaps)	Adults: 0.5–1 mg IV or PO in divided doses in 24-h period	0.125–0.5 mg IV or PO qd (average dose, 0.25 mg)
deslanoside (Cedilanid-D)	1.2–1.6 mg IM or IV in 2 divided doses in 24-h period	(Not used for maintenance therapy)

condition warrants. During maintenance treatment, assess the patient each day. Teach patients and caregivers the adverse effects and the appropriate assessments for them. They should know how to assess the radial pulse for rate and rhythm.

N U R S I N G   A L E R T

▼▼▼▼▼▼▼▼▼▼▼▼▼▼▼▼▼▼▼▼▼▼▼▼▼▼▼▼▼▼▼▼▼

Digitalis toxicity can occur at any time during therapy.

▲▲▲▲▲▲▲▲▲▲▲▲▲▲▲▲▲▲▲▲▲▲▲▲▲▲▲▲▲▲▲▲▲

Before each dose of a cardiac glycoside, take the pulse for a full minute and document the rate and rhythm. Assess the apical and radial pulses. If the rate is below 60 beats per minute or if there is a difference of more than a few beats between the apical and radial pulses (called a pulse deficit), do not administer the dose until the physician is contacted for further orders. (This is often referred to as holding the drug.) Sometimes the physician specifies in the drug order a different heart rate (other than 60) at which the drug is to be held. Also hold the drug and notify the physician if any of the other signs or symptoms of digitalis toxicity are noticed.

Weigh the patient each day or as ordered. Monitor intake and output, edema, cough, sputum, respiratory rate, and lung sounds. If the patient is also receiving a diuretic, monitor for signs and symptoms of hypokalemia because this may precipitate an episode of digitalis toxicity.

Many drugs interact with the cardiac glycosides, so the physician should be aware of all drugs taken by the patient, including over-the-counter medications. Many antibiotics, diuretics, and corticosteroids may predispose the patient to hypokalemia. Use of calcium and the thiazides may cause hypercalcemia and hypomagnesemia and predispose patients to digitalis toxicity. Antacids and antidiarrheals decrease absorption of oral forms of cardiac glycosides. These preparations should be taken 2 to 3 hours before or after the glycoside. Phenobarbital, phenytoin, and rifampin cause increased metabolism and a decrease in the duration of the action of the glycoside. The physician may order an increased dosage of the cardiac glycoside.

Patients with hypothyroidism are especially susceptible to the effects of glycosides and may experience toxic effects more rapidly. Patients with hyperthyroidism may require increased dosages of glycosides. Patients with renal and hepatic impairment may require decreased dosages.

If the physician orders intravenous administration of a cardiac glycoside, it must be administered slowly. Intramuscular injections cause muscle soreness, so the injection sites must be rotated. Teach patients to take medications at the same time each day.

Lanoxicaps are liquid preparations contained in capsules. This form is absorbed more rapidly, so dosages are usually lower than for the tablet form of the drug.

EVALUATION Take vital signs, weigh the patient, and ▲▲▲▲▲▲▲▲▲▲ compare findings with baseline data. Monitor for a decrease in edema, improved lung sounds, slower heart rate, and improved rhythm of the heart beat. Patients will usually state an improvement in their energy level. Monitor laboratory values for hypokalemia. Monitor digitalis levels to determine whether the blood levels of the drug are within therapeutic ranges. Monitor ECG results.

CARDIAC DEPRESSANTS (ANTIARRHYTHMICS)

Cardiac depressants (antiarrhythmics) are used to treat disturbances in the rate and rhythm of the heart. Some arrhythmias (also called dysrhythmias) are mild and do not cause the patient any difficulty; others are severe and life-threatening. The patient may be unaware of the disturbance.

Arrhythmias may be caused by electrolyte imbalances (such as hypokalemia or hypercalcemia), myocardial infarctions, hyperthyroidism, pheochromocytoma, and cardiotonic medications.

If the cause of the arrhythmia can be determined, it will be treated by the physician. In addition, the physician may order medications to decrease the myocardial response to the electrical stimuli of the conduction impulse. As the muscle response to some of the stimuli decreases, the heart rate decreases and becomes more rhythmical.

Although all of the cardiac depressant drugs are used to treat arrhythmias, their modes of action may vary. The drugs are grouped here according to their actions. Typical dosage ranges for each group are listed in Table 41–2.

Group I Antiarrhythmics

ACTION AND USES Group I antiarrhythmic drugs include disopyramide (Rhythmodan), disopyramide phosphate (Norpace, Norpace CR), lidocaine hydrochloride (Xylocaine), phenytoin (Dilantin, Infatabs), phenytoin sodium (Dilantin), procainamide hydrochloride (Pronestyl, Procan, Procan SR), quinidine sulfate, and quinidine gluconate (Duraquin, Quinaglute). These medications act to decrease myocardial excitability and lengthen the refractory (or rest) period of the heart. This means that although the heart may be receiving many impulses or stimuli, it responds more slowly to the responses received and does not conduct them as quickly throughout the cardiac tissue.

Adverse actions of most drugs in this group include hypotension, dizziness, blurred vision, headache, nausea, vomiting, diarrhea, and tinnitus.

Group I antiarrhythmics are used to treat premature atrial contractions, premature atrial tachycardia, atrial fibrillation or flutter, premature ventricular contractions, and premature ventricular tachycardia.

ASSESSMENT Assessment of the patient is the same for all groups of cardiac depressant drugs. Assess vital signs, skin color, orientation, level of consciousness, and any signs and symptoms described by the patient. Document as baseline data.

PLANNING AND IMPLEMENTATION If the patient is experiencing a cardiac emergency, cardiac depressants are often initiated with an intravenous (IV) bolus. This dose may continue until the arrhythmia disappears or adverse effects occur. The physician may then order the dose reduced somewhat but continued as an IV loading dose for the first 24 hours. This is followed by a decrease to a maintenance dose given by the oral route.

Monitor vital signs and cardiac function continuously during administration of the IV bolus and until the patient's condition stabilizes. During maintenance treatment, assess the patient each day.

Teach patients and their caregivers how to store and administer the drugs, the adverse effects, and the appropriate assessments to make. Before giving each dose, patients or caregivers should assess the radial pulse for the rate and rhythm. They should report to the physician if the rate drops below 60 or increases above 120 beats per minute. Reinforce the fact that adverse effects can occur at any time during therapy.

Teach patients to change positions slowly and to dangle before rising because dizziness and hypotension pose the threat of injury. Caution patients not to drive or operate hazardous machinery if dizziness and nausea are present.

For complaints of dry mouth or bitter taste, relief may be obtained through use of mouthwash, chewing gum, or hard candy. Measure intake and output (I & O) of patients who experience vomiting and diarrhea, and monitor for electrolyte disturbances.

Maintenance doses should be distributed throughout a 24-hour period. Teach patients to set an alarm clock for nighttime doses.

EVALUATION Monitor the patient's vital signs and compare findings with the baseline data and normal values. Monitor signs and symptoms and compare with baseline assessments. Question the patient about changes in subjective complaints. Monitor laboratory values to determine whether blood levels of the drug are within therapeutic ranges.

Disopyramide

Teach patients who are taking disopyramide (Rhythmodan) or disopyramide phosphate (Norpace, Norpace CR) and their caregivers to monitor for the additional adverse effects of blurred vision, constipa-

Table 41–2. Typical Dosage Ranges for Cardiac Depressants

DRUG	DOSAGE
Group I Cardiac Depressants	
disopyramide (Rhythmodan)	Adults: 150–200 mg PO q6h
disopyramide phosphate (Norpace, Norpace CR)	Patients weighing less than 50 kg or those with renal, hepatic, or cardiac impairment: 100 mg PO q6h Sustained-release capsules: 200 mg q12h
lidocaine hydrochloride (Xylocaine)	Adults: 50–100 mg (1–1.5 mg/kg) by IV bolus, given at a rate of 25–50 mg/min; repeat bolus every 3–5 min until arrhythmias subside or until adverse effects occur (maximal dose, 300 mg total during a 1-h period)
phenytoin (Dilantin, Infatabs) phenyoin sodium (Dilantin)	Oral loading dose for adults: 1 g PO divided in a 24-h period, followed by 500 mg qd for 2 days IV loading dose: 100 mg IV every 15 min until adverse effects develop or arrhythmias are controlled (maximal dose, 1 g); may be diluted in normal saline solution Maintenance dose: 200–400 mg PO qd in divided doses
procainamide hydrochloride (Procan, Procan SR, Pronestyl)	Loading dose: IV and IM loading doses are specific to the condition being treated; consult other references Maintenance dose (adults): SR tablets 500 mg to 1 g q6h

Table 41–2. Typical Dosage Ranges for Cardiac Depressants *Continued*

DRUG	DOSAGE
quinidine sulfate	Test dose to determine possible allergy (adults): 200 mg (or 2 mg/kg) Maintenance dose: 300–400 mg PO q6h
quinidine gluconate (Quinaglute)	Sustained-release tablets: 324–648 mg q8–12h IV and IM preparations: IV and IM doses are specific to the condition being treated; consult other references
Group II Cardiac Depressants	
propranolol hydrochloride (Inderal)	IV dose: 1–3 mg diluted in 50 mg 5% dextrose in water or dextrose in normal saline (no faster than 1 mg/min); may repeat in 2 min if needed; subsequent doses q4h Maintenance dose (adults): 10–30 mg PO tid–qid
Group III Cardiac Depressants	
bretylium tosylate (Bretylol)	Adults: 5–10 mg/kg IM or IV q1–2h Maintenance dose: 5–10 mg/kg IM or IV q6–8h
Unclassified Cardiac Depressants	
atropine sulfate	Adults: 0.5–1 mg IV push; may repeat q5min to a maximum of 2 mg

tion, nausea, vomiting, diarrhea, jaundice, urinary retention, and hesitancy.

Teach patients to manage constipation with proper diet and bulk laxatives, if approved by their physician. Teach them to avoid sunlight to prevent photosensitivity reactions.

Monitor the pattern of bowel movements, color of the skin and sclera, and I & O. Compare findings with baseline data. Question patients about changes in visual acuity.

Lidocaine

Lidocaine (Xylocaine) is an emergency drug used for life-threatening arrhythmias. Administration requires constant cardiac monitoring and observation for vertigo, visual disturbances, nausea, vomiting, convulsions, hypotension, and cardiac or respiratory arrest.

Administer intramuscular (IM) doses *only* in the deltoid muscle. Patients may complain of muscle soreness. Patients who have received IM doses will have elevated creatine kinase (CK) levels (formerly called creatine phosphokinase [CPK] levels), up to seven times the normal value. The elevated levels are due to trauma to the skeletal muscle.

Infusion pumps or microdrip devices must be used for IV administration. Airways and suction equipment must be at the bedside in the event of respiratory arrest or convulsions. If bradycardia occurs, the physician may order atropine or isoproterenol (Isuprel) to increase the heart rate, so these drugs should be readily available. Elderly or small patients and those patients with congestive heart failure or hepatic disease are given lower doses. *Solutions for IV and IM administration must be marked "for cardiac arrhythmias."* Do not use preparations containing preservatives, which are intended for use as local anesthetics.

Monitor for toxic signs and symptoms. Convulsions may be the first sign. If dizziness occurs, stop the drug and notify the physician.

Lidocaine interacts with a number of other drugs. Barbiturates cause decreased responses, so the dose of lidocaine may need to be increased. Beta-blockers such as propranolol (Inderal) cause decreased metabolism of lidocaine and make the occurrence of toxic effects and adverse effects more likely. Phenytoin causes additive effects when it is given with lidocaine. Monitor carefully for adverse effects. Procainamide may increase the neurological effects of lidocaine, so monitor the patient carefully for these.

Monitor the patient's laboratory reports for electrolyte levels, blood urea nitrogen concentration, and creatinine levels. Notify the physician if abnormal results are present. Remember that CK (CPK) levels will be elevated if IM doses have been given.

Phenytoin

Additional adverse effects of phenytoin include blood dyscrasias such as anemia, leukopenia, thrombocytopenia, and agranulocytosis. Neurological symptoms include ataxia, slurred speech, insomnia, nystagmus, blurred vision, and diplopia. Gingival hyperplasia, rash, and Stevens-Johnson syndrome are also possible.

Patients who are to receive phenytoin should have a baseline complete blood count (CBC). Also, assess the skin and document bruising and petechiae or rashes.

Monitor the patient for bruising and signs and symptoms of infection. Protect patients from trauma and infection. Monitor neurological signs and symptoms, such as level of consciousness and visual difficulties. Rash may be the beginning of the life-threatening Stevens-Johnson syndrome and should be reported immediately. Document and report bleeding gums. Teach patients to use a soft toothbrush and to brush gently.

To avoid drug interactions, monitor the patient's entire drug regimen. Alcohol, barbiturates, and folic acid may decrease blood levels of phenytoin. Oral anticoagulants, antihistamines, chloramphenicol, diazepam, disulfiram, isoniazid, and salicylates may increase blood levels of phenytoin. Phenytoin potentiates other antiarrhythmics. Monitor for hypotension and bradycardia.

The conditions of heart block, sinus bradycardia, and Adams-Stokes syndrome are contraindications for the use of phenytoin. Elderly persons and those with congestive heart failure, hepatic or renal impairment, hypotension, myocardial insufficiency, respiratory depression, or hyperthyroidism may need to receive lower dosages.

Caregivers administering IV medications should be aware that phenytoin will crystallize if it is mixed with 5% dextrose. Flush IV lines with saline after dose administration.

Shake oral suspensions until particles are evenly distributed before pouring dosages. Oral preparations should be taken with food and a large glass of liquid to decrease gastric irritation.

Avoid IM administration if possible because of the potential for bruising and bleeding.

Monitor blood levels for therapeutic levels. Blood levels above 20 mcg/mL indicate toxicity.

Procainamide

Patients receiving procainamide infusions require the use of infusion pumps or microdrip devices to regulate dosage. Procainamide infusions should be given only through a secondary line. Constant cardiac monitoring is necessary to note the onset of other disturbances of rhythm, such as ventricular fibrillation.

Keep patients supine for the infusion. If hypotension occurs, discontinue the procainamide infusion, keep the primary infusion running, and notify the physician.

IM injections of procainamide should be given only into the gluteus medius muscle. Rotate sites and monitor for pain and irritation.

Do not administer procainamide to patients who are allergic to procaine. Administration is also contraindicated in patients with second- or third-degree heart block or complete heart block unless they have a pacemaker. Administration is also contraindicated in patients with myasthenia gravis. Administer the drug cautiously if the patient has congestive heart failure or renal or hepatic impairment. Lower doses may be ordered for these patients.

Monitor patients for thromboemboli. Physicians may order anticoagulation therapy to prevent this from occurring.

Agranulocytosis may occur after repeated doses. Teach patients to report fever, rash, muscle pain, diarrhea, or chronic pain.

If sustained-release tablets are used, the wax matrix is not absorbed by the body and may be noted in the stool. Tell patients and caregivers of this to prevent them from becoming alarmed.

Monitor CBC results and assess for signs and symptoms of infection, unusual bleeding, or bruising.

Quinidine

Quinidine is an alkaloid derived from the bark of the *Cinchona* tree. This drug is related to but not to be confused with the drug called quinine, which is used to treat malaria.

Discard quinidine solutions for IV or IM use if they are discolored. Teach patients to take this medication with food to avoid gastrointestinal upset. Also teach the patient to avoid excessive intake of citrus fruits and juices, which may increase the alkalinity of the urine. The increased alkalinity may slow excretion of quinidine and increase the likelihood of adverse effects.

Monitor for the toxic signs of *cinchonism*. The symptoms include tinnitus, headache, nausea, vomiting, diarrhea, visual disturbances, abdominal pain, cardiac arrhythmias, pruritus, confusion, and delirium. Immediately report to the physician any changes in the electrocardiogram (ECG) pattern and changes in pulse rate and rhythm.

Teach patients and caregivers that antacids may increase alkalinity of the urine. Review the patient's entire drug regimen for possible drug interactions. Barbiturates, phenytoin, and rifampin may antagonize quinidine and decrease therapeutic effects. Verapamil may cause hypotension if it is used with quinidine to treat patients with cardiac myopathy. Digitalis may increase the likelihood of quinidine toxicity.

Report changes in objective and subjective symptoms. Monitor the pH of the urine for increased alkalinity. Monitor laboratory reports for therapeutic blood levels of the drug (above 8 mcg/mL is toxic). The dose is titrated by signs, symptoms, and blood levels.

Group II Cardiac Depressants

Propranolol Hydrochloride

ACTIONS AND USES Propranolol hydrochloride (Inderal) is a beta-adrenergic blocker with actions similar to those of quinidine. It blocks the myocardial response to the adrenal neurohormones epinephrine and norepinephrine, which are secreted by the sympathetic nervous system. As a result, the pulse rate is decreased. This drug is used to treat paroxysmal atrial tachycardia, atrial flutter and fibrillation, and ventricular tachycardia. After an acute myocardial infarction, propranolol decreases the patient's risk of repeated myocardial infarction and death. It is also used for control of tachycardia in patients with pheochromocytoma, migraines, angina, or hyperthyroidism and during anesthesia.

Adverse actions of propranolol include bradycardia, hypotension, dizziness, vertigo, bronchospasm, congestive heart failure, peripheral vascular disease, visual disturbances, confusion, hallucinations, headache, rash, pruritus, hyperglycemia or hypoglycemia, chest pain, joint pain, nausea, vomiting, and diarrhea.

ASSESSMENT Obtain baseline assessments and record the data, as you would for all patients receiving cardiac depressants. Assess for a history of asthma and allergic rhinitis because these may be contraindications to use. Assess for a history of any heart block above first degree because this contraindicates use. Caution should be exercised if the patient has a history of congestive heart failure, diabetes mellitus, or respiratory disease.

PLANNING AND IMPLEMENTATION Monitor the apical
▲▲▲▲▲▲▲▲▲▲▲▲▲▲▲▲▲▲▲▲▲▲▲▲ pulse and blood
pressure before dosage administration. If these assessments are not within normal ranges or the
parameters indicated by the physician, hold the dose
and notify the physician. If propranolol is used with
other antihypertensives, monitor the patient's blood
pressure in lying, sitting, and standing positions
because the patient will be at increased risk for
development of postural hypotension.

If administration of propranolol is by the IV route,
monitor the ECG and heart rate and rhythm frequently. IV doses are much smaller than oral doses.
Monitor for increased signs and symptoms of congestive heart failure, such as increased weight, peripheral edema, and signs of pulmonary edema.

Monitor for signs and symptoms of thromboembolic
disorders and report these to the physician.

Do not discontinue propranolol suddenly. If the
patient is scheduled for surgery, notify the surgeon
and anesthesiologist if the patient is receiving propranolol. If the patient has hyperthyroidism or pheochromocytoma, abrupt withdrawal may precipitate a
crisis.

Teach the patient to take this medication with food
unless the physician orders otherwise. The patient
should avoid hazardous activities until the response to
the drug is determined.

Diabetics should monitor for signs and symptoms of
hypoglycemia or hyperglycemia. Frequent finger-stick
blood glucose or urine monitoring should be done
because the hypoglycemic agent may need to be
adjusted.

Many drugs have adverse effects when they are
administered to a patient who is also taking propranolol. Cardiac glycosides potentiate the actions of
propranolol. Aminophylline and propranolol have
antagonistic effects, so they should be used together
only with caution. Epinephrine may cause severe
vasoconstriction, so the patient must be carefully
monitored for the occurrence of hypertension, changes
in the color of the extremities, or chest pain. Report
these symptoms to the physician immediately.

EVALUATION Monitor the vital signs and ECG and
▲▲▲▲▲▲▲▲▲▲ compare findings with the baseline data.
Monitor for improvement in the patient's condition.

hibits the release of norepinephrine from the sympathetic nervous system. The action of this drug is not
clear. It is used in emergency treatment of ventricular
fibrillation and also in the prevention and treatment
of ventricular tachycardia that does not respond to
other antiarrhythmic drugs.

Adverse actions of bretylium include hypotension,
vertigo, dizziness, and angina. Nausea and vomiting
may occur with rapid infusion.

ASSESSMENT Assess the patient in the same manner as
▲▲▲▲▲▲▲▲▲▲ for all patients taking cardiac depressant
medications. Assess for a history of renal impairment
because the physician will usually order a decreased
dose.

PLANNING AND IMPLEMENTATION To administer brety-
▲▲▲▲▲▲▲▲▲▲▲▲▲▲▲▲▲▲▲▲▲▲▲▲▲▲▲▲▲▲ lium by the IM or IV
route, place the patient in the supine position. If the
patient has been diagnosed to have ventricular fibrillation, the physician usually orders the dose to be
administered rapidly IV. Monitor the ECG and vital
signs continuously during IV administration. Anticipate nausea and vomiting during rapid IV administration. Have suction equipment available and turn
the patient's head to maintain an airway and prevent
aspiration.

Monitor for severe hypotension. Request parameters for the blood pressure and report to the physician
as ordered. Have the patient avoid sudden position
changes.

If the drug is ordered to be given by the IM route,
rotate the injection sites and monitor them for
irritation. IM administration is not recommended for
children.

If there is renal impairment, there is an increased
risk for adverse effects. The physician may order a
lower dose.

The actions of bretylium are potentiated by all
antihypertensives. Observe the patient for symptoms
of angina.

EVALUATION Monitor the vital signs and ECG record-
▲▲▲▲▲▲▲▲▲▲ ings and compare findings with the baseline data. Monitor for improvement in the patient's
condition.

Group III Cardiac Depressants

Bretylium Tosylate

ACTIONS AND USES Bretylium tosylate (Bretylol) is an
▲▲▲▲▲▲▲▲▲▲▲▲▲▲▲▲▲ adrenergic blocking agent that in-

Unclassified Cardiac Depressants

Atropine Sulfate

Atropine sulfate blocks vagal stimulation of the
sinoatrial node. It relieves severe sinus bradycardia

and atrioventricular block. As the impulses are conducted more rapidly through the atrioventricular node, the heart rate increases.

Adverse actions include mydriasis (dilated pupils), blurred vision, dry mucous membranes, thirst, constipation, nausea, vomiting, urinary retention, and flushed skin.

Assess the chart for documentation of administration of other anticholinergic drugs because they potentiate the blocking of vagal stimulation. Assess elderly men for a history of benign prostatic hypertrophy because an increase in urinary retention may result.

When atropine is used as a cardiac depressant, the physician usually orders it to be administered by IV push. Doses are repeated until the signs and symptoms are relieved or until the maximal dose of 2 mg is reached. Monitor the patient's I & O, especially for elderly men with a history of benign prostatic hypertrophy.

EXERCISES

LEARNING ACTIVITIES

1. A 49-year-old man has been admitted to the hospital with severe congestive heart failure. The physician plans to digitalize him and then start maintenance therapy. Prepare a teaching plan for them, then role play your teaching.

2. In the clinical area: Choose a patient with a cardiac condition. Prepare a chart of the patient's medications that the patient can use at home to remember dosage, type of drug, the reason it is prescribed, and any special precautions or interventions of which to be aware.

DRUGS THAT AFFECT THE BLOOD VESSELS

L E A R N I N G   O B J E C T I V E S

After studying this chapter, you should be able to:

1. Describe the action of drugs in each classification included in this chapter.

2. Identify the use of drugs given as examples in each classification.

3. List the adverse effects of the drugs given as examples of each classification.

4. Prepare an appropriate plan of care for a patient receiving one of these drugs.

DRUGS YOU WILL LEARN ABOUT IN THIS CHAPTER

Antilipidemics

cholestyramine (Questran)

clofibrate (Atromid-S)

colestipol HCl (Colestid)

gemfibrozil (Lopid)

lovastatin (Mevacor)

niacin (Nicobid, Nicolar)

probucol (Lorelco)

Antianginals (Coronary Vasodilators)

Nitrates

erythrityl tetranitrate (Cardilate)

isosorbide dinitrate (Iso-Bid, Iso-D, Isordil, Sorbitrate)

nitroglycerin (Nitro-Bid, Nitro-Dur, Nitro-stat, Transderm-Nitro)

Non-nitrates (beta-adrenergic blockers)

nadolol (Corgard)

propranolol HCl (Inderal, Inderal LA)

Calcium Antagonists (Calcium Channel Blockers)

diltiazem (Cardizem)

nifedipine (Procardia)

verapamil (Calan, Isoptin)

Three major groups of drugs that affect the blood vessels are included in this chapter: the antilipidemics, the antianginals (coronary vasodilators), and the calcium antagonists (calcium channel blockers). Other groups are included in Chapter 43, Antihypertensive Drugs.

Table 42–1 lists dosages of these groups of drugs that affect the blood vessels.

ANTILIPIDEMICS

For blood to flow through the system of blood vessels, the vessels must be open or patent. The size of the opening or lumen of a blood vessel normally varies with its location and function. Arteries have larger lumens than arterioles and capillaries, and veins have larger lumens than venules and capillaries. Arteries have a smooth inner lining with muscular elastic walls that alter the force of the blood within the vessel. When this muscle layer contracts, it constricts the lumen, which increases the pressure within the vessel. When this happens, the heart must pump with more force to move the blood through the system.

Table 42–1. Drugs that Affect the Blood Vessels

DRUG	DOSAGE
Antilipidemics	
clofibrate (Atromid-S)	500 mg PO qid
gemfibrozil (Lopid)	1200 mg PO, administered in 2 divided doses; usual range, 900–1500 mg qd
cholestyramine (Questran)	Usual dose: 4 g PO before meals and at hs (maximal dose, 32 g qd)
colestipol hydrochloride (Colestid)	15–30 g PO qd in 2 to 4 divided doses
niacin (Nicobid, Nicolar, Tega-Span	1.5–6 g PO qd in 2–4 divided doses taken with or after meals
probucol (Lorelco)	500 mg PO bid with meals
lovastatin (Mevacor)	Initial dose: 20 mg qd with evening meal; maintenance dose: 20–80 mg in a single dose or divided doses
Antianginals (coronary vasodilators)	
Nitrates erythrityl tetranitrate (Cardilate)	5 mg SL tid, 10 mg chewable tid; dose may be increased in 2–3 days if needed
isosorbide dinitrate (Iso-Bid, Iso-D, Isordil, Sorbitrate)	2.5–10 mg SL; repeat q2–3h for acute angina, q4–6h to prevent angina Chewable form: 5–10 mg prn; repeat q2–3h to prevent angina Oral tablets: 5–30 mg PO qid to prevent angina Slow-release tablets: 40 mg PO q6–12h

Table 42–1. Drugs that Affect the Blood Vessels
Continued

DRUG	DOSAGE
nitroglycerin (Nitro-Bid, Nitro-Dur, Nitrostat, Transderm-Nitro)	Sublingual forms: 1 tablet at onset of attack; may repeat every 5 min × 3; if no relief, summon medical personnel Slow-release capsules: 1 q8–12h Dermal patches: 1 qd in doses ranging from 2.5–15 mg
Non-nitrates (beta-adrenergic blockers) nadolol (Corgard)	40 mg PO once qd, increased as needed Usual maintenance dose: 80–240 mg once qd
propranolol hydrochloride (Inderal, Inderal LA)	10–20 mg PO tid–qid Slow-release capsule: 80 mg once qd; dosage may be increased to 160 mg
Calcium Antagonists (calcium channel blockers)	
diltiazem (Cardizem)	30 mg PO qid before meals and at hs; may be increased gradually to 240 mg qd in divided doses
nifedipine (Procardia)	10 mg PO tid; may be increased gradually to 180 mg qd in divided doses
verapamil (Calan, Isoptin)	80 mg PO tid–qid; may be increased weekly to 480 mg qd in divided doses

When the muscle layer relaxes, it dilates the lumen, which decreases the pressure within the vessel. The heart does not need as much force to move blood through dilated vessels.

Veins do not have as much muscle in their walls. They do, however, have valves on the inside to keep the blood moving toward the heart. Contraction and relaxation of the skeletal muscles surrounding the veins assist in propelling the blood back toward the heart.

The lumen of a blood vessel can be altered by pathological changes that impair the vessel wall's elasticity, cause abnormal vasodilation or vasoconstriction, or promote formation of plaque on the lining of arterial walls.

The formation of plaque on the lining of the arterial walls is called atherosclerosis. In this disease, fatty acids in the blood, called lipids, are deposited along the artery walls. If there are unusually high levels of lipids in the blood, the plaque formation increases and hardens (called arteriosclerosis). Atherosclerosis and arteriosclerosis narrow the lumen of the vessel, alter the elasticity of the vessel walls, and promote formation of clots as the blood flows over the roughened patches of plaque. This seriously impairs peripheral circulation and increases risks of thromboembolic disorders.

Low-density lipoproteins (LDL) have large particles. These are associated with an increased risk of atherosclerosis and coronary artery disease.

High-density lipoproteins (HDL) have smaller particles. These promote mobilization and metabolism of cholesterol and thereby protect against atherosclerosis.

Those who smoke, those who eat a high-calorie diet and consume foods high in saturated fat and cholesterol, and those who lack a regular exercise regimen are susceptible to hyperlipidemia and atherosclerosis. Genetics and hormone levels also affect progression of this disease.

ACTIONS AND USES Research continues to find medications that can safely decrease hyperlipidemia, but a number of medications are currently in use for this purpose. These drugs are discussed individually because their actions vary. Examples include clofibrate (Atromid-S), gemfibrozil (Lopid), cholestyramine (Questran), colestipol hydrochloride (Colestid), niacin (Nicobid, Nicolar), probucol (Lorelco), and lovastatin (Mevacor).

Common adverse actions include gastrointestinal disturbances such as increased or decreased appetite, nausea, vomiting, diarrhea or constipation, and flatulence. Skin rashes and pruritus are also common.

ASSESSMENT Inform female patients that some antilipidemic medications are contraindicated during pregnancy and lactation and that ovulation control pills interfere with the action of some other preparations. Offer information about alternative birth control measures.

Review histories for the presence of non–insulin-dependent diabetes mellitus treated with oral hypoglycemics and for the presence of renal or hepatic disease; the antilipidemics may be contraindicated in these patients. Review the chart for results of renal or hepatic function tests. Determine the patient's normal bowel pattern and document this with the baseline data. Ask the patient and family to assist with documentation of the patient's diet history and daily exercise regimen.

Assess the chart for total serum levels of cholesterol (<200 mg/dL), triglycerides (40–190 mg/dL), LDL (<130 mg/dL), and HDL (>35 mg/dL). (Remember that normal values of these tests vary with age and gender.) Verify desired parameters with the physician.

PLANNING AND IMPLEMENTATION Teach the patient to recognize and avoid foods with a high fat (especially animal fat) and calorie content. Encourage consumption of dietary sources of bulk-forming foods, increased intake of liquids, and development of patterns of activities of daily living that promote regular bowel patterns. Emphasize the advantages of an exercise regimen that is practiced three to five times a week and the importance of achieving and maintaining a healthy weight for height and age. Review the options for birth control other than the ovulation control pills. Emphasize also the importance of regular checkups and laboratory tests for cholesterol, triglycerides, LDL, and HDL. Teach the adverse effects of medications that should be reported to the physician.

EVALUATION Laboratory tests denoting total serum levels of cholesterol, triglycerides, LDL, and HDL indicate effectiveness of medications, daily diet, and exercise regimens.

Clofibrate

Clofibrate (Atromid-S) acts to inhibit the synthesis of cholesterol at an early stage. It is used when the triglyceride level is increased and the cholesterol level is only moderately elevated.

Additional adverse actions include leukopenia, decreased libido, impotence and gynecomastia in men, gallstones, myalgias and arthralgias, fever, and weight gain.

Assess for symptoms of infection or abdominal pain. Monitor the complete blood count (CBC). Weigh the patient at every visit.

Teach the patient to report the signs and symptoms

of adverse effects along with any increase in bruising or bleeding.

This drug is contraindicated in pregnancy and lactation and in severe renal or hepatic disease. Monitor laboratory test results.

Monitor the laboratory results of renal and hepatic function tests and the CBC. The physician discontinues the drug if there is a steady rise in these values or if a decrease in lipids is not apparent in 3 months.

Gemfibrozil

Gemfibrozil (Lopid) lowers lipid levels by decreasing serum triglycerides and increasing HDL. Additional adverse actions include anemia, leukopenia, headache, and dizziness.

Monitor for signs and symptoms of infection and for subjective complaints of adverse actions.

Gemfibrozil may be teratogenic. Teach the patient to strictly follow chosen birth control measures. The drug should be discontinued several months before attempts at pregnancy.

Take this drug ½ hour before morning and evening meals. There is increased risk of gallstones, heart disease, and cancer with gemfibrozil therapy. Teach patients the signs and symptoms of these conditions.

Monitor the CBC and results of liver function tests to evaluate effectiveness of therapy.

Cholestyramine and Colestipol Hydrochloride

Cholestyramine (Questran) and colestipol hydrochloride (Colestid) combine with bile acids in the intestine to prevent their absorption and to increase their excretion. An additional adverse action of these drugs is that they interfere with the absorption of fat-soluble vitamins A, D, and K.

Assess for a history of gout and peptic ulcer. Obtain and document a baseline lipid profile.

Mix the powdered medication with 6 ounces of the liquid of the patient's choice. If a carbonated beverage is chosen, the foaming action will be increased, so place it in a large glass to prevent spillage. Allow the mixture to stand for 2 to 3 minutes to absorb the liquid. The powder can also be sprinkled on wet food. Teach the patient to take all other medications at least 1 hour before or 4 to 6 hours after these products so that absorption of the medications is not blocked.

Observe the patient for signs of deficiencies of vitamins A, D, and K. Monitor for toxic effects of cardiac glycosides and monitor serum levels of glyco-

sides. The physician may need to prescribe lower doses of the glycoside.

Teach the patient to report epistaxis, bleeding gums, hematuria, increased bruising, and other signs of bleeding tendencies.

Evaluate effectiveness of therapy by monitoring the lipid profile for signs of improvement.

Niacin

Niacin (Nicobid, Nicolar) decreases synthesis of LDL. Adverse actions include flushing, which usually subsides in a few weeks. However, in 10% to 15% of patients, flushing persists throughout therapy. Some patients complain of dry skin and scaling. Peptic ulcers may be reactivated. Hyperuricemia, hyperglycemia, and cholestatic jaundice may occur.

Assess for a history of diabetes mellitus, liver disease, and gout. Monitor results of glucose tolerance tests (GTT) and results of hepatic function tests.

Teach patients to take niacin with meals to decrease gastrointestinal problems. Therapy is usually begun with a lower dose and gradually increased according to the physician's orders. Aspirin is often ordered with the niacin to decrease the initial problems with flushing.

To evaluate therapy, compare serum glucose levels and results of liver function tests with normal values. Monitor serum levels of niacin.

Probucol

Probucol (Lorelco) is used to decrease cholesterol levels. Additional adverse actions include the possibility of arrhythmias.

Assess the patient and the chart for a history of arrhythmia or blood dyscrasias. Obtain a baseline CBC level. Assess the patient's apical heart rate and rhythm and document the data.

Teach patients to take probucol with meals to decrease gastrointestinal irritation. Also teach them to monitor the pulse daily and to report changes in rate and rhythm to the physician. Tell them to report increased bruising, bleeding gums, and any other signs of bleeding. Alcoholic beverages should be avoided because they may increase the chance of gastrointestinal irritation and bleeding.

Evaluate the effectiveness of probucol therapy by monitoring CBC levels and comparing the results with normal and with baseline values. Compare the pulse rate and rhythm with documented baseline information.

Lovastatin

Lovastatin (Mevacor) is the first of an effective new classification of lipid-lowering drugs called hydroxymethylglutaryl–coenzyme A (HMG-CoA) reductase inhibitors. HMG-CoA is an enzyme necessary for the synthesis (production) of cholesterol.

The drug decreases the total plasma cholesterol, LDL, and total triglyceride levels. It does not affect HDL levels. LDL levels should begin to decrease in 2 weeks, with maximal effect reached after 6 weeks of therapy. Other drugs, such as cholestyramine and colestipol, may be used to enhance the effects of lovastatin.

Because this is a new medication, safety with long-term use has not yet been determined. Adverse effects include mild gastrointestinal disturbances, headache, and rashes. Hepatotoxic effects and myopathy may occur. Lovastatin may be teratogenic.

Lovastatin is available as 10-mg, 20-mg, and 40-mg tablets.

Caution patients to avoid alcohol. Offer counseling about birth control measures, if the patient desires. Tell women not to breast-feed while taking this drug.

To evaluate the effectiveness of lovastatin, monitor the serum cholesterol and triglyceride levels. Creatine kinase levels may be elevated if myopathy occurs.

ANTIANGINALS (CORONARY VASODILATORS)

Diseases of the coronary arteries cause diminished blood flow to the myocardium. This results in chest pain or angina, a symptom of myocardial ischemia, and may lead to a myocardial infarction if the blockage in the coronary vessel is not relieved. Various drugs are given to relax the smooth muscle layer of the coronary vessels. These drugs dilate the blood vessels and allow increased blood flow to the myocardium. Two main groups of drugs are used to relieve angina, the nitrates and the non-nitrates.

Nitrates

ACTIONS AND USES Nitrates act directly on the smooth ▲▲▲▲▲▲▲▲▲▲▲▲▲▲▲ muscle of the coronary vessels to produce vasodilation. They also decrease the heart's demand for oxygen. They are used to treat acute angina attacks or to prevent further angina attacks.

Examples of the nitrates include erythrityl tetranitrate (Cardilate), isosorbide dinitrate (Iso-Bid, Iso-D, Isordil, Sorbitrate), and nitroglycerin (Nitro-Bid, Nitro-Dur, Nitrostat, Transderm-Nitro).

Adverse actions are headache (especially early in treatment), postural hypotension, hypotension, dizziness, vertigo, weakness, flushing, tachycardia, palpitations, nausea, vomiting, and sublingual irritation or burning. These often subside with continued use, but if they worsen, the physician may decrease the dose until signs or symptoms are relieved. Hypersensitivity reactions may also occur, so any other adverse signs or symptoms should be reported to the physician.

ASSESSMENT Perform a complete cardiovascular as-
▲▲▲▲▲▲▲▲▲▲▲ sessment and assess vital signs after the patient has been at rest for 10 minutes. Document baseline information. Be certain to include subjective data, such as the patient's description of the type of pain, whether it radiates, and to what area it radiates. Also include any known precipitating causes for the pain and any known relief measures.

Assess the chart for history of hypersensitivity to nitrates, head trauma, cerebral hemorrhage, severe anemia, or hypertension. Use is contraindicated in these patients.

PLANNING AND IMPLEMENTATION Monitor the pa-
▲▲▲▲▲▲▲▲▲▲▲▲▲▲▲▲▲▲▲▲▲▲▲▲▲▲▲▲▲▲ tient's safety because of the possibility of postural hypotension. Teach the patient to sit or dangle before ambulation and to change positions slowly. Alcohol ingestion should be avoided. Capsules or tablets should be taken 1 hour before meals or 2 hours after meals, unless otherwise specified by the physician. Store medications in their original containers in a cool, dry place away from light. Also, keep medication containers tightly closed because the nitrates deteriorate quickly.

Tell the patient to avoid ambulation or hazardous occupations until dizziness and pain subside. Teach the patient to record the date and time of the angina attack, including a description of the pain and any relief measures. Encourage the patient to share this information with the physician. Report to the physician if episodes increase in frequency or intensity.

Teach patients and caregivers the proper method of administration for the form of drug prescribed for them. Tablets should be swallowed whole. Chewable tablets must be thoroughly chewed before swallowing. To facilitate absorption of the drug, the mouth may be moistened before taking a sublingual tablet.

Sublingual tablets are the only form used for relief of acute pain. These tablets should be kept accessible at all times, either on the person or in the immediate vicinity. They should be taken at the first sign of an attack or before increased stress or a strenuous activity. Place sublingual tablets under the tongue until they are completely absorbed. A burning sensation indicates potency. If a tingling sensation is noted, the patient may place the tablet in the buccal cavity instead.

The patient should lie, sit, or rest until the pain is relieved. If pain is unrelieved in 10 to 15 minutes, repeat the dosage until a maximum of three doses have been taken. If pain is still unrelieved, the patient should seek emergency care. Because these tablets deteriorate rapidly, it is best to purchase small amounts and discard unused tablets on the expiration date.

Transdermal patches may be applied to any hairless area of the trunk or proximal extremities, such as the upper arms or thighs. The area should be clean and dry. Sites must be rotated. Teach patients and caregivers to read the instructions enclosed in the box. Remove the patch from the previous day's dose and cleanse the area. Do not touch the medicated side of the patch. Discard patches properly to avoid injury to small children or pets who may find them. Wash hands after handling patches.

EVALUATION Monitor vital signs and compare findings
▲▲▲▲▲▲▲▲▲▲ with the baseline documentation. Monitor the subjective complaints of the patient. Monitor the patient's log of angina attacks.

Non-nitrates (Beta-Adrenergic Blockers)

Non-nitrates or beta-adrenergic blockers such as nadolol (Corgard) and propranolol hydrochloride (Inderal, Inderal LA) decrease the heart's demand for oxygen. They do this by blocking increases in heart rate, blood pressure, and force of contraction that are stimulated by the adrenergic neurohormones epinephrine and norepinephrine. (See Chapter 38 for more information on propranolol hydrochloride.)

CALCIUM ANTAGONISTS (CALCIUM CHANNEL BLOCKERS)

Calcium antagonists (also called calcium channel blockers) decrease oxygen demand by decreasing the amount of calcium in the muscle cell. This decrease means that there is less calcium available for transmission of nerve impulses. As a result, the coronary arteries dilate to increase the blood flow and the amount of oxygen available to the cardiac muscle.

Examples of the calcium antagonists are diltiazem (Cardizem), nifedipine (Procardia), and verapamil (Calan, Isoptin). These medications are used in patients with angina when they cannot tolerate nitrates or beta-blockers. Verapamil also affects the conduction system of the heart and is used to treat some arrhythmias.

Adverse actions include peripheral edema, hypotension, arrhythmia, nausea, vomiting, diarrhea or constipation, rash, pruritus, fever, chills, headache, drowsiness, dizziness, nocturia, and polyuria. Notify the physician if adverse effects occur.

Diltiazem should be used with caution in patients with impaired ventricular function or conduction abnormalities and in those with renal or hepatic impairment. Use diltiazem with caution with propranolol and other beta-blockers because they may prolong the conduction time.

Nifedipine should be used with caution in patients with congestive heart failure (CHF) or hypotension. Use may worsen angina in some patients. If used with propranolol and other beta-blockers, nifedipine may cause CHF. Dose must be reduced slowly. Do not withdraw this drug suddenly. Capsules should be swallowed whole.

Verapamil should be used with caution with advanced heart failure, atrioventricular block, severe hypotension, and myocardial infarction. In older patients, intravenous doses must be given slowly. Hepatic function should be monitored periodically because liver enzyme activity may become elevated. Use of beta-blockers with verapamil may cause CHF. Severe hypotension may occur if verapamil is given with quinidine.

E X E R C I S E S

LEARNING ACTIVITIES

1. A 46-year-old man has recently been given a diagnosis of hyperlipidemia. The physician has prescribed cholestyramine (Questran) in an attempt to lower his cholesterol levels. With a classmate, roleplay the teaching that the patient should receive about his medication.

2. Prepare a teaching plan for a patient receiving isosorbide dinitrate for a diagnosis of angina pectoris.

ANTIHYPERTENSIVE DRUGS

LEARNING OBJECTIVES

After studying this chapter, you should be able to:

1. Describe the action of drugs in each classification of antihypertensives included in this chapter.

2. List the adverse effects of the antihypertensives.

3. Prepare an appropriate plan of care for a patient receiving one or more of the antihypertensive agents.

DRUGS YOU WILL LEARN ABOUT IN THIS CHAPTER

Adrenergic Blockers

Alpha-adrenergic blockers

prazosin (Minipress)

terazosin (Hytrin)

Beta-adrenergic blockers

atenolol (Tenormin)

metoprolol tartrate (Betaloc, Lopressor)

nadolol (Corgard)

pindolol (Visken)

propranolol HCl (Inderal, Inderal LA)

timolol maleate (Biocadren)

Indirect-acting adrenergic blockers

rauwolfia serpentina (Raudixin)

reserpine (Serpasil)

Centrally acting adrenergic blockers

clonidine (Catapres)

Peripheral Vasodilators

diazoxide (Hyperstat)

sodium nitroprusside (Nitropress)

hydralazine (Apresoline)

minoxidil (Loniten)

Calcium Channel Blockers

diltiazem (Cardizem)

nifedipine (Adalat, Procardia)

nicardipine (Cardene)

verapamil (Calan, Isoptin)

Angiotensin-converting Enzyme (ACE) Inhibitors

captopril (Capoten)

enalapril (Vasotec)

lisinopril (Prinivil, Zestril)

Hypertension (high blood pressure) is a diagnosis made when the mean arterial blood pressure of an adult is above 140/90 mm Hg on two or more measurements taken on two or more different occasions. The etiology (cause) of hypertension can be primary or secondary.

Primary hypertension (also called essential hypertension) is the most common type. There is a familial tendency, but the actual cause is unknown. Certain factors contribute to acquiring primary hypertension, such as gender (more common in females), aging, and obesity. The high intake of sodium, caffeine, and alcohol is also a contributing factor.

Secondary hypertension is a symptom of an underlying disease, such as heart disease or a renal tumor. When the underlying disease is treated, the hypertension may be reduced.

ACTIONS AND USES Several different classifications ▲▲▲▲▲▲▲▲▲▲▲▲▲▲▲ and subclassifications of medications are used in the control of hypertension. These must be discussed separately because their modes of action and related information vary considerably.

ASSESSMENT Assess the patient's vital signs, especially the blood pressure. If this is an initial contact with the patient, or if the patient was involved in a physical activity before the assessment, obtain additional readings after the patient has been at rest for 5 to 10 minutes. If the result is abnormal, obtain readings with the patient lying, sitting, and standing. Document results as baseline data.

Assess for a family history of hypertension. Assess the patient's history of peripheral vascular disease, hepatic disease, or renal disease.

Review the patient's history for contributing factors, such as stress, obesity, high sodium intake, and physical inactivity. Document your findings.

PLANNING AND IMPLEMENTATION Individual responses ▲▲▲▲▲▲▲▲▲▲▲▲▲▲▲▲▲▲▲▲▲▲▲▲▲▲▲ to treatment vary considerably. It is not unusual to see some patients with mild hypertension treated with one drug, and others with severe problems treated with two or more drugs. By combining complementary types of drugs, therapy may be successful with smaller doses than if only one type of drug is ordered. Regimens of this type may avoid the adverse effects produced when large doses of drugs are used. Table 43–1 lists dosages of the antihypertensive drugs.

Teach the patient to modify sodium intake. Clarify the difference between sodium and table salt. Provide a list of foods that are high in sodium. Encourage the patient to omit salting food as it is being cooked and to decrease the amount of salt used at meals. Encourage the patient to experiment with the use of various herbs to enhance the flavors of the foods.

If the patient is obese, teach the effects of the excess workload on the heart and blood vessels. Encourage the use of a dietary log to record the types and amounts of food ingested. Provide literature and explanations of the caloric values of specific foods. Teach the patient to avoid ingestion of alcohol because it provides only calories without nutritional value and because it may interact with the medications. Refer the patient to a dietitian for ongoing education and reinforcement of teaching.

Table 43–1. Antihypertensive Drugs

DRUG	DOSAGE
Alpha-Adrenergic Blockers	
prazosin (Minipress)	Initial dose: 1 mg bid–tid; may be increased gradually to a maximal dose of 20–40 mg qd in divided doses. Maintenance dose: 6–15 mg qd in divided doses
terazosin (Hytrin)	Initial dose: 1 mg at hs, gradually increase to a maximal dose of 20 mg. Maintenance dose: 1–5 mg qd in a single dose or 2 divided doses
Beta-Adrenergic Blockers	
atenol (Tenormin)	50 mg qd PO; may be increased to 100 mg qd (after 7–14 days)
metoprolol tartrate (Betaloc, Lopressor)	50 mg bid, or 100 mg qd PO; may be increased to 200–400 mg qd PO in 2–3 divided doses
nadolol (Corgard)	40 mg qd PO initially; may be increased by 40- to 80-mg increments to a maximal dose of 240 mg qd
pindolol (Visken)	10 mg bid PO q 2–3 weeks; may be increased by 10 mg/qd to a maximal dose of 60 mg qd

Table continued on following page

Table 43–1. Antihypertensive Drugs *Continued*

DRUG	DOSAGE
propranolol hydro-chloride (Inderal, Inderal LA)	10–20 mg tid or qid or one 80-mg sustained-release capsule qd; may be increased to 160 mg qd
timolol maleate	10 mg bid PO; may be increased to a maximal dose of 60 mg PO
Indirect-Acting Adrenergic Blockers	
rauwolfia serpentina (Raudixin)	Initially and for 1–3 weeks: 200–400 mg qd PO in single or 2 divided doses Maintenance dose: 50–300 mg qd
reserpine (Serpasil)	0.5 mg qd PO for 1–2 weeks Maintenance dose: 0.1–0.5 mg qd PO IM initial dose: 0.5–1 mg followed by doses of 2–4 mg q2h
Centrally Acting Adrenergic Blockers	
clonidine (Catapres)	0.1 mg bid PO; increase by 0.1–0.2 mg qd on a weekly basis Maintenance dose: 0.2–0.8 mg qd in divided doses
Peripheral Vasodilators	
diazoxide (Hyperstat)	300 mg IV bolus push, administered in 30 seconds or less into a peripheral vein; repeat in 4–24 h

Table 43–1. Antihypertensive Drugs *Continued*

DRUG	DOSAGE
sodium nitroprusside (Nitropress)	50-mg vial diluted with 2–3 mL of 5% D/W, then added to 250–1000 mL 5% D/W; infuse at 0.5–10 mcg/kg/min
hydralazine (Apresoline)	10 mg PO qid; increase gradually to maxi-mal dose of 300–400 mg qd 20–40 mg slow IV or IM, repeat q4–6h prn; change to oral antihy-pertensives as soon as possible
minoxidil (Loniten)	5 mg PO, once qd; gradually increase to 10–40 mg qd in 1–2 doses
Angiotensin-Converting Enzyme (ACE) Inihibitors	
captopril (Capoten)	25 mg PO tid; may be increased in 1–2 weeks to 50 mg tid; may add diuretics and increase to maximal dose of 150 mg tid
enalapril (Vasotec)	5 mg PO qd; may be increased to 40 mg qdIV doses are avail-able to treat hyper-tensive crises
lisinopril (Prinivil, Zestril)	5–10 mg PO qd; may be increased to 20 mg

Table continued on following page

Table 43–1. Antihypertensive Drugs *Continued*

DRUG	DOSAGE
Calcium Antagonists (calcium channel blockers)	
diltiazem (Cardizem)	30 mg PO quid before meals and at hs; may be increased gradually to 240 mg qd in divided doses
nifedipine (Procardia)	10 mg PO tid; may be increased gradually to 180 mg qd in divided doses
verapamil (Calan, Isoptin)	80 mg PO tid-qid; may be increased weekly to 480 mg qd in divided doses

Whether or not the patient is obese, participation in regular physical activity is a significant factor in the reduction of hypertension. Walking is an excellent exercise because it requires no special equipment, it does not overly stress the joints, and the pace is easily regulated. In addition, outside activity provides distraction and relaxation.

Teach the patient that hypertension is a chronic illness. Ordered medications should be taken at the same time each day. Patients should continue taking the medication even after the blood pressure returns to normal levels. Emphasize the importance of follow-up with the physician because many patients omit their medications and cancel appointments when they feel better.

EVALUATION Monitor the patient and the chart for ▲▲▲▲▲▲▲▲▲▲ reduction in the blood pressures and the weight.

ADRENERGIC BLOCKERS

Adrenergic blockers help to decrease blood pressure by dilating the blood vessels. Dilating arteries directly reduces blood pressure by reducing the pressure within the artery. Dilating veins indirectly lowers blood pressure because the venous return to the heart is decreased and, as a result, the cardiac output is diminished. (More information on adrenergic blockers can be obtained in Chapter 38.)

Alpha-Adrenergic Blockers

Alpha$_1$-blockers (antagonists) act to lower blood pressure by blocking the alpha$_1$-receptors on arterioles and veins. Vasodilation occurs as a result. Prazosin (Minipress) and terazosin (Hytrin) are examples of this group.

The adverse effects of alpha$_1$-blockers are orthostatic hypotension, reflex tachycardia, nasal congestion, and inhibition of ejaculation in men.

Orthostatic hypertension is the most serious of these adverse effects. Warn the patient to change positions slowly and to avoid hazardous activities, such as driving and operating other machinery, until the response to the medication can be determined.

Prazosin

Prazosin (Minipress) may cause a "first-dose effect" in patients. Warn them that they may lose consciousness 30 to 60 minutes after the first dose is taken. Driving and other hazardous activities must be avoided for at least the first 24 hours. This first-dose effect can often be minimized by initiation of therapy with a 1-mg dose and gradual increases in the dose. Administration of the first dose at bedtime may also be beneficial in reducing this effect.

Beta-Adrenergic Blockers

Beta$_1$ and beta$_2$-blockers are widely used to treat mild to moderate hypertension. They reduce the heart rate, force of contraction, and cardiac output. Impulse conduction through the atrioventricular (AV) node is decreased. Beta-blockers also suppress renal production of the hormone renin. Renin plays a major role in maintaining blood pressure and in elevating the pressure when it falls as a result of certain conditions, such as anemia and hypovolemic shock.

Adverse effects of beta$_1$-blockers include bradycardia, diminished cardiac output, AV block, and possibly congestive heart failure. Beta$_2$-blockers may also cause bronchoconstriction and inhibition of glycogenolysis (the breakdown of glycogen into glucose).

Atenolol (Tenormin), metoprolol tartrate (Betaloc, Lopressor), nadolol (Corgard), pindolol (Visken), propranolol hydrochloride (Inderal, Inderal LA), and timolol maleate (Biocadren) are examples of beta-blockers.

Indirect-Acting Adrenergic Blockers

The rauwolfia alkaloids act peripherally, affecting norepinephrine release and storage in adrenergic nerve endings. An example is rauwolfia serpentina (Raudixin).

Adverse effects include severe depression, bradycardia, orthostatic hypotension, gastrointestinal stimulation, and nasal congestion. Because of the severity of the adverse effects and the current availability of other effective drugs, the use of the rauwolfia alkaloids to treat hypertension has declined.

Centrally Acting Adrenergic Blockers

Centrally acting adrenergic blockers act within the central nervous system to reduce the flow of impulses through the sympathetic nerves to the blood vessels and the heart. Clonidine hydrochloride (Catapres) is an example of this group. It is widely used to treat hypertension because it is generally free of adverse effects.

Rebound hypertension occasionally occurs, especially in connection with sudden discontinuation of clonidine. Other adverse effects include sedation, dry mouth, and constipation. Localized skin reactions may follow use of transdermal preparations. Safe use in pregnancy has not been determined.

PERIPHERAL VASODILATORS

ACTIONS AND USES Peripheral vasodilators, such as
▲▲▲▲▲▲▲▲▲▲▲▲▲▲▲▲ diazoxide (Hyperstat) and sodium nitroprusside (Nipride, Nitropress), lower blood pressure by relaxing the smooth muscle of the arterioles, which decreases resistance to blood flow. They may also relax the venules, thereby causing a decreased return cardiac flow.

Chronic hypertension may be treated with hydralazine (Apresoline) or minoxidil (Loniten).

Peripheral vasodilators act directly on the smooth muscle of the vascular system to produce vasodilation. Many are administered by the oral route and are used for long-term management of hypertension. Others can be administered intravenously (IV) and are used to treat hypertensive crises.

Peripheral vasodilators are absorbed and metabolized by the liver, distributed throughout the body for action, and excreted by the kidneys.

Adverse actions of drugs in this classification commonly include postural hypotension (especially early in treatment), water and sodium retention, flushing, headache, dizziness, sweating, weakness, tachycardia and palpitations, nausea, vomiting, diarrhea, and cramps.

ASSESSMENT Assess the patient's history for evidence
▲▲▲▲▲▲▲▲▲▲▲▲ of hepatic or renal impairment, coarctation of the aorta, and atrioventricular shunt. Use is contraindicated in these conditions. Assess for risk factors related to the illness.

Assess the vital signs, especially the blood pressure. Document the patient's signs and symptoms. If the patient has peripheral vascular disease, be certain to perform a circulatory assessment and document findings as baseline data.

PLANNING AND IMPLEMENTATION Physicians often be-
▲▲▲▲▲▲▲▲▲▲▲▲▲▲▲▲▲▲▲▲▲▲▲▲▲▲▲▲▲▲ gin treatment with lower dosages and progressively increase the dose as the patient's response is evaluated. Use caution in patients with hepatic and renal impairment. Monitor for signs and symptoms of increased cardiac workload. Advise the patient to avoid gastrointestinal disturbance by taking medications with meals or antacids. Teach safety measures, such as to change position or rise slowly, and to avoid driving and operating hazardous equipment until response is evaluated. Teach the patient about the medication regimen and to take the medications at the same time each day.

EVALUATION Compare the patient's vital signs with
▲▲▲▲▲▲▲▲▲▲▲▲ baseline documentation. Note whether the patient is expressing improvement of subjective symptoms. Note whether circulatory assessment indicates improvement of the condition.

Diazoxide

ACTIONS AND USES Diazoxide (Hyperstat) is used *only*
▲▲▲▲▲▲▲▲▲▲▲▲▲▲▲▲ in hypertensive crises. Additional adverse effects include euphoria, angina, arrhythmia, myocardial ischemia, hyperglycemia, hyperuricemia, pain, and inflammation at the IV site if it infiltrates.

ASSESSMENT Assess for a history of diabetes mellitus,
▲▲▲▲▲▲▲▲▲▲▲▲ cardiac disease, or uremia because there may be additional complications. Assess vital signs and weight, and document your findings as baseline data. Assess fasting blood glucose and uric acid levels. Review the patient's medication regimen.

PLANNING AND IMPLEMENTATION Administration is by
▲▲▲▲▲▲▲▲▲▲▲▲▲▲▲▲▲▲▲▲▲▲▲▲▲▲ the IV route only. An
initial bolus is given undiluted, by rapid IV push
within 30 seconds or less. The treatment is changed to
oral medication as soon as the patient is stabilized.

Review the medication regimen. Use caution if the
patient also takes thiazide diuretics because these
may potentiate diazoxide. Have norepinephrine available to reverse severe hypotension.

Monitor intake and output for signs of fluid retention. Daily weights are important. Monitor the IV site
carefully. Monitor vital signs as ordered or as the
situation warrants. Be aware of parameters ordered
and notify the physician if they are not maintained.

Observe patients with diabetes mellitus for symptoms of severe hyperglycemia, which may require
insulin.

EVALUATION Compare the patient's vital signs and
▲▲▲▲▲▲▲▲▲▲ weight with baseline data. Evaluate fluid
intake for balance. Monitor laboratory values of uric
acid and blood glucose for abnormal values.

Sodium Nitroprusside

ACTIONS AND USES Sodium nitroprusside (Nitropress)
▲▲▲▲▲▲▲▲▲▲▲▲▲▲▲▲ is used *only* to treat hypertensive
emergencies. It lowers blood pressure rapidly.

Adverse effects usually indicate an overdose and
should be reported immediately. These adverse signs
include dizziness, ataxia, loss of consciousness or
coma, weak pulse, absence of reflexes, dilated pupils,
restlessness, muscle twitching, diaphoresis, dyspnea, shallow respirations, and signs of metabolic
acidosis.

ASSESSMENT Assess the patient for a history of thy-
▲▲▲▲▲▲▲▲▲▲ roid, renal, and hepatic diseases because
these may be contraindications for use. Assess the
entire medication regimen for other antihypertensive
drugs because they may potentiate each other. Assess
vital signs and document as baseline data.

PLANNING AND IMPLEMENTATION Fresh solution has a
▲▲▲▲▲▲▲▲▲▲▲▲▲▲▲▲▲▲▲▲▲▲▲▲▲▲▲▲▲ faint brownish tint.
Discard solution after 24 hours. Dilute medication in
5% dextrose in water *only*. Do *not* use bacteriostatic
water or sterile saline to prepare the solution. Infuse
the solution by pump into a secondary line. Wrap the
IV solution container in foil to protect it from light. Be
aware of ordered parameters for blood pressure and
report to the physician if these are not maintained.
Take the vital signs every 5 minutes at the start of

administration and every 15 minutes after. Discontinue use if severe hypotension occurs, then notify the
physician.

N U R S I N G   A L E R T
▼▼▼▼▼▼▼▼▼▼▼▼▼▼▼▼▼▼▼▼▼▼▼▼▼▼▼▼▼▼▼▼▼▼▼▼

Sodium nitroprusside can cause cyanide poisoning.
Monitor serum thiocyanate levels every 72 hours
(results above 10 mcg/dL indicate toxicity).

▲▲▲▲▲▲▲▲▲▲▲▲▲▲▲▲▲▲▲▲▲▲▲▲▲▲▲▲▲▲▲▲▲▲▲▲

If adverse effects occur, discontinue the medication,
maintain the primary IV line, and notify the physician.

EVALUATION Compare vital signs with the parameters
▲▲▲▲▲▲▲▲▲▲ ordered by the physician. Monitor thiocyanate levels.

Hydralazine

ACTIONS AND USES The adverse effects of hydralazine
▲▲▲▲▲▲▲▲▲▲▲▲▲▲▲▲ hydrochloride (Apresoline) include
the lupus erythematosus (LE)–like syndrome.

ASSESSMENT Assess the laboratory results of the
▲▲▲▲▲▲▲▲▲▲ complete blood count (CBC), LE cell
prep, and antinuclear antibody titer as baseline
findings.

PLANNING AND IMPLEMENTATION Observe for signs
▲▲▲▲▲▲▲▲▲▲▲▲▲▲▲▲▲▲▲▲▲▲▲▲▲▲▲▲▲ and symptoms that
resemble LE, such as sore throat, fever, muscle or joint
aches, and rash. Notify the physician immediately if
these become apparent.

EVALUATION Periodically during therapy, the CBC,
▲▲▲▲▲▲▲▲▲▲ LE cell prep, and antinuclear antibody
titer are measured. Compare results with baseline
findings.

Minoxidil

Adverse actions of minoxidil (Loniten) include edema,
tachycardia, pericardial effusion and tamponade, congestive heart failure, electrocardiographic changes,
Stevens-Johnson syndrome, increase in body hair, and
breast tenderness.

This drug is contraindicated if there is a history of pheochromocytoma. Assess for history of this condition.

Minoxidil is used when other antihypertensive medications have failed. Reassure the patient that the increase in body hair will disappear 1 to 6 months after stopping the drug. Caution the patient to follow the entire medication regimen. Minoxidil is usually ordered with a beta-blocker to control the tachycardia, and a diuretic may be ordered to control fluid retention.

DIURETICS

Diuretics assist in lowering blood pressure by increasing the excretion of sodium and water. As the circulating blood volume decreases, the cardiac output also decreases. Diuretics also act to decrease the resistance in the peripheral blood vessels by dilating the arterioles.

Examples of the thiazide diuretics are chlorothiazide (Diuril), hydrochlorothiazide (HydroDIURIL, Esidrix), and cyclothiazide (Anhydron). The loop diuretics include furosemide (Lasix) and bumetanide (Bumex). Spironolactone (Aldactone) and triamterene (Dyrenium) are potassium-sparing diuretics. Mannitol (Osmitrol) is an osmotic diuretic.

Each type of diuretic acts by a different mechanism. Consult Chapter 47 for additional information.

CALCIUM CHANNEL BLOCKERS

ACTIONS AND USES Calcium channel blockers lower ▲▲▲▲▲▲▲▲▲▲▲▲▲▲▲▲ blood pressure by blocking the movement of calcium in the cells of smooth muscles, which inhibits contraction of the muscles and causes dilation of the arterioles. The decreased peripheral resistance causes the blood pressure to drop.

Examples are diltiazem (Cardizem), nifedipine (Adalat, Procardia), nicardipine (Cardene), and verapamil (Calan, Isoptin).

Patients who experience adverse effects from diuretics and beta-blockers can often benefit from the calcium channel blockers. At times, they are prescribed with a diuretic for additional antihypertensive effects. (See Chapter 42, where these drugs are discussed as antianginals.)

Adverse effects vary with the type of drug. Commonly occurring symptoms include headache, dizziness, fainting, lethargy, dry mouth, orthostatic hypotension, weakness, trembling, sweating, depression, male impotence, rashes, nausea, vomiting, and constipation or diarrhea.

ASSESSMENT For patients receiving any type of anti-▲▲▲▲▲▲▲▲▲▲▲ hypertensive therapy, obtain vital signs and document them as baseline information. Obtain blood pressure measurements with the patient lying, then sitting, then standing.

Assess for a history of cardiovascular disease, renal or hepatic disorders, allergies, or bronchitis. These conditions may be contraindications for use of some types of medications. Assess for a history of diabetes mellitus because some of these medications alter requirements for hypoglycemic agents.

PLANNING AND IMPLEMENTATION Monitor vital signs ▲▲▲▲▲▲▲▲▲▲▲▲▲▲▲▲▲▲▲▲▲▲▲▲▲▲▲▲▲▲▲ frequently and compare with baseline findings. Monitor blood pressure in lying, sitting, and standing positions to detect orthostatic hypotension.

Teach the patient to change positions slowly to prevent orthostatic hypotension and to avoid driving and other hazardous activities until response to the medication has been determined.

Always teach the patient about the ordered drug regimen because this may increase compliance with therapy. Encourage patients to discuss with the physician any adverse effects or any thoughts about changes in the ordered regimen. Discourage the patient from altering dosage or any part of the regimen without first consulting the physician. Severe hypertension may result from abrupt discontinuation of many of these medications. Encourage the patient to discuss all medications being taken with the physician; some will interact with the antihypertensive medications.

Patients should weigh themselves daily and observe for signs of edema. If possible, teach patients how to monitor the blood pressure at home. Instruct patients to report abnormal findings to the physician.

Teach the signs and symptoms of hypokalemia if a diuretic is part of the regimen. Include information about dietary sources of potassium, if the antihypertensive or diuretic is not potassium sparing. Some patients will also be prescribed a potassium supplement to replace amounts of the electrolyte lost through urination.

Mouth dryness may be relieved by chewing sugarless gum or by sucking ice chips or sour hard candy.

Encourage persons who also have diabetes mellitus to monitor fingerstick blood glucose levels at regular intervals. Advise them to report to the physician if abnormal results occur.

EVALUATION Monitor blood pressure at regular inter-▲▲▲▲▲▲▲▲▲▲ vals and compare with parameters specified by the physician. Monitor for adverse effects versus therapeutic effects. Monitor laboratory values for evidence of renal or hepatic disorders. Ask the patient for subjective reports of effectiveness of therapy.

ANGIOTENSIN-CONVERTING ENZYME INHIBITORS

ACTIONS AND USES When renin is released from the ▲▲▲▲▲▲▲▲▲▲▲▲▲▲▲▲ kidney, it is converted into angiotensin I, which is then changed by angiotensin-converting enzyme (ACE) into the vasoconstrictor angiotensin II. Because vasoconstrictors increase blood pressure, drugs that inhibit or block the production of ACE may lower blood pressure.

Examples of ACE-inhibiting drugs are captopril (Capoten), enalapril (Vasotec), and lisinopril (Prinivil, Zestril).

ACE inhibitors are also believed to increase the production of the prostaglandins, which cause vasodilation. This, plus the fact that they decrease the production of aldosterone and reduce salt and water retention, makes them effective as antihypertensives. They can be used alone or in combination with diuretics, calcium channel blockers, or other antihypertensives. They are often first-choice drugs because they are not contraindicated in diabetes mellitus, gout, congestive heart failure (CHF), and asthma, as are many other antihypertensives and diuretics.

Adverse actions are less than those produced by other antihypertensives. General side effects include dizziness, fainting, hypotension, tachycardia, CHF, diarrhea, vomiting, hyperkalemia, rash and pruritus, fever, transient increase in liver enzyme activity, leukopenia, and agranulocytosis. A dry, irritating, nonproductive cough is the most common adverse effect noted.

ASSESSMENT Review the patient's history for preg-▲▲▲▲▲▲▲▲▲▲ nancy, lactation, or heart block. Use is contraindicated in these patients. Obtain a baseline complete blood count (CBC), platelet count, renal and hepatic function test results, and electrolyte determinations. Review the patient's entire medication regimen for other antihypertensives or diuretics.

PLANNING AND IMPLEMENTATION Monitor electrolytes. ▲▲▲▲▲▲▲▲▲▲▲▲▲▲▲▲▲▲▲▲▲▲▲▲▲▲▲▲▲▲ Be aware that serious hypotension may occur after the first dose in pa-tients taking diuretics and those who have severe salt depletion.

Store oral preparations in a cool, dry area. Give oral medications 1 hour before meals. Administer intravenous medications slowly, as directed.

Monitor vital signs frequently. Monitor intake and output and weight daily. Teach patients to change position slowly, dangle before ambulation, and avoid hazardous activities until their individual response is evaluated. Caution patients that dizziness and fainting may occur for the first few days of treatment.

Emphasize that medications should be taken at the same time each day and that over-the-counter preparations should not be used unless approved by the physician.

Monitor for signs of infection and encourage patients to report fever, sore throats, and other symptoms to the physician.

EVALUATION Monitor vital signs and compare with ▲▲▲▲▲▲▲▲▲▲ baseline data. Monitor the CBC, electrolyte levels, and results of renal and hepatic function tests. Monitor for improvement in signs and symptoms of CHF.

E X E R C I S E S

LEARNING ACTIVITIES

1. Mr. K.S., a 53-year-old social worker, has recently been diagnosed as having hypertension. As you are caring for him, he tells you that he dislikes taking medications and plans to discontinue his antihypertensive medications as soon as his blood pressure gets under control. What is your response to him?

2. Ms. A.D. has moderate to severe hypertension that is being controlled by an adrenergic blocker, a peripheral vasodilator, and a diuretic. She is also taking a potassium replacement. She objects to taking all these medications and is questioning why her roommate is only taking the ACE inhibitor captopril (Capoten). Ms. A.D. wants to know why her physician does not change her to the Capoten, if it is a better drug. Role play this interaction with a classmate as you explain to Ms. A.D.

ANTIHYPOTENSIVE DRUGS

L E A R N I N G   O B J E C T I V E S

After studying this chapter, you should be able to:

1. Discuss the use of the adrenergic drugs to maintain blood pressure.

2. List possible adverse effects of these medications.

3. Discuss ways to assess effectiveness of the medication.

4. Prepare an appropriate plan of care for a patient receiving one of these medications.

DRUGS YOU WILL LEARN ABOUT IN THIS CHAPTER

epinephrine (Adrenalin)

dopamine HCl (Intropin, Dopastat)

ephedrine sulfate

metaraminol bitartrate (Aramine)

norepinephrine (Levophed)

If dilation of blood vessels lowers blood pressure and constriction of blood vessels increases blood pressure, then it would seem that vasoconstrictors should be used to treat all hypotension and shock. This is true to some extent, but we must remember that shock has many causes, and treatment must be aimed at the specific cause. For example, hypovolemic shock is treated with volume replacement and control of blood and fluid loss; bacteremic shock is treated with antibiotics and supportive therapy.

ACTIONS AND USES Adrenergic or sympathomimetic drugs increase or simulate the effects of epinephrine and norepinephrine on alpha-adrenergic and beta-adrenergic receptors in the sympathetic nervous system. Actions include bronchodilation, increased heart rate and contractility, stimulation of the central nervous system, dilation of skeletal blood vessels, constriction of peripheral blood vessels, and release of glycogen from the liver.

Sympathomimetic or adrenergic drugs that increase cardiac output or increase peripheral resistance are often used to treat shock that results from inappropriate dilation of peripheral blood vessels, such as in patients with shock due to anaphylaxis and neurogenic causes. They are also used to treat orthostatic or postural hypotension when the hypotension is caused by spinal anesthesia.

Adverse actions depend on the specific product used. Typical effects include headache, dizziness, nervousness, apprehension, tremors, arrhythmias, severe hypertension, hyperglycemia, diminished renal output, and irritation or necrosis if the intravenous (IV) solutions infiltrate. With those products used to increase blood pressure, excessive cardiac stimulation may occur. Also, sympathetic stimulation may cause renal vasoconstriction and the possibility of renal ischemia.

Examples of antihypotensive drugs are epinephrine (Adrenalin), dopamine hydrochloride (Intropin, Dopastat), ephedrine sulfate, metaraminol bitartrate (Aramine), and norepinephrine (Levophed). Table 44–1 lists dosages for the antihypotensive drugs.

ASSESSMENT Assess the vital signs and compare your findings with the normal range recorded in the chart for this patient. Perform a complete cardiovascular assessment, noting especially the color and temperature of the skin and the capillary refill. Do a general assessment to determine the possible cause of the shock, such as trauma, a source of bleeding, an infection, or an allergic reaction. Document all of the information as baseline data for comparisons.

Table 44-1. Antihypotensive Drugs

DRUG	DOSAGE
epinephrine (Adrenalin)	0.1–0.5 mL of 1:1000 SC, IM; repeat q 10–15 min, prn 0.1–0.25 mL of 1:1000 IV
dopamine hydro-chloride (Intropin, Dopastat)	2–5 mcg/kg/min IV; titrated by response (maximal dose, 50 mcg/kg/min)
ephedrine sulfate	25–50 mg IM, SC; 10–25 mg IV Maximal dose, 150 mg/24 h
metaraminol bitar-trate (Aramine)	Severe shock: 0.5–5 mg IV push, followed by infusion of 15–100 mg in 500 mL normal saline or 5% D/W Flow rate is adjusted to maintain blood pressure parameters
norepinephrine (Levophed)	8–12 mcg/min initial IV infusion Flow rate is adjusted to maintain blood pressure parameter

PLANNING AND IMPLEMENTATION Initiate nursing care ▲▲▲▲▲▲▲▲▲▲▲▲▲▲▲▲▲▲▲▲▲▲▲▲▲▲▲▲▲▲▲▲ to support the body systems during shock. Initiate measurement of intake and output (I & O) because this information is needed to determine the amount of fluid replacement and to monitor for renal impairment. An indwelling catheter may be ordered to measure urinary output each hour. The physician may order specific parameters for the amount of output and the rate and volume of the IV infusion. Specific gravity tests may also be ordered to monitor renal function. Note and document the color and consistency of the urine.

Monitor the vital signs frequently as ordered by the physician or as the patient's condition indicates. Be aware of any specific parameters that the physician may have ordered and report readings outside of these parameters.

Place the patient flat to maximize blood flow throughout the body, unless another position is or-

dered by the physician or indicated by the condition. Position the head to maintain the airway and prevent aspiration if vomiting occurs.

Administer oxygen as ordered to prevent tissue and organ ischemia. Keep the patient warm to minimize expenditure of energy and oxygen to generate heat.

Monitor the IV site frequently to prevent infiltration with resultant irritation or necrosis and sloughing of tissue.

Use caution with sympathomimetics in the treatment of the elderly or those with cardiovascular disease, hypertension, diabetes mellitus, or hyperthyroid conditions. Use extreme caution in patients with bronchial asthma or emphysema. Sympathomimetics may also be contraindicated in patients with brain damage or coronary insufficiency.

EVALUATION Monitor for alteration in level of con-
▲▲▲▲▲▲▲▲▲▲ sciousness. Monitor vital signs until they are stable and within normal limits. Monitor I & O measurements until they are within normal limits. Compare general assessment findings with baseline data until results are within previous limits and stable.

EPINEPHRINE

Additional adverse effects of epinephrine (Adrenalin) are anxiety, palpitations, weakness, and hyperglycemia. Chest pain is more common in patients with hyperthyroidism.

Assess the chart for a history of diabetes mellitus and glaucoma because these are contraindications to the use of epinephrine. Assess the medication regimen for the use of tricyclic antidepressants because these may precipitate a hypertensive crisis.

Small doses are required, so use a tuberculin syringe for accuracy. Medications are prepared in light-resistant vials. The solution should be clear. Discard the solution if it is discolored or precipitated.

If an intramuscular dose is ordered, aspirate after inserting the needle because epinephrine may be toxic if it is accidentally administered intravenously. Rotate injection sites to prevent tissue necrosis. Avoid using the buttocks as a site. Massage the injection site after administration to disperse effects.

For intravenous administration, mix solutions immediately before use. Normal saline, 5% dextrose in water, or a combination of these may be used. Monitor the patient's blood pressure constantly until it stabilizes, then every 5 minutes after that until the physician orders otherwise.

Monitor for restlessness or anxious behaviors, which may indicate an excessive dose. Monitor the patient's blood glucose level for hyperglycemia.

DOPAMINE HYDROCHLORIDE

Dopamine hydrochloride (Intropin, Dopastat) can dilate renal vessels, so it is preferred in patients with renal impairment. Additional adverse actions include ectopic beats, tachycardia, hypotension, bradycardia, and vasoconstriction. Tissue necrosis may occur if the intravenous (IV) solution infiltrates.

Administer dopamine IV into a large vein with a microdrip device or an infusion pump. Monitor frequently for infiltration. If it occurs, stop the drug and notify the physician. Mix solutions immediately before use with 5% dextrose in water, normal saline, or a combination of these. Discard the solution after 24 hours or sooner if it is discolored. Do not mix other medications in the same IV container. Do not infuse alkaline drugs in the same IV line.

Do not use dopamine with ergot alkaloids because of the possibility of extreme hypertension. This drug may cause further hypotension in patients taking phenytoin. Also use caution in patients taking monoamine oxidase (MAO) inhibitors, pregnant patients, and those with peripheral vascular disease.

Watch for sudden hypotension after the medication is discontinued.

EPHEDRINE SULFATE

Ephedrine sulfate is used to correct hypotension. Additional adverse effects include insomnia, dizziness, muscle weakness, diaphoresis, euphoria, confusion, delirium, urinary retention, and painful spasms of the urinary sphincter.

Give ephedrine intramuscularly, subcutaneously, or by slow intravenous injection. This drug is contraindicated if the patient also takes monoamine oxidase (MAO) inhibitors or tricyclic antidepressants because severe hypertension may result. Use caution if the patient is also receiving methyldopa because it may inhibit the effects of ephedrine.

METARAMINOL BITARTRATE

N U R S I N G   A L E R T

▼▼▼▼▼▼▼▼▼▼▼▼▼▼▼▼▼▼▼▼▼▼▼▼▼▼▼▼▼

Antidotes to have on hand during administration of metaraminol include atropine for bradycardia, phentolamine mesylate (Regitine) to reverse vasopressor effects, and propranolol hydrochloride (Inderal) for arrhythmias.

▲▲▲▲▲▲▲▲▲▲▲▲▲▲▲▲▲▲▲▲▲▲▲▲▲▲▲▲▲

Metaraminol bitartrate (Aramine) is used to prevent or treat hypotension and severe shock. Additional adverse effects include tachycardia, bradycardia, flushing or pallor, convulsions, increased body temperature, respiratory distress, metabolic acidosis, and irritation if the intravenous (IV) solution infiltrates.

Administer metaraminol by IV infusion in 5% dextrose in water or normal saline with a pump into a secondary IV line and a large vein. If infiltration occurs, stop the drug and notify the physician. Do not mix other drugs in the same container or IV line. Do not discontinue the IV infusion suddenly. Gradually decrease the dose. Monitor for recurrence of hypotension.

Metaraminol is contraindicated if the patient is also taking a monoamine oxidase (MAO) inhibitor. Its use is also contraindicated in patients with pulmonary edema or acidosis and during anesthesia with cyclopropane.

Monitor the patient's blood pressure every 5 minutes until it stabilizes, then every 15 minutes.

Monitor intake and output. The output may initially decline and then increase as the blood pressure stabilizes. Report to the physician if the output remains persistently low.

NOREPINEPHRINE

N U R S I N G   A L E R T

▼▼▼▼▼▼▼▼▼▼▼▼▼▼▼▼▼▼▼▼▼▼▼▼▼▼▼▼▼

Emergency drugs to have on hand during administration of norepinephrine include atropine, phentolamine mesylate (Regitine), and propranolol hydrochloride (Inderal).

▲▲▲▲▲▲▲▲▲▲▲▲▲▲▲▲▲▲▲▲▲▲▲▲▲▲▲▲▲

Norepinephrine (Levophed) is used to treat acute hypotension. Adverse actions include ventricular tachycardia, ventricular fibrillation, and metabolic acidosis.

Constant attendance is necessary during administration. Do not administer norepinephrine if the patient is also receiving monoamine oxidase (MAO) inhibitors or tricyclic antidepressants because severe hypertension may occur. Monitor blood pressure every 2 minutes until stable, then every 5 minutes.

Prepare intravenous (IV) norepinephrine solutions with dextrose/normal saline, not with normal saline alone. Infuse with a microdrip device or infusion pump. Change the IV site frequently.

Report decreased output immediately.

E X E R C I S E S

LEARNING ACTIVITIES

Prepare a plan of care for a 70-year-old woman whois receiving norepinephrine IV to maintain her blood pressure.

DRUGS THAT AFFECT COAGULATION

LEARNING OBJECTIVES

After studying this chapter, you should be able to:

1. Identify the actions and uses of anticoagulant medications.

2. List adverse effects of anticoagulants.

3. Name the drug that may be used to reverse the effects of heparin and also the effects of the oral anticoagulants.

4. Identify the laboratory tests that are used to monitor anticoagulant therapy.

5. Discuss/demonstrate the procedure for subcutaneous heparin administration.

6. Prepare an appropriate teaching plan for a patient who is receiving either an oral or injectable anticoagulant.

DRUGS YOU WILL LEARN ABOUT IN THIS CHAPTER

Antiplatelet Drugs

aspirin (ASA, acetylsalicylic acid)

sulfinpyrazone (Anturan, Anturane)

dipyridamole (Persantine)

ticlopidine (Ticlid)

Anticoagulants

Injectable anticoagulants

heparin calcium (Calciparine)

heparin sodium (Liquaemin Sodium)

Oral anticoagulants

warfarin potassium (Athrombin-K)

warfarin sodium (Coumadin)

dicumarol (Dicoumarol)

Antagonists of the Anticoagulants

protamine sulfate

phytonadione (vitamin K_1, AquaMEPHYTON, Konakion, Mephyton)

Thrombolytic Enzymes

streptokinase (Kabikinase, Streptase)

urokinase (Abbokinase, Breokinase)

tissue plasminogen activator (TPA, Activase)

Blood clotting, or coagulation, is a protective device to prevent excess blood loss when a blood vessel is injured. Many substances are involved in the process. These factors that prevent clotting are called *anti*coagulants; *pro*coagulants promote clotting. The balance of these factors determines whether blood will coagulate.

For blood to flow smoothly through the vessels without clotting, we must have more circulating anticoagulant factors. However, when there is an injury to a blood vessel, we need more procoagulants to prevent hemorrhage.

When a blood vessel incurs an injury, there is a rough spot on the normally smooth lining. Some of the thrombocytes/platelets disintegrate as they flow over the rough spot. This causes clumping (also called agglutination or aggregation). The disintegrating thrombocytes release a chemical called thromboplastin, which triggers the clotting mechanism.

Thromboplastin combines with proteins or platelet factors and calcium to form prothrombin. The pro-

Box 45-1. Clot Formation

Injury
Stage 1 Thrombocytes release thromboplastin
Stage 2 Thromboplastin + Calcium = Prothrombin
Prothrombin + Calcium = Thrombin
Stage 3 Thrombin + Fibrinogen (from the liver) = Fibrin
Fibrin = Clot

thrombin then combines with calcium to form thrombin. Thrombin reacts with the protein fibrinogen, which is manufactured in the liver. This changes the fibrinogen from a liquid to a gel called fibrin, which traps the red cells and forms a clot (Box 45–1).

Several classifications of medications are used in the prevention and treatment of clotting disorders. Dosages of common anticoagulant medications are listed in Table 45–1.

ANTIPLATELET DRUGS

When a condition is diagnosed in which platelets are likely to clump or aggregate to form clots, the physician often prescribes a medication to prevent platelet aggregation. Examples are aspirin (ASA), sulfinpyrazone (Anturan, Anturane), dipyridamole (Persantine), and ticlopidine (Ticlid).

Aspirin

ACTIONS AND USES Aspirin (ASA, acetylsalicylic acid)
▲▲▲▲▲▲▲▲▲▲▲▲▲▲▲▲ is discussed elsewhere in this text as an analgesic, anti-inflammatory, and antipyretic agent. It also acts to inhibit platelet aggregation, so it is used to prevent further clotting in patients who have had myocardial infarction (MI), stroke, transient ischemic attacks (TIAs), and other vascular problems.

Adverse actions include gastrointestinal irritation and bleeding, salicylism, blurred vision, allergic reactions, tinnitus, and confusion.

ASSESSMENT Before use, assess the patient for a
▲▲▲▲▲▲▲▲▲▲ history of gastrointestinal ulcers or bleeding, bleeding tendencies of any type, and allergy to aspirin. Review the patient's current medication regimen for the presence of anticoagulant therapy.

PLANNING AND IMPLEMENTATION Teach the patient
▲▲▲▲▲▲▲▲▲▲▲▲▲▲▲▲▲▲▲▲▲▲▲▲▲▲▲▲▲ to take aspirin with meals or to use an enteric coated product to minimize

Table 45-1. Drugs that Affect Coagulation

DRUG	DOSAGE
Antiplatelet Drugs	
aspirin (ASA, acetylsalicylic acid)	1½–5 gr PO qd
sulfinpyrazone (Anturan, Anturane)	200 mg PO qid
dipyridamole (Persantine)	Angina: 50 mg PO tid at least 1 h before meals TIA: 100 mg PO qd To prevent clotting with prosthetic valves (used with warfarin): 100–400 mg PO qd
ticlopidine (Ticlid)	250 mg PO bid with food
Anticoagulants	
Injectable forms heparin calcium (Calciparine) heparin sodium (Liquaemin Sodium)	Deep vein thrombosis/ myocardial infarction: Initial dose: 5000–7500 units IV push, then adjust dose according to PTT results and give IV dose q4h (average 5000–7500 units), followed by 1000 units/hr by IV pump; wait 8 h after bolus dose and adjust hourly rate according to PTT Pulmonary embolus: Initial dose: 5000–10,000 units IV push, then adjust dose by PTT and give dose IV q4h (average 5000–10,000 units) IV bolus, then 1000 units hourly by IV infusion pump; wait 8 h after bolus and adjust hourly rate according to PTT taken q4–6h

Table continued on following page

Table 45–1. Drugs that Affect Coagulation
Continued

DRUG	DOSAGE
	Prophylaxis of embolus: Dose: 5000 units SC q12h Heparin locks (heparin sodium only): prepared in syringes/cartridges 10–100 units/mL for use in heparin locks; too weak to produce systemic anticoagulation effects

Oral forms
  warfarin potassium (Athrombin-K)
  warfarin sodium (Coumadin)
	Initial dose: 10–15 mg PO for 3 days, then adjust dose according to PT
	Maintenance dose: 2–10 mg PO qd

dicumarol (Dicoumarol)	Initial dose: 200–300 mg PO Maintenance dose: 25–200 mg PO qd based on PT
Anticoagulant Antagonists	
protamine sulfate	1 mg to dilute 78–95 units of heparin Dilute to 10 mg/mL and give by slow IV push in 1 to 3 min (maximal dose, 50 mg every 10 min)
phytonadione (vitamin K$_1$, AquaMEPHYTON, Konakion, Mephyton)	2.5–10 mg PO, SC, or IM based on prothrombin time
Thrombolytic Enzymes	
streptokinase (Kabikinase, Streptase)	Venous thrombosis, pulmonary embolus, arterial thrombosis, embolism: Loading dose: 1.5 million IU per IV infusion over 60 min

Table 45–1 Drugs that Affect Coagulation
Continued

DRUG	DOSAGE
	Maintenance: 100,000 IU/h per IV infusion pump × 72 h For myocardial infarction: Loading dose: 20,000 IU per coronary catheter Maintenance: 2000 IU/min × 60 min
urokinase (Abbokinase, Breokinase) (mixed with normal saline)	Pulmonary embolus: Loading dose: 4400 IU/kg/h given over 10 min Maintenance dose: 4400 IU/kg/h for 12–24 h (total volume not to exceed 200 ml solution.); follow with continuous IV infusion of heparin, then PO anticoagulants.
tissue plasminogen activator (TPA, Activase)	100 mg IV infusion over 3 h (1st h, 60 mg; 2nd h, 20 mg; 3rd h, 20 mg)

the gastrointestinal irritation. If the patient is taking other anticoagulant medications, aspirin should not be taken unless it is prescribed by a physician because chances of hemorrhage are increased.

EVALUATION Monitor platelet counts and compare ▲▲▲▲▲▲▲▲▲▲ with normal ranges. Monitor for adverse effects, and monitor patients for symptoms of the condition being treated.

Sulfinpyrazone

Sulfinpyrazone (Anturan, Anturane) inhibits platelet aggregation (clumping) and increases platelet survival time. It is used to treat patients who have TIAs or MI.

Assess the patient for a history of renal or hepatic problems, gastrointestinal ulcers, and diabetes. Review the patient's entire medication regimen.

Patients with diabetes mellitus who are taking oral hypoglycemics may have increased frequency of hypoglycemia. Be certain physicians are aware of all medications being taken. Review the symptoms of hypoglycemia and appropriate interventions with the patient. Encourage frequent monitoring of fingerstick blood glucose levels.

Encourage the patient to take medications with meals to minimize gastric disturbance. Encourage fluid intake of 2500 to 3000 cc every day unless contraindicated by the physician.

Dipyridamole

ACTIONS AND USES Dipyridamole (Persantine) is used
▲▲▲▲▲▲▲▲▲▲▲▲▲▲▲▲ to prevent postoperative complications in patients who have a history of thromboembolic disease, especially in association with prosthetic heart valves.

ASSESSMENT Review the history for evidence of preg-
▲▲▲▲▲▲▲▲▲▲ nancy or lactation (which are contraindications to use), hypotension, or recent MI. Also note whether there is a history of aspirin sensitivity because this may be a contraindication to use of the drug. Document baseline vital signs.

PLANNING AND IMPLEMENTATION Postural hypoten-
▲▲▲▲▲▲▲▲▲▲▲▲▲▲▲▲▲▲▲▲▲▲▲▲▲▲▲▲▲▲ sion may occur, so teach the patient to change positions slowly. Monitor vital signs. Medication should be taken on an empty stomach, 1 hour before meals or 2 hours after meals. If gastric irritation occurs and persists, then the medication should be taken with food or milk.

EVALUATION Monitor platelet counts and compare
▲▲▲▲▲▲▲▲▲▲ with normal ranges. Know the parameters desired and notify the physician if they are not maintained. Evaluate vital signs for evidence of hypotension.

Ticlopidine

Ticlopidine (Ticlid) has been approved only for the prevention of thrombolytic cerebrovascular accident. Its action begins approximately 48 hours after ingestion and reaches maximal effects in approximately 1 week. The effects last a week or more after the drug is discontinued.

Adverse effects include gastrointestinal upsets, such as nausea, diarrhea, pain, and dyspepsia. A rash and pruritus may also occur. There is a risk of neutropenia and agranulocytosis.

Monitor the patient's complete blood count (CBC) with differential every 2 weeks. Ticlopidine should be discontinued if neutropenia or agranulocytosis develops.

Monitor for signs of infection. Teach patients to report symptoms of infection to the physician. Patients and caregivers should wash their hands frequently. Tell patients to avoid contact with persons with infection, if possible.

ANTICOAGULANTS

Anticoagulant medications are used to interfere with clot formation. They do not "thin the blood" but are often referred to in this manner. These medications are available as injectable preparations and as oral preparations. They are discussed individually because their manner of action and the appropriate antidotes differ. *Injectable forms* of anticoagulants include heparin calcium (Calciparine) and heparin sodium (Liquaemin). *Oral forms* of anticoagulants include warfarin potassium (Athrombin-K), warfarin sodium (Coumadin), and dicumarol (Dicoumarol).

Injectable Anticoagulants

Heparin

ACTIONS AND USES Heparin inactivates thromboplas-
▲▲▲▲▲▲▲▲▲▲▲▲▲▲▲▲ tin and interferes with the conversion of prothrombin to thrombin. This prevents fibrinogen from forming fibrin and thus prevents clotting. Heparin also keeps the platelets from clumping to enhance the formation of a clot. It has a rapid onset of action, which makes it useful in emergencies. The duration of action is relatively short compared with that of the oral preparations.

Heparin is used to treat a blood clot, such as in deep venous thrombosis, myocardial infarction, and pulmonary embolism. It may be used to prevent clotting of blood during vascular and heart surgery or during any major surgery of the chest or abdomen. It also prevents clotting of blood removed from the body, such as during renal dialysis and use of the heart-lung bypass machines. Small doses are also used to "flush" central lines, heparin-locked intravenous catheters, and ports or reservoirs used to administer chemotherapeutic medications.

Hemorrhage, the chief complication, results from prolonged clotting time and thrombocytopenia. Other adverse actions include irritation of the injection site and sensitivity reactions manifested by chills, fever, pruritus, and hives.

ASSESSMENT Question the patient about and review the chart for a history of bleeding disorders such as hemophilia, gastrointestinal ulcers, threatened abortion, end-stage renal disease, liver disease, or others that are possible contraindications to use. Continuous gastrointestinal suctioning may also be a contraindication to use. The physician must weigh the benefits of therapy in each patient. Review the laboratory tests in the chart for results of the complete blood count (CBC) that may indicate thrombocytopenia. Note results of the partial thromboplastin time (PTT) as a baseline value. Assess the patient for signs of bruising or petechiae and document the location and size of the areas. Question the patient about presence of epistaxis, bleeding gums, hematuria, and blood in stools and document your findings. Assess vital signs and document them as baseline data.

PLANNING AND IMPLEMENTATION Dosage is highly individualized, depending on the reason for use, the age and weight of the patient, and the status of the renal and hepatic function. Initial doses are usually larger; the dose is then decreased when therapeutic ranges are documented by laboratory tests.

Heparin is measured in units. Strengths range from 250 units to 40,000 units per milliliter. *Read labels and dosages carefully!* Dosages are based on the results of the venous clotting times or PTTs. Therapeutic ranges are 1.5 to 2 times the control values. Notify the laboratory of dosing times because the laboratory results must be available in time for the physician to order the next dose. If heparin is being given intravenously (IV), blood draws should be taken from the opposite arm for greater accuracy of test results.

Heparin is given by injection because it is inactivated by gastric secretions. Intramuscular (IM) injections are not given because of the likelihood of hematoma formation at the site. Injections may be given as intermittent IV bolus doses or as continuous IV infusions. For safety, the use of an infusion pump is recommended with continuous IV infusions. Other drugs should not be mixed with or administered piggyback into a heparin infusion because incompatible mixtures will result. Heparin may also be administered by subcutaneous injection, but certain precautions must be observed (Box 45–2).

Because the patient will be predisposed to the formation of hematomas, pressure must be applied to the site after all venipunctures. If possible, IM injections should be avoided.

N U R S I N G   A L E R T

The antidote, protamine sulfate, should be available for the physician's use in the event that hemorrhage occurs or is likely to occur.

IV heparin therapy is usually not discontinued abruptly. It is often followed by subcutaneous injection therapy or oral anticoagulation therapy.

Many drugs increase the effectiveness of heparin. Some examples are aspirin, quinidine, indomethacin, phenothiazines, allopurinol, thyroid preparations, and oral anticoagulants. Many drugs also decrease the effectiveness of heparin, such as alcohol, estrogen, rifampin, phenytoin, and barbiturates. Teach the patient to always be certain that the prescribing physician is aware of all prescription and nonprescription medications being taken.

If the patient is to self-administer heparin by the subcutaneous route, be certain that all of the precautions for injection are understood. Have the patient verbalize the precautions, demonstrate the procedure, and administer the injection with supervision until it is performed accurately.

The following interventions are for patients receiving injectable or oral forms of anticoagulants:

Teach the patient to wear a Medic-Alert device and to inform physicians, dentists, therapists, and anyone else who may be ordering medications or performing procedures that an anticoagulant is being taken.

Box 45–2. Precautions for Subcutaneous Heparin Injections

1. Always inject into the abdomen, unless ordered otherwise.

2. Appropriate sites are between the iliac crests, but 2 inches away from the umbilicus.

3. A 25-gauge needle, $\frac{1}{2}$- to $\frac{5}{8}$-inch in length, is used.

4. Inject at a 90-degree angle.

5. Do not aspirate before injection.

6. Wait 10 seconds before withdrawing the needle.

7. Do not massage the site before or after the injection.

8. Alternate sites from the right to the left abdomen every 12 hours. Keep an accurate record of sites used.

Alert women that menstrual bleeding may be heavier than normal. Advise them to notify the physician if this occurs.

Teach the patient to carry identification to alert caregivers of the possibility of hemorrhage in the event of injury. Contact sports and activities that may induce trauma are to be discouraged. Encourage the patient or significant others to inspect the skin for bruising and bleeding and to notify the physician if they occur. To decrease trauma, the patient should use an electric razor for shaving and a soft toothbrush for oral hygiene. Bowel movements and urine should be monitored for changes in color, and these should be reported to the physician immediately.

EVALUATION Monitor the PTT results and the heparin ▲▲▲▲▲▲▲▲▲▲ dosage for therapeutic ranges. Monitor the patient for signs and symptoms of hemorrhage and compare with baseline assessments. Report abnormal symptoms or vital signs.

Oral Anticoagulants

ACTIONS AND USES Oral anticoagulants reduce the ▲▲▲▲▲▲▲▲▲▲▲▲▲▲▲ blood's ability to clot by interfering with the synthesis of clotting factors II, VII, IX, and X in the liver. The use of vitamin K is prevented, which causes the circulating prothrombin levels to drop (hypoprothrombinemia). Oral anticoagulants are used to treat pulmonary emboli and to prevent and treat deep venous thromboses, myocardial infarctions, rheumatic heart disease with valve damage, and atrial arrhythmias. Examples are warfarin potassium (Athrombin-K), warfarin sodium (Coumadin), and dicumarol (Dicoumarol).

Adverse actions include hemorrhage, nausea, vomiting, anorexia, ulcerations of the mouth, diarrhea, rash, and dermatitis.

ASSESSMENT Baseline assessments are the same as ▲▲▲▲▲▲▲▲▲▲ those for injectable anticoagulants, except that the blood test used to monitor therapeutic levels is the prothrombin time (PT).

PLANNING AND IMPLEMENTATION Effects of oral anti- ▲▲▲▲▲▲▲▲▲▲▲▲▲▲▲▲▲▲▲▲▲▲▲▲▲▲ coagulants are not apparent for 4 to 7 days. Treatment begins with a larger dose for 1 or 2 days, then a decreased dose is administered according to the PT. Oral medications are usually administered once a day. If the patient is receiving heparin, the oral anticoagulant is often initiated several days before discontinuation of the heparin. (See injectable forms for other interventions.)

Emphasize that the medication should be taken at the same time each day to maintain consistent blood levels of the drug. Encourage the patient to obtain PT tests when ordered by the physician and to keep appointments for follow-up visits.

Teach the patient which foods are high in vitamin K and encourage a moderate, consistent intake of these foods. Sporadic intake of these food items influences the prothrombin levels, and increased amounts counteract the effects of the anticoagulant.

Teach nursing mothers to monitor their infants for signs and symptoms of bleeding. The medication may cross through with the breast milk and affect the infant's prothrombin levels.

Many drugs alter the prothrombin level. Some examples of those that increase prothrombin levels are heparin, salicylates, disulfiram, steroids, glucagon, danazol, and the sulfonamides. Some examples of those that decrease prothrombin levels are rifampin, griseofulvin, and haloperidol.

N U R S I N G   A L E R T
▼▼▼▼▼▼▼▼▼▼▼▼▼▼▼▼▼▼▼▼▼▼▼▼▼▼▼▼▼▼▼▼

In the hospital, vitamin K should be kept available to reverse the effects of the anticoagulant medication in the event of hemorrhage or the likelihood that it will occur.

▲▲▲▲▲▲▲▲▲▲▲▲▲▲▲▲▲▲▲▲▲▲▲▲▲▲▲▲▲▲▲▲

It takes several hours to reverse the effects of oral anticoagulants.

EVALUATION Monitor the prothrombin levels in the ▲▲▲▲▲▲▲▲▲▲ chart. Therapeutic range is 1.5 to 2 times the control values. Notify the physician if the levels become too high. Compare the baseline assessments with the daily assessments and document the data. Report abnormalities to the physician.

ANTAGONISTS OF THE ANTICOAGULANTS

Protamine Sulfate

Protamine sulfate is a "base" chemical. Heparin sulfate is an "acid" chemical.

ACTION AND USES Protamine acts to block or neutral- ▲▲▲▲▲▲▲▲▲▲▲▲▲▲▲ ize the effects of heparin. It is used when the coagulation times become too high and the patient is likely to hemorrhage. Adverse actions include hypotension, bradycardia, flushing, and dyspnea.

ASSESSMENT See assessment for heparin. Protamine ▲▲▲▲▲▲▲▲▲▲ sulfate is given when laboratory values indicate a potential problem or when adverse signs and symptoms occur.

PLANNING AND IMPLEMENTATION Protamine sulfate is ▲▲▲▲▲▲▲▲▲▲▲▲▲▲▲▲▲▲▲▲▲▲▲▲▲ administered by a physician through a slow intravenous (IV) push to decrease the adverse effects. Monitor vital signs frequently. Observe for signs of spontaneous bleeding, such as hematuria, epistaxis, bleeding gums, and gastrointestinal bleeding. Patients whose status is post cardiac surgery and patients on renal dialysis are at higher risk than others.

EVALUATION Monitor laboratory values, which should ▲▲▲▲▲▲▲▲▲▲▲ reverse and approximate the control values.

Phytonadione

Vitamin K is a fat-soluble vitamin that is required by the liver to manufacture prothrombin and other clotting factors.

ACTIONS AND USES Vitamin K is used as an antagonist ▲▲▲▲▲▲▲▲▲▲▲▲▲▲▲ when the prothrombin levels of a patient receiving anticoagulant therapy are greater than 2.5 times the control value (Box 45–3). This drug is also given to neonates by the subcutaneous (SC) or intramuscular (IM) route immediately after birth to prevent hemorrhage. An example of vitamin K is phytonadione (vitamin K$_1$, AquaMEPHYTON, Konakion, Mephyton).

Adverse actions include nausea, vomiting, headache, flushing, tachycardia, pain, and nodule formation at the site of injection. Anaphylactic reactions may occur after parenteral administration.

ASSESSMENT See assessment for the oral anticoagu- ▲▲▲▲▲▲▲▲▲▲▲ lants. Vitamin K is given when laboratory values indicate a potential problem.

> **Box 45–3. Acceleration of Blood Clotting by Vitamin K**
>
> Vitamin K stimulates the liver cells to increase the synthesis of **prothrombin.**
>
> Increased prothrombin in the blood causes faster **thrombin** formation and faster **clot** formation.

PLANNING AND IMPLEMENTATION Administration to ▲▲▲▲▲▲▲▲▲▲▲▲▲▲▲▲▲▲▲▲▲▲▲▲▲ adults may be orally, SC, or IM. The oral dose may be repeated 12 to 48 hours later. The parenteral dose may be repeated in 6 to 8 hours. The drug may be administered IV in an emergency, but it is given slowly. Infusion is not to exceed 1 mg per minute. The dose may be repeated in 4 hours. Protect parenteral products from light.

Observe for signs of spontaneous bleeding, such as hematuria, epistaxis, bleeding gums, hematemesis, and tarry stools.

EVALUATION Monitor laboratory values, which should ▲▲▲▲▲▲▲▲▲▲▲ reverse and approximate the control values.

THROMBOLYTIC ENZYMES

A different approach for clotting disorders has been developed in recent years. Streptokinase (Kabikinase, Streptase) is a water-soluble protein produced by beta-hemolytic streptococci. Another thrombolytic enzyme, urokinase (Abbokinase, Breokinase), is present in human urine. Tissue plasminogen activator (TPA, Activase) is a synthetic protein.

ACTIONS AND USES The thrombolytic enzymes act to ▲▲▲▲▲▲▲▲▲▲▲▲▲▲▲▲ break up the fibrin and fibrin deposits that provide hemostasis or clotting. They are used to treat acute myocardial infarction, pulmonary emboli, and deep venous thromboses.

Adverse actions include hemorrhage and anaphylaxis. Fever may occur but should not be treated with aspirin, which interferes with platelet formation. Phlebitis sometimes occurs at the intravenous site. Blood pressure may be decreased or elevated.

ASSESSMENT Review the patient's history for evidence ▲▲▲▲▲▲▲▲▲▲ of recent trauma, such as surgery, delivery of an infant, intra-arterial diagnostic procedures, liver or kidney biopsy, gastrointestinal bleeding, active tuberculosis, or hypertension. These are contraindications to thrombolytic therapy. Recent cerebral hemorrhage or emboli and predisposition to infection are other contraindications, so the patient or family should be questioned in this regard. Review the chart for the initial partial thromboplastin time (PTT) and prothrombin time (PT) because these help determine the infusion rate.

PLANNING AND IMPLEMENTATION If therapy is to be ▲▲▲▲▲▲▲▲▲▲▲▲▲▲▲▲▲▲▲▲▲▲▲▲▲▲▲▲ effective, these enzymes must be initiated within the first few hours after onset of the condition being treated.

N U R S I N G   A L E R T

These medications should be used only by physicians who are widely experienced with treatment of thromboses.

A larger "loading" dose is given initially; the dose is then reduced. Infusion pumps are used for safety. Caregivers must monitor the infusion pumps and infusion site. Monitor the patient for signs of bleeding. Avoid unnecessary handling of the patient and pad side rails to minimize bruising. Avoid intramuscular injections and other invasive procedures, if possible. Apply pressure to venipuncture sites for 15 minutes, then follow with a pressure bandage and monitor the site frequently. Monitor vital signs and do circulation checks to the extremity hourly or more often as necessary.

EVALUATION The therapeutic range for PTT and PT will be 2 to 5 times the normal values. Monitor laboratory reports carefully and notify the physician when therapeutic range has been achieved so that the infusion rate can be adjusted.

E X E R C I S E S

LEARNING ACTIVITIES

1. Mr. M.B. has been hospitalized for 2 weeks and is receiving IV heparin therapy for a severe thrombophlebitis in his right thigh. The physician has just informed him that he will need to take SC heparin at home. Mr. M.B. wishes to learn to administer his own injections. Prepare a teaching plan that includes the information he needs to know about his medication, injection techniques, and diet.

UNIT NINE

DRUGS THAT AFFECT THE URINARY SYSTEM

The urinary system is composed of two kidneys, two ureters, one urinary bladder, and one urethra. The kidneys are bean shaped and located in the back below the chest. They lie on either side of the spine and behind the peritoneum. Each kidney is approximately 2 inches wide, 4 to 5 inches long, and 1 inch thick.

A kidney has many parts to it. The outer rim of the kidney is called the renal cortex; the inner tissue is referred to as the renal medulla. Within the renal medulla are the renal pyramids. The pyramids gather the waste fluid and direct them to the calyces, the openings to the renal pelvis. The inner border of the kidney is the hilum. The hilum is where the renal artery, vein, and ureter are all connected. Inside the kidney is a collecting space, the renal pelvis (Fig. IX–1).

The microscopic filtering system of the kidney is a structure called the nephron. Parts of the nephron are found in both the cortex and the medulla. One part of the nephron, the Bowman's capsule, is the point at which waste and water are filtered from the blood-

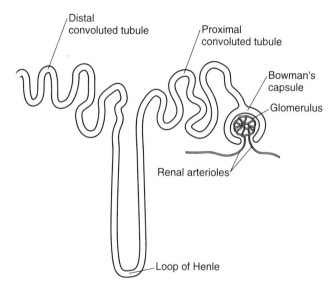

Figure IX–2. Waste and water are filtered from the bloodstream in the Bowman's capsule. Selective reabsorption of substances that the body still needs occurs farther along the tubule.

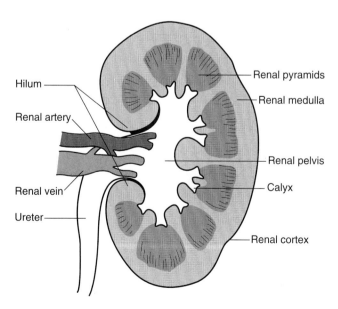

Figure IX–1. The human kidney.

stream. The Bowman's capsule lies above a glomerulus, a small network of tiny capillaries that have branched off from the renal artery. This is the blood supply to the kidney from which waste and water are filtered.

After the Bowman's capsule is the convoluted tubule. Certain parts of the convoluted tubule have specialized names. First comes the proximal convoluted tubule, meaning it is closest to the Bowman's capsule. Next comes the loop of Henle; it is referred to as a loop because of its shape. Last comes the distal convoluted tubule, meaning it is farthest from the Bowman's capsule. Along this twisted and curved tube, selective reabsorption occurs. Selective reabsorption, influenced by aldosterone and antidiuretic hormone, causes those substances that the body still needs to be reabsorbed (Fig. IX–2).

After the convoluted tubules, the filtrate flows into the calyx and finally into the renal pelvis.

The kidneys are responsible for the excretion of water and nitrogenous waste (the products of protein metabolism). These nitrogenous wastes are mainly uric acid, urea, ammonia, and creatinine. The kidneys also help maintain fluid and electrolyte balance, especially for potassium, chloride, sodium, and bicarbonate. Acid-base balance in the body is also influenced by the kidneys.

The kidneys produce the enzyme renin, which may act to raise the blood pressure. They also produce erythropoietin, which may act to stimulate the bone marrow to produce more red blood cells.

Approximately 1 quart of blood flows through the kidneys each minute. Although the kidneys actually filter out approximately 50 gallons of liquid a day, only about 1 quart (or 1 liter) is excreted by the body. The rest of the filtrate is reabsorbed along the convoluted tubule.

One ureter leads downward from each kidney. This is a muscular tube capable of peristaltic action. The ureters are lined with mucous membrane. Each ureter is 10 to 12 inches long and approximately the size of a pencil lead in diameter. These tubes connect to the urinary bladder.

The urinary bladder is a hollow muscular organ found in the pelvic cavity. It, too, is lined with mucous membrane. This organ acts as a reservoir until urine builds up to about 250 cc. At this point, the person feels the urge to void. The bladder contracts to force the urine out.

The urethra is a tube leading from the bladder to the outside of the body. It is lined with mucous membrane also. In women, the urethra is about 1 and 1/2 inches long; in men, it is about 8 inches long. In men, the urethra is surrounded by the prostate gland.

Two sphincters, or circular muscles, are located on the urethra. One is at the top of the urethra where it connects to the bladder, and one is at the bottom of the urethra where it opens to the outside. This outside opening is often referred to as the meatus. Both sphincters must relax for the person to void.

The urine is sterile. If microbes invade, a urinary tract infection (UTI) can develop. Signs and symptoms of a UTI depend on which area of the tract, upper or lower, is involved. In general, lower UTIs can produce burning on urination, pain, muscle spasms of the bladder, frequency, and urgency. If the infection is of the upper tract, add malaise, fever, chills, and lower flank pain.

In Chapter 46, we discuss the need for and purpose of fluid and certain electrolytes in the body. The drugs or solutions used to treat deficits or excesses of each of these are addressed. Chapter 47 describes the diuretic classification. These drugs are used for a variety of purposes and achieve their action by a variety of different mechanisms, but each alters how the kidney deals with fluid and electrolytes. Chapter 48 discusses drugs that may be used to treat the causes or symptoms of UTIs. Other drugs that may be prescribed for treatment of UTI are discussed in Unit IV.

FLUIDS AND ELECTROLYTES

LEARNING OBJECTIVES

After studying this chapter, you should be able to:

1. State nursing responsibilities for the patient with an intravenous line.

2. Name common fluid preparations administered by IV.

3. Name common medications used to treat increased or decreased levels of each electrolyte.

4. Identify the actions and uses of and adverse reactions to electrolyte supplements.

5. State appropriate nursing implications for the patient receiving an electrolyte supplement.

6. Evaluate a patient for the effectiveness of IV fluids and electrolytes.

7. Demonstrate how to administer PO or IM preparations of electrolyte supplements by use of the nursing process.

8. State what electrolytes are contained in specific fluid solutions.

9. Define phosphate binder.

10. Identify actions and uses of and adverse reactions to phosphate binders.

11. State nursing responsibilities for the patient receiving phosphate binders

DRUGS YOU WILL LEARN ABOUT IN THIS CHAPTER

For Hypovolemia

0.9% sodium chloride (normal saline).

dextrose 5% in water (D5W)

6% dextran 70 (Macrodex)

10% dextran 40 (Rheomacrodex)

For Hyperkalemia

sodium polystyrene (Kayexalate)

For Hypokalemia

potassium chloride (KCl-IV, K-Dur extended-release tablets, K-TaB extended-release tablets, Kaon-CL, Micro-K Extencaps, Kay Ciel, Slow-K controlled-release tablets)

potassium chloride and potassium bicarbonate (Klorvess)

potassium citrate and potassium bicarbonate (K-Lyte)

For Metabolic Acidosis (Bicarbonate Deficit)

sodium bicarbonate ($NaHCO_3$)

tromethamine (Tham)

sodium citrate

sodium lactate

For Hypocalcemia

calcium chloride (CaCl)

calcium gluconate

calcium phosphate

calcium lactate

calcium citrate

calcium carbonate

For Hypomagnesemia

magnesium sulfate ($MgSO_4$)

magnesium gluconate

magnesium lactate

magnesium oxide

For Hyponatremia

0.9% sodium chloride (normal saline)

0.45% sodium chloride (half-strength saline)

Combination Solutions

600 mg sodium chloride, 310 mg sodium lactate, 20 mg calcium chloride, 30 mg potassium chloride, 100 mL sterile distilled water (lactated Ringer's or Ringer's lactated solution)

Phosphate Binders

aluminum hydroxide (Amphojel, Dialume)

Think just for a moment of all the patients you have taken care of so far, or if you have not yet started clinical experience, remember the times you have visited in the hospital. How many of the patients had an intravenous infusion (an IV) running? Do you remember what types of solutions were in the IVs? Were there any other substances added?

There are many different types of solutions. They are made up of fluid and different electrolytes. Two of the most common are sodium chloride (NaCl) and dextrose 5% in water (D5W).

Recall your duties for a patient with an IV. They include assessing for signs and symptoms of infection (redness, warmth, pain) and of infiltration (swelling, coolness to touch, redness, pain). You should also note the solution hanging and compare it with the order. Also compare the actual drip rate with the timed drip rate.

FLUID IMBALANCE

Hypervolemia

If a patient receives an overload of fluid, for example, from an intravenous (IV) infusion, symptoms of hypervolemia may occur. Look for edema of three general body spaces: circulatory edema, pulmonary edema, and peripheral edema.

If a patient has circulatory edema, symptoms may include increased and bounding pulse, increased blood pressure, distended neck veins, and increased body weight. On chest x-ray, an enlarged heart may be noted.

If a patient has an IV, carefully monitor the blood pressure and pulse and weigh the patient daily. Look for distended neck veins when the patient reclines.

If a patient has pulmonary edema, symptoms may include abnormal breath sounds (especially rales—bubbling or popping sounds), dyspnea, and altered respiratory rate. The patient's arterial blood gases may also be altered. Therefore, in any patient who has an IV, frequently assess breath sounds and respiratory rate. Monitor reports of any blood gas analyses and report abnormalities immediately.

If a patient has peripheral edema, periorbital edema (around the eyes) is often the first sign. This is especially prevalent first thing in the morning or just after a nap, when the patient has been lying down. Other areas where peripheral edema is detected include dependent areas. This means any part of the body that is held lower than the heart. After the patient has been standing or sitting for a time, ankle edema is noted. Fluid may accumulate to the degree that pitting occurs. Pitting is described as an indentation that is left by gently pressing the fingers on the skin. Methods of grading pitting are usually imprecise. Sacral or coccygeal edema may also be position-related peripheral sites. Ascites is the accumulation of fluid in the abdominal cavity and may or may not be positional.

If a patient has an IV, assess all dependent areas for edema routinely. Pitting is a later sign. Ascites may be detected by weight gain and by measuring the patient's abdominal girth at the same place, in the same position, and at the same time of day, every day.

Hypovolemia

Hypovolemia means a lack of fluid circulating in the body systems. It is most often seen in cases of shock or hemorrhage. This fluid imbalance may be treated with IV infusions. Many different types of solutions may be used, depending on the cause of the problem.

In some cases of extreme loss of fluids, plasma volume expanders may be used. One of the most common is dextran. Dextran is available in different percentages, including 6% of dextran 70 and 10% of dextran 40. Trade names for these are Macrodex and Rheomacrodex, respectively. Adverse reactions to dextran are rare but may include anaphylactic shock.

POTASSIUM

Potassium (K^+) is needed by your body to conduct nerve impulses and to produce muscle contractions. This affects all the muscles in your body, both voluntary and involuntary. The normal serum level of potassium is 3.5 to 5.0 mEq per liter.

Potassium is found in generous supplies in our daily diet. Foods high in potassium include citrus fruits, bananas, milk, tomatoes, potatoes, bran, and chocolate.

Hyperkalemia

An increased level of potassium in the body may be seen in patients with kidney disease and damage. Potassium levels may also be increased through supplemental overdose. The patient may begin to experience weakness of voluntary muscle movement. The pulse weakens and may become irregular. Respirations become labored and irregular, and cardiac arrhythmias occur. The patient can die of respiratory paralysis or cardiac arrest.

The most commonly used drug to treat hyperkalemia is sodium polystyrene (Kayexalate). The trade name has been designed to tell you exactly what it does: it makes the K exit. Sodium polystyrene causes the body to release the excess potassium.

Sodium polystyrene can be given either orally or by rectal enema. Monitor the patient's serum potassium levels carefully. An overdose of sodium polystyrene can lead to hypokalemia.

Hypokalemia

Patients with too little potassium circulating in their body may have signs and symptoms of hypokalemia. These include muscle weakness and even paralysis as well as decreased blood pressure and muscle tetany.

Hypokalemia may be caused by diuretic therapy (a medication that causes the body to lose fluid). Any disorder that causes the loss of gastrointestinal (GI) fluids can also cause hypokalemia, such as vomiting, diarrhea, or GI suctioning. Malnutrition, diabetic coma, and congestive heart failure may also be factors.

Potassium supplements are given for treatment of hypokalemia. Potassium chloride (KCl) is one of the most common. There are numerous trade names for potassium chloride, including K-Dur extended-release tablets, K-TaB extended-release tablets, Kaon-CL (extended-release), Micro-K Extencaps, Kay Ciel, and Slow-K controlled-release tablets. Klorvess effervescent granules are a combination of potassium chloride and potassium bicarbonate. K-Lyte effervescent tablets are made from potassium citrate and potassium bicarbonate. All of these are oral preparations. Potassium chloride can also be given in solution intravenously (IV).

When given orally, potassium supplements can cause gastric upset and, in severe cases, GI bleeding with black stools or even bowel perforation.

If potassium chloride is given too quickly IV, it can cause cardiac arrhythmias.

BICARBONATE

Bicarbonate (HCO_3^-) is an anion, an electrolyte that carries a negative charge. It is vital for maintaining the body's acid-base balance.

The normal serum bicarbonate level is 22 to 26 mEq per liter. The body's pH (and therefore indirectly the bicarbonate level) can be monitored with the plasma pH (normal is 7.35 to 7.45) or the urine pH (normal is 4.8 to 7.5).

Metabolic Acidosis

If the body loses bicarbonate ions, it enters a state called metabolic acidosis. The patient becomes weak, may become stuporous, and begins having Kussmaul respirations. Metabolic acidosis is most often seen in renal diseases such as end-stage renal disease, cardiac arrest, shock, and diabetic coma.

To treat metabolic acidosis, the physician may order sodium bicarbonate ($NaHCO_3$) orally, intramuscularly, or intravenously. Be sure you are aware of the rationale for an order for sodium bicarbonate because it may also be used to make the urine alkaline to decrease the risk of crystalluria in a patient receiving sulfonamides. You may also see other medications used to treat metabolic acidosis, such as tromethamine (Tham), sodium citrate, or sodium lactate.

Whenever a patient has a bicarbonate imbalance, monitor results of serum electrolyte determinations and arterial blood gas analyses. An overdose of the medication can lead to alkalosis.

Three main blood gas determinations can be used to analyze the acid-base balance of the patient: plasma pH, partial pressure of carbon dioxide (Pco_2) and bicarbonate level (HCO_3^-). You need to know the normal values to determine whether each is acidic or alkaline:

plasma pH 7.35–7.45 low = acidic high = alkaline

HCO_3^- 22–26 low = acidic high = alkaline

P_{CO_2} 35–45 low = alkaline high = acidic

The patient's acid-base balance is detected by the plasma pH. If it is too low, the patient is in acidosis. If it is too high, the patient is in alkalosis. If the pH is in normal limits but one or both of the other two blood gases is abnormal, use 7.40 as your cutoff point. If the reading is below 7.40, the patient is in acidosis. If the reading is above 7.40, the patient is in alkalosis. We will explain why we do this in a moment.

The other two blood gases tell us the origin of the imbalance. Determine which of the two matches the pH for acid-base status. If HCO_3^- and pH are both acidic or both alkaline, then the source of the imbalance is said to be metabolic. If the P_{CO_2} and pH are both acidic or both alkaline, then the source of the imbalance is said to be respiratory.

The blood gas that did not match the pH for acid-base status tells us the level of compensation. If the pH is abnormal but the unmatching blood gas is normal, then the body is not attempting to compensate for the acid-base imbalance.

If the pH is abnormal and so is this last blood gas (but in an opposite direction), then the body is attempting to compensate. Full compensation has not yet occurred, though, or the pH would be normal. This is referred to as partial compensation.

If the pH is normal (you used 7.40 as your cutoff point) but this last blood gas is abnormal, then the body has fully compensated for its acid-base imbalance. This is called complete compensation.

Metabolic Alkalosis

If the body has an excess of bicarbonate, this is called metabolic alkalosis. It can lead to slow respirations, quickened reflexes, and muscle tetany.

Metabolic alkalosis is most often seen in overdoses of sodium bicarbonate therapy. However, also suspect the ingestion of baking soda if a patient presents with metabolic alkalosis. Some people use baking soda ($NaHCO_3$) in water for indigestion. This should be strongly discouraged.

N U R S I N G   A L E R T
▼▼▼▼▼▼▼▼▼▼▼▼▼▼▼▼▼▼▼▼▼▼▼▼▼▼▼▼▼▼

Besides disguising symptoms that should be brought to the physician's attention, the practice of ingesting baking soda may also lead to alkalosis.

Gastrointestinal (GI) perforation may also occur if the patient has any weakening of the GI system, such as a peptic ulcer or ulcerative colitis.

▲▲▲▲▲▲▲▲▲▲▲▲▲▲▲▲▲▲▲▲▲▲▲▲▲▲▲▲▲▲▲▲▲▲▲▲▲

The sodium bicarbonate releases carbon dioxide in the stomach. Instead of release of the gas by belching, the GI system may burst. This is why preparations such as Amphojel or Gelusil and many other antacids are preferred to sodium bicarbonate. Instruct your patients about the dangers of this practice and refer them to their physicians for thorough evaluation.

CALCIUM

Calcium (Ca^{2+}) is used by your body to produce bones, teeth, nerve, and muscle tissue and for the process of blood clotting. Vitamin D helps the body use the calcium. High amounts of calcium and vitamin D are found in the diet in foods from the dairy group (milk, cheeses, yogurt, ice cream) and in dark green leafy vegetables. Normal dairy dietary requirements should be met. Sunshine is also an excellent source of vitamin D because it changes a substance in the skin to vitamin D precursor.

Serum calcium levels can be measured in two ways. The normal levels are 8.8 to 10.4 mg per 100 mL, or 4.4 to 5.2 mEq per liter. It is easy to remember the second once you learn the first if you notice it is just half of the first (the numbers are, that is, not the amounts). Serum calcium levels vary because of dietary intake and activity.

Parathormone, the hormone produced by the parathyroid glands, increases the serum calcium levels by promoting the release of calcium from the bones. Calcitonin from the thyroid gland is the antagonist of parathormone. It decreases the amount of serum calcium by inhibiting the release of calcium from the bones. A third hormone, hydroxycholecalciferol, also regulates calcium. It is produced from vitamin D after first being modified by the liver and the kidney. It regulates the absorption of calcium by the intestine. These three hormones work together to maintain the balance or homeostasis of calcium levels in the body.

Hypocalcemia

Primary hypofunction of the parathyroid glands is rare. Because the parathyroids are embedded in the posterior capsule of the thyroid, it is difficult to remove the thyroid without inadvertently removing the parathyroids. Therefore, it is more common to have hypofunction occurring secondary to thyroidectomy. This results in a calcium deficiency. Hypocalcemia is also seen in patients with renal failure, cardiac arrest, rickets, osteomalacia, and pregnancy.

The calcium levels that can cause symptoms of deficiency or hypocalcemia vary with the person. The patient may complain of tingling of fingers and toes, muscle and abdominal cramping, or muscle tetany and may even experience convulsions. Tetany is the term given to the collection of symptoms resulting from irritability of the neuromuscular system. Calcium is necessary for normal muscle response to stimuli from the nervous system. Tetany usually begins with numbness and tingling of the lips, then the extremities. Cardiac arrhythmias, tremors, spasms, and convulsions follow if the condition is untreated.

If dietary measures are insufficient to treat a patient's calcium deficit, supplements must be used. Some of the more common forms include calcium chloride, calcium gluconate, calcium phosphate, calcium lactate, calcium citrate, and calcium carbonate.

When administered orally, calcium supplements can cause gastric upset and constipation. Intramuscular (IM) injections of calcium supplements can cause local inflammation. Given intravenously (IV), calcium can cause irritation of the vein, with tingling, warmth, and pain along its pathway.

If you are to administer calcium IM, warm the solution to body temperature to decrease the risk of inflammation. IV solutions should also be warmed before infusion and given slowly. Oral calcium supplements may be hampered if the patient's diet is high in fiber and, ironically, dairy products.

Calcium gluconate is the product most often administered IV if an emergency condition such as tetany exists and immediate action is crucial. Duration of action is 1/2 to 2 hours. If treatment is begun before any emergency exists, calcium lactate is administered orally. When normal serum calcium levels are restored, neuromuscular response should return to normal. Calcium lactate is continued as maintenance therapy.

Before administration of a calcium product, assess the patient for neuromuscular irritability. This is done with Chvostek's sign. The presence of Chvostek's sign indicates low calcium levels. To assess Chvostek's sign, tap the cheek near the ear. The facial nerve is located in this area. If the nose, mouth, and eye twitch on the side tapped, the sign is present. Report findings to the physician immediately. Compare serum calcium levels with normal values.

Emergency treatment requires the use of 500 mg to 1 g IV calcium, but there can be serious adverse reactions. Hypotension, syncope, bradycardia, arrhythmias, and cardiac arrest may result. The drug is administered slowly. The physician may order cardiac monitoring during administration. Personnel should be prepared to begin cardiopulmonary resuscitation

(CPR) if necessary. Monitor vital signs and compare findings with baseline assessments. Patients may complain of heat waves during IV administration. Reassurance should be given.

N U R S I N G   A L E R T

If the IV solution infiltrates, necrosis and sloughing of tissues often result. Monitor the IV site frequently and document assessments.

If infiltration occurs, stop the drip (unless your institutional policy forbids this) and notify your supervisor immediately.

The patient should remain recumbent for a short while after administration. Further dosage is based on serum calcium levels.

The IM route is used only if the patient's condition has deteriorated to circulatory collapse and no IV site is accessible. In adults, the site should be the gluteus medius muscle. In infants, the site is the lateral thigh (vastus lateralis muscle).

N U R S I N G   A L E R T

Burning, necrosis and sloughing of tissues, cellulitis, and soft tissue calcification may result. Monitor the site of injection and document assessments. Notify the physician of adverse reactions.

With oral ingestion, gastrointestinal complaints often result. Administer calcium 60 to 90 minutes after meals. Monitor patients for complaints of indigestion, constipation, or gastrointestinal hemorrhage. Teach patients to monitor stools for color change that may indicate bleeding.

Calcium may interact with cardiotonic glycosides and increase toxic effects of the glycosides. Monitor vital signs and compare with baseline assessments. Encourage the patient to maintain follow-up appointments and obtain blood tests ordered by the physician. Monitor the patient for relief of the symptoms of tetany. Continue to assess Chvostek's sign. Monitor serum calcium levels.

Hypercalcemia

Cases of too high levels of calcium in the bloodstream are called hypercalcemia. These are fairly rare and generally seen only in overdoses of calcium supplements.

If your patient takes calcium supplements, assess for lack of appetite, nausea, muscle weakness, and dehydration.

N U R S I N G   A L E R T

Do not be complacent with calcium supplements. Overdoses can lead to coma and death.

Serious arrhythmias may also occur if calcium levels become too high. Teach patients to monitor the pulse daily and report irregularities and changes in rate to the physician.

Renal calculi may result if serum calcium levels become too high. Monitor intake and output. Encourage intake of 2000 to 3000 mL of fluid per day unless this is contraindicated because of another medical condition. Physical activity is also encouraged to prevent formation of calculi. Encourage patients to report diminished output to the physician.

MAGNESIUM

Magnesium (Mg^{2+}) is a cation, which means it carries a positive charge. It is used by the body for the transmission of nerve impulses and for the complete metabolism of carbohydrates. The normal serum magnesium level is 1.4 to 2.0 mEq per liter.

Hypomagnesemia

When a patient loses excessive amounts of magnesium, this is called hypomagnesemia. The patient may experience muscle weakness, tremors, personality changes, quickened reflexes, and even seizures. It is most commonly seen in renal failure and in eclampsia, a disorder that causes seizures during pregnancy.

Treatment is initiated with magnesium sulfate ($MgSO_4$). This supplement may be given intramuscularly or slowly by intravenous infusion. Magnesium sulfate may also be added to total parenteral nutrition (TPN) mixtures to enhance the metabolism of the carbohydrates.

Magnesium supplements can also be given orally. Preparations include magnesium sulfate, magnesium gluconate, magnesium lactate, and magnesium oxide.

The most common adverse reactions to magnesium supplements are hypotension, nausea and vomiting, drowsiness, weakness, and slowed respirations. In severe hypomagnesemia, respiratory arrest has occurred.

Hypermagnesemia

Hypermagnesemia, a high level of magnesium in the bloodstream, does not usually produce symptoms until the levels are 3.0 mEq per liter or higher. It is most often seen in cases of overdose of magnesium supplements but is also common in renal failure.

SODIUM

Sodium (N^+) is as common as your salt shaker, yet it is essential in maintaining the body's fluid balance. Sodium helps the kidneys determine the amount of fluid to be excreted or reabsorbed. It also helps regulate the heart rhythm. Normal serum sodium level is 135 to 145 mEq per liter.

Hyponatremia

Loss of sodium is commonly seen in diuretic therapy, water intoxication, renal disease, vomiting and diarrhea, fever, and diaphoresis. It is called hyponatremia.

In general, symptoms of hyponatremia do not appear until the sodium level is very low, less than 125 mEq per liter. Symptoms may include lethargy, confusion, coma, tachycardia, and hypotension.

Severe cases of hyponatremia are treated with intravenous sodium chloride (NaCl). The most common solutions are 0.9% NaCl and 0.45% NaCl. The 0.9% NaCl solution is often referred to as normal saline. This is because it closely resembles the amount of NaCl in the body. The 0.45% NaCl solution, because it is exactly half of normal saline, is referred to as half-strength saline.

These solutions are often used in combination with other solutions or electrolytes. Because of sodium's role in fluid balance, be aware of any signs or symptoms of circulatory edema, pulmonary edema, or peripheral edema.

Hypernatremia

Hypernatremia is an overload of sodium in the body and is usually seen only in supplemental overdose. Symptoms may include dehydration, thirst, oliguria, and stupor.

COMBINATION SOLUTIONS

In addition to the combination of saline and dextrose 5% in water with other electrolytes, a solution that combines several electrolytes is used. Ringer's lactated (or lactated Ringer's) solution is used to replace both fluid and electrolytes for extracellular volume depletion. It is made of 600 mg sodium chloride, 310 mg sodium lactate, 20 mg calcium chloride, 30 mg potassium chloride, and 100 mL of sterile distilled water.

Because of the large amounts of electrolytes, Ringer's lactated solution should not be used for patients with kidney failure, congestive heart failure, or hypoproteinemia. Assess the patient frequently for signs of fluid and electrolyte overload.

PHOSPHATE BINDERS

Phosphate binders are not electrolytes but rather work to remove a particular electrolyte. Patients with end-stage renal disease often retain phosphates. Phosphates are plentiful in our daily diets and are virtually impossible to eliminate. Aluminum hydroxide is used to bind with the phosphate in foods.

N U R S I N G   A L E R T

▼▼▼▼▼▼▼▼▼▼▼▼▼▼▼▼▼▼▼▼▼▼▼▼▼▼▼▼▼▼▼▼

Aluminum hydroxide must be given with meals, however, or it will not be present when absorption of the phosphates occurs. Giving the medication to the patient immediately after eating is too late.

▲▲▲▲▲▲▲▲▲▲▲▲▲▲▲▲▲▲▲▲▲▲▲▲▲▲▲▲▲▲▲▲

Aluminum hydroxide is found in Amphojel and Dialume. These are also classed as antacids.

E X E R C I S E S

CASE STUDIES

1. Your patient is taking a diuretic. The physician prescribes a potassium supplement to be given orally. The physician also states to encourage high-potassium foods. What foods could you include in the patient's diet if he dislikes oranges and bananas? What assessments would you make while the patient is receiving this medication?

2. Your patient has periodic arterial blood gas determinations. What would your analysis of the following results be?

   a. pH   7.51
      P_{CO_2} 54
      HCO_3^- 31
   b. pH   7.22
      P_{CO_2} 55
      HCO_3^- 32
   c. pH   7.41
      P_{CO_2} 32
      HCO_3^- 20
   d. pH   7.27
      P_{CO_2} 36
      HCO_3^- 19
   e. pH   7.33
      P_{CO_2} 133
      HCO_3^- 33

3. Mr. T.U. has been admitted with a diagnosis of fluid and electrolyte imbalance. He has an IV running with Ringer's lactated solution infusing. What assessment responsibilities do you have?

4. Ms. C.F. had a thyroidectomy 4 days ago. Today, as you are doing your morning assessment, Ms. C.F. casually mentions that her lips "feel funny." What is an appropriate response? Explain your rationale.

MENTAL AEROBICS

1. Demonstrate to a classmate the assessment of Chvostek's sign. Explain the rationale for assessing this sign. Discuss the meaning of the sign's presence.

2. Role play a patient experiencing the beginning signs of hypokalemia. Have a classmate role play advanced signs of hypokalemia. Discuss interventions that might be used.

3. Role play the teaching you would do for a patient who is taking baking soda at home for indigestion. Have a classmate role play the patient who is having difficulty comprehending your teaching. Have your study group critique the interaction. Was the teaching thorough? Do they have any suggestions for alternative approaches to use in a situation similar to this?

DIURETICS

L E A R N I N G   O B J E C T I V E S

After studying this chapter, you should be able to:

1. Define diuretic, osmotic, thiazide, carbonic anhydrase inhibitor, potassium sparing, acidifying agent, xanthine, and loop.

2. Identify the actions and uses of and adverse reactions to diurectics in general and each specific subclassification.

3. State common examples of each subclassification of diuretics.

4. State appropriate nursing implications for patients receiving diuretics in general and each specific subclassification.

5. Demonstrate how to administer diuretics by use of the nursing process.

DRUGS YOU WILL LEARN ABOUT IN THIS CHAPTER

Osmotic Diuretics

mannitol (Osmitrol)

urea (Urevert)

Thiazide Diuretics

chlorothiazide (Diuril)

hydrochlorothiazide (HydroDIURIL, HCTZ, Esidrix)

methyclothiazide (Enduron)

Carbonic Anhydrase Inhibitors

acetazolamide (Diamox)

Potassium-Sparing Diuretics

spironolactone (Aldactone)

triamterene (Dyrenium)

Acidifying Agents

ammonium chloride

Xanthines

aminophylline

theophylline

Loop Diuretics

bumetanide (Bumex)

ethacrynic acid (Edecrin)

furosemide (Lasix)

Combination Drugs

amiloride and hydrochlorothiazide (Moduretic)

spironolactone and hydrochlorothiazide (Aldactazide)

triamterene 50 mg and hydrochlorothiazide 25 mg (Dyazide)

triamterene 75 mg and hydrochlorothiazide 50 mg (Maxzide)

triamterene 37.5 mg and hydrochlorothiazide 25 mg (Maxzide-25)

ACTIONS AND USES Diuretics are a class of drugs that ▲▲▲▲▲▲▲▲▲▲▲▲▲▲▲▲ promote elimination of excess fluid. Most diuretics act on the convoluted tubule. They are generally used to help treat diseases associated with fluid retention, such as kidney disease, hypertension, congestive heart disease, liver disease, eclampsia in pregnancy, and certain types of toxic drug effects (such as with steroids).

Mild edema is usually treated with milder oral diuretics. More severe edema often needs more potent diuretics delivered by different routes. These are generalized statements, and like all generalized statements, they cannot be assumed to be correct in all cases.

ASSESSMENT Many diuretics can cause electrolyte imbalances. For this reason, the nurse administering diuretics must be familiar with signs and symptoms of disturbances of electrolyte levels (see Chapter 46). Also monitor serum electrolyte reports as they come in.

Whenever a patient is prescribed a diuretic, automatically initiate intake and output monitoring. Weigh the patient daily at the same time, in the same type of clothing, and on the same scale. Also assess the patient for any signs of dehydration. Teach the patient what symptoms to look for because many patients go home on diuretic therapy.

PLANNING AND IMPLEMENTATION Caution your patient who is receiving diuretic therapy that the urge to void will occur more frequently. Many people do not understand this when they are prescribed a "water pill." If the patient has an indwelling catheter, be prepared to empty the collection bag more often. It should be emptied no later than when it is half-full.

Some of the diuretics can cause postural or orthostatic hypotension, leading to dizziness and falls. Make sure that your patient knows where the call light is, that the call light is close to the patient, and that you answer the call light promptly.

Some diuretics can cause a loss of potency. Be sure you address the subject of sexuality with your patients. Many patients are embarrassed to raise the subject but will gladly ask questions if you bring it up.

If your assessment of the patient indicates possible electrolyte imbalance, withhold the drug at its next dose and contact the physician. Be prepared to relay pertinent serum electrolyte reports to the physician.

If a diuretic is being given intravenously (IV), assess not only the rate but also the rhythm of the heart. IV diuretics can cause arrhythmias, some of them fatal.

Many diuretics are scheduled to be taken just once a day. Stress the importance of taking the medication exactly as directed. Some patients stop taking the medication when visible signs of edema are lessened. You can recommend methods to help the patient remember to take the medication. Calendars can be marked when the pill has been taken. Pill boxes are available with spaces marked for each day of the week.

The correct dosage is placed into each cavity at the beginning of the week. The patient need only look at the day's space to see if a pill still remains to be taken. Some pill boxes even come with alarms that sound if the box is not opened by a certain time each day!

Some patients experience sleep disturbances when diuretic therapy is initiated. This reaction often goes away on its own; but you may need to use methods to promote sleep until it does. Also, schedule the medication early in the day to prevent or reduce sleep disturbance due to nighttime voiding.

EVALUATION You can evaluate the effectiveness of diuretic therapy by continuing assessments of the patient's weight, blood pressure, heart rate, ease of breathing, breath sounds, abdominal girth, and dependent edema. You should also be evaluating for any signs of adverse reactions, including electrolyte imbalance.

OSMOTIC DIURETICS

Mannitol and Urea

ACTIONS AND USES The osmotic diuretics mannitol (Osmitrol) and urea (Urevert) prevent selective reabsorption of water, sodium, and chloride. They are used most often in the treatment of oliguria and anuria as well as for increased intracranial pressure.

ASSESSMENT Monitor the patient's intake and output. In the case of oliguria or anuria, a device placed on the catheter above the collection bag is necessary to measure the urine exactly.

Assess your patient's level of consciousness and orientation if the drug is being used to treat increased intracranial pressure.

PLANNING AND IMPLEMENTATION Patients requiring treatment for oliguria, anuria, or increased intracranial pressure are most often in a critical care unit. Frequent monitoring of the patient's condition is vital. Serum electrolyte levels must be reported promptly.

Also report any signs of electrolyte imbalance or adverse reactions, such as headache, nausea, or changes in the blood pressure.

EVALUATION Evaluation of effectiveness of the drug depends on the disorder being treated. If the patient was oliguric or anuric, continued assessment of output establishes effectiveness. Improved alertness and orientation show effectiveness if increased intracranial pressure was the problem.

THIAZIDE DIURETICS

Chlorothiazide, Hydrochlorothiazide, and Methyclothiazide

ACTIONS AND USES Thiazide diuretics depress the ▲▲▲▲▲▲▲▲▲▲▲▲▲▲▲ ability of the convoluted tubules to reabsorb sodium and chloride. A saying will help you to remember that this also means fluid will be excreted. "Where goes water, so goes sodium. Where goes sodium, so goes water."

N U R S I N G   A L E R T
▼▼▼▼▼▼▼▼▼▼▼▼▼▼▼▼▼▼▼▼▼▼▼▼▼▼▼▼▼▼▼▼▼▼

Thiazide diuretics are likely to cause electrolyte imbalances, especially loss of potassium, bicarbonate, and magnesium, and retention of calcium. Serum uric acid levels and serum glucose levels can also be elevated.

▲▲▲▲▲▲▲▲▲▲▲▲▲▲▲▲▲▲▲▲▲▲▲▲▲▲▲▲▲▲▲▲▲▲

The patient may complain of gastrointestinal upset, urticaria, muscle spasm, blurred vision, and headache. You may note an elevated temperature, signs of dehydration, and a rash. Thiazide diuretics may also cause blood dyscrasias and renal dysfunction.

ASSESSMENT In addition to the assessments recom-
▲▲▲▲▲▲▲▲▲▲ mended for all diuretics, assess the patient's ability to produce urine before initiating thiazide diuretics. Anuria is a contraindication to use of thiazide diuretics.

N U R S I N G   A L E R T
▼▼▼▼▼▼▼▼▼▼▼▼▼▼▼▼▼▼▼▼▼▼▼▼▼▼▼▼▼▼▼▼▼

Also be aware of the patient's medical history. Patients with bronchial asthma are more likely to be sensitive to thiazide diuretics.

▲▲▲▲▲▲▲▲▲▲▲▲▲▲▲▲▲▲▲▲▲▲▲▲▲▲▲▲▲▲▲▲▲

PLANNING AND IMPLEMENTATION Chlorothiazide (Di-
▲▲▲▲▲▲▲▲▲▲▲▲▲▲▲▲▲▲▲▲▲▲▲▲▲ uril) is supplied as tablets and liquid and is administered orally. The usual dose is 0.5 to 1.0 g every other day, every day, or twice a day. Hydrochlorothiazide (HydroDIURIL, Esidrix, HCTZ) is supplied as tablets and given orally. (HCTZ is the abbreviation for the generic hydrochlo-

rothiazide.) The dosage is about 1/10 that of chlorothiazide or about 50 to 100 mg every other day, every day, or twice a day. Methyclothiazide (Enduron), also supplied as tablets and given orally, is generally prescribed at 2.5 to 10 mg every day.

If the patient is taking insulin or oral hypoglycemics, be sure the physician is aware of this. The dosage of these medications may need to be adjusted when a patient is prescribed thiazides.

If tests of parathyroid function are ordered for your patient who is taking thiazides, the thiazides must be discontinued. Be sure to notify the physician so this order can be given.

EVALUATION Effectiveness of the drug is established
▲▲▲▲▲▲▲▲▲▲ by decreased blood pressure, clear breath sounds, absence of edema, and adequate urine output.

Thiazide diuretics interact with many medications. When thiazides are given with other antihypertensive agents, the effects of both are potentiated. Concurrent use with alcohol, barbiturates, and other narcotics may increase the chances of orthostatic hypotension. Electrolyte loss, especially of potassium, is more likely if thiazides are given with steroids or corticotropin. Skeletal muscle relaxants have increased effectiveness.

N U R S I N G   A L E R T
▼▼▼▼▼▼▼▼▼▼▼▼▼▼▼▼▼▼▼▼▼▼▼▼▼▼▼▼▼▼▼▼▼

When given with lithium, a thiazide diuretic may increase the patient's chances for lithium toxicity.

▲▲▲▲▲▲▲▲▲▲▲▲▲▲▲▲▲▲▲▲▲▲▲▲▲▲▲▲▲▲▲▲▲▲

Concomitant use of nonsteroidal anti-inflammatory drugs (NSAIDs) may reduce the effects of the thiazide diuretic.

As thiazide therapy continues, monitor serum cholesterol and triglyceride levels. These may be increased with thiazide therapy. Also monitor serum uric acid levels. Hyperuricemia or symptoms of acute gout may be precipitated by thiazides. Evaluate your patient for signs and symptoms of systemic lupus erythematosus because activation or exacerbation of this disorder is possible.

CARBONIC ANHYDRASE INHIBITORS

Acetazolamide

ACTIONS AND USES Carbonic anhydrase is an enzyme
▲▲▲▲▲▲▲▲▲▲▲▲▲▲▲▲ that prevents the excretion of sodium by the kidneys. Therefore, medications that

inhibit this enzyme promote the excretion of sodium, and water is excreted with it. Potassium and bicarbonate are also lost.

Carbonic anhydrase inhibitors are usually used for glaucoma, seizures, and alkalosis.

These drugs may cause complaints of anorexia, nausea, and vomiting. The patient may experience drowsiness, numbness or tingling of extremities, blurred vision, and blood dyscrasias. Renal stone formation can be precipitated by this drug. Serum glucose and serum uric acid levels may be elevated. Metabolic acidosis may occur with acetazolamide therapy because it does not allow carbonic acid to break down.

ASSESSMENT If the drug is being given for increased ▲▲▲▲▲▲▲▲▲▲ intraocular pressure, assess your patient's vision for clarity. Ask about the level of eye discomfort.

If the drug is being given as an anticonvulsant, be aware of the type of seizures the patient experiences. Ask the patient about events that precipitate the seizure. Assess the level of consciousness and orientation.

N U R S I N G   A L E R T
▼▼▼▼▼▼▼▼▼▼▼▼▼▼▼▼▼▼▼▼▼▼▼▼▼▼▼▼▼▼

Because this drug is a sulfonamide, be sure to ask your patient about allergies to "sulfa" drugs.

▲▲▲▲▲▲▲▲▲▲▲▲▲▲▲▲▲▲▲▲▲▲▲▲▲▲▲▲▲▲

If the patient has a history of respiratory disorders or diabetes mellitus, bring this to the attention of the physician because these disorders can be affected by the drug.

PLANNING AND IMPLEMENTATION Acetazolamide (Di-▲▲▲▲▲▲▲▲▲▲▲▲▲▲▲▲▲▲▲▲▲▲▲▲▲ amox) can be given orally, intramuscularly (IM), or intravenously (IV). The usual oral dose is 250 to 1000 mg. The usual dose for the IM or IV route is 250 to 500 mg. Regardless of the route of administration, the dose can be divided into as many as four doses. Oral preparations may need to be given with food to decrease gastrointestinal upset. Tablets may not be crushed or chewed. IM injection of this drug is painful. Therefore, the IV route is more often used, and the drug is often diluted in another solution, such as dextrose 5% in water.

Be sure the patient knows to report any adverse reactions. If drowsiness occurs with use of the drug, caution the patient to avoid the use of hazardous machinery or driving until the effect is alleviated.

If the drug is being used for treatment of seizures, initiate seizure precautions. Caution the patient to continue therapy and not to stop taking the drug without consulting the physician. Seizures will recur, and sudden stoppage can lead to status epilepticus.

EVALUATION Evaluate the patient for increased or ▲▲▲▲▲▲▲▲▲▲ decreased eye discomfort and visual acuity. Document any seizure activity and report it immediately. Monitor serum electrolyte and blood gas levels.

POTASSIUM-SPARING DIURETICS

We address the potassium-sparing diuretics separately because they achieve their actions in different ways.

Spironolactone

ACTIONS AND USES Spironolactone (Aldactone) is an ▲▲▲▲▲▲▲▲▲▲▲▲▲▲▲▲ antagonist of aldosterone. Aldosterone is a steroid that promotes sodium reabsorption. Therefore, spironolactone causes sodium to be excreted, taking the water with it.

Fluid and electrolyte imbalances are common with spironolactone, but it does not cause hypokalemia. Gastric upset, headache, drowsiness, and rash are fairly common adverse reactions. It is also possible that the patient may experience blood dyscrasias and hyperkalemia. Sexuality may be altered in the patient receiving spironolactone. This can include impotence, irregular menses, postmenopausal bleeding, gynecomastia, and other abnormal secondary sexual characteristics.

N U R S I N G   A L E R T
▼▼▼▼▼▼▼▼▼▼▼▼▼▼▼▼▼▼▼▼▼▼▼▼▼▼▼▼▼▼

Spironolactone has been demonstrated to cause tumors. Therefore, it is used only when deemed absolutely necessary.

▲▲▲▲▲▲▲▲▲▲▲▲▲▲▲▲▲▲▲▲▲▲▲▲▲▲▲▲▲▲

Spironolactone may be used for primary hyperaldosteronism, hypokalemia, and hypertension. It may also be used to prevent hypokalemia in patients taking digitalis because this can precipitate digitalis toxicity.

ASSESSMENT Be familiar with the patient's medical history. Spironolactone is contraindicated in acute renal insufficiency, hyperkalemia, and anuria. Assessments could include perusal of the chart, monitoring of serum electrolyte levels, and assessment of the patient's ability to produce urine.

PLANNING AND IMPLEMENTATION At a usual dose of 25 to 400 mg daily, spironolactone is supplied in tablets and given orally.

N U R S I N G   A L E R T

Spironolactone should not be given with potassium supplements or with other potassium-sparing diuretics.

Be sure your patient is familiar with the signs and symptoms of hyperkalemia. Teach the patient how to take the pulse and evaluate for irregularity.

EVALUATION Effectiveness of this drug can be demonstrated by improved blood pressure and dependent edema. Monitor serum potassium levels.

N U R S I N G   A L E R T

If the patient is taking digoxin, monitor the serum levels of this drug because concurrent use of digoxin and spironolactone may precipitate digitalis toxicity.

Spironolactone also potentiates other diuretics and antihypertensives. Hyperkalemia may be more pronounced if spironolactone is given together with indomethacin (Indocin).

Triamterene

ACTIONS AND USES Triamterene (Dyrenium) is used to treat many of the same disorders as spironolactone is. However, it achieves its actions by depressing sodium reabsorption, potassium excretion, and hydrogen ion excretion. Therefore, the body loses sodium and water while retaining potassium and hydrogen.

N U R S I N G   A L E R T

This can lead to hyperkalemia and metabolic acidosis. Triamterene can also cause the serum glucose level to rise.

The patient may complain of a rash, gastrointestinal upset, weakness, dizziness, and headache. Laboratory reports may show blood dyscrasias.

ASSESSMENT Assess the patient's ability to produce urine before initiating triamterene because anuria, kidney disease, and kidney dysfunction are contraindications. Triamterene should also not be given if the patient has a history of liver disease or laboratory reports demonstrate hyperkalemia. Monitor serum potassium levels frequently. Also monitor blood gas levels to note metabolic acidosis.

PLANNING AND IMPLEMENTATION Triamterene is supplied in capsules and given orally. The usual dose is 100 mg twice a day.

N U R S I N G   A L E R T

Do not give triamterene with potassium supplements or other potassium-sparing diuretics.

Be especially alert to hidden sources of potassium, such as potassium-containing medications (penicillin G, for example) or any potassium-containing foods (salt substitutes and low-salt products, for example).

If the patient receiving triamterene is also diabetic, be sure to notify the physician. Adjustment of insulin or oral hypoglycemics may be necessary while this diuretic is being taken.

EVALUATION Effectiveness of this drug is demonstrated by improved blood pressure, decreased evidence of edema from all body cavities, and stabilization of potassium levels.

N U R S I N G   A L E R T

Careful evaluation of the patient's status is necessary if triamterene is given in conjunction with lithium. Monitor the serum lithium levels frequently because lithium toxicity may be precipitated.

Use of triamterene with indomethacin may cause acute renal failure. Evaluate the patient's ability to produce urine or any signs or symptoms of renal failure. Use with chlorpropamide increases the risk of hyponatremia. Add sodium to the serum electrolyte levels you monitor.

ACIDIFYING AGENTS

Ammonium Chloride

ACTIONS AND USES Ammonium chloride causes a temporary diuresis that lasts approximately 1 to 2 days. The kidney excretes greater than normal amounts of sodium and water, but body mechanisms compensate for the actions of ammonium chloride and reverse after the 1 to 2 days.

Ammonium chloride is more often used to acidify the urine. It may be useful to prevent the adverse reaction of crystalluria when the patient is receiving sulfonamide drugs. Ammonium chloride may also be used to cause expectoration.

Ammonium chloride can cause gastrointestinal upsets. It is also possible that the patient may exhibit symptoms of electrolyte imbalances, especially of potassium, calcium, and magnesium. Acidosis can result from prolonged use or overdosage.

ASSESSMENT In addition to the usual baseline assessments you make for all diuretics, be aware of the patient's latest laboratory results of electrolyte and blood gas levels.

N U R S I N G   A L E R T

Monitor for signs of acidosis, such as shortness of breath and respiratory depression.

PLANNING AND IMPLEMENTATION Ammonium chloride is given orally. Monitor electrolyte and arterial blood gas levels throughout ammonium chloride therapy. Keep careful track of intake and output. Immediately report when a decrease of output occurs.

EVALUATION Effectiveness of this drug is demonstrated by increased urine output and decreased fluid retention in all body cavities.

If the patient is also receiving aspirin therapy, monitor the patient's level of pain. Concurrent administration can slow the use of aspirin and can also lead to crystalluria.

Be especially alert for signs of acidosis if the patient is also taking spironolactone. The effectiveness of both drugs is decreased if ammonium chloride is used together with tricyclic antidepressants or amphetamines.

XANTHINES

Theophylline and Aminophylline

Xanthines are primarily classified as bronchodilators. Because they increase the blood flow through the kidneys and increase sodium and chloride excretion, xanthines also produce a mild diuresis. Therefore, you will often see them used for pulmonary edema or congestive heart failure, when they perform two duties at once—that of diuresis and that of bronchodilation.

The xanthines can cause gastric upset, diarrhea, irritability, restlessness, dehydration, and postural hypotension. Persons who are prescribed these drugs may need to be provided with an outlet for excess energy.

Theophylline and aminophylline are closely related. Theophylline is supplied as capsules or liquid and given orally. Aminophylline is supplied as tablets given orally or is administered by intravenous injection.

N U R S I N G   A L E R T

Monitor serum theophylline levels as they return from the laboratory. The therapeutic range is 10 to 20 µg/mL. Levels above 20 µg/mL can cause toxicity.

If additional laboratory tests are done while the patient is receiving a xanthine, be aware that these drugs can cause false-positive serum uric acid elevations. Uric acid is used for the diagnostic test of gouty arthritis (or gout).

For additional information on these drugs, see Chapter 50.

LOOP DIURETICS

Furosemide, Ethacrynic Acid, and Bumetanide

ACTIONS AND USES The loop diuretics are the strongest acting drugs of this classification. In fact, they are sometimes referred to as the high-potency diuretics. They are also very fast acting. For example, furosemide (Lasix) has its maximal effect about 1 hour after an oral dose is given and lasts about 4 hours. Intravenous doses act even faster.

The loop diuretics work on the loop of Henle and inhibit the reabsorption of sodium. As our saying goes, the water goes along with the sodium.

Because these diuretics are quick and strong, they are often used in emergency situations, such as severe exacerbations of congestive heart failure symptoms. By decreasing edema, especially pulmonary edema, they ease breathing.

The loop diuretics can also cause severe adverse reactions.

N U R S I N G   A L E R T
▼▼▼▼▼▼▼▼▼▼▼▼▼▼▼▼▼▼▼▼▼▼▼▼▼▼▼▼▼▼▼▼▼

Electrolyte imbalances are common, especially of potassium and sodium.

▲▲▲▲▲▲▲▲▲▲▲▲▲▲▲▲▲▲▲▲▲▲▲▲▲▲▲▲▲▲▲▲▲

Serum calcium concentration can also be decreased and cause tetany.

The loss of fluid from the loop diuretics can be dramatic.

N U R S I N G   A L E R T
▼▼▼▼▼▼▼▼▼▼▼▼▼▼▼▼▼▼▼▼▼▼▼▼▼▼▼▼▼▼▼▼▼

Dehydration so severe can arise that the patient is at risk for development of a thrombus or an embolus or of going into hepatic coma.

▲▲▲▲▲▲▲▲▲▲▲▲▲▲▲▲▲▲▲▲▲▲▲▲▲▲▲▲▲▲▲▲▲

The loop diuretics can also cause gastrointestinal upsets, jaundice, dizziness, rash, headache, blurred vision, blood dyscrasias, hyperglycemia, photosensitivity, orthostatic hypotension, and weakness.

The loop diuretics are also ototoxic. The patient may complain of tinnitus and experience hearing loss.

ASSESSMENT Know the purpose of the drug being
▲▲▲▲▲▲▲▲▲▲ given. Is the patient experiencing dyspnea? Is severe hypertension the problem? Take baseline assessments related to the patient's problem.

In addition, check the patient's history for any liver dysfunction or abnormal liver function test results. The loop diuretics are to be used with caution if the patient has cirrhosis. Check also for a history of diabetes or hyperglycemia because of the effects of the loop diuretics on the serum glucose level.

PLANNING AND IMPLEMENTATION Furosemide (Lasix)
▲▲▲▲▲▲▲▲▲▲▲▲▲▲▲▲▲▲▲▲▲▲▲▲▲▲▲▲ can be given orally, as either tablets or liquid, or intramuscularly (IM) or intravenously (IV). Ethacrynic acid (Edecrin) is given either orally or IV. Bumetanide (Bumex) can be given by mouth, IM, or IV. Table 47–1 lists usual doses of the loop diuretics.

Plan to encourage a diet high in potassium-rich foods. Explain to the patient the importance of eating these foods every day while taking a loop diuretic. The physician may also order potassium supplements or an aldosterone antagonist, such as triamterene. Use of these can decrease the risk of hypokalemia as well as of metabolic alkalosis.

Caution your patient about the risk of falling because of postural hypotension. Have the call light close at hand and urge the patient to use it before getting up. Answer the light promptly to prevent the patient from trying to get out of bed alone.

Table 47–1. Usual Doses of Loop Diuretics

DRUG	DOSAGE		
	PO	IM	IV
bumetanide (Bumex)	0.5–2.0 mg/day	0.5–1.0 mg/day	0.5–1.0 mg/day
ethacrynic acid (Edecrin)	50–200 mg/day	—	50–100 mg/day
furosemide (Lasix)	20–80 mg/day	20–80 mg/day	20–80 mg/day

EVALUATION To evaluate the effectiveness of these
▲▲▲▲▲▲▲▲▲▲ drugs, reassess and compare your findings with the baseline data. Are breath sounds clearer? Is the patient breathing more easily? Has the blood pressure come down? Is dependent edema decreased? Again, these evaluative observations are individualized to the patient and the presenting problem.

Monitor the patient's serum electrolyte, carbon dioxide, blood urea nitrogen, and serum glucose levels.

Look for interactions with other drugs the patient may be prescribed. The loop diuretics given together may produce adverse reactions that are more intense, especially ototoxic effects. Given with salicylates, they may lead to salicylism. With aminoglycoside antibiotics, the patient is again at higher risk for ototoxic effects. Toxic effects of lithium may develop sooner in the patient receiving lithium and a loop diuretic. Antihypertensives and the loop diuretics potentiate each other. The effect of the loop diuretics is decreased if they are given with indomethacin or other nonsteroidal anti-inflammatory drugs (NSAIDs). In addition, bumetanide is antagonistic to probenecid, a drug used to treat gout.

COMBINATION DRUGS

Many diuretics are combinations of the subgroups. They are given together to supplement each other's actions or to decrease the chance of adverse reactions.

Aldactazide

Aldactazide is a combination of spironolactone and hydrochlorothiazide (HCTZ) in equal proportions. Remember that spironolactone is tumorigenic. Aldactazide is supplied in tablets.

Dyazide

Dyazide is a combination of 50 mg of triamterene and 25 mg of HCTZ. These are given together to decrease the risk of hypokalemia, but the patient then has an increased risk of hyperkalemia. Dyazide is given orally.

Maxzide

Maxzide is also a combination of triamterene and HCTZ, but it comes in two different doses. Maxzide is 75 mg of triamterene and 50 mg of HCTZ. Maxzide-25 is 37.5 mg of triamterene and 25 mg of HCTZ.

Moduretic

Moduretic is a combination of HCTZ and amiloride hydrochloride. Amiloride is a weak diuretic classed as a potassium sparer.

Assess your patient for urine output because anuria is a contraindication to the use of this drug. It should also not be used with other potassium-sparing diuretics or if the patient has hyperkalemia.

Use caution, and monitor the patient more closely, if there is a history of diabetes, electrolyte imbalances, respiratory or metabolic acidosis, or an increased blood urea nitrogen concentration.

Adverse reactions include hyperkalemia, weakness, gastrointestinal upset, headache, rash, and dizziness.

E X E R C I S E S

CASE STUDIES

1. Your patient has recently been prescribed a diuretic. When you approach her at 8 AM, she states that she wants to wait until lunchtime to take her medication. What would be your best response to this? Why?

2. Your patient explains that the reason she wants to take her medication at lunchtime is because she did not sleep well last night. In fact, she has not slept well for the last few nights. What is your best response to this?

3. The diuretic your patient has been prescribed can cause hypokalemia. The physician has suggested a high-potassium diet. What foods can you recommend to her?

4. Your patient mentions that she had an episode of gout about a year ago. What would you expect to be the least likely diuretic that she is taking?

5. Your patient begins having trouble with hypokalemia. What assessments should you make? What diuretics might you expect the physician to try if the decision is made to change her medication?

MENTAL AEROBICS

The following poem can be used to help you remember some of the information about diuretics. The authors invite you to add stanzas of your own and suggest that you say the poem to a "rap" beat.

The Water Pill Blues

I was sitting in my schoolroom chair.
I was learning my lessons, really, I swear!
Then I heard a voice explain a way
To remember diuretics on examination day.

So many types, so many facts!
A trick to make up for what my memory lacks.
These water pills, they aren't so bad
They help you get rid of all the fluid you had.

"Whither thou goest, I'll go too."
Sodium and water, two by two.
Potassium says, "I'll tag along,
Out of the body," but that's all wrong.

Thiazides and loops help kick the K out
Don't take these if you have the gout.
Aldactone, Dyrenium, they spare the K
But they each work in their own special way.

Don't take your pill late in the day
It'll keep you up in three different ways.
Enuresis and nocturia, they're not the same
And insomnia comes, but it goes away.

This pill might also let a guy down
When he's near his lady in a low-cut gown.
He's got the will, he's got the desire,
But this water pill put out his fire.

Lasix and theophylline will get the water out
  of your lungs so then you can sing and shout.
But be careful of theophylline, she doesn't work
  before 10
And at 20 she can poison the strongest of men.

His blood sugar's up but you say "never mind"
It's all because of your chlorothiazide.
Hydro packs a bigger punch
But it's still related to the entire bunch.

If you've got some swelling in your head
Mannitol might keep you from being dead.
When your kidneys stop, you need them fixed quick
Osmotic diuretics might do the trick.

Dyrenium and Diamox don't fiddle around
They kick the base out 'til he can't be found.
Ammonium chloride will do it too
But you only void a lot for a day or two.

These aren't so bad, they aren't so hard
I just needed my memory jarred.
You take it from here, I'm out of time
But worse than that, I'm out of rhymes.

*   *   *

CHAPTER 48

URINARY ANALGESICS AND URINARY ANTISEPTICS

Urinary analgesics relieve the symptoms of urinary tract infection (UTI), and urinary antiseptics are aimed specifically at treating the cause of a UTI. Combination drugs address both the symptoms and the cause of the UTI.

URINARY ANALGESICS

Phenazopyridine Hydrochloride

ACTIONS AND USES Phenazopyridine hydrochloride (Pyridium), a form of azo dye, is the most common urinary analgesic. It does not decrease the bacterial count but does lessen the pain and burning associated with a urinary tract infection. Urinary analgesics may also be prescribed after urinary tract surgery, trauma, or endoscopy and after removal of a urinary catheter.

Adverse reactions are usually mild but include a headache, rash, pruritus, gastric upset, and red-orange urine.

ASSESSMENT Be aware of what symptoms the patient has had. You should also check the chart for and ask the patient about decreased kidney function. Renal insufficiency is a contraindication to the use of azo dyes.

PLANNING AND IMPLEMENTATION Phenazopyridine hydrochloride is supplied in tablets. The usual dose is 200 mg given three times a day. It exhibits a topical action. You will often see it prescribed with antibacterial agents, especially sulfa drugs, but its use is recommended for only 2 days—the time interval before antibacterial agents begin to control infection and the symptoms. If the patient has been receiving the drug for longer than this, bring it to the physician's attention.

Because azo dyes can cause red-orange urine and other body fluids, remember to warn the patient about this.

It can be frightening to experience this reaction without prior knowledge of the cause. Warn patients, too, that this drug can stain fabrics, so they should wear protection between themselves and clothing in the perineal area. Azo dye can also stain contact lenses. Caution your patient to wear glasses until after the reaction is gone.

Be aware also that the drug can skew the results of a urinalysis. Many of these tests are based on color readings. Because the drug is a dye, it can change these colors. If urinalysis is ordered, bring this to the attention of the physician.

EVALUATION Ask your patient often about the continuation of presenting symptoms. Is there still urgency, burning, or pain? How often is the patient voiding?

Observe the patient's skin carefully. A yellow cast to the skin may mean that the drug is not being excreted.

If this occurs, the physician will stop the drug. This problem happens more frequently in older age groups.

URINARY ANTISEPTICS

Methenamine Mandelate

ACTIONS AND USES Methenamine mandelate (Mandelamine) is an antibacterial agent. It is used to treat different types of urinary tract infections (UTIs), such as pyelonephritis and cystitis, and chronic UTIs. It can also be prescribed prophylactically to prevent recurrences. It is effective against both gram-positive and gram-negative organisms.

This drug works best in an acidic urine. The pH of the urine needs to be 5.5 or less.

Adverse reactions from methenamine mandelate are unusual but also usually mild. They can include gastrointestinal upset, rash, or rarely hematuria. Large doses can lead to dysuria. Elderly and debilitated patients are at risk for lipid pneumonia from this drug.

ASSESSMENT Maintain accurate intake and output records for the patient. Check the chart for and ask the patient about kidney dysfunction because the drug is contraindicated in renal insufficiency.

Assess breath sounds frequently. Ask about pain on urination. Monitor the pH of the patient's urine.

PLANNING AND IMPLEMENTATION Methenamine mandelate is supplied as tablets, suspension, and granules. Granules are to be dissolved, 1 packet in 2 to 4 ounces of water. Do not make up the solution ahead of time. Mix just before administration. The solution should be cloudy. Always shake the solution well before administration.

To maintain an acidic urine, restrict alkalinizing foods from your patient's diet. Encourage instead foods that are known to acidify the urine, such as meats, eggs, cheese, cranberries, plums, prunes, nuts, legumes, and cereals. Be careful to note any contraindications to any of these foods. (For example, you would not encourage eggs for a patient on a low-cholesterol diet.)

The physician will no doubt restrict the use of alkalinizing medications. It may be necessary with some patients for the physician to prescribe an acidifying agent. A common one is ammonium chloride. Remember that this drug also acts as a temporary diuretic.

EVALUATION Ask the patient about relief of symptoms. Monitor results of microscopic urinalysis for improvement.

Be aware that methenamine mandelate can interact with sulfamethizole (Thiosulfil Forte) and is usually not given with it.

Potassium Permanganate

Potassium permanganate ($KMnO_4$) is an oxidizing agent. (Remember that hydrogen peroxide is also an oxidizing agent.)

Potassium permanganate should be purple before you use it.

It exhibits its action by losing an oxygen molecule to become $KMnO_3$. When it loses the oxygen molecule, the solution turns brown. It is the free oxygen that is antibacterial. Therefore, if a solution of potassium permanganate has turned brown on the shelf, it is useless.

Potassium permanganate is occasionally used for bladder irrigations.

N U R S I N G   A L E R T

▼▼▼▼▼▼▼▼▼▼▼▼▼▼▼▼▼▼▼▼▼▼▼▼▼▼▼▼▼▼▼▼▼▼▼▼▼

Potassium permanganate should not be used in solutions stronger than 1:5000 ratio.

▲▲

Warn patients that the solution will stain clothing and other inanimate objects. They should wear protection.

Benzalkonium Chloride

Benzalkonium chloride (Zephiran) is a surface-acting agent. (Soap is also a surface-acting agent.) It is occasionally used for bladder irrigations, but it is no longer used regularly.

COMBINATION MEDICATIONS

Azo-Mandelamine

Azo-Mandelamine combines the analgesic qualities of azo dye and the antiseptic qualities of methenamine mandelate. Adverse reactions include gastrointestinal upsets, rash, headache, pruritus, and red-orange urine. Your responsibilities include those for both drugs.

E X E R C I S E S

CASE STUDIES

1. Mr. R.T. is your patient and has been prescribed Azo-Mandelamine for a urinary tract infection. What are your responsibilities?

2. A bladder irrigation using potassium permanganate has been ordered for your patient. Review the procedure for a bladder irrigation. Describe your responsibilities specific to the use of potassium permanganate.

UNIT TEN

DRUGS THAT AFFECT THE RESPIRATORY SYSTEM

The respiratory system consists of the

- Lungs, alveoli, pleura, and bronchi (Fig. X–1)
- Diaphragm and intercostal muscles
- Pharynx, larynx, tonsils, nose, and mouth

Respiration involves the exchange of oxygen and carbon dioxide between the alveoli and the blood. Each alveolus is surrounded by tiny capillaries, arterioles, and venules. Once oxygen enters the bloodstream, it is carried on a portion of the blood called hemoglobin. Carbon dioxide is carried in the blood as bicarbonate and carbonic acid. Control of respirations is centered in the medulla oblongata. This center reacts to changes in the concentration of carbon dioxide and oxygen in the blood.

The internal areas of the respiratory system are lined with mucous membrane. This mucous membrane produces mucus, which helps moisten the air as it passes through the system. The mucus also helps rid the system of unwanted intruders, such as bacteria, dust, and other airborne materials.

Many different drugs affect the respiratory system. Because several of these drugs are over-the-counter medications, people tend to think of them as "harmless." Far from being harmless, these drugs affect the whole body. Many are from one of the autonomic nervous system classifications. As you have read, these drugs affect the functioning of every part of the body.

Some of the drugs in this unit are administered by inhalation. Some of the methods of inhalation are outlined along with the medications you are likely to see given in this manner.

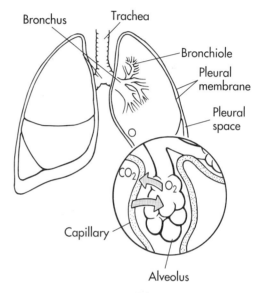

Figure X–1. Important parts of the respiratory system include the bronchus, bronchiole, pleural membrane, pleural space, and alveolus.

In Chapter 51, we will debunk the myth that all cough medicines are alike. You will learn why some cough medicines are good for one type of cough but not for another, and you will learn what you as a nurse should do to help a cough medicine work best.

Chapter 52 outlines the antitubercular drugs. This chapter is not intended to replace your medical-surgical textbook or to make you an expert on tuberculosis, but some background information is necessary before the medications for testing or treatment of tuberculosis are discussed.

CHAPTER 49

ANTIHISTAMINES AND DECONGESTANTS

LEARNING OBJECTIVES

After studying this chapter, you should be able to:

1. Define antihistamine, decongestant, and rebound phenomenon.

2. State actions and uses of and adverse reactions to antihistamines and decongestants.

3. Identify common examples of antihistamines and decongestants.

4. State appropriate nursing implications for patients receiving antihistamines or decongestants.

5. Prepare an appropriate teaching plan for a patient receiving antihistamines or decongestants.

6. Demonstrate how to administer antihistamines and decongestants to a patient by use of the nursing process.

DRUGS YOU WILL LEARN ABOUT IN THIS CHAPTER

Antihistamines

brompheniramine (Dimetane)

chlorpheniramine (Chlor-Trimeton)

triprolidine

clemastine (Tavist, Tavist-1)

clemastine with phenylpropanolamine HCl, a decongestant (Tavist-D)

diphenhydramine HCl (Benadryl)

promethazine HCl (Phenergan)

terfenadine (Seldane)

astemizole (Hismanal)

dimenhydrinate (Dramamine)

meclizine (Antivert, Bonine)

Decongestants

pseudoephedrine HCl (an ingredient of Sudafed, Sine-Aid, Dristan, Actifed, Comtrex, CoAdvil, Rondec, Novahistine, Deconamine)

phenylpropanolamine HCl (an ingredient of Entex, Naldecon, Ornade, Triaminic, Comtrex, Tavist-D)

phenylephrine HCl (an ingredient of Neo-Synephrine, Dristan, Entex, Extendryl, Naldecon, Congespirin)

oxymetazoline HCl (Dristan Long Lasting Nasal Spray, 4-Way Long Lasting Nasal Spray)

ANTIHISTAMINES

ACTIONS AND USES The prefix anti- means to work against. Therefore, this classification works against the actions of histamine. Histamine is a substance released by the body any time there is a chemical or physical injury. It acts to dilate the arterioles, which causes the area to become red. Histamine increases the permeability of capillaries and venules, which allows fluid to escape into surrounding tissues and cause swelling. The combined effects cause warmth in the area. It may be easier for the student to remember that histamine release causes the inflammatory process. In addition, histamine dilates smooth muscles and increases exocrine secretions of the gastrointestinal system (GI) and respiratory tract (Box 49–1). Antihistamines there-

---

Box 49-1. Histamine Actions

Redness
Warmth
Swelling
Opened air passages
Increased respiratory mucus secretion
Decreased gastrointestinal motility
Increased gastrointestinal mucus secretion

Box 49-2. Uses of Antihistamines

Allergies
Common cold
Conjunctivitis
Nausea and vomiting
Itching
Blood transfusion reaction
Pain
Parkinsonism
Anaphylactic shock

---

fore work against each of these actions of histamine. Many of the antihistamines are anticholinergics.

Because antihistamines dry secretions, they have obtained the nickname "driers." They dry secretions of the respiratory tract and may be used to treat nasal congestion, allergies that cause rhinitis and rhinorrhea, and coryzo (the common cold). Antihistamines dry secretions of the GI system and may be useful in the management of nausea and vomiting or even motion sickness. They may be used to treat itching from pruritus or urticaria. They are effective in producing sedation. Some symptoms of transfusion reaction, a reaction to blood products, respond to antihistamines, as does allergic conjunctivitis, which causes red, itchy, and watery eyes. Box 49-2 lists the uses of antihistamines.

Antihistamines may be used in conjunction with other drugs to treat pain, parkinsonism, and anaphylactic shock. In each of these cases, the antihistamine is used because it increases the effectiveness of the other drugs.

Because of the many diverse effects of antihistamines, there are also many diverse adverse effects. One of the most common is drowsiness. The patient may complain of lethargy, fatigue, muscle weakness, dizziness, and ataxia. Antihistamines may also cause GI distress, dry mouth, or excessive dryness of other mucous membranes. This can lead to blurred vision. The patient's blood pressure may drop, which contributes to the dizziness and ataxia, or the patient may complain of a headache.

As the antihistamine dries secretions, it causes normal bronchial secretions to thicken and become difficult to produce. A paradoxical excitation with nervousness and hyperactivity is possible when antihistamines are used for children and the elderly.

ASSESSMENT Antihistamines are often found in over-the-counter medications. Always ask your patients what medications they are taking at home. Stress to them to include prescription as well as nonprescription drugs.

N U R S I N G   A L E R T

Be aware of the patient's medical history. Caution is to be used with antihistamines if there is a history of asthma, cardiovascular disease, hypertension, hyperthyroidism, closed-angle glaucoma, or benign prostatic hypertrophy.

A warning about these conditions appears on the label of over-the-counter antihistamines, but patients often do not read it.

Antihistamines are contraindicated in infants and therefore also nursing mothers because they do pass through the mother's milk.

PLANNING AND IMPLEMENTATION One of the most important steps you must take for the patient receiving antihistamines is to ensure safety. The patient is much more susceptible to falls and injury because of the dizziness and drowsiness from the drug. Instruct your patients about these possible side effects. Ask them to call for help whenever getting out of bed. Be sure to answer the call light promptly to ensure that patients do not try to get up alone. Walk with patients keeping a hand on their arm until you are sure they are steady. Keep walkways clear of clutter and well lit. While a patient is in bed, keep side rails up and the bed in low position and locked at the wheels. If sources of heat or cold are being used for therapy, check the sites often; the patient may be too drowsy to awaken from pain. Explaining the rationale for each of these precautions will encourage the patient's compliance and provide a better sense of well-being.

If the patient complains of a dry mouth from the antihistamine, frequent sips of water will ease the dryness better than larger amounts at one time. Be sure to check whether the patient is allowed to have fluids. Ice chips may also feel like more liquid than they are. The patient whose fluid intake is restricted may use candy or gum as allowed. Brushing the teeth and rinsing with mouthwash also help ease the dryness.

Because the bronchial secretions become thicker, encourage fluid intake to keep them more mobile. Failure to do so could result in hypostatic pneumonia.

If the patient complains of GI upset with antihistamines, they can be given with meals. This reduces the adverse effect in most people.

The patient may be undergoing treatment and diagnosis at the same time. Be sure to discontinue the use of all antihistamines for at least 3 to 4 days before allergy skin testing. The use of antihistamines during these tests may cause false-negative results.

Caution the patient not to overuse any antihistamine, whether prescription or over-the-counter. Overuse leads to increased adverse reactions and a lessening of effectiveness.

If the antihistamine is provided in an extended-release form, it may not be crushed or opened but must be swallowed whole. If the patient has difficulty swallowing medications, another form may need to be ordered. Consult the physician.

EVALUATION Effectiveness of these drugs is measured ▲▲▲▲▲▲▲▲▲▲ by increased airway patency and decreased symptoms. The patient is the best judge of these.

N U R S I N G   A L E R T
▼▼▼▼▼▼▼▼▼▼▼▼▼▼▼▼▼▼▼▼▼▼▼▼▼▼▼▼▼▼▼▼

Evaluate the patient for signs of overdose, which are atropine-like effects: fixed dilated pupils, flushing, nausea and vomiting, and palpitations.

▲▲▲▲▲▲▲▲▲▲▲▲▲▲▲▲▲▲▲▲▲▲▲▲▲▲▲▲▲▲▲▲

Be alert, too, for any symptoms of drug interactions (Box 49–3). It is known that antihistamines have an additive effect with other anticholinergics. Use of

Box 49–3. Drug Interactions with Antihistamines

Additive effects with anticholinergics
Increased effects with monoamine oxidase inhibitors
Increased effects of central nervous system depressants

antihistamines with monoamine oxidase (MAO) inhibitors increases the effects and duration of the antihistamines. Antihistamines potentiate the effects of central nervous system depressants, such as tricyclic antidepressants, tranquilizers, sedative-hypnotics, narcotics, and alcohol. Warn your patients to avoid all sources of these substances when they return home.

Brompheniramine

Brompheniramine (Dimetane) is used for allergic rhinitis and urticaria, transfusion reaction, and anaphylactic shock. It is provided in oral, subcutaneous, intramuscular (IM), and intravenous (IV) forms. The usual dosage is 4 to 8 mg three or four times a day orally, or 5 to 20 mg every 6 to 12 hours parenterally.

Chlorpheniramine

Chlorpheniramine (Chlor-Trimeton) is similar to brompheniramine and has the same uses. It is also available in oral, subcutaneous, IM, and IV forms. It is often used in combination with decongestants. The usual dosage is 4 mg every 4 to 6 hours orally or every 8 to 12 hours in the extended-release form, or 5 to 20 mg parenterally.

Triprolidine

Triprolidine is similar to brompheniramine and has the same uses. It is given orally and is often combined with decongestants. The usual dosage is 2.5 mg every 4 to 6 hours or 5 mg in the extended-release form.

Clemastine

Clemastine (Tavist) is used for allergic rhinitis with sneezing, rhinorrhea, pruritus, and lacrimation. It can also be used for urticaria. Clemastine is available in several common forms. The syrup provides 0.5 mg in every 5 mL. Tavist-1 is available in tablets of 1.34-mg strength. Tavist is 2.68-mg tablets. Tavist-D tablets combine clemastine with phenylpropanolamine hydrochloride (a decongestant).

In addition to the symptoms listed for overdose of all antihistamines, clemastine can produce hallucinations, convulsions, and death.

Diphenhydramine Hydrochloride

Diphenhydramine hydrochloride (Benadryl) is a commonly used over-the-counter medication as well as a prescription drug. It is prescribed for allergic conjunctivitis, for urticaria, before chemotherapy, and for transfusion reactions. It is given for both short-term and prophylactic treatment of motion sickness. In combination with epinephrine diphenhydramine is used to treat anaphylactic shock. It may be used to treat mild parkinsonism, but usually in combination with other anticholinergic agents.

Diphenhydramine is given orally, IV, or deep IM. Its effects occur quickly, with the maximal effect in about 1 hour.

Evaluate your patient for the adverse reactions listed for all antihistamines as well as for chills, perspiration, photosensitivity, palpitations, and irregular pulse. Check the laboratory results of blood work-ups for signs of blood dyscrasias. The symptoms of an overdose are the same as for clemastine.

The usual dosage for diphenhydramine is 25 to 50 mg three or four times a day orally, or 10 to 50 mg IM or IV.

Promethazine Hydrochloride

ACTIONS AND USES Promethazine (Phenergan) has numerous uses. It can be prescribed for allergic rhinitis, allergic conjunctivitis, urticaria, transfusion reactions, and motion sickness or other nausea and vomiting. It is effective in producing sedation.

Promethazine may also be used with epinephrine to treat anaphylactic shock. It may be used as an adjunct to analgesics.

In addition to the adverse reactions listed for all antihistamines, promethazine may lead to jaundice, false-positive pregnancy test results, elevated serum glucose level, and extrapyramidal movements of the muscles and tongue. Extrapyramidal movements are especially likely to occur with IM or IV administration or in the case of an overdose.

ASSESSMENT Be aware of your patient's history. Patients with seizures may have an increased risk for seizures when they are given promethazine. Also check for a history of allergic reactions to other phenothiazines (antipsychotics) because pro-methazine is in this classification.

PLANNING AND IMPLEMENTATION Promethazine can be ordered orally (tablets or syrup), rectally (suppository), deep IM, or IV.

N U R S I N G   A L E R T

Do not give promethazine subcutaneously because this will cause tissue necrosis.

When promethazine is given IV, the instillation must be slow to prevent vein irritation.

N U R S I N G   A L E R T

Avoid intra-arterial administration of promethazine because this will cause gangrene of the extremity fed by the artery.

The dosage of promethazine depends on its intended use. The range is 12.5 to 25 mg.

EVALUATION The effectiveness of this drug is judged on the basis of its use. In addition to evaluating the patient for improvement of symptoms, watch for signs of an overdose. Depression of both the central nervous system and the cardiovascular system, respiratory depression, low blood pressure, and even unconsciousness indicate an overdose.

Also evaluate for any drug interactions. Promethazine is known to interact with barbiturates. The dose of the barbiturate often needs to be lowered. Consult the physician.

Terfenadine

Terfenadine (Seldane) is used for seasonal allergies with allergic rhinitis, pruritus, and lacrimation. It produces much less drowsiness because it does not cross the blood-brain barrier. Signs of an overdose are also much milder, including headache, nausea, and confusion.

This oral drug in tablet form is given twice a day, 60 mg each time. The effects begin in 1 to 2 hours, with maximal effectiveness in 3 to 4 hours, but it is a twice-a-day drug because the effects can last 12 hours or more.

Astemizole

Astemizole (Hismanal) is similar to terfenadine in that it does not cross the blood-brain barrier. It, too, is much less sedating. It is useful for allergic rhinitis and urticaria.

Astemizole is given orally. Because food decreases its absorption, it should be given on an empty stomach, 1 hour before or 2 hours after a meal. The usual dosage is 10 mg per day.

Caution the patient that astemizole may increase the appetite and thus cause weight gain. The patient may need to increase physical activity to offset this response.

Dimenhydrinate

ACTIONS AND USES Dimenhydrinate (Dramamine) is
▲▲▲▲▲▲▲▲▲▲▲▲▲▲▲ useful for vertigo, dizziness, nausea, vomiting, and motion sickness. It is therefore classified not only as an antihistamine but also as an antiemetic and anticholinergic. Dimenhydrinate achieves its actions by decreasing stimulation of the vestibule in the inner ear.

ASSESSMENT Be aware of the reason dimenhydrinate
▲▲▲▲▲▲▲▲▲▲ is being used for your patient. Assess for baseline information about those symptoms. Ask the patient to rate the level of vertigo or the level of nausea on a scale of 1 to 10 because these are subjective symptoms.

Know the patient's medical history. Dimenhydrinate has the same precautions as for other antihistamines. Patients with seizure disorders are at a higher risk for seizure during therapy with this medication.

PLANNING AND IMPLEMENTATION Dimenhydrinate is
▲▲▲▲▲▲▲▲▲▲▲▲▲▲▲▲▲▲▲▲▲▲▲▲▲▲▲ given orally, IM, or IV. The usual dosage is 50 to 100 mg every 4 to 6 hours. It is recommended that the drug be given 1 to 2 hours before activity that causes motion sickness so the drug will be at its peak effectiveness. If the drug is to be given IM, the needle must be placed deep into a large muscle. Massage the injection site to relieve the pain.

EVALUATION Because of the action on the vestibule,
▲▲▲▲▲▲▲▲▲▲ ototoxic effects may not be readily recognized if dimenhydrinate is given with ototoxic drugs. Be especially alert to even slight changes in symptoms or complaints from the patient in these circumstances.

If dimenhydrinate is being given for vomiting, evaluate the patient's hydration status and monitor intake and output. Continue to evaluate bowel sounds and abdominal pain because this drug may mask major symptoms of other abdominal conditions.

Meclizine

Meclizine (Antivert, Bonine) is classified as an antihistamine, antiemetic, and anticholinergic. It is used for short-term and prophylactic treatment of motion sickness and vertigo, labyrinthitis, and Meniere's disease. Its actions are achieved by decreasing stimulation to both the vestibule and the labyrinth of the inner ear.

This oral drug is given 1 hour before activity in a dose of 25 to 50 mg. For labyrinthitis or Meniere's disease, it is given in divided doses of 25 to 100 mg daily.

DECONGESTANTS

ACTIONS AND USES Decongestants are sympathomi-
▲▲▲▲▲▲▲▲▲▲▲▲▲▲▲▲ metic amines or adrenergics. They stimulate the alpha- and beta-receptors. This produces vasoconstriction of the nasal mucosa, which then decreases edema and increases nasal patency. For this reason, decongestants have earned the nickname "drainer."

Decongestants are often prescribed for rhinorrhea and nasal congestion from the common cold, sinusitis, allergic rhinitis (hay fever), and other upper respiratory allergies. When used with antihistamines, decongestants also relieve eustachian tube congestion, such as that associated with serous otitis media.

N U R S I N G   A L E R T
▼▼▼▼▼▼▼▼▼▼▼▼▼▼▼▼▼▼▼▼▼▼▼▼▼▼▼▼▼

Decongestants can cause an epinephrine-like reaction, producing central nervous system stimulation with seizures, severe hypotension, and even cardiac collapse.

▲▲▲▲▲▲▲▲▲▲▲▲▲▲▲▲▲▲▲▲▲▲▲▲▲▲▲▲▲▲▲▲

Common adverse reactions include nervousness, excitation, restlessness, insomnia, anxiety reactions, tremors, dizziness, weakness, headache, nausea and vomiting, pallor, dry mouth, metallic taste in the mouth, dysuria, thickened respiratory secretions, and respiratory distress.

N U R S I N G   A L E R T
▼▼▼▼▼▼▼▼▼▼▼▼▼▼▼▼▼▼▼▼▼▼▼▼▼▼▼▼▼

Rebound phenomenon is possible with the use of topical decongestants. The medication is used or even overused to reduce symptoms. After use for several days, the symptoms return with greater intensity. This encourages the patient to use the medication sooner and in greater quantity. In this way, the patient becomes "addicted" to the drug because more and more of it is needed to maintain patency of the passageways.

▲▲▲▲▲▲▲▲▲▲▲▲▲▲▲▲▲▲▲▲▲▲▲▲▲▲▲▲▲▲

Excessive drying and even epistaxis are also possible if the medication is overused.

ASSESSMENT Check the patient's chart for a history of
▲▲▲▲▲▲▲▲▲▲ cardiovascular disease. Decongestants must be used with caution if the patient has hypertension. The blood pressure can go even higher and contribute to a cerebrovascular accident (CVA). The blood pressure can also go higher in patients with hyperthyroidism. Decongestants can cause further vasoconstriction of the coronary arteries in those with ischemic heart disease. The risk of complications from decreased blood flow is higher in diabetics. Intraocular pressure in those with glaucoma can increase. Hypertrophy increases in patients with benign prostatic hypertrophy.

N U R S I N G   A L E R T
▼▼▼▼▼▼▼▼▼▼▼▼▼▼▼▼▼▼▼▼▼▼▼▼▼▼▼▼▼▼▼

Also check the medication orders for any monoamine oxidase (MAO) inhibitors. Use of decongestants with these drugs may precipitate hypertensive crisis.

▲▲▲▲▲▲▲▲▲▲▲▲▲▲▲▲▲▲▲▲▲▲▲▲▲▲▲▲▲▲

Decongestants should not be given to pregnant women or nursing mothers because of the potential effects on the fetus.

PLANNING AND IMPLEMENTATION When decongestants
▲▲▲▲▲▲▲▲▲▲▲▲▲▲▲▲▲▲▲▲▲▲▲▲▲▲▲▲ are given orally, caution the patient that extended-release tablets or capsules are to be swallowed whole. If the patient has difficulty swallowing medications, the capsules can be opened and mixed with a small amount of food, but the medication must still be swallowed without chewing.

In scheduling a decongestant, give the last dose of the medication at least 2 hours before bedtime. This decreases difficulty sleeping.

Instruct the patient not to try to "catch up" if a dose of decongestant is missed after returning home. Advise the patient to omit the missed dose unless it is remembered within just 1 or 2 hours.

Teach the patient to reduce caffeine intake if decongestants cause symptoms of central nervous system stimulation. Describe hidden sources of caffeine, such as in other medications, and identify sources with which the patient is unfamiliar. Common sources include coffee, tea, chocolate, colas and other soft drinks, and certain over-the-counter pain relievers.

If the decongestant is being given topically, teach the patient how to use the medication. When drops are to be instilled nasally, the patient should be sitting with the head tilted back. If the drops are ordered for the sinuses, the patient should be lying down with the shoulders up on pillows so the head is allowed to fall back.

If the decongestant is being given with a spray bottle, ask the patient to blow the nose gently before instillation, then to inhale on spraying the medication. Teach the patient to remove the tip of the spray bottle from the nose before releasing to prevent nasal mucus from being suctioned into the spray bottle and contaminating the solution (Fig. 49–1). The patient should rinse the tip of the bottle with hot water after each use to prevent recontamination at the next use.

If the decongestant is being given with a metered dose pump, the procedure is similar to that for use of a spray bottle. Prime the pump before use by depressing once or twice until a spray of medication comes from the tip. It is not necessary to remove the tip of a metered dose pump before releasing because the pump does not produce suctioning action (Fig. 49–2).

Caution the patient not to use any decongestant for more than 3 days. Bottles should not be shared with others because cross-contamination will occur.

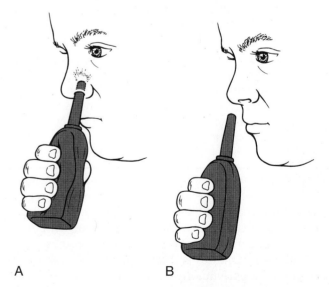

Figure 49–1. *A.* Instruct the patient to inhale on spraying the medication. *B.* Remove the tip of the spray bottle from the nose before releasing to prevent contamination.

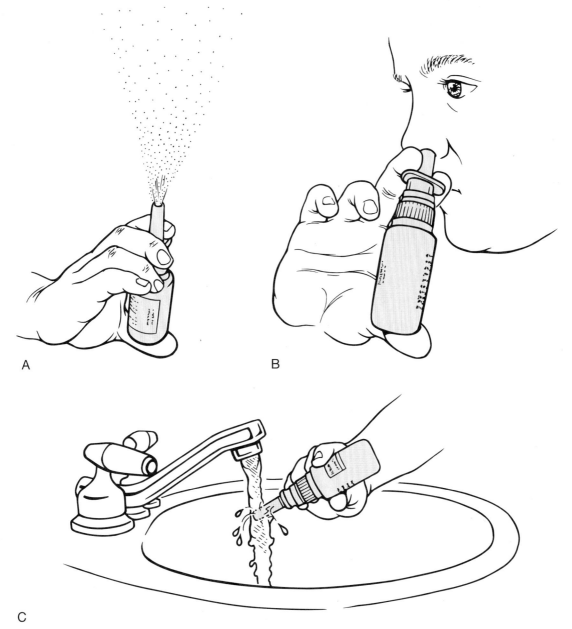

A

B

C

Figure 49-2. *A.* A metered dose pump must be primed before use by depressing once or twice until a spray of medication comes from the tip. *B.* Insert the tip into the naris, with fingers on "wings" and thumb on the bottom of the bottle. *C.* Wash the bottle after use.

EVALUATION Effectiveness of decongestants can be de-
▲▲▲▲▲▲▲▲▲▲ termined by evaluating for presence of symptoms. Ask the patient to rate the level of congestion on a scale of 1 to 10. Ask the patient to breathe through each nostril while the other is blocked.

To determine possible adverse reactions, evaluate the patient's blood pressure and pulse (rate and rhythm) throughout drug therapy. Listening to lung sounds is also important because secretions may become viscous and hard to expel. Note whether the patient is maintaining a normal fluid intake.

Evaluate the patient for any drug interactions (Box 49–4). Concomitant use of decongestants reduces the effectiveness of methyldopa (Aldomet), reserpine and other rauwolfia alkaloids, veratrum alkaloids (antihypertensives), and mecamylamine (Inversine, an oral antihypertensive agent).

The effects of the decongestant can be increased when it is used with beta-adrenergic blockers. This combination can also lead to bradycardia and hypertension.

When given with other sympathomimetics (adrenergics), the decongestants are more likely to have an adverse effect on the cardiovascular system.

The pH of the body also affects the actions of decongestants. When acidifying agents, such as ammonium chloride or cranberries, are used with decongestants, the effects of the decongestant are decreased. When alkalinizing agents, such as sodium bicarbonate or cheese, are used with decongestants, the effects of the decongestant are increased.

Evaluate your patient for improvement of symptoms, which should occur within 3 to 5 days. If symptoms do not improve or if fever develops, notify the physician.

Also consult the physician if any signs or symptoms of overdose occur. These may include central nervous system stimulation, difficulty urinating, flushing, palpitations, arrhythmias, or hypertension and then hypotension followed by possible cardiovascular collapse.

Pseudoephedrine Hydrochloride

Pseudoephedrine hydrochloride is an oral medication given to reduce nasal congestion. It is an ingredient of Sudafed, Sine-Aid, Dristan, Actifed, Comtrex, CoAdvil, Rondec, Novahistine, and Deconamine. The usual dosage is 30 to 60 mg three or four times a day or 120 mg every 12 hours if the sustained-release form is used. Pseudoephedrine causes little or no drowsiness.

Phenylpropanolamine Hydrochloride

Phenylpropanolamine hydrochloride is used as a decongestant. It is also used as an anorexiant in treatment of obesity. Phenylpropanolamine is contained in Entex, Naldecon, Ornade, Triaminic, Comtrex, and Tavist-D.

Phenylpropanolamine causes considerable central nervous system stimulation. It increases both the heart rate and the cardiac output. It is subject to overuse because it is readily available in over-the-counter diet aids.

This oral drug is given to persons older than 12 years at a dosage of 20 to 40 mg every 3 to 4 hours. Dosages for younger children are age dependent.

Phenylephrine Hydrochloride

Phenylephrine hydrochloride is used as a decongestant, but it causes little or no central nervous system stimulation. There is no stimulation of heart muscle receptors. It acts to slow the heart rate when it is used in usual doses.

Phenylephrine can be administered orally, subcutaneously, intramuscularly, and ophthalmically. It is found in Neo-Synephrine, Dristan, Entex, Extendryl, Naldecon, and Congespirin.

Parenteral phenylephrine may be used to maintain the blood pressure during spinal and inhalation anesthesia, in shock, and with hypotension caused by other drugs.

Hypertensive patients may have even higher blood pressure readings when they are given parenteral phenylephrine with oxytocics (obstetrical medications). Be sure the physician is aware of the concurrent use because the risk of CVA is increased.

Cautious use of parenteral phenylephrine is also recommended for the elderly, those with heart disease, and those with arteriosclerosis.

The dose of phenylephrine depends on the action desired. An overdose may lead to arrhythmias, a sense of fullness in the head, and tingling of the extremities. It may be necessary to give an alpha-adrenergic blocker such as phentolamine mesylate (Regitine) to counteract an overdose of phenylephrine.

Oxymetazoline Hydrochloride

Oxymetazoline hydrochloride (Dristan Long Lasting Nasal Spray, 4-Way Long Lasting Nasal Spray) is a topical decongestant given for temporary relief. Its effects last up to 12 hours. The usual dose for persons older than 6 years is 2 or 3 sprays in each nostril twice a day.

Box 49–4. Drug Interactions with Decongestants

Decreased effects of
methyldopa
rauwolfia alkaloids
veratrum alkaloids
mecamylamine (Inversine)

Increased effects of decongestants with
other adrenergics
beta-adrenergic blockers
alkalinizing agents

Decrease effects of decongestants with
acidifying agents

E X E R C I S E S

CASE STUDIES

1. Ms. A.D., your patient, is 22 years old and has been prescribed an antihistamine. What safety precautions should you institute? What other nursing actions would be appropriate for her?

Ms. A.D. tells you that after she leaves the hospital, her friends intend to "throw her a party." Because she will probably still be taking the antihistamine, what should you teach her?

2. S.I., age 8 years, has been prescribed an antihistamine. Her mother tells you that she seems irritable and anxious. What is the reason for this reaction?

S.I.'s mother mentions that her daughter cannot swallow pills and must chew them. What do you need to know next to properly advise S.I.'s mother about this practice?

S.I. is scheduled for skin testing to determine whether she has allergies that cause her symptoms. What precaution needs to be taken before the test?

3. A friend of yours mentions that he uses a nasal spray often but still seems to have congestion "all the time." What teaching is appropriate for your friend?

4. Mr. J.A. has been prescribed a topical decongestant. What are the three main ways in which this form of drug is delivered? What patient teaching needs to be done for each?

Mr. J.A. has also been prescribed an oral decongestant. He complains of nervousness. What could you teach him that may reduce his nervousness?

MENTAL AEROBICS

1. Go to your own medicine cabinet and read the labels of any cold remedy packages you have there. (If you do not have any, go to a store and read several labels from different brands.)

2. Observe at a physician's office (preferably during "cold season"). What medications are most commonly prescribed? What teaching is done? What differences would you expect if the office was for a pediatrician?

BRONCHODILATORS, CROMOLYN SODIUM, AND DNase

LEARNING OBJECTIVES

After studying this chapter, you should be able to:

1. Define bronchodilator and cromolyn.

2. State actions and uses of and adverse reactions to bronchodilators and cromolyn.

3. Identify common examples of bronchodilators.

4. State appropriate nursing implications for patients receiving bronchodilators or cromolyn sodium.

5. Prepare an appropriate teaching plan for patients receiving bronchodilators or cromolyn sodium.

6. Demonstrate how to administer bronchodilators or cromolyn sodium to a patient by use of the nursing process.

DRUGS YOU WILL LEARN ABOUT IN THIS CHAPTER

Bronchodilators

Sympathomimetics

epinephrine (Sus-Phrine, Primatene Mist)

albuterol (Proventil, Ventolin)

metaproterenol sulfate (Alupent, Meta-prel)

terbutaline sulfate (Brethine)

isoproterenol HCl (Isuprel)

ephedrine (an ingredient of Primatene tablets, Marax)

isoetharine (Bronkosol)

Xanthine derivatives

aminophylline, theophylline (Slo-bid, Theo-Dur, Elixophyllin)

oxtriphylline (Choledyl)

dyphylline (Lufyllin)

Anticholinergics

ipratropium bromide (Atrovent)

Adrenergics

salmeterol xinafoate (Serevent)

Cromolyn

cromolyn sodium (Intal, Nasalcrom)

DNase

dornase alfa (Pulmozyme)

Bronchodilators are medications that can relax the smooth muscle of the bronchi, resulting in more open airways, eased breathing and comfort for the patient, and improved gas exchange. The bronchodilators are often used to treat diseases or conditions associated with nonmechanical (reversible) airway obstruction. This could include asthma, chronic bronchitis, emphysema, and other chronic obstructive pulmonary diseases (COPDs).

There are three main subclasses of bronchodilators:

• Sympathomimetics (adrenergics)

- Xanthine derivatives
- Parasympathomimetic blockers (anticholinergics).

SYMPATHOMIMETICS

ACTIONS AND USES Although sympathomimetics are useful in reversing bronchospasms, they are also associated with all of the effects of sympathetic nervous system stimulation. (The student may wish to review Chapter 37.) The patient may complain of nervousness and insomnia. You may observe tremors. Drowsiness is also possible in some patients. The patient using a sympathomimetic often experiences a dry mouth, sweating, and increased pulse and blood pressure—all from the sympathetic stimulation. Gastrointestinal effects may include nausea, vomiting, and diarrhea. Some patients also complain of palpitations and headaches.

ASSESSMENT Before beginning therapy with a sympathomimetic bronchodilator, thoroughly assess the patient's health status to establish baseline information. You need to know the underlying reason the drug was ordered. Check the blood pressure, pulse, and respirations as well as lung sounds so these may be compared with later data. Ask the patient to show you any secretions produced so the character can be documented.

If the patient has a history of a cardiovascular disease, such as hypertension, angina, or coronary artery disease, assess for any chest pain, what brings on the pain, and the severity of the pain. The physician often orders electrocardiograms (ECGs) frequently throughout therapy. Be sure to monitor reports of these tests for any changes.

Caution is advised for the patient who has a history of diabetes mellitus, hyperthyroidism, or seizures and for the patient who is prescribed other sympathomimetics. Sympathomimetics are contraindicated if the patient has tachycardia.

N U R S I N G   A L E R T

Consult the physician if the pulse is above 100 beats per minute.

PLANNING AND IMPLEMENTATION In planning the schedule for a sympathomimetic bronchodilator, remember that it is to be given in evenly spaced doses around the clock to maintain therapeutic drug levels. For the best compliance after discharge, the patient needs to understand the rationale for this.

Eliminate sources of caffeine from the patient's diet because these may contain xanthines, which increase both the effects of and the adverse reactions to the bronchodilator. Common sources of caffeine include colas, coffee, tea, and chocolate. Ask the patient about the amount of each of these taken each day.

Because many cold preparations contain anticholinergics (antihistamines), these can counteract the effects of a sympathomimetic bronchodilator. Ask patients about over-the-counter medications they may be taking.

Advise any patient, but especially ones with pulmonary conditions, to stop smoking and to avoid those who do. This may be difficult for the patient and requires careful intervention. Help may be elicited from the American Lung Association, which sponsors programs to stop smoking. The patient must also become aware of air pollutants. Discuss with the physician what measures may be necessary for the individual patient, including simple avoidance techniques or air purifier devices for the home.

Encourage the patient to drink at least 2000 cc of a variety of fluids each day. Sympathomimetics can cause secretions to thicken. By increasing the fluid intake, the viscosity of the fluid will lessen. Be sure that no contraindications exist.

Teach the patient the effects expected from the drug. Be sure the patient knows signs and symptoms of toxic effects. It is often best to write a list of these for the patient to keep. If toxic effects occur, or if symptoms worsen or are not as controlled by the medication, instruct the patient to call the physician immediately.

Many bronchodilators, both sympathomimetics and the other subclasses, may be administered by inhalation. If the patient will be using a hand-held inhaler (or nebulizer), the nurse must provide instruction on the proper use of the inhaler. Have the patient make a return demonstration before discharge to ensure understanding of the process.

Instruct the patient to shake any inhaler first. The mouthpiece of the inhaler is held downward for use. Ask the patient to exhale completely and place the lips around the mouthpiece, making a good seal (Fig. 50–1). Simultaneously, the patient should take a deep breath and depress the inhaler, which releases the medication. By this method, the mist will be drawn fully into the lungs. Ask the patient to hold the breath for a few seconds (counting to 3 or 5 slowly may help) and then to exhale slowly through the nose.

After use, the mouthpiece of the inhaler should be rinsed and recovered with its cap. Once a day, the patient should wash the inhaler apparatus with soap and water, rinse it thoroughly to remove all residue, and then dry it. Because any contaminants on the

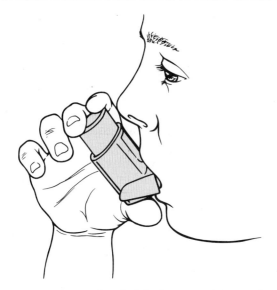

Figure 50–1. A good seal of the lips around the mouthpiece is necessary for proper administration of bronchodilators.

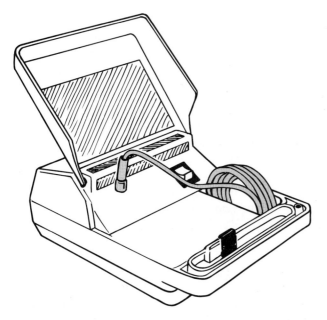

Figure 50–2. Nebulizers are attached to an air compressor by tubing. The compressor delivers the bronchodilators in a fine mist.

cleansed thoroughly after each use. A good home solution to use is white vinegar (Fig. 50–4).

EVALUATION Effectiveness of the sympathomimetic
▲▲▲▲▲▲▲▲▲▲ bronchodilators can be determined best by asking the patient about ease of breathing. A decreased number of bronchospasm attacks also indicates effectiveness. The nurse can use clear breath sounds as a more objective evaluation tool.

While the patient is taking the medication, be alert for signs of drug interactions. The effects of both the bronchodilator and a beta-blocker medication are decreased if these are used together. Additive effects occur if sympathomimetics are used with other adrenergics, including vasopressors and decongestants.

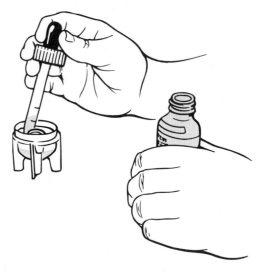

Figure 50–3. The medication is measured carefully with a dropper and placed in the cup.

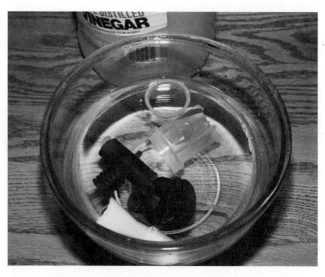

Figure 50–4. The nebulizer should be cleaned thoroughly after each use. White vinegar is a good home solution.

mouthpiece may potentially be drawn into the lungs, the apparatus should be dried with a lint-free material only.

Bronchodilators may also be administered with a nebulizer. This machine delivers the medication in a fine mist in a period of 10 to 15 minutes. The nebulizer is attached by tubing to an air compressor (Fig. 50–2). The medication is placed in the well of the nebulizer (Fig. 50–3). The patient must once again make a good seal around the mouthpiece. Normal breaths are taken through the mouth with occasional deep breaths throughout the specified time. The nebulizer should be

Use with monoamine oxidase (MAO) inhibitors or tricyclic antidepressants increases the risk of cardiovascular adverse reactions.

Also be alert for signs or symptoms of drug overdose or overuse. In addition to heightened adverse reactions, the patient may experience fatigue, malaise, cardiac arrhythmias, angina, increased or decreased blood pressure, paradoxical bronchospasms, cardiac arrest, and even death. Teaching about the dangers of overuse of these drugs may help prevent the occurrence.

Epinephrine

Epinephrine (Sus-Phrine, Primatene Mist, and others) is considered an emergency drug. As a bronchodilator, it is used for acute asthma attacks or other causes of acute bronchospasms.

Sus-Phrine is a subcutaneous form of epinephrine. A test dose is often used to check for an allergic reaction to epinephrine before a full therapeutic dose is given. Be sure to shake the vial thoroughly before drawing up the medication because it is a suspension. The usual dose is small, 0.1 to 0.3 mL, given subcutaneously only once in a 6-hour period. Because of the small dose, use a tuberculin syringe, preferably with a 26-gauge, 1/2-inch needle.

When epinephrine is given subcutaneously, it may cause urticaria, a wheal, and hemorrhage at the injection site. Be sure to assess previous injection sites often.

N U R S I N G   A L E R T

Also rotate the sites. Repeated injections into the same site may cause tissue necrosis because of extreme constriction of the blood vessels.

N U R S I N G   A L E R T

After the patient has received an injection of epinephrine, be sure to watch for signs of an overdose. The patient's blood pressure can climb to dangerous levels and cause a cerebrovascular accident, pulmonary edema, and resultant death. These outcomes may also result from accidental intravenous injection of the solution.

Primatene Mist is an inhalant form of epinephrine. Be sure the patient fully understands how to use the inhaler. A single inhalation is considered a dose. It can be repeated if symptoms are not relieved, but the patient must wait at least 1 full minute between doses. This is to ensure that the patient has allowed enough time for the medication to work with the first dose.

After the second inhalation, Primatene Mist is not to be repeated for at least 3 hours. If the patient did not experience relief after the second dose and 20 minutes, medical attention should be sought.

Albuterol

Albuterol (Proventil, Ventolin) is used to treat acute bronchospasms and as a prophylactic drug in maintenance therapy. Albuterol is available in many forms, including tablets, extended-release tablets, syrup, inhalation solution, aerosol, and capsules from which the powder is used in an inhaler. The average dose depends on the form of the drug, but it can be given as often as four times a day or as little as twice a day for extended-release forms.

While the patient is receiving albuterol, be alert for the same drug interactions as relate to all sympathomimetic bronchodilators.

Metaproterenol Sulfate

Metaproterenol sulfate (Alupent, Metaprel) is used for treatment of acute bronchospasms and for prophylactic therapy. It is supplied as tablets, syrup, inhalation solution, or inhalers.

After use of metaproterenol, the patient experiences an improvement of pulmonary function test results. This effect will last up to 6 hours.

When metaproterenol is given as a tablet or syrup, the usual dose is 20 mg three or four times a day. Inhalation solution is supplied to the client with intermittent positive-pressure breathing (IPPB) or a hand-held nebulizer. The solution must be diluted in saline or a similar solution (possibly even another medication, such as cromolyn). The dose is then titrated to the patient's individual needs. Two or three inhalations from an inhaler are considered a single dose. This can be repeated every 3 to 4 hours. Caution the patient not to exceed 12 inhalations a day (24 hours).

Terbutaline Sulfate

Terbutaline sulfate (Brethine) can be used for short-term or prophylactic therapy. Its effects occur in about

30 minutes. These effects last up to 8 hours, but effectiveness is maximal at about 3 hours.

Terbutaline is given orally, 5 mg every 6 hours, but only three times a day. Subcutaneously, it is given at a dose of 0.25 mg. If relief does not follow the injection within 30 minutes, it may be repeated once. After the second dose, however, the drug must not be repeated again for at least 4 hours.

Isoproterenol Hydrochloride

Isoproterenol hydrochloride (Isuprel) can be delivered orally, by inhalation, or by injection. As an injectable, it is used to treat bronchospasms during anesthesia. The student may also review its uses as a cardiac drug. It may be administered for treatment of heart block or during cardiac arrest. It may also be used as an adjunct to fluid and electrolyte replacement.

The injectable forms of isoproterenol are associated with the same side effects as other sympathomimetics are. In addition, they may lead to pulmonary edema and ventricular tachycardia.

Before initiating the medication, assess the blood pressure, pulse, urine output, and results of any ECG. In an emergency, these assessments must obviously be performed quickly. Extreme caution must be used with isoproterenol if the patient's heart rate is above 130 beats per minute. This may lead to arrhythmias.

Isoproterenol is contraindicated in patients with tachyarrhythmias, ventricular arrhythmias, digitalis toxicity, or angina pectoris.

N U R S I N G   A L E R T
▼▼▼▼▼▼▼▼▼▼▼▼▼▼▼▼▼▼▼▼▼▼▼▼▼▼▼▼▼▼▼▼

Isoproterenol is also contraindicated in patients who are allergic to sulfites because the injectable forms contain sulfites. Persons susceptible to other allergies may also react to sulfites.

▲▲▲▲▲▲▲▲▲▲▲▲▲▲▲▲▲▲▲▲▲▲▲▲▲▲▲▲▲▲▲▲

The dose used for the patient depends on the reason for use. The drug can be administered subcutaneously, intramuscularly, intravenously, or even by intracardiac injection by a physician.

After isoproterenol injectable has been used for a patient, carefully monitor the blood pressure. An overdose of the drug can cause either an increase or a decrease of blood pressure. Evaluate, too, for increased pulse, palpitations, or angina.

Isoproterenol can also be given orally or by inhalation. Inhalation administration can be used to treat acute bronchospasms with a single dose. It should not be repeated more than three times in a 24-hour period without notifying the physician before further use. Inhalation of isoproterenol has been associated with throat irritation as well as with the other adverse reactions of sympathomimetics.

Oral or inhalation isoproterenol should not be given at the same time as an epinephrine-containing drug. This can lead to cardiac arrhythmias. The two drugs can be alternated but must be separated by at least 4 hours.

Ephedrine

Ephedrine (an ingredient of Primatene tablets and Marax) can be used as a bronchodilator. It stimulates both alpha- and beta-receptors of the respiratory system. In Primatene tablets, ephedrine is combined with theophylline, another bronchodilator. (Other forms contain additional drugs.) In Marax, ephedrine is combined with theophylline, hydroxyzine (Atarax), and alcohol. Both drugs are used in maintenance therapy for bronchospasms. They tend to have slower onset of actions and longer duration of actions than other sympathomimetics do.

Isoetharine

Isoetharine (Bronkosol) can be administered by inhalation for rapid relief of acute bronchospasms. Adverse reactions to the drug are rare unless the patient overuses it.

Before administration, check the patient's history for hypertension and asthma. Both conditions warrant extra caution in use of isoetharine.

N U R S I N G   A L E R T
▼▼▼▼▼▼▼▼▼▼▼▼▼▼▼▼▼▼▼▼▼▼▼▼▼▼▼▼▼▼▼▼

Asthmatics are especially susceptible to allergic reactions to isoetharine because it contains sulfites.

▲▲▲▲▲▲▲▲▲▲▲▲▲▲▲▲▲▲▲▲▲▲▲▲▲▲▲▲▲▲▲▲

Other precautions associated with sympathomimetics also apply to this drug.

With administration by an inhaler, 1 to 2 inhalations are considered a single dose. Caution the patient to wait a full minute between the inhalations to allow the first dose to work. Isoetharine may also be administered by IPPB or aerosolization. In this case, it must be diluted with saline or another solution.

XANTHINE DERIVATIVES

ACTIONS AND USES The xanthine derivatives work by
▲▲▲▲▲▲▲▲▲▲▲▲▲▲ relaxing the smooth muscles of the
airways and also the pulmonary blood vessels. As a
result, they can be classified as bronchodilators,
vasodilators, diuretics, smooth muscle relaxants, cardiac
stimulants, cerebral stimulants, and skeletal
muscle stimulants. The xanthines are often used to
treat asthma and chronic obstructive pulmonary
disease (COPD) as well as other causes of bronchospasms.

Xanthines can cause gastric distress with nausea,
vomiting, and diarrhea. The patient may complain
of dizziness, headache, nervousness and insomnia,
or agitation. The xanthines can also have cardiovascular
effects, such as increased or irregular
pulse, palpitations, and flushing. The respiratory
rate may also increase. Some patients experience
urticaria.

ASSESSMENT Before use, assess the patient's pulse,
▲▲▲▲▲▲▲▲▲▲ respirations, and blood pressure. Ask
the patient about frequency of bronchospasms, usual
causes, how long they usually last, and whether
anything relieves them.

Check for a history of any cardiac disease, such as
congestive heart failure, or an acute myocardial
infarction. Other conditions that warrant precaution
include hypertension, hyperthyroidism, hypoxemia,
liver impairment, and alcoholism. Also use care when
administering the drug to either the elderly or
neonates.

N U R S I N G   A L E R T
▽▽▽▽▽▽▽▽▽▽▽▽▽▽▽▽▽▽▽▽▽▽▽▽▽▽▽▽▽▽▽

Xanthines are contraindicated if the patient has a
history of seizures because these drugs can lower
the seizure threshold.

▲▲▲▲▲▲▲▲▲▲▲▲▲▲▲▲▲▲▲▲▲▲▲▲▲▲▲▲▲▲▲▲▲

Because the xanthines increase the output of gastric
secretions, an active peptic ulcer also precludes
their use.

PLANNING AND IMPLEMENTATION Xanthines are provided
▲▲▲▲▲▲▲▲▲▲▲▲▲▲▲▲▲▲▲▲▲▲▲▲▲▲▲▲ vided in a variety of
forms, including oral, inhalation, and intravenous.
Whenever a patient is receiving a xanthine derivative,
frequent blood samples should be drawn to determine
therapeutic serum levels. To provide maximal effectiveness,
this level should be 10 to 20 µg per milliliter.

Levels above 20 µg may be toxic and produce untoward
effects.

Encourage your patient to refrain from eating or
drinking sources of caffeine or acetaminophen before
a blood sample is drawn for therapeutic serum level
determinations. Both caffeine and acetaminophen can
cause falsely high test results.

As a nurse, you should encourage the patient to stop
smoking. Those who continue to smoke may require
larger doses of xanthines to be prescribed by the
physician.

Instruct patients who are taking oral doses of
xanthines to take the medication at the same time
each day to ensure even blood levels. Administer
intravenous aminophylline by infusion pump to prevent
accidental overdose or underdose.

EVALUATION Effectiveness of the drug is determined
▲▲▲▲▲▲▲▲▲▲ by decreased dyspnea, decreased frequency
of bronchospasms, and clear lung sounds. The
patient is the best judge of ease of breathing, but
objective signs can include audible wheezes, nasal
flaring, sternal and intercostal retractions, and agitation.

Throughout therapy, be alert for signs of toxic
effects. These can include gastric distress, diarrhea,
bloody emesis, quickened reflexes, seizures, hypotension,
increased respirations, circulatory failure, and
respiratory arrest. Monitor blood levels of the xanthines
for toxic results.

Also continue to evaluate for signs of drug interactions.
The xanthines are known to interact with
many drugs (Box 50–1). Blood levels of the xanthines
may be increased if they are used with allopurinol,
cimetidine, erythromycin, lithium, or oral contraceptives.
The effectiveness of lithium is also decreased.
Xanthine levels are decreased if they are
used with rifampin, phenobarbital, or phenytoin. The
effects of phenytoin are also decreased. When xanthines
are used with propranolol, propranolol loses
effectiveness. Xanthine toxicity is more likely with
use of ephedrine or other sympathomimetic bronchodilators.
Finally, use with halothane anesthesia
may lead to tachycardia and even ventricular arrhythmias.

Aminophylline and Theophylline

One of these two closely related drugs is the single
ingredient of Slo-bid, Theo-Dur, and Elixophyllin.
They are considered to be the prime drugs of the
xanthine derivatives. The information presented for
xanthines relates directly to both aminophylline and
theophylline. In testing for blood levels of either drug,

Box 50–1. Drug Interactions with Xanthines

Xanthine blood levels increased with
allopurinol
cimetidine
erythromycin
lithium
oral contraceptives
ephedrine
other sympathomimetics

Xanthine blood levels decreased with
rifampin
phenobarbital
phenytoin

Decreased effectiveness of other drug with
lithium
phenytoin
propranolol

Additional severe adverse reactions with
halothane anesthetics

the form in the serum is theophylline. The test is therefore called a theophylline level.

Aminophylline or theophylline is also one of the ingredients of Marax, Primatene tablets, and Theo-Organidin, among others.

Elixophyllin is an elixir form of the drug. Slo-bid and Theo-Dur are both capsules. When an order is written to give Theo-Dur Sprinkle, a special form of the drug is required. This is supplied in a capsule. The capsule is opened and the medication granules are sprinkled over a small amount (generally a teaspoon) of food. Aminophylline is also given intravenously. Drug forms include enteric coated tablets, sustained-release tablets, chewable tablets, syrups, suspension, and rectal solution.

The serum levels of aminophylline may be increased if it is used at the same time as influenza vaccination. This is important to note because many of the patients receiving aminophylline are at risk for respiratory infection and are therefore candidates for the vaccination.

Oxtriphylline

Oxtriphylline (Choledyl) releases theophylline when it enters the bloodstream. Therefore, information listed for the xanthines is pertinent to this drug. Oxtriphylline is given orally. Dosages for the medica-

tion are higher than for theophylline, however, because oxtriphylline does not release an amount of theophylline equal to itself.

Dyphylline

Dyphylline (Lufyllin) is chemically related to theophylline. However, laboratory testing will not evaluate serum dyphylline levels. Dyphylline is given orally or intramuscularly. Increased effects of dyphylline are experienced if the drug is used with probenecid.

ANTICHOLINERGICS

Ipratropium Bromide

Ipratropium bromide (Atrovent) is used as a maintenance treatment of bronchospasms only. It does not treat acute attacks. It is useful for chronic obstructive pulmonary disease (COPD), chronic bronchitis, emphysema, and other causes of recurrent bronchospasms.

Ipratropium relaxes smooth muscles by antagonizing acetylcholine. It has a local effect and not a systemic one. It does not cross the blood-brain barrier.

Patients may complain of nervousness, dizziness, gastrointestinal upset, headache, palpitations, dry mouth, and nausea or vomiting. You may note a rash or a cough also as an adverse reaction to the drug.

Before initiating an order for ipratropium, check the patient's history for glaucoma or prostatic hypertrophy. This drug is used with caution in both conditions.

N U R S I N G   A L E R T

Also check for an allergy to atropine. Use of ipratropium is contraindicated in such patients.

Ipratropium is provided as an aerosol for inhalation. The average dose is 2 inhalations four times a day. Warn the client not to exceed 12 inhalations a day.

Effectiveness of the drug is determined by a lessened occurrence of bronchospasms over time. Listen to lung sounds and evaluate respiratory rate and effort frequently. Interactions with other drugs have not been reported. As always, be alert to individual responses to the drug. An overdose is unlikely because the drug does not exhibit systemic effects.

ADRENERGICS

Salmeterol Xinafoate

Salmeterol xinafoate (Serevent) is a relatively new bronchodilator. It is used to treat asthma and other causes of bronchospasms on a long-term basis. It is considered a maintenance drug only because bronchospasms that are currently occurring will not be affected by the drug.

Adverse reactions associated with salmeterol are similar to those found with other bronchodilators.

Salmeterol is given by inhalations 12 hours apart. Because this drug lasts longer than others in the classification, it is considered especially useful in preventing nocturnal bronchospasms. Some patients will require a short-acting bronchodilator between these doses. Each inhalation delivers 21 µg of salmeterol.

Salmeterol should not be used by patients taking monoamine oxidase (MAO) inhibitors or tricyclic antidepressants unless extreme caution is practiced.

CROMOLYN SODIUM

ACTIONS AND USES Cromolyn is classified as an antiallergic or antiasthmatic drug. It is available as Intal inhalation solution, Intal inhaler, Intal capsules, or Nasalcrom nasal spray. It inhibits the release of histamine by the body but does not counteract any histamine already released. Therefore, cromolyn is effective only as a maintenance drug for prevention of allergic reactions or asthmatic bronchospasms. It cannot be used to treat acute allergic reactions or asthma attacks. In fact, cromolyn has been demonstrated to interfere with treatment when it is given during acute episodes.

The most common adverse reactions to cromolyn have been nausea, cough or wheezing, nasal congestion, and sneezing. Some patients also experience drowsiness, gastrointestinal upset, nasal irritation or epistaxis, bronchospasms, difficulty urinating, tearing, rash, or urticaria.

ASSESSMENT Assess the patient's lung sounds and respiratory rate and effort. Also question the patient about frequency of symptoms and what symptoms are experienced. Ask about events or substances that may increase or initiate these symptoms.

Use caution when administering the medication to persons with either kidney or liver impairment. Both the kidney and the liver are routes of biotransformation or excretion of the drug.

PLANNING AND IMPLEMENTATION Cromolyn may be given by inhaler, spinhaler (a capsule that is broken apart so the powder may be inhaled with a special inhaler), nebulization, ophthalmic drops, or nasal spray. Ensure that the patient knows how to use the medication correctly. Cromolyn can be given before exposure to allergens or before exercise to persons in whom these would predictably cause an attack. It should be given approximately 10 to 15 minutes before contact with an allergen to allow the best results.

Because throat or mouth irritation may occur with the use of inhaled cromolyn, advise the patient to rinse the mouth with water after inhalation.

EVALUATION It generally takes about 2 to 4 weeks for cromolyn to become effective in preventing allergic reactions or asthmatic episodes. Evaluate for decreased nasal irritation, sniffling, nasal drainage, and bronchospasms, depending on the reason for use and the route of administration.

DNase

Dornase Alfa

Dornase alfa (Pulmozyme) is a relatively new drug developed specifically for the treatment of cystic fibrosis. Although not truly a bronchodilator, it nevertheless provides opened respiratory passageways by decreasing the viscosity of the pulmonary secretions. This improves the clearance of the secretions, removing the environment that allows the growth of pathogenic organisms. It is thought that antibiotics are also able to penetrate the lungs easier and are therefore more effective.

Dornase is a grown form of the human pancreatic enzyme DNase. Because it is a human product, it is thought that allergic reactions will be fewer. The most common adverse reactions have been hoarseness, pharyngitis, and a rash.

Dornase is given by nebulization. The usual dose is 2.5 mg one time a day. It is not yet approved for children younger than 5 years. Dornase is also being studied for possible use with chronic obstructive pulmonary diseases, including chronic bronchitis.

This is an expensive drug. The nurse may be involved in helping the patient obtain funding and services. Referral to a social worker can also be useful.

E X E R C I S E S

CASE STUDIES

1. P.L., age 8 years, is asthmatic. He receives the following drugs: Proventil syrup, 1 tsp tid; Tavist-1, 1 tablet tid; Nasalcrom, 2 sprays each nostril tid; Intal, 20 mg by inhalation nebulizer tid; Ventolin, 0.25 cc by inhalation nebulizer tid. He also has a Ventolin inhaler for acute bronchospasms.

Because P.L. receives albuterol from more than one source each day, what adverse reactions is he more likely to experience?

If P.L.'s physician orders the Ventolin inhaler to be given before contact with an allergen, when would you advise the parents to give the medication?

What ongoing assessments would be expected of the nurse who sees P.L. in the clinic?

What foods, medications, or other substances would you advise the parents to remove from P.L.'s environment because he is receiving a sympathomimetic bronchodilator?

How would you teach P.L. and his family to use the inhaler?

What tools would you use to evaluate the effectiveness of his drug regimen?

2. Ms. R.M., age 57 years, has COPD. She has been prescribed Theo-Dur, 1 tablet bid; Theo-Organidin, 1 tbsp tid; Ventolin inhaler, 1 inhalation as needed for acute bronchospasms; and Ventolin, 0.25 cc by inhalation nebulizer tid.

Because Ms. R.M. has been prescribed a xanthine derivative, for what symptoms should the nurse observe that may indicate toxic effects?

What testing will probably be performed for Ms. R.M. to evaluate the use of the xanthine? What precautions should you give the patient before the testing?

If Ms. R.M. contracts an infection, why is it less likely that she will be prescribed erythromycin?

Ms. R.M. mentions to you that her stomach is upset but it is a chronic condition for her. Why is this information important to report to the physician?

Ms. R.M. is concerned because since she has started taking aminophylline, she urinates much more often and in greater amounts. What is your best response to her on the basis of your knowledge of aminophylline?

MENTAL AEROBICS

1. Visit the office or clinic of a pulmonary specialist. What kinds of conditions are treated there? What medications are commonly used? What teaching is done? What diagnostic testing is performed?

2. Observe a respiratory therapist treating patients for one day. What conditions do the patients have? What medications did the therapist administer? What teaching did the therapist do? What equipment was used to administer the medications?

3. Interview patients with a chronic respiratory disease. How does the disease interfere with activities of daily living? What special precautions do the patients need to include in their lifestyle? How does the treatment affect their lives?

CHAPTER 51

ANTITUSSIVE DRUGS

LEARNING OBJECTIVES

After studying this chapter, you should be able to:

1. Define antitussive, suppressant, mucolytic, and expectorant.

2. State actions and uses of and adverse reactions to each type of antitussive.

3. Identify common examples of each type of antitussive.

4. State appropriate nursing implications for the patient receiving each type of antitussive.

5. Prepare an appropriate teaching plan for patients receiving each type of antitussive.

6. State contraindications to the use of suppressants, expectorants, and mucolytics.

7. Demonstrate how to administer each type of antitussive to a patient by use of the nursing process.

DRUGS YOU WILL LEARN ABOUT IN THIS CHAPTER

Cough Suppressants

  narcotics

    codeine

    hydrocodone (Hycodan)

    hydromorphone (Dilaudid)

  non-narcotics

    dextromethorphan

    diphenhydramine (Benadryl, Benylin, Nytol, Sominex)

    promethazine HCl (Phenergan)

    benzonatate (Tessalon)

Expectorants

  guaifenesin (Robitussin)

Mucolytics

  acetylcysteine (Mucomyst, Mucosol)

Antitussives are medications that treat a cough. Not all antitussive drugs work in the same way, nor are they all given for the same type of cough or cause. Three main types of antitussives are suppressants, expectorants, and mucolytics.

COUGH SUPPRESSANTS

ACTIONS AND USES Cough suppressants are given to treat acute or chronic dry (or nonproductive) coughs. Most act by depressing the cough center of the medulla.

NURSING ALERT

Cough suppressants should not be used for a productive cough.

A patient with a productive cough is raising mucus from the lungs. If this action by the body is stopped, mucus will build up in the lungs and lead to a worsened condition. Patients with chronic respiratory diseases, such as chronic obstructive pulmonary disease, should not be given a suppressant either because our goal for the patient is to clear the lungs.

Some coughs are not useful to the body. They are merely irritating, causing a sore throat and restlessness. This type of cough may be suppressed without ill effects. For this reason, cough suppressants are often found in over-the-counter cough and cold remedies. They should not be used for prolonged periods, however. If a cough lasts longer than 5 to 7 days, encourage the patient to seek medical attention. Cough suppressants should not be used for smoker's cough or similar problems. In this instance, suppressing the cough would discourage the patient from seeking help when a much greater problem may be the cause.

Because of the action on the medulla and other areas of the central nervous system (CNS), some cough suppressants may cause dizziness, drowsiness, or nausea.

ASSESSMENT Before giving the first dose of an ordered ▲▲▲▲▲▲▲▲▲▲ cough suppressant, assess the client thoroughly. Note the type of cough. Is it productive or nonproductive? If it is productive, assess the sputum. Note the color, amount, consistency, and frequency. Assess the respiratory status of the patient. Note the rate and rhythm of respirations as well as respiratory effort. Listen carefully to breath sounds in all lobes,

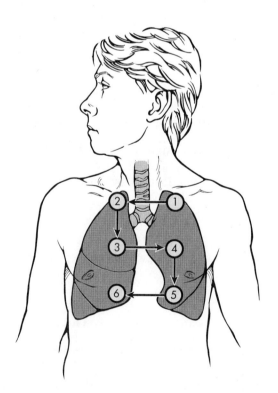

Figure 51–1. Using an S formation, listen carefully to breath sounds in all lobes.

using an S formation (Fig. 51–1). Note the presence of abnormal sounds and when they occur (inspiration, expiration, or both). Do the lungs clear with a cough?

PLANNING AND IMPLEMENTATION When a patient is ▲▲▲▲▲▲▲▲▲▲▲▲▲▲▲▲▲▲▲▲▲▲▲▲▲▲▲▲▲▲▲ prescribed a cough suppressant, the medication is often ordered on an as-needed basis. Be sure to warn the patient not to eat or drink immediately after taking the medication. Many of the cough suppressants also act to soothe the throat.

Help the patient avoid respiratory irritants that may be causing or increasing the cough. This includes cigarette smoke. If the patient is a smoker, encourage him to quit. You can offer helpful suggestions for dealing with the withdrawal symptoms of quitting, or you can refer your patient to organizations such as the American Lung Association or the American Cancer Society for help. Other irritants may include both indoor and outdoor air pollutants. Help the patient identify pollutants in the environment and then develop strategies to decrease exposure.

Teach the patient effective methods of deep breathing and coughing exercises (Box 51–1). This may help change a dry, hacky cough to a productive one. In some conditions, you would encourage deep breathing only because coughing may irritate.

Encourage the patient to drink between 1500 and 2000 cc of fluids every day. Depending on the condition and the physician's orders, this amount may be increased to 2500 or even 3000 cc. Give the patient a choice of fluids and offer them frequently. Small sips and the use of ice chips may also help quiet an irritating cough.

Institute safety precautions. The patient may be dizzy, drowsy, or both. Keep side rails up on the bed if the patient is in a health care facility. Be sure the call light is close and that the patient knows how to use it. Be sure the patient understands the importance of calling for help. Many times, patients believe they are bothering the nurse and attempt to get up by themselves. Be sure your attitude when answering a call light never gives the patient this impression or you may not receive the call the next time. Walk with the patient at least until it is known how the patient will react to the medication. If the patient is going home on the medication, warn against driving or operating hazardous machinery at home or at work. The dizziness is often caused by orthostatic hypotension. Teach the patient to sit up and dangle before standing. Keep items the patient may want close at hand so that reaching will be eliminated.

EVALUATION Determine the effectiveness of a cough ▲▲▲▲▲▲▲▲▲▲ suppressant by evaluating the frequency and intensity of the cough. Listen also to breath

Box 51–1. Instructions for Deep Breathing and Coughing

1. Position the patient sitting up. You may wish to use the tripod position.

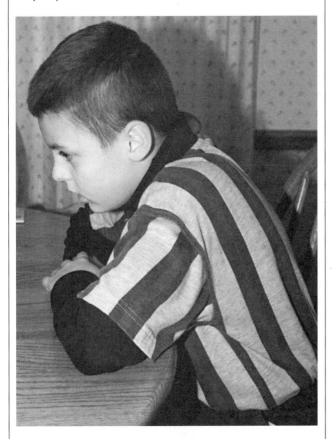

2. Have the patient breathe in deeply through the nose and exhale through the mouth several times. You may wish to demonstrate for a patient who does not seem to fill the lungs.

Box 51–1. Instructions for Deep Breathing and Coughing *Continued*

3. If coughing is to be used, ask the patient to hold the third breath for a count of 3, then cough forcibly. You may wish to provide a pillow to hold against the patient's chest or abdomen. Have tissues handy. Assess any production for color, consistency, and amount. Listen to breath sounds after these exercises to determine whether the lungs are clearer.

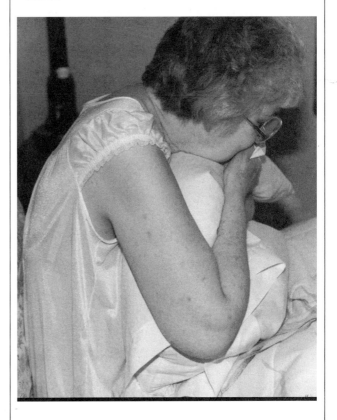

sounds for abnormalities. The lungs should remain clear but not diminished.

Be sure to check the patient's other medications for any CNS depressants in the ingredients, including alcohol, and warn the patient not to mix these drugs at home. The combination may produce added CNS depression.

Types of Suppressants

Suppressants are further divided into two types: narcotics and non-narcotics. The non-narcotic suppressants are most often found in over-the-counter medications; the preceding information also applies to them.

Narcotic suppressants are classified as scheduled drugs. In larger amounts, they are often used as analgesics. In addition to the information for cough suppressants in general, narcotic suppressants can cause the patient to experience confusion, low blood pressure, nausea and vomiting, constipation, headache, euphoria, hallucinations, blurred vision, respiratory depression, urinary retention, sweating, and flushing. Use narcotic drugs only with caution in patients who have any type of pulmonary disease, increased intracranial pressure (such as from a head injury), hypothyroidism, adrenal insufficiency, or prostatic hypertrophy and in the alcoholic or elderly patient. Assess the additional areas of bowel function, blood pressure, and pulse before initiating this medication.

Check the patient's other medications. Narcotics should not be given with monoamine oxidase (MAO) inhibitors or with narcotic antagonists.

Codeine

Codeine is an ingredient in many medications. It is classified as a narcotic, analgesic, and antitussive suppressant. When given as an antitussive, it can be administered orally, subcutaneously, or intramuscularly, although the most common route by far is orally. The usual dose is 10 to 20 mg every 4 to 6 hours. Codeine is classified as a Schedule V drug in amounts given for its antitussive qualities.

Hydrocodone

Hydrocodone (Hycodan) is a narcotic, analgesic, and antitussive suppressant. As an antitussive, it is usually given in combination with decongestants. For antitussive effect, it is administered orally at 5 to 10 mg every 4 to 6 hours; 10-mg and long-acting preparations are administered every 12 hours.

Hydromorphone

Hydromorphone (Dilaudid) is also a narcotic, analgesic, and antitussive suppressant. It can be administered orally, rectally, subcutaneously, or intramuscularly. As an antitussive, the most common route is oral. The antitussive dose is 1 mg every 3 to 4 hours.

Dextromethorphan

Dextromethorphan is a non-narcotic antitussive suppressant. As a non-narcotic, it is one of the most common over-the-counter cough remedies. It does not have any analgesic qualities.

Dextromethorphan is available as tablets, chewables, lozenges, syrups, and suspensions. The usual dose is 10 to 20 mg every 4 hours or 60 mg every 12 hours for extended-release formulas. Be sure the patient understands how to take the preparation. Any suspension needs to be shaken before dispensing. Chewable tablets of this medication cannot be swallowed whole or the effects will be greatly diminished.

Diphenhydramine

Information on diphenhydramine (Benadryl, Benylin, Nytol, Sominex) appears in Chapter 49 because this drug can be classified as either an antihistamine or an antitussive suppressant.

Promethazine Hydrochloride

Promethazine hydrochloride (Phenergan) is a phenothiazine that can be given in syrup form as a non-narcotic antitussive suppressant for coughs and allergy relief. It is also classified as an antihistamine, sedative, and antiemetic. Information about this medication appears in Chapters 49 and 54.

Benzonatate

Benzonatate (Tessalon) is a non-narcotic antitussive suppressant, but its actions differ from those of the previous drugs. This drug anesthetizes the receptors in the respiratory system that trigger the cough reflex. In addition to the adverse reactions mentioned for other non-narcotics, benzonatate can cause pruritus, nasal congestion, numbness in the chest, and burning in the eyes.

The usual dose of benzonatate is 100 mg three times a day. It is given orally. Because this is a local anesthetic, there is usually no interaction with other medications or any major systemic effects.

EXPECTORANTS

ACTIONS AND USES Expectorants reduce the viscosity of the patient's sputum by increasing production of watery respiratory secretions. These secretions mix with the thick mucus and become easier to expel.

Expectorants can also cause drowsiness, nausea and vomiting, diarrhea, and abdominal pain.

ASSESSMENT Assessments that are appropriate for the patient receiving a cough suppressant are also appropriate for the patient receiving an expectorant. This includes assessing the type of cough, production, respiratory status, and breath sounds.

PLANNING AND IMPLEMENTATION The goal for the patient receiving an expectorant is to improve production and reduce abnormal breath sounds. To do this, initiate interventions that further thin the mucus. Encourage the patient to drink plenty of fluids, 1500 to 2000 cc or even more if it is not contraindicated by the condition. However, do not allow the patient to eat or drink immediately after taking the medication. Some medications combine expectorants and suppressants to decrease nonproductive coughs while improving production when the patient does cough.

Instruct the patient to seek medical attention if the cough is prolonged or if other symptoms appear. This could indicate the need for additional medications or a worsening of the condition.

Safety concerns are again a primary focus. Be sure the patient understands that many of the medications can cause drowsiness. Discourage driving or the operation of other hazardous machinery until the patient's individual response to the drug is known.

EVALUATION Evaluate the effectiveness of an expectorant by easier production, increased production, a change from a dry or hacky cough to a productive cough, and improved breath sounds.

Guaifenesin

Guaifenesin (Robitussin) is an expectorant found in many over-the-counter cough remedies. Because it is available over-the-counter, be sure the patient understands the dangers of self-medication. Advise the patient to consult the physician if the cough is not relieved in 5 to 7 days.

Guaifenesin is available as a syrup, tablet, and capsule. In capsule form, the patient needs to swallow the medication whole. Guaifenesin is also available in combination medications. The usual dose is 200 to 400 mg every 4 hours.

MUCOLYTICS

ACTIONS AND USES Mucolytics combine with viscous sputum in the lungs, add moisture, and cause the breakup of microdroplets, thereby thinning the mucus. This allows easier expectoration. Because of this, many reference books classify the mucolytics with the expectorants.

The effects of the mucolytic are local only. The medication is inhaled, usually by nebulization, and acts directly on the mucus.

N U R S I N G   A L E R T

Check for any allergy to iodine before initiating an order for a mucolytic. Many contain potassium iodide.

Mucolytics are also used only with caution in patients with asthma or other chronic respiratory diseases and in the elderly.

ASSESSMENT Assess the patient's breath sounds, ability to produce sputum, and type of cough before initiating the medication.

PLANNING AND IMPLEMENTATION Instruct the patient to cough before treatment with a mucolytic. This helps clear the air passages and allows the medication to come into contact with as much mucus as possible.

N U R S I N G   A L E R T

It is possible, after treatment with a mucolytic, that the patient may experience difficulty handling the excess secretions. The patient may choke. Keep emergency equipment nearby in case this happens.

EVALUATION Evaluate the effectiveness of the mucolytic by production after the treatment and clearer breath sounds.

Acetylcysteine

Acetylcysteine (Mucomyst, Mucosol) is a mucolytic delivered by inhalation. It is also an antidote for the overdose of acetaminophen (it prevents liver damage). As adverse side effects, acetylcysteine can produce drowsiness, a runny nose, nausea and vomiting, hives and itching, fever, and chills.

When giving acetylcysteine, instruct the patient that the medication has an unpleasant odor. This odor generally decreases as the treatment progresses, however.

Do not administer this medication with any equipment containing rubber or metals. The ingredients react with these products and alter what the patient is receiving.

If the medication has changed color to a light purple, it is still all right to use. This insignificant color change does not affect the potency of the drug.

After the treatment has finished, allow the patient to rinse the mouth to help remove any medication residue and unpleasant taste.

The usual dose for acetylcysteine is 1 to 10 cc of the 10% solution or 2 to 20 cc of the 20% solution by inhalation or nebulization, repeated every 2 to 6 hours. The action is nearly immediate.

E X E R C I S E S

CASE STUDIES

1. Your patient has been prescribed a medication to suppress a cough. What nursing assessments should you perform? What teaching could you do that would improve the effectiveness of this drug?

2. Your patient's cough has changed to a productive one, and his medication has been changed to an expectorant. Why would the physician make this change?

3. Mr. J.H. has been prescribed a mucolytic. What allergies should you check his chart for? Why should emergency equipment be kept nearby?

MENTAL AEROBICS

DIRECTED RESEARCH Use a medication reference book to look up the ingredients and their classifications for the following drugs.

1. Vicks Formula 44
2. Tussionex
3. Guaifed
4. Naldecon
5. Triaminic
6. Novahistine
7. Tussi-Organidin
8. Comtrex
9. Codimal
10. Ru-Tuss DE

ANTITUBERCULAR DRUGS

LEARNING OBJECTIVES

After studying this chapter, you should be able to:

1. Describe the actions and uses of antitubercular drugs.

2. State potential adverse reactions to antitubercular drugs.

3. Describe nursing care related to the use of antitubercular drugs by use of the nursing process.

4. State appropriate patient teaching for patients receiving antitubercular drugs.

DRUGS YOU WILL LEARN ABOUT IN THIS CHAPTER

First-Line Drugs

isoniazid (INH)

rifampin (Rimactane, Rifadin)

isoniazid and rifampin (Rifamate)

pyrazinamide (PZA)

ethambutol HCl (EMB, Myambutol)

streptomycin

Second-Line Drugs

kanamycin

cycloserine (Seromycin)

capreomycin sulfate (Capastat Sulfate)

ethionamide (Trecator-SC)

p-aminosalicylic acid (PAS)

Tuberculosis is a disease, primarily pulmonary, caused by the tubercle bacillus, or *Mycobacterium tuberculosis* (MTB). MTB is transmitted by droplets sprayed through the air when an infectious person talks, coughs, sneezes, or sings. If the bacillus is then breathed into the alveoli of a susceptible person, this person can become infected with tuberculosis.

This does *not* mean that the person has tuberculosis disease, however. The patient is said to be infected. The tubercle bacillus can live in the body in a dormant stage for years, or it can produce tuberculosis disease immediately. If it stays in a dormant stage, the patient is not contagious but has the potential to "break down" with tuberculosis disease later in life. Most often, this happens when the immune system is no longer as strong as it once was, perhaps because of other disease processes or the aging process.

The person in whom tuberculosis disease results, whether immediately or later in life, is said to be infectious and is contagious. The infectious patient releases more MTB into the air of the immediate environment.

Tuberculosis infection can be detected with a skin test. The Mantoux or PPD (purified protein derivative) skin test is considered the most accurate. A small amount of altered MTB (0.1 cc) is injected just under the skin. Much practice is required to perfect the technique. The nurse must insert the needle with the bevel up and nearly parallel to the skin. A small wheal must form as the liquid is injected or the process was done incorrectly. It is best not to place a bandage over the site to prevent irritation. The patient is cautioned not to scratch the area, but otherwise normal use and washing of the arm are permitted.

The patient must return to the clinic or office between 48 and 72 hours later to have the test read. This is done by palpating for the edges of induration (a knot under the skin). The nurse carefully measures the size of any induration in millimeters. Any erythema (redness) is ignored because this is most likely caused by a minor reaction to the preservative in the fluid and is not an indication of MTB infection.

In most cases, a tuberculin skin test result is considered positive if the induration is more than 15

Box 52–1. Guidelines for Reading a Tuberculin Skin Test

Consider a skin test result positive at 5 mm of induration for

- Recent converters
- Known close contacts of a patient with an active case
- Persons with abnormal chest radiograph findings that may suggest either previous or current tuberculosis
- Persons who are known to be or are suspected of being positive for human immunodeficiency virus (HIV)
- Persons who inject drugs but for whom the HIV status is unknown

Consider a skin test result positive at 10 mm of induration for

- Health care workers
- Workers from institutions such as correctional facilities
- Persons who were born in or lived in areas of the world where tuberculosis is endemic, such as Asia, Africa, and Latin America
- Persons from medically underserved low-income populations including high-risk racial and ethnic groups, such

as Asians, Pacific Islanders, blacks, Hispanics, and Native Americans

- Children younger than 4 years of age
- Persons who are or have been homeless or migrant workers
- Persons with certain conditions, such as diabetes mellitus, silicosis, low body weight (10% or more below the ideal), malignant diseases, hematological diseases, reticuloendothelial diseases, end-stage renal disease, intestinal bypass or gastrectomy, chronic malabsorption syndromes, and others
- Persons who use corticosteroids in large doses or receive immunosuppressive therapy
- Some northern states consider 10 mm a positive response for all categories except those mentioned at 5 mm

Consider a skin test result positive with 15 mm of induration for

- All others
- Some southern states use only 15 mm of induration as a positive response except for those mentioned at 5 mm

---

mm. However, in special cases, smaller induration sizes are considered a positive reaction, such as in residents of nursing homes, health care workers, or prison inmates. Box 52–1 presents guidelines for reading skin tests in these and other special cases.

If the result of a skin test is determined to be positive, it should be reported to the physician and to the local health department. State laws regulate mandatory reporting and contact investigation. Persons spending considerable time in a shared airspace are contacts.

The physician will order a chest x-ray to determine whether the patient has active tuberculosis at present. If the x-ray shows changes characteristic of tuberculosis (usually granulomatous changes, or other changes in the elderly), a sputum specimen is obtained. The sputum specimen is tested for MTB. Depending on the techniques used by the laboratory, results may be preliminary but nonspecific for MTB. That is, the test may show that there is some type of *Mycobacterium* present, but it may not be MTB. The final culture may take many more days or even weeks (up to 8 weeks). The physician often prescribes medication on the basis of a positive preliminary report (sometimes called a smear). Because of the occurrence of multidrug-resistant strains of tuberculosis, a sensitivity test should also be done before initiation of the

medication. The order may then need to be changed on the basis of the results of this test.

If chest x-ray findings were negative, it is presumed the patient is infected but not yet infectious. It is now recommended by the Centers for Disease Control that such patients receive preventive therapy to lessen their risk for development of tuberculosis disease later.

ANTITUBERCULAR DRUGS

ACTIONS AND USES In general, the antitubercular
▲▲▲▲▲▲▲▲▲▲▲▲▲▲▲▲ drugs can be divided into two groups, the first-line drugs and the second-line drugs. The first-line drugs tend to be more effective. Second-line drugs are usually more difficult to use because of major adverse reactions. They are therefore held in reserve until use is absolutely necessary, and the patient must be monitored more often while taking them.

As preventive medication, a single drug is usually prescribed, and this is most often isoniazid (INH). If the patient cannot tolerate this medication, the second drug of choice is rifampin.

For treatment of tubercular disease, however, it is recommended that no fewer than two, and preferably three or even more, medications be prescribed. The latest recommendation from the Centers for Disease Control is that four medications be prescribed until sputum culture and sensitivity studies are complete. The rationale for multiple-drug therapy is to prevent the development of resistant strains of MTB. Most often, the drug regimen consists of INH, rifampin, ethambutol, and pyrazinamide.

Preventive therapy should be taken for 6 to 12 months or even longer in some cases, such as human immunodeficiency virus (HIV)–positive patients. Antitubercular drug therapy for tuberculosis disease should be taken for 6, 9, 12, or even 18 months, depending on the circumstances of the patient. Most of these medications can be ordered daily or, later in therapy, twice weekly.

ASSESSMENT Before the initiation of drug therapy, ensure that the patient has had a chest x-ray. If the chest x-ray findings were positive or questionable, the patient should have had a sputum specimen collected. The specific drug therapy depends on the results of both the chest x-ray and the sputum culture and sensitivity.

N U R S I N G   A L E R T

Many of the antitubercular drugs cause toxic liver effects. Check the medical history for any liver dysfunction or hepatitis. This necessitates a baseline liver function test (alanine transaminase, aspartate transaminase, serum and urine bilirubin) and repeated tests every 1 to 3 months.

Check also for any history of neuropathies because these may be precipitated by some antitubercular drugs.

PLANNING AND IMPLEMENTATION Inform the patient of the importance of compliance with the drug regimen. Noncompliance, whether with preventive or therapeutic medications, can lead to resistance of the MTB the patient has and render medication ineffective.

The patient should see the physician frequently during the course of drug therapy. The American Thoracic Society of the American Lung Association recommends that the patient be seen by the physician monthly. Inform the patient of the need for frequent visits and possible blood tests.

The physician will order repeated examination of the sputum and chest x-ray frequently during drug therapy. A chest x-ray may be ordered often during preventive therapy or at the beginning and at the end of therapy. Most physicians then recommend an x-ray examination every year thereafter.

Many of the antitubercular drugs are toxic to the neurological system. The physician often prescribes pyridoxine (vitamin B_6) along with the antitubercular agents to prevent neuropathies. The patient may need teaching and encouragement to continue taking medication seen as "only a vitamin."

If a patient is not compliant with the ordered drug regimen, directly observed therapy may be ordered. A tuberculosis specialty nurse or other personnel must watch the patient take the medication. This may be at the clinic or the patient's home. It may also require finding the patient every day. In extreme cases, the health commissioner of the local health district (city, county, or region) has the option to order forced hospitalization of the patient.

EVALUATION Monitor the patient frequently for any changes in liver function test results. If the patient has significant changes in the results of liver function tests (in the healthy person, medications may be continued with test levels up to three times the normal values) or any signs of hepatitis (fever, gastrointestinal upset, abdominal pain, fatigue, weakness, malaise, or even prostration), the physician will immediately remove the patient from the medication. It is possible that the patient will be prescribed the drug again after liver function test results return to normal, or the physician may opt to try a different drug.

N U R S I N G   A L E R T

Because of possible neurological effects of these drugs, assess the patient for any pain in the extremities, visual disturbances, decreased hearing acuity, or even dizziness.

FIRST-LINE DRUGS

Isoniazid

ACTIONS AND USES Isoniazid (INH) is used in the treatment of tuberculosis that is susceptible to it and for preventive therapy. It is commonly given in the following circumstances:

• As preventive therapy for patients who are close contacts of someone with active tuberculosis disease

(share the same airspace, such as family members or carpool partners)

• For those with a positive skin test result (especially if they recently converted from negative to positive or if they have an abnormal chest x-ray)

• For positive reactors receiving steroids or immunosuppressive drugs; with certain blood disorders that can lower the immune system, diabetes, or silicosis; and after a gastrectomy. Other reactors without these special circumstances may also be prescribed INH for preventive therapy in the absence of contraindications. Because of recent increases in tuberculosis cases, the Centers for Disease Control is now recommending that all positive reactors be prescribed some type of preventive medication.

N U R S I N G   A L E R T
▼▼▼▼▼▼▼▼▼▼▼▼▼▼▼▼▼▼▼▼▼▼▼▼▼▼▼▼▼▼▼▼

INH can cause numerous adverse reactions, including severe and even fatal hepatitis.

▲▲▲▲▲▲▲▲▲▲▲▲▲▲▲▲▲▲▲▲▲▲▲▲▲▲▲▲▲▲▲▲

This reaction can occur at any time during therapy. The risk of hepatitis increases with the patient's age and with alcohol consumption.

INH can lead to vitamin B_6 (pyridoxine) deficiency in large doses. For this reason, many physicians choose to prescribe this vitamin adjunctively with INH.

Other side effects include neuropathies with paresthesia of the feet and hands, optic neuritis, encephalopathy, optic atrophy, convulsions, toxic psychosis, loss of memory, and gastrointestinal upset. Blood dyscrasias, febrile reactions, rash, hyperglycemia, metabolic acidosis, gynecomastia (the development of breasts in men or increased breast size in women), rheumatic syndrome (swollen joints), and systemic lupus erythematosus may also occur but are less common.

ASSESSMENT Because the risk of hepatitis increases ▲▲▲▲▲▲▲▲▲▲ with alcohol consumption, ask questions about the patient's intake. Several questions designed to elicit this information may be required because a patient may not appropriately answer a direct question about daily intake.

Visual acuity should be assessed before initiation of the drug. The physician may recommend a thorough ophthalmological examination before the drug is started and periodically thereafter.

Before the first dose of the drug, obtain the sputum specimen. Assess the patient for any history of hepatitis or other liver disease. Precaution is also

recommended if the patient is currently receiving phenytoin (Dilantin, an anticonvulsant) because both drugs can cause liver dysfunction.

PLANNING AND IMPLEMENTATION INH is most com-
▲▲▲▲▲▲▲▲▲▲▲▲▲▲▲▲▲▲▲▲▲▲▲▲▲▲▲ monly prescribed by the physician at a dose of 300 mg every day. If it is used for treatment of disease, it should *not* be used alone. Caution the patient not to stop and start the medication because this can cause the development of a resistant strain of MTB.

Because of the high frequency of gastrointestinal disturbance, encourage the patient to take INH with food.

Teach the patient the signs of hepatitis and instruct the patient to report these signs immediately to the physician. If the drug is not stopped, hepatitis can be fatal.

Contact the local health department's tuberculosis nurse. This health care professional will follow-up on the patient's care and see that any contacts are tested for possible infection. The tuberculosis nurse will assess the patient's compliance and keep the physician informed of occurrences.

EVALUATION The patient receiving INH should be
▲▲▲▲▲▲▲▲▲▲ interviewed at least monthly and have frequent liver function tests. The nurse is responsible for monitoring results of these tests. Report any increases or any prodromal symptoms of hepatitis to the physician immediately.

N U R S I N G   A L E R T
▼▼▼▼▼▼▼▼▼▼▼▼▼▼▼▼▼▼▼▼▼▼▼▼▼▼▼▼▼▼▼▼

Overdose of INH is possible. Evaluate the patient for gastrointestinal upset, blurred vision, slurred speech, hallucination, or dizziness. It is possible with severe overdose to have respiratory distress, central nervous system depression, seizures, and even coma and death.

▲▲▲▲▲▲▲▲▲▲▲▲▲▲▲▲▲▲▲▲▲▲▲▲▲▲▲▲▲▲▲▲

If these signs occur, report them immediately. The patient may require physician orders for gastric lavage, intravenous barbiturates for the convulsions, intravenous pyridoxine (vitamin B_6), and respiratory support. Monitor the blood gas levels and blood pH. Acidosis may need to be controlled. The physician will probably order sodium bicarbonate. Osmotic diuretics and hemodialysis may also be ordered. Accurate intake and output measurements are required.

Repeated examination of the sputum will be ordered

periodically throughout INH therapy to determine whether the medication is effective for the patient with active disease. Monitor reports of these smears and cultures.

Rifampin

ACTIONS AND USES Rifampin (Rimactane, Rifadin) is a ▲▲▲▲▲▲▲▲▲▲▲▲▲▲▲▲ rifamycin type of antibiotic. It inhibits bacterial reproduction. It can be used for pulmonary tuberculosis disease or MTB preventive therapy and for exposure to or asymptomatic carriers of *Neisseria meningitidis*. It cannot be used for current *N. meningitidis* infection. When used for either bacterium, this drug should not be used alone.

Rifampin can cause adverse reactions. In addition to those listed for INH, it can turn body fluids red-orange. This includes urine, feces, saliva, sputum, tears, and sweat. Rifampin can also cause headaches, drowsiness, muscle weakness, and menstrual disturbances. In addition to numbness in the extremities from neuropathy, there may also be pain.

Rifampin can lead to renal dysfunction. Increases can be seen in the blood urea nitrogen and serum uric acid levels. Hypersensitivity reactions are usually a rash and itching.

ASSESSMENT In addition to those assessments for INH, ▲▲▲▲▲▲▲▲▲▲ assess the patient prescribed rifampin for a history of hypersensitivity to rifamycins.

PLANNING AND IMPLEMENTATION The dose generally ▲▲▲▲▲▲▲▲▲▲▲▲▲▲▲▲▲▲▲▲▲▲▲▲▲▲▲ prescribed for rifampin is 600 mg every day for tuberculosis. This should be given to the patient 1 to 2 hours after eating to decrease the risk of gastric upset. It is also recommended to be given 1 to 2 hours after any other antitubercular drugs.

N U R S I N G   A L E R T

Because of the unusual coloration of body fluids that is likely, warn the patient ahead of time. It can be frightening to the patient to experience this adverse reaction if it is unexpected.

Also caution the patient that the body fluids will stain clothing and other objects, including soft contacts. Therefore, protection may be worn for the period of time, and soft contacts should not be used.

EVALUATION In addition to those points listed for INH, ▲▲▲▲▲▲▲▲▲▲ evaluate the patient receiving rifampin for possible drug interactions. Those drugs that can interact with rifampin include oral contraceptives, which will become less effective. Warn the patient to use another form of protection during drug therapy.

The dose of coumarin (anticoagulant) may need to be increased. Monitor the prothrombin time closely.

The effects of methadone are decreased by the use of rifampin. The physician may need to increase the dose of methadone by as much as double to obtain the same effects. Other drugs that may need increased doses are oral hypoglycemics, corticosteroids, digitalis, and verapamil.

p-aminosalicylic acid (PAS, a drug sometimes used as an adjunct in the treatment of tuberculosis) lowers the effectiveness of rifampin. For this reason, give them at least 4 hours apart.

N U R S I N G   A L E R T

An overdose of rifampin can cause gastrointestinal upset, lethargy, unconsciousness, red-orange skin, liver enlargement, and liver tenderness.

If you evaluate the patient and detect any of these signs, they must be reported immediately. The physician will often need to order gastric lavage, activated charcoal, antiemetics, diuretics, and even hemodialysis.

Rifamate

Rifamate is the trade name for a combination drug of both rifampin and isoniazid. This oral drug is actually giving the patient the benefits of both of these drugs. Be aware of this and do not make the mistake of thinking only one drug is being used.

Pyrazinamide

ACTIONS AND USES Pyrazinamide (PZA) is a bacteri-▲▲▲▲▲▲▲▲▲▲▲▲▲▲ cidal agent that is useful against active tuberculosis only. It cannot be used as a preventive drug.

Common adverse reactions in addition to those of INH include increased serum uric acid levels and development of symptoms of gout, arthralgias, and gastrointestinal upset.

ASSESSMENT In addition to those assessments for INH, check the patient's history for gout. PZA could aggravate a pre-existing condition.

PLANNING AND IMPLEMENTATION The average dose of PZA is 750 to 1000 mg given twice a day. This is an oral drug. The drug may need to be given after eating to reduce gastrointestinal upset.

EVALUATION Continue to monitor for abnormal results of liver function tests, as with INH. Also check for increased serum uric acid levels and evaluate the patient for any symptoms of gout. If any of these occur, report them immediately. It is possible that the physician may want to order rifampin to be given with the PZA because this can reduce the effects on uric acid levels.

The effectiveness of PZA is decreased if it is given concomitantly with probenecid (an antigout agent). Conversely, the effects of probenecid are increased.

Ethambutol Hydrochloride

ACTIONS AND USES Ethambutol hydrochloride (EMB, Myambutol) is useful against MTB for pulmonary tuberculosis, but as with the other drugs, it should not be used alone.

In addition to the common adverse reactions listed for INH, EMB can decrease visual acuity and change color perception as well as cause a rash and itching, joint pain, gastrointestinal upset, malaise, headache, and confusion. Serum uric acid levels may increase or precipitate symptoms of gout.

ASSESSMENT Other assessments to perform for the patient prescribed EMB include checking for a history of optic neuritis or renal dysfunction. EMB should not be used with optic neuritis. The dose of EMB needs to be decreased if the patient has kidney disease.

PLANNING AND IMPLEMENTATION EMB is an oral drug generally given once a day. The average dose is 1000 mg.

N U R S I N G   A L E R T

Because of the effect on the patient's vision, a baseline eye examination and color vision examination are necessary.

These examinations should be repeated approximately every month while the patient is receiving the medication. Report significant changes to the physician promptly because the drug will need to be stopped. The vision usually returns to normal after the medication is stopped. Tell the patient to report any blurred vision between visits.

EVALUATION In addition to monitoring results of liver function tests, monitor serum uric acid levels and symptoms of gout. Report these immediately.

Streptomycin

ACTIONS AND USES Streptomycin was the first drug discovered to be effective against tuberculosis. It is a bactericidal aminoglycoside anti-infective. It is useful against active MTB infection but not as a preventive medication. As with other antitubercular drugs, streptomycin should not be used alone.

Streptomycin can also be used for some types of endocarditis in conjunction with penicillin as well as for tularemia and the plague.

Streptomycin is associated with severe adverse reactions. In addition to those listed for INH, it is ototoxic, nephrotoxic, and neurotoxic. The patient may experience hearing loss, vertigo, tinnitus, kidney dysfunction with edema, electrolyte imbalances, liver dysfunction, and respiratory paralysis.

ASSESSMENT Assess the patient to be given streptomycin for any signs of renal dysfunction. The physician orders baseline kidney function tests. Neuromuscular diseases also necessitate precaution while the patient is taking this medication. Because streptomycin can cause deafness in the fetus if it is used during pregnancy, assess the patient for sexual activity and use of birth control. The physician often orders a pregnancy test before initiating this drug.

PLANNING AND IMPLEMENTATION Streptomycin is given intramuscularly.

It should be placed deep into a large muscle. Rotate sites to prevent excoriation. The average dose is 1000 mg per day for tuberculosis.

Caution the patient not to become pregnant during drug therapy. Teach effective methods of birth control and emphasize the importance of using birth control with every sexual intercourse.

N U R S I N G   A L E R T

▼▼▼▼▼▼▼▼▼▼▼▼▼▼▼▼▼▼▼▼▼▼▼▼▼▼▼▼▼▼▼▼▼

Teach signs and symptoms of ototoxic, nephrotoxic, and neurotoxic effects. Instruct the patient to report these signs to the physician immediately.

▲▲▲▲▲▲▲▲▲▲▲▲▲▲▲▲▲▲▲▲▲▲▲▲▲▲▲▲▲▲▲▲▲

EVALUATION Monitor the patient's kidney function test results as well as serum electrolyte levels. Evaluate respiratory rate and effort frequently. Initiate intake and output monitoring. Check the hearing acuity often.

Be aware that streptomycin can interact with other medications. It can be antagonistic to penicillin. The risk of respiratory paralysis is greatly increased if the patient must have anesthetic. Ototoxicity is increased if streptomycin is given with the loop diuretics.

SECOND-LINE DRUGS

Kanamycin

See aminoglycosides in Chapter 19.

Cycloserine

ACTIONS AND USES Cycloserine (Seromycin) is a broad-spectrum antibiotic effective against gram-positive and gram-negative bacteria. It is useful in the management of both pulmonary and extrapulmonary tuberculosis caused by MTB. As with other antitubercular drugs, it should not be used alone for MTB.

In addition to those adverse reactions listed for INH, cycloserine can cause neurological dysfunction, congestive heart failure, and a rash.

ASSESSMENT Before initiating the first dose of cycloserine, assess for a history of epilepsy, depression, severe anxiety, psychosis, renal insufficiency, and alcoholism. Each of these is a contraindication to the use of cycloserine.

PLANNING AND IMPLEMENTATION Cycloserine is an oral medication. The average dose is 500 to 1000 mg per day. This is given in two divided doses.

EVALUATION Carefully monitor your patient who is receiving cycloserine. This drug must be stopped immediately if any of the following signs or symptoms of toxic effect occur: rash, seizure, psychosis, drowsiness, confusion, headache, depression, dizziness, tremors, joint pain, or paresthesia.

In addition, cycloserine is known to interact with several medications or substances. The neurotoxic adverse reactions are more likely to occur if cycloserine is given with either ethionamide or INH, both antitubercular agents. The risk of seizures during cycloserine therapy is dramatically increased if the patient drinks alcohol. Check all medications given to the patient for alcohol content.

Capreomycin Sulfate

ACTIONS AND USES Capreomycin sulfate (Capastat Sulfate) is an antibiotic that can be used against MTB, but not alone. It is known to be ototoxic and nephrotoxic. It can also cause hypokalemia, liver dysfunction, blood dyscrasias, rash, hives, and itching.

ASSESSMENT Before initiating capreomycin, check the patient's history for kidney or liver dysfunction. Perform a baseline hearing test. Monitor results of tests of kidney function, serum potassium concentration, and liver function and the complete blood count (CBC).

PLANNING AND IMPLEMENTATION Capreomycin is given intramuscularly or intravenously only.

N U R S I N G   A L E R T

▼▼▼▼▼▼▼▼▼▼▼▼▼▼▼▼▼▼▼▼▼▼▼▼▼▼▼▼▼▼▼▼▼

Capreomycin must be placed deep into a large muscle. Sterile abscesses may occur if the injection is too shallow.

▲▲▲▲▲▲▲▲▲▲▲▲▲▲▲▲▲▲▲▲▲▲▲▲▲▲▲▲▲▲▲▲▲

Also be aware of the possibility of pain, induration, and excessive bleeding at the site of an intramuscular injection. If capreomycin is given intravenously, the rate of flow must be slow. Too rapid instillation can lead to muscle weakness and respiratory paralysis.

EVALUATION Continue to monitor results of all labo-
▲▲▲▲▲▲▲▲▲▲ ratory tests performed. Perform frequent hearing tests.

Ethionamide

ACTIONS AND USES Given in conjunction with other
▲▲▲▲▲▲▲▲▲▲▲▲▲▲▲ drugs, ethionamide (Trecator-SC) is effective against MTB. However, it can cause seizures, gastrointestinal upset, mood disturbances, orthostatic hypotension, rash, and impotence in addition to those adverse reactions already mentioned for INH.

ASSESSMENT Check your patient's history for diabetes
▲▲▲▲▲▲▲▲▲▲ mellitus. Diabetes can increase the risk for liver dysfunction while the patient is taking this drug.

PLANNING AND IMPLEMENTATION Ethionamide is an
▲▲▲▲▲▲▲▲▲▲▲▲▲▲▲▲▲▲▲▲▲▲▲▲▲▲▲▲▲▲▲ oral medication. It is recommended to be given together with pyridoxine to reduce adverse reactions.

EVALUATION See evaluation for INH.
▲▲▲▲▲▲▲▲▲▲

p-Aminosalicyclic Acid

ACTIONS AND USES p-Aminosalicylic acid (PAS) is
▲▲▲▲▲▲▲▲▲▲▲▲▲▲▲▲ most often used for children in treatment of MTB infection. It is less expensive than some other antitubercular drugs. It can cause many of the adverse reactions of INH as well as severe gastrointestinal upset, kidney dysfunction, hypokalemia, and fluid and sodium retention.

N U R S I N G   A L E R T

▼▼▼▼▼▼▼▼▼▼▼▼▼▼▼▼▼▼▼▼▼▼▼▼▼▼▼▼▼▼▼▼▼

In addition to the assessments to be made common to all antitubercular drugs, assess this patient for a history of hypersensitivity to INH or rifampin because the allergy may cross over.

▲▲

PLANNING AND IMPLEMENTATION It may be difficult
▲▲▲▲▲▲▲▲▲▲▲▲▲▲▲▲▲▲▲▲▲▲▲▲▲▲▲▲▲▲▲ to elicit cooperation from the pediatric patient to take this oral medication. Suggestions are offered in Chapter 11.

EVALUATION Continue to monitor results of renal
▲▲▲▲▲▲▲▲▲▲ function tests and serum potassium levels. Report any abnormalities immediately.

E X E R C I S E S

CASE STUDIES

1. Ms. M.W., age 42 years, was tested at your clinic with a tuberculin skin test. Now, 2 days later, the skin test result is read as positive. What would be the next step?

It is determined that Ms. M.W. does not now have active tuberculosis. Why, then, did her physician prescribe her medication? What baseline information should you look for before her first dose of medication?

2. Mr. S.J., age 37 years, has a positive finding on chest x-ray examination. His sputum smear and culture are positive for MTB. He has active tuberculosis with symptoms. How can you best explain to Mr. S.J. the need for his family to be tested?

Mr. S.J. tells you at his next appointment that he did not like taking all those medications so he now takes only one. How can you best address his statement?

What symptoms would you tell Mr. S.J. to be aware of and report to the physician if he is prescribed INH?

MENTAL AEROBICS

Ask to observe at a local health department clinic, in the tuberculosis clinic if they have one. Watch the technique used to administer a tuberculin skin test. Listen for questions the nurses routinely ask patients taking tuberculosis medications.

UNIT ELEVEN

DRUGS THAT AFFECT THE DIGESTIVE SYSTEM

The classifications of drugs that affect the digestive system contain many over-the-counter medications. Just as the drugs that affect the respiratory system are "serious medicine," so too are the drugs used for the digestive system.

Recall some basic information about digestion. Food is taken in and broken down by a series of mechanical and chemical processes. Mechanical processes include mastication with the teeth and the churning action of the stomach. Chemical processes involve digestive enzymes and digestive juices. Digestive juices are produced in the mouth (saliva), the stomach (gastric juice), the small intestine (intestinal juice), the pancreas (pancreatic juice), and the gallbladder (bile). Digestive enzymes are contained in these fluids. Problems of the digestive system often involve an overproduction of digestive juice or enzymes or the inability of the digestive enzymes to reach the intended site of action.

In the small and large intestine, some digestion and absorption take place. As the material passes farther along the colon, it contains less usable material and more waste. It is moved along by the peristaltic action of the colon. Problems of the intestines are often due to either hyperactivity or hypoactivity of peristalsis.

When digestion occurs normally, the body is given the nutrients it needs for daily function. However, the body must first receive the raw material (food) with which to work. If a patient does not ingest the proper nutrients in the daily diet, malnutrition can result. Nutritional supplements may then become necessary.

In Chapter 53, you will learn the difference between an antacid and an antiflatulent and why they are often found in combinations. We discuss the histamine H_2-receptor antagonists often used for ulcer patients.

Although the antiemetics and the emetics have opposite actions, we discuss them together in Chapter 54. Public teaching is discussed when we talk about the emetics. Some information about potential poisoning is presented as background material.

Five types of laxatives are discussed in Chapter 55. Although they produce a similar action, their modes of action are different. Antidiarrheals are discussed in the same chapter. You will learn that some of these drugs are not only serious medicine but even addicting.

Digestants and their proper use are covered in Chapter 56. A detailed discussion of vitamins and minerals is included. This chapter is not intended to replace your nutrition textbook, but some nutritional information is necessary for discussing deficits and nursing actions.

ANTACIDS AND RELATED DRUGS

LEARNING OBJECTIVES

After studying this chapter, you should be able to:

1. Describe the actions and uses of antacids and related drugs.

2. Identify the side effects of and contraindications to antacids and related drugs.

3. Describe appropriate nursing care relating to antacids and related drugs.

4. Describe appropriate patient teaching for patients receiving antacids and related drugs.

DRUGS YOU WILL LEARN ABOUT IN THIS CHAPTER

Antacids

aluminum hydroxide (Amphojel, Dialume, Maalox [one ingredient])

magnesium hydroxide (milk of magnesia, Maalox [one ingredient])

magaldrate (Riopan)

sodium bicarbonate (Alka-Seltzer Effervescent Antacid, baking soda)

calcium carbonate (Rolaids, Tums)

sucralfate (Carafate)

omeprazole (Prilosec)

Antiflatulents

simethicone (ingredient of Maalox Plus, Mylanta, Riopan Plus)

Histamine H_2-Receptor Antagonists

cimetidine HCl (Tagamet)

ranitidine HCl (Zantac)

famotidine (Pepcid)

For nearly every gastrointestinal problem there is, we have something to treat it. The antacids and related drugs are given for treatment of increased gastric secretions and gas. The patient is one who is complaining of an "upset stomach" or "heartburn." Although these may seem like innocuous symptoms, they can be indicators of much more serious problems. The drugs used to treat these symptoms also cannot be discounted as harmless.

ANTACIDS

Aluminum Hydroxide

ACTIONS AND USES Aluminum hydroxide is used alone or as one ingredient of many over-the-counter antacids. It is the main ingredient of Amphojel and Dialume and one ingredient of Maalox. It works by counteracting the hydrochloric acid in the stomach. Physicians may prescribe aluminum hydroxide for patients with peptic ulcer, gastritis, hiatal hernia, esophagitis, or other gastrointestinal disorders.

Aluminum hydroxide may also be used as a phosphate binder to prevent the absorption of phosphate in patients with renal failure.

This ingredient can cause constipation. Most other adverse reactions are associated with prolonged use or overuse.

ASSESSMENT Assess the patient's symptoms of gas-
▲▲▲▲▲▲▲▲▲▲ trointestinal distress. When do they occur? How would the patient rate them on a scale of 1
to 10 (or 1 to 100 for even greater accuracy)? Does
anything that the patient has tried relieve the symptoms?

Be aware of all of the patient's disorders. Caution is
warranted with aluminum hydroxide for patients with
renal failure or on renal dialysis. Patients with renal
failure are at an increased risk for osteomalacia when
they are taking this antacid. Renal dialysis patients
are at increased risk for encephalopathy.

PLANNING AND IMPLEMENTATION The usual dose of
▲▲▲▲▲▲▲▲▲▲▲▲▲▲▲▲▲▲▲▲▲▲▲▲▲▲▲ aluminum hydroxide is 600 to 650 mg five or six times a day. The patient
should not exceed 3600 mg in a 24-hour period.
Encourage the patient to drink plenty of water with
this drug.

This antacid and most others are best taken on an
empty stomach. Other oral medications should not be
taken at the same time because aluminum hydroxide
interferes with their absorption. Be sure to separate
administration of these drugs by at least 1 hour.

N U R S I N G   A L E R T
▼▼▼▼▼▼▼▼▼▼▼▼▼▼▼▼▼▼▼▼▼▼▼▼▼▼▼▼▼▼▼▼▼▼▼▼▼▼▼

It is important to teach the patient signs of
gastrointestinal bleeding. Instruct the patient to immediately report to the physician any bright red
blood in the stool, black tarry stools, or emesis of
blood or coffee grounds–like substances.

▲▲▲▲▲▲▲▲▲▲▲▲▲▲▲▲▲▲▲▲▲▲▲▲▲▲▲▲▲▲▲▲▲▲▲▲▲

EVALUATION The patient is the best judge of improve-
▲▲▲▲▲▲▲▲▲▲ ment of symptoms. The same rating scale
you used in assessing symptoms will show changes in
the condition by going up or down.

Remember to ask the patient about constipation.
Often, if you do not ask, the patient may be too
embarrassed to mention the problem.

Check for any interactions with other drugs. Use of
aluminum hydroxide with aspirin may decrease the
effects of the aspirin, but it can increase the effects of
amphetamines. In addition to decreasing the absorption of all oral medications, aluminum hydroxide
especially decreases absorption of iron, phenothiazines, and isoniazid (an antitubercular drug). Aluminum hydroxide and most other antacids should not be
taken with tetracycline antibiotics.

Watch the patient for signs of hypophosphatemia,
which can occur with prolonged use. Signs and
symptoms of hypophosphatemia include anorexia,
muscle weakness, malaise, and osteomalacia.

Magnesium Hydroxide

Magnesium hydroxide is another common over-the-
counter antacid that can be used alone or as one
ingredient. It is the main ingredient of milk of
magnesia and one of the ingredients of Maalox. It
tends to be less constipating than aluminum hydroxide. It should not be used for patients with renal
failure. Watch the patient for signs of hypermagnesemia, which occurs with overuse.

Magaldrate

Magaldrate (Riopan) is an over-the-counter preparation of aluminum and magnesium hydroxides bound
together. It can cause either constipation or diarrhea.
Other information is the same as that listed for
aluminum hydroxide and magnesium hydroxide.

Sodium Bicarbonate

ACTIONS AND USES Sodium bicarbonate (Alka-Seltzer
▲▲▲▲▲▲▲▲▲▲▲▲▲▲▲▲▲ Effervescent Antacid, baking soda)
is a commonly used over-the-counter antacid. Readily
available, it lends itself easily to overuse.

Sodium bicarbonate is an alkalinizing agent. As
such, it neutralizes stomach acid, relieving acid
indigestion and heartburn.

ASSESSMENT
▲▲▲▲▲▲▲▲▲▲

N U R S I N G   A L E R T
▼▼▼▼▼▼▼▼▼▼▼▼▼▼▼▼▼▼▼▼▼▼▼▼▼▼▼▼▼▼▼▼▼▼▼▼▼▼▼

In addition to the assessments listed under aluminum hydroxide for gastrointestinal distress, also
note whether the patient has any symptoms of abdominal pain. The use of sodium bicarbonate in any
form when the patient has such pain is contraindicated. If the patient has a condition that resulted in
a weakened area of the stomach, the gas (carbon
dioxide) forming from the neutralization process
could perforate the stomach at this spot. This
includes peptic ulcers, ulcerative colitis, and others.

▲▲▲▲▲▲▲▲▲▲▲▲▲▲▲▲▲▲▲▲▲▲▲▲▲▲▲▲▲▲▲▲▲▲▲▲▲▲▲

Other contraindications include alkalosis, hypocalcemia, and renal failure. Use is also contraindicated in
any patient on a sodium-restricted diet. Those with
congestive heart failure should be monitored closely
during use of this drug.

PLANNING AND IMPLEMENTATION The usual dose for
▲▲▲▲▲▲▲▲▲▲▲▲▲▲▲▲▲▲▲▲▲▲▲▲▲ sodium bicarbonate
is 1 teaspoon to 3 to 4 ounces of water. If an
effervescent tablet is used, the dose is 1 to 2 tablets
every 4 hours as needed. Place each effervescent tablet
in 3 to 4 ounces of water. The dose for children and the
elderly is decreased.

Caution the patient not to take more than 8 tablets
or 8 teaspoons in a 24-hour period. Inform the patient
that belching is normal after use of this drug.

EVALUATION Because this drug is so easily overused,
▲▲▲▲▲▲▲▲▲▲ evaluate the patient for signs of metabolic alkalosis.

Calcium Carbonate

Calcium carbonate (Tums, Rolaids) is an over-the-
counter antacid used for gastric distress. It may also
be used to treat a calcium deficiency or hyperphosphatemia. It should not be given to the patient with a
history of calcium kidney stones. Greater monitoring
of the patient is warranted with a history of either
kidney or heart disease. It should not be taken with
the tetracycline antibiotics or with digitalis. The most
common adverse reactions are constipation, renal
calculi, and hypercalcemia.

Sucralfate

ACTIONS AND USES Sucralfate (Carafate) has little if
▲▲▲▲▲▲▲▲▲▲▲▲▲▲▲▲ any systemic effect. Its localized
action is to adhere to the ulcer site, forming a film-like
barrier and allowing healing. It also inhibits pepsin
activity and adsorbs bile salts. A single gram of
sucralfate can neutralize up to 16 mEq of acid.
Sucralfate is used for short-term treatment of duodenal ulcers and to maintain a healed state after the
initial term of treatment. The most common adverse
reaction is constipation.

ASSESSMENT Although there are no true contraindica-
▲▲▲▲▲▲▲▲▲▲ tions to the use of sucralfate, assess the
patient for a history of renal failure or current
decreased renal function. Because sucralfate causes
the absorption of a small amount of aluminum, these
patients could be put at risk if they were to use it.

PLANNING AND IMPLEMENTATION This oral drug is
▲▲▲▲▲▲▲▲▲▲▲▲▲▲▲▲▲▲▲▲▲▲▲▲▲▲ generally used for 4
to 8 weeks to heal an ulcer. The patient may become
asymptomatic within 1 to 2 weeks. It is the nurse's

responsibility to teach the patient the importance of
continuing the medication even when symptoms subside.

The usual dose prescribed for healing of an acute
ulcer is 1 g four times a day on an empty stomach. If
the drug is to be given for maintenance, the usual dose
is 1 g twice a day. Do not give the drug with other oral
medications. Give sucralfate 2 hours before other
drugs.

EVALUATION To determine the effectiveness of the
▲▲▲▲▲▲▲▲▲▲ drug, ask the patient about comfort level.
Be sure to include questions about discomfort when
the stomach is empty as well as after eating.

Be alert for any signs of decreased effectiveness of
other oral medications the patient may also be taking.
Sucralfate is known to decrease the absorption of
cimetidine, ciprofloxacin, digoxin, norfloxacin, phenytoin, ranitidine, tetracycline, and theophylline. It is
possible that it could interfere with any oral drug.

Omeprazole

Omeprazole (Prilosec) is not an antacid in the strictest
definition of the word. It could be termed an antisecre-
tory agent. Omeprazole suppresses the secretion of
gastric acid by the parietal cells by blocking the final
step of production. This final step is called the
pumping mechanism. For this reason, omeprazole
may be called a pump blocker.

Omeprazole is prescribed for short-term treatment
of severe erosive esophagitis and for symptomatic
gastroesophageal reflux. It is usually reserved for
patients who do not respond to other treatment
because of its adverse reactions. Omeprazole is not
used as a maintenance drug.

N U R S I N G   A L E R T
▼▼▼▼▼▼▼▼▼▼▼▼▼▼▼▼▼▼▼▼▼▼▼▼▼▼▼▼▼▼▼▼

Omeprazole has been shown to cause the growth
of tumors in laboratory animals. For this reason,
it is used with great caution and only for short
periods.

▲▲▲▲▲▲▲▲▲▲▲▲▲▲▲▲▲▲▲▲▲▲▲▲▲▲▲▲▲▲▲▲▲▲▲▲

Other adverse reactions may include a headache,
gastrointestinal distress, constipation, rash, cough,
and asthenia.

Omeprazole is supplied in delayed-release capsules
with enteric coated granules inside. For this reason,
caution the patient not to open the capsule, chew it, or
crush it. It must be swallowed whole.

Watch for signs of increased effectiveness of other drugs used by the patient. It may become necessary for the physician to decrease the dose of diazepam, warfarin, and phenytoin.

ANTIFLATULENTS

Simethicone

Antiflatulents are often used in conjunction with antacids to help the patient with relief of gas. You may see these combination medications used to treat patients with dyspepsia or peptic ulcer and postoperative patients.

Simethicone (an ingredient of Maalox Plus, Mylanta, and Riopan Plus) is not absorbed systemically. Therefore, it does not exert systemic side effects. It does help induce either belching or flatus by encouraging the passing of gas trapped in the gastrointestinal system.

HISTAMINE H$_2$-RECEPTOR ANTAGONISTS

Cimetidine Hydrochloride

ACTIONS AND USES Cimetidine hydrochloride (Tagamet) is chemically related to histamine but without the same actions as histamine. As a result of this close relation, it can take up space at a receptor site and effectively block histamine from the site. This inhibits gastric acid secretion. Therefore, cimetidine is used to treat ulcers for a short term and can be used to prevent the formation of new ulcers.

Cimetidine is rarely associated with serious adverse reactions. When it is, these can include cardiac arrhythmia, hypotension, and blood dyscrasias. It is more common to find the patient experiencing diarrhea, headache, dizziness, confusion, or even gynecomastia or impotence.

ASSESSMENT A thorough gastrointestinal assessment is warranted for the patient receiving cimetidine. Assess the symptoms associated with the condition. Include baseline vital signs in this assessment.

PLANNING AND IMPLEMENTATION Cimetidine is available as tablets, as a liquid, and for intramuscular (IM) or intravenous (IV) injection. The usual oral dose is 800 mg at bedtime. IM and IV doses are 300 mg every 6 to 8 hours.

Teach the patient that cigarette smoking decreases the effectiveness of cimetidine and lengthens the amount of time necessary to heal the ulcer.

EVALUATION Caution the patient that between 4 and 8 weeks is needed to completely heal an ulcer. Although the patient may be feeling better much sooner than this, the medication (and dietary prescriptions) must be continued to prevent relapse.

Watch for any drug interactions. Cimetidine can lengthen the effects of anticoagulants, phenytoin (an anticonvulsant), lidocaine (a cardiovascular drug), and theophylline (a bronchodilator). Doses of these drugs may need to be adjusted by the physician.

Ranitidine Hydrochloride

Ranitidine hydrochloride (Zantac) is a drug similar to cimetidine, but it is associated with fewer drug interactions. It is available as tablets, as a syrup, and in injectable form. It is known to cause a false-positive response for urinary protein with use of the Multistix brand dipstick.

The usual oral dose is 150 mg twice a day or 300 mg once a day. Given IM or IV, the dose is 50 mg every 6 to 8 hours.

Famotidine

ACTIONS AND USES Famotidine (Pepcid) inhibits gastric secretion of acid in much the same way as cimetidine does. It has no other common systemic effects.

Famotidine is used for short-term treatment of gastric and duodenal ulcers and as a method of preventing future ulcers.

The adverse reactions associated with famotidine are not common but include headache, dizziness, constipation, or diarrhea. If the IV route is used, irritation at the injection site can occur.

ASSESSMENT Check for renal insufficiency in the patient's medical examination. Severe renal insufficiency causes the drug to stay in the system longer and can cause adverse reactions to be more likely.

PLANNING AND IMPLEMENTATION The usual oral dose of famotidine is 40 mg every day for up to 8 weeks. Once the ulcer has healed, a maintenance dose of 20 mg every day is often ordered. Oral forms include both tablets and suspension.

If famotidine is ordered IV, the usual dose is 20 mg every 12 hours. Dilute it in 5 to 10 mL of normal saline and inject it for at least a 2-minute period. Famotidine can also be given by IV drip, diluted in 100 mL of dextrose in water. Set it to drip for at least a 15- to 30-minute period.

EVALUATION Famotidine is not commonly associated ▲▲▲▲▲▲▲▲▲▲ with drug interactions.

CHOLINERGIC BLOCKERS

Several cholinergic blocking drugs are prescribed by the physician for treatment of gastrointestinal upset. These can include propantheline bromide (Pro-Banthine), scopolamine, glycopyrrolate (Robinul), hyoscyamine sulfate (Anaspaz), and anisotropine methylbromide (Valpin 50). See Chapters 40 and 54 for more information on these drugs.

E X E R C I S E S

CASE STUDIES

1. On admission, Ms. S.W., age 67 years, tells you to be sure to give her some baking soda after lunch each day. She assures you that she has been using this to reduce stomach upset for several months and refers to it as an "old home remedy my mother used." What would be your best actions as a nurse for Ms. S.W.? What could her need for the baking soda for such a length of time indicate?

2. Your patient has been prescribed Ecotrin every 4 hours and Maalox every 4 hours. What would be the best schedule for both of these drugs? If the drug prescribed with Maalox is tetracycline, what would your best action be?

3. During a clinic visit, a patient mentions to you that he has stopped taking his cimetidine now because his stomach problems have stopped. What would be your best nursing actions?

4. This same patient is starting cimetidine therapy again. During a subsequent clinic visit, you smell cigarette smoke on his clothes. What teaching does your patient need?

MENTAL AEROBICS

Write a care plan to address the major problems that could be associated with a peptic ulcer patient who is receiving cimetidine.

ANTIEMETICS AND EMETICS

LEARNING OBJECTIVES

After studying this chapter, you should be able to:

1. Describe the action and use of antiemetics.

2. Give examples of antiemetics.

3. Identify the adverse reactions and nursing responsibilities relating to the use of antiemetics.

4. State the appropriate method of administration of antiemetics.

5. Prepare an appropriate teaching plan for patients receiving antiemetics.

6. Describe the action and use of emetics.

7. Identify two emetics.

8. Describe adverse reactions to emetics and appropriate nursing responsibilities for patients given an emetic.

9. State the appropriate method of administration of emetics.

DRUGS YOU WILL LEARN ABOUT IN THIS CHAPTER

Antiemetics

hydroxyzine pamoate (Vistaril)

hydroxyzine HCl (Atarax)

benzquinamide HCl (Emete-con)

phosphorated carbohydrate solution (Emetrol)

metoclopramide HCl (Reglan)

trimethobenzamide HCl (Tigan)

scopolamine (Transderm Scōp)

Emetics

syrup of ipecac

apomorphine

Many different types of drugs exert an antiemetic effect on the body. Some are phenothiazines, like promethazine (Phenergan), chlorpromazine (Thorazine), and prochlorperazine (Compazine). Refer to Chapter 32 for more information on this classification of drugs. Other drugs that can be called antiemetics are certain antihistamines, such as meclizine (Antivert, Bonine), diphenhydramine (Benadryl), and dimenhydrinate (Dramamine). Refer to Chapter 49 for more information on this classification of drugs.

ANTIEMETICS

Hydroxyzine Pamoate and Hydroxyzine Hydrochloride

ACTIONS AND USES Hydroxyzine pamoate (Vistaril) ▲▲▲▲▲▲▲▲▲▲▲▲▲▲▲▲ and hydroxyzine hydrochloride (Atarax) are closely related drugs with similar actions and uses. They suppress areas of the central nervous system (CNS) and are therefore useful for a variety of disorders. The physician may prescribe them to treat nausea, anxiety, and pruritus or to produce sedation. They are frequently prescribed for potentiation of narcotic analgesics postoperatively to decrease the amount and frequency with which narcotics must be administered.

Hydroxyzine has only a few common adverse reactions: dry mouth, drowsiness, and, on rare occasions, tremor or even convulsions.

ASSESSMENT When hydroxyzine is being used to treat nausea, be sure to assess for any contributing factors to the nausea. Ask the patient when nausea occurs, how often it occurs, and if anything seems to bring it on. If the patient does produce emesis, be sure to assess the color, amount, and consistency.

Because hydroxyzine should not be used during pregnancy, be sure to ask the patient about this possibility.

PLANNING AND IMPLEMENTATION Hydroxyzine is given orally at doses of 50 to 100 mg four times a day. If the drug is ordered to be given by intramuscular injection, the dose is 25 to 100 mg.

N U R S I N G   A L E R T

An intramuscular injection of hydroxyzine is painful and poses the risk of abscess formation. If the injection is not deep enough or is accidentally given subcutaneously, the tissue in the area will slough. Be sure to use a large muscle, such as the upper outer quadrant of the gluteus medius muscle. Inject deeply by the Z-track method to prevent the escape of the solution into subcutaneous tissues.

To help the patient deal with the dry mouth so common with hydroxyzine, offer sips of water frequently or ice chips. Hard candy or gum may also help the patient feel more comfortable. Let the patient rinse the mouth as desired.

Be sure to institute safety precautions for this potentially drowsy patient. Do not allow the patient to perform actions that could cause a fall, such as ambulating alone. If the patient is discharged with this medication, caution against driving or operating hazardous machinery, such as lawn mowers or machines at work. Caution should also be taken with smoking or with sources of heat, such as a heating pad.

EVALUATION The effectiveness of this drug is determined by the decreased frequency of vomiting and decreased sensation of nausea. Watch for adverse reactions throughout drug therapy.

Watch also for any drug interactions. Hydroxyzine can potentiate the effects of narcotics, analgesics, barbiturates, and alcohol, producing increased CNS depression. Warn the patient to avoid sources of alcohol after discharge.

Benzquinamide Hydrochloride

ACTIONS AND USES Primarily used to treat nausea and vomiting associated with anesthesia and surgery, benzquinamide hydrochloride (Emete-con) is an antiemetic and antihistamine. It shares some adverse reactions with hydroxyzine, including drowsiness, dry mouth, and tremors. It is also associated with dizziness, blurred vision, salivation, and headache. Other adverse reactions are route dependent.

ASSESSMENT In addition to those assessments listed for hydroxyzine, take baseline blood pressure and pulse readings.

Check the patient's history for any cardiovascular disease. Be especially alert also to any factors that could cause increased intracranial pressure or paralytic ileus.

PLANNING AND IMPLEMENTATION Benzquinamide can be given intramuscularly (IM) or intravenously (IV). The usual IM dose is 50 mg, which can then be repeated in 1 hour and again every 3 to 4 hours as necessary. Use a large muscle, inject deeply, and preferably use the Z-track method.

Given IV, the usual dose is 25 mg. Instill the solution for at least a 2-minute period or longer. The next doses should then be IM. The IV route can be used only if no cardiovascular disease pre-exists. Watch the patient for any sudden increase of blood pressure or cardiac arrhythmias.

Any route of benzquinamide administration may mask the symptoms of increased intracranial pressure or those of paralytic ileus. If your patient is at risk for these problems, you must be especially alert to even slight indicators, such as vital sign changes, level of consciousness changes, or abdominal discomfort.

Maintain the nursing interventions discussed with hydroxyzine.

EVALUATION See hydroxyzine for evaluation of effectiveness.

Phosphorated Carbohydrate Solution

ACTIONS AND USES Phosphorated carbohydrate solution (Emetrol) contains dextrose, fructose, and phosphoric acid. It has localized actions only and works by reducing the hyperactivity of the smooth muscle of the gastric wall. It works immediately to relieve nausea.

ASSESSMENT See hydroxyzine for assessments of
▲▲▲▲▲▲▲▲▲▲ nausea.

Check your patient's history for diabetes or hereditary fructose intolerance. Because of the ingredients of this drug, these patients could be compromised.

PLANNING AND IMPLEMENTATION This drug is com-
▲▲▲▲▲▲▲▲▲▲▲▲▲▲▲▲▲▲▲▲▲▲▲▲▲ monly used for both
adults and children. The adult dose is 1 to 2 tablespoons every 15 minutes until relief, but caution the patient not to take more than five doses. The children's dose is 1 to 2 teaspoons on the same schedule. Instruct the patient not to dilute the drug or to take it with, immediately before, or after fluids.

EVALUATION The patient should experience the anti-
▲▲▲▲▲▲▲▲▲▲ emetic effects of this drug immediately. If the patient experiences nausea even after the fifth dose, discontinue use and notify the physician. Another more serious problem may be the cause of the nausea.

Metoclopramide Hydrochloride

ACTIONS AND USES Metoclopramide hydrochloride
▲▲▲▲▲▲▲▲▲▲▲▲▲▲▲▲ Reglan) is an antiemetic primarily
because it is a dopamine antagonist and, to a lesser degree, because it increases the rate at which the stomach empties. It is therefore useful in treating gastroesophageal reflux and general vomiting.

Metoclopramide is unfortunately associated with many adverse reactions. It can cause either restlessness or drowsiness. The patient may experience a headache, confusion, hypotension or hypertension, tachycardia or bradycardia, various endocrine disturbances, and urinary frequency. Metoclopramide has also been shown to cause mental depression and suicide, extrapyramidal movements, and tardive dyskinesia.

ASSESSMENT In addition to assessments associated
▲▲▲▲▲▲▲▲▲▲ with nausea and vomiting, be sure to
make a careful check of the patient's history. Those with mental depression episodes in the history must be periodically evaluated throughout therapy.

Take baseline vital signs to compare with those you will take during drug therapy.

The use of metoclopramide is contraindicated in any patient in whom the following are present or suspected: gastrointestinal hemorrhage, perforation, or obstruction; epilepsy; or pheochromocytoma.

PLANNING AND IMPLEMENTATION The usual dose of
▲▲▲▲▲▲▲▲▲▲▲▲▲▲▲▲▲▲▲▲▲▲▲ metoclopramide is
10 to 15 mg orally four times a day. It is also possible to see the drug regimen of 20 mg orally once a day prescribed. Oral forms include tablets or syrup.

Given IM or IV, the dose is 10 mg. Administer the IV solution for at least a 15-minute period.

N U R S I N G   A L E R T
▼▼▼▼▼▼▼▼▼▼▼▼▼▼▼▼▼▼▼▼▼▼▼▼▼▼▼▼▼▼▼▼▼▼

Institute safety measures appropriate for drowsiness and mental depression. Take the patient's blood pressure and pulse frequently.

▲▲▲▲▲▲▲▲▲▲▲▲▲▲▲▲▲▲▲▲▲▲▲▲▲▲▲▲▲▲▲▲▲▲

Caution the patient to avoid alcohol sources.

EVALUATION In addition to relief of nausea and vom-
▲▲▲▲▲▲▲▲▲▲ iting, evaluate for the presence of adverse
reactions. Watch for any drug interactions. The effects of metoclopramide are decreased if it is used with anticholinergics or the narcotic analgesics. The sedative effect of this drug increases if it is used with any other CNS depressants, such as alcohol, sedative-hypnotics, narcotics, or tranquilizers.

The dose and timing of insulin for the diabetic patient may need to be adjusted because of the change in gastric emptying time. This also applies to all oral drugs because their absorption is decreased from the stomach but increased from the small intestine.

It is not recommended that this drug be used with any monoamine oxidase (MAO) inhibitors.

Trimethobenzamide Hydrochloride

ACTIONS AND USES The actions of trimethobenzamide
▲▲▲▲▲▲▲▲▲▲▲▲▲▲▲▲ hydrochloride (Tigan) are not
clearly understood, but it is useful in the treatment of nausea and vomiting.

Trimethobenzamide is associated with drowsiness and dizziness, blurred vision, headache, diarrhea, and low blood pressure. It may also cause parkinsonism-like symptoms, blood dyscrasias, convulsions, and even coma.

ASSESSMENT
▲▲▲▲▲▲▲▲▲▲

Trimethobenzamide should not be given to children with viral illnesses by any route. This drug is suspected of leading to Reye's syndrome under these circumstances. The drug should not be used for children in the injectable form for any reason or for newborns in the suppository form.

Check your patient's allergies. Trimethobenzamide contains benzocaine.

PLANNING AND IMPLEMENTATION The usual oral dose is 250 mg three or four times a day. Rectal suppositories and IM injections are given at a dose of 200 mg three or four times a day.

The IM injection is painful and can cause tissue destruction. Be sure to use a large muscle and inject deeply. The Z-track method is preferred.

Institute appropriate safety precautions for this patient because of potential drowsiness, dizziness, blurred vision, low blood pressure, tremors, and convulsions.

EVALUATION Evaluate for the effectiveness of the drug and for the presence of adverse reactions. The most likely drug interaction is with alcohol. Warn the patient to avoid sources of alcohol at home.

Scopolamine

ACTIONS AND USES Refer to Chapter 40 for more information on this anticholinergic drug because it is a belladonna derivative. Information here relates solely to the transdermal form (Transderm Scōp) and its use as an antiemetic for motion sickness.

Side effects most often experienced with the transdermal route are a dry mouth, drowsiness, pupil dilation, and blurred vision.

ASSESSMENT Check the patient's history for glaucoma, liver disease, or kidney disease. Each of these is a contraindication to the use of this drug. See Chapter 40 for other assessments.

PLANNING AND IMPLEMENTATION Delivery of the transdermal form of this drug is by use of a "patch" that adheres to the skin. The drug is then absorbed into the skin and into the blood system. The patch or disk is applied only to the postauricular (behind the ear) area. It should be applied 4 hours before the need for its actions. The same disk remains in place for 3 days unless it is lost or loosened by water. A new one can then be used.

When applying and removing the disk, wear gloves and wash your hands afterward to avoid inadvertent absorption of the drug into your system. Wash the area after removal of the disk.

Caution the patient to avoid all sources of alcohol while using the transdermal disk. Other drugs should be used only on the advice of a physician.

Inform the patient of the possibility of blurred vision and possible discomfort from bright sunlight. Sunglasses may help. Driving is not recommended if the patient's vision is blurred.

EVALUATION See evaluation for hydroxyzine.

EMETICS

An emetic is a drug used to cause vomiting in the case of poisoning or overdose. One should never be given unless the nurse or patient has been instructed to do so by a physician or the poison control center. Some poisons should be diluted rather than removed from the stomach. Caustics, for example, can do as much tissue damage during vomiting as they did during swallowing.

Teach this to all patients, especially those with small children or grandchildren. Encourage the patients to keep an emetic at home. This usually takes the form of syrup of ipecac because it is oral and nonprescription.

Instruct the patient to determine what the victim has taken, if possible. Keep the label and take it with you if the victim must be transported. Be able to tell personnel about symptoms the victim is experiencing. General symptoms of poisoning can include abdominal pain, nausea, vomiting, and diarrhea. Symptoms of central nervous system (CNS) depression include respiratory depression, shock, and coma.

The best treatment for poisoning is prevention. Teach all patients at every opportunity measures to

---

Box 54–1. Measures to Prevent Poisoning

- Keep all poisons locked away or out of the reach of small children.

- Never assume that a child understands the dangers of poisons. Although the usual age for poisoning victims is 4 years or younger, this does not preclude the problem in older children.

- Thoroughly investigate the four most common sites of poisoning in your home—kitchen, bedroom, bathroom, and garage—for any poisons left unattended.

- Evaluate your home for sources of the most frequently swallowed poisons: aspirin and acetaminophen, caustics (such as lye and drain cleaners), and lead hydrocarbons (such as gasoline, paint thinner, and kerosene).

---

prevent this common tragedy. Box 54–1 describes some of these measures.

Syrup of Ipecac

If the poison control center instructs the use of syrup of ipecac, the usual dose is 1 to 2 teaspoons with at least 1 to 2 glasses of water. Caution the patient to be prepared for vomiting. Many laypersons do not understand the purpose of the medication and are therefore unprepared for its action. Also caution the patient to observe the victim carefully because of the risk of aspiration. Instruct the patient to be sure the victim can turn the head to breathe. Syrup of ipecac should never be given to a victim who is unconscious or semiconscious. It should also not be administered to a patient who is suspected of having taken a caustic substance or a petroleum product.

The dose of syrup of ipecac can be repeated once after 20 minutes if no emesis was produced, but it should not be used again after this. Caution the patient that the victim may experience the symptoms of CNS depression. Syrup of ipecac has also been associated with feelings of euphoria or depression.

Apomorphine

Apomorphine is an emetic related to morphine. See Chapter 30 for more information on this drug. Apomorphine is given subcutaneously. It can also produce CNS depression, including respiratory depression.

E X E R C I S E S

CASE STUDIES

1. Your patient has been prescribed hydroxyzine IM. How is this drug administered? What patient teaching is important? For what adverse reactions would you watch the injection site?

2. Your next-door neighbor and friend calls you on the phone and is frantic. Her 3-year-old son has swallowed "something" from under the sink. What should you do? What information must you know? What teaching will you do for your neighbor after this crisis is over?

3. Your patient has been prescribed a scopolamine "patch" to prevent motion sickness while on vacation on a cruise. Your patient says to you, "With this patch, I won't have to worry about getting seasick. I can just eat, drink, and be merry all vacation long." What teaching does your patient require? Of what adverse reactions should the patient be cautioned?

MENTAL AEROBICS

Offer to present a program to a parent's group (such as a parent-teacher group, scouting leaders and parents, or a church group). Teach these parents about poisoning safety and what to do if a poisoning occurs in their home. Be prepared to answer their questions about how often poisoning happens and what syrup of ipecac can do.

LAXATIVES AND ANTIDIARRHEAL DRUGS

LEARNING OBJECTIVES

After studying this chapter, you should be able to:

1. Classify laxatives according to methods of action.

2. Contrast the effects of stimulants, bulk-forming laxatives, saline laxatives, lubricants, and stool softeners related to peristalsis.

3. Give examples of laxatives in each classification.

4. Identify contraindications to the use of laxatives.

5. Determine the presence of adverse reactions and appropriate nursing responsibilities relating to the use of laxatives.

6. State appropriate patient teaching for the use of laxatives.

7. Identify two major antidiarrheal classifications.

8. Identify adverse reactions and appropriate nursing responsibilities relating to the use of antidiarrheals.

9. Prepare an appropriate teaching plan for a patient receiving an antidiarrheal.

DRUGS YOU WILL LEARN ABOUT IN THIS CHAPTER

Laxatives

Stimulant laxatives

castor oil

bisacodyl (Dulcolax)

polyethylene glycol with electrolytes (GoLYTELY)

Saline laxatives

dibasic sodium phosphate and monobasic sodium phosphate (Fleet Phospho-Soda)

lactulose (Chronulac, Cephulac)

Bulk-forming laxatives

psyllium hydrophilic mucilloid (Metamucil)

methylcellulose (Citrucel)

senna (Senokot)

Lubricant laxatives

glycerin suppositories (Fleet Babylax)

mineral oil

Stool softeners

docusate sodium (Colace, Dialose)

casanthranol and docusate sodium (Peri-Colace)

Antidiarrheal drugs

pectin and kaolin (Kaopectate)

pectin, kaolin, and paregoric (Parepectolin)

diphenoxylate HCI with atropine sulfate (Lomotil)

loperamide HCI (Imodium)

LAXATIVES

ACTIONS AND USES Laxatives are medications, either over-the-counter or prescription, that produce a bowel movement. Laxatives produce this action in different ways. They can be divided into groups according to these types of actions (Table 55–1).

The adverse reactions of laxatives differ according to the group. In general, all laxatives can cause intestinal discomfort or cramping.

ASSESSMENT Before giving a laxative, be sure you understand your patient's condition and the purpose of the laxative. Do not give laxatives to a patient with nausea and vomiting or with abdominal pain. These symptoms may indicate a condition that would increase the risk of rupture of the bowel if a laxative were used.

PLANNING AND IMPLEMENTATION If the laxative is being used to treat temporary constipation, be sure to teach your patient other methods to produce regular stools. Also be sure to include in your teaching that a daily stool is not necessarily normal in all persons. The elderly may not have daily stools because of decreased intake and activity, even if daily stools were normal for them at one time. Teach the patient to increase intake of fruits, vegetables, whole grains, seeds, and nuts to help establish a more normal routine. Be sure to assess the patient's fluid intake and do remedial teaching if a problem is determined. Encourage the patient to increase daily activity levels. This can be accomplished in simple ways. A patient who will not take an aerobics course may take a daily walk. Even something as simple as walking to the store instead of driving may be helpful.

Teach the patient that a laxative meant to treat temporary constipation should not be used for longer than a week. If the patient continues to use it, the bowel may become dependent on the laxative to produce stool. The peristaltic action and the defecation reflex are diminished.

Teach the patient to seek advice if bleeding occurs, if no stool is produced by the use of a laxative, or if a

Table 55–1. Common Examples of Laxatives

TYPE	ACTION	EXAMPLES
Stimulant or irritant laxatives	Increase peristalsis by stimulating the bowel wall	castor oil bisacodyl (Dulcolax) polyethylene glycol with electrolytes (GoLYTELY)
Saline laxatives	Increase amount of liquid in the large intestine	dibasic sodium phosphate and monobasic sodium phosphate (Fleet Phospho-Soda, Fleet Enema) Milk of magnesia lactulose (Chronulac, Cephulac)
Bulk-forming laxatives	Form a jelly-like substance and soften the stool	psyllium hydrophile mucilloid (Metamucil) methylcellulose (Citrucel) senna (Senokot) bran
Lubricant laxatives	Soften the exterior of a fecal mass to ease passage	glycerin suppositories mineral oil
Stool softeners	Allow liquid to enter a fecal mass	docusate sodium (Colace, Dialose) casanthranol and docusate sodium (Peri-Colace) docusate calcium (Surfak)

change in the stool lasts 2 weeks or longer. Each of these indicates more serious problems and should be evaluated by a physician. The overuse of a laxative may mask these other problems and make diagnosis difficult.

EVALUATION Evaluate whether the laxative produced
▲▲▲▲▲▲▲▲▲ a stool. Note the color, amount, and consistency of the stool. Note whether the bowel movement was accompanied by excessive discomfort or bleeding.

N U R S I N G   A L E R T
▼▼▼▼▼▼▼▼▼▼▼▼▼▼▼▼▼▼▼▼▼▼▼▼▼▼▼▼▼▼▼▼

If the patient has nausea and vomiting or abdominal pain during the course of laxative therapy, consult the physician at once and do not give the laxative. Monitor serum electrolyte values and watch for symptoms of imbalance.

▲▲▲▲▲▲▲▲▲▲▲▲▲▲▲▲▲▲▲▲▲▲▲▲▲▲▲▲▲▲▲▲▲

Stimulant Laxatives

Castor Oil

Castor oil, an over-the-counter laxative, can be dangerous to some patients. It can cause dehydration and the loss of electrolytes with regular use.

Castor oil is available as an emulsion. Be sure to shake the bottle well before administering this form. You may wish to chill the medication to improve the palatability. It works best on an empty stomach followed by a full glass of water (8 ounces).

Castor oil may be given to relieve constipation. The adult dose is 3 tablespoons. It may be ordered to empty the bowel, such as before x-ray examination of the gastrointestinal tract. The adult dose then is 6 tablespoons.

Bisacodyl

Although bisacodyl (Dulcolax) can be administered orally (tablets), it is not readily absorbed systemically. The tablets must be swallowed whole and not within 1 hour of receiving an antacid or drinking or eating a milk product. Bisacodyl is also available as a suppository.

The usual dose as a laxative is 10 to 15 mg (2 to 3 tablets) or 1 suppository. If the patient needs an empty bowel, up to 6 tablets (30 mg) may be prescribed.

Polyethylene Glycol with Electrolytes

Polyethylene glycol with electrolytes (GoLYTELY) is an oral solution that induces diarrhea within 4 hours of administration. It is often prescribed to cleanse the bowel before surgery or diagnostic testing. It can cause the patient to experience nausea and vomiting, anal irritation, bloating or distention, and cramping.

Because this drug has caused vomiting in some patients, it should not be given if the patient's consciousness is impaired or if the gag reflex is not fully present.

The patient must drink at least 3 liters of the solution, although 4 liters work more effectively. Because the patient may find this onerous, chill the solution before administration to improve the palatability. Encourage your patient to drink at least 8 ounces every 10 minutes. Slower administration has been found to decrease the effectiveness of the drug.

No solid food should be eaten for at least 3 to 4 hours before the solution is given. Any oral drugs the patient must use should be given more than 1 hour before this solution. Any taken within 1 hour of GoLYTELY may be flushed out and not fully absorbed.

Saline Laxatives

N U R S I N G   A L E R T
▼▼▼▼▼▼▼▼▼▼▼▼▼▼▼▼▼▼▼▼▼▼▼▼▼▼▼▼▼▼▼▼

Saline laxatives are likely to cause fluid and electrolyte imbalances, such as hypernatremia, dehydration, and others. Therefore, they should not be given to patients with kidney disease, congestive heart failure, or congenital megacolon or to patients on a low-salt diet. Be alert to any signs or symptoms that could indicate such an imbalance and encourage an adequate fluid intake.

▲▲▲▲▲▲▲▲▲▲▲▲▲▲▲▲▲▲▲▲▲▲▲▲▲▲▲▲▲▲▲▲▲

Dibasic Sodium Phosphate and Monobasic Sodium Phosphate

Give this liquid laxative (Fleet Phospho-Soda) at least 30 minutes before a meal or at bedtime. Dilute 20 mL of the solution in 4 ounces of cool water. Be sure the patient follows this with at least 8 ounces of clear liquid. If the laxative is being given to empty the bowel, 45 mL is used.

Lactulose

Lactulose (Chronulac, Cephulac) is given as an oral syrup when it is administered for treatment of constipation. The usual dose is 1 to 2 tablespoons daily. The patient may experience distention with flatus, belching and abdominal cramps, and diarrhea. It is not generally used as a laxative for diabetics because it contains galactose and lactose.

Lactulose can also be prescribed for the treatment of hepatic coma or for pre-coma states. It lowers the patient's blood urea nitrogen concentration, thus reducing central nervous system symptoms. When lactulose is prescribed for hepatic coma, the dose is larger. The oral syrup dose is 2 to 3 tablespoons three or four times a day. Lactulose can also be given as an enema for those in a coma; 300 mL of lactulose is given with 700 mL of water or saline. The patient should retain the solution for 30 to 60 minutes if possible. The procedure can be repeated every 4 to 6 hours.

Lactulose should not be used with other laxatives. Also be cautious of using lactulose with certain anti-infectives. These, especially neomycin, can interfere with the actions of lactulose.

Bulk-Forming Laxatives

Bulk-forming laxatives are nonaddictive and are therefore often prescribed for more chronic conditions, such as irritable bowel syndrome, chronic constipation, hemorrhoids, or diverticulitis. Because the laxative forms a jelly-like substance in the stool, it should not be given if the patient has an intestinal obstruction or impaction. Allowed to set in the bowel, the bulk-forming laxatives can become hard and rock-like.

NURSING ALERT

▼▼▼▼▼▼▼▼▼▼▼▼▼▼▼▼▼▼▼▼▼▼▼▼▼▼▼▼▼▼▼▼

While mixing the powder forms of these laxatives, be careful to make only deliberate movements. If the powder is stirred or handled carelessly, it can become airborne. The inhalation of this powder can cause an allergic reaction in the health care worker.

▲▲▲▲▲▲▲▲▲▲▲▲▲▲▲▲▲▲▲▲▲▲▲▲▲▲▲▲▲▲▲▲

Most forms of these laxatives require 1 teaspoon to 1 tablespoon mixed in 8 ounces of cool water, fruit juice, milk, or other beverage. This must be followed by an additional glass of water or liquid. Without this amount of liquid intake, the patient is at increased risk for impaction. The laxative may be ordered 1 to 3 times a day. Reassure the patient that gas or bloating may occur at first but usually decreases as the bowel becomes accustomed to the laxative.

Psyllium Hydrophilic Mucilloid

Psyllium hydrophilic mucilloid (Metamucil) is available in different flavors, in a sugar-free form, and as an effervescent.

Methylcellulose

Methylcellulose (Citrucel) is similar to psyllium. Also available in different flavors and a sugar-free form, methylcellulose has what some patients consider a more pleasant texture than the somewhat gritty psyllium.

Senna

Senna (Senokot) is available in tablets or granules. It is a natural vegetable derivative that produces a bowel movement in 6 to 12 hours. It is associated with few if any adverse reactions if it is used according to directions.

Encourage the patient to take senna at bedtime. The usual dose is 2 tablets a day or 2 to 3 teaspoons of granules a day.

Lubricant Laxatives

Lubricant laxatives do not have systemic or local actions. They simply coat the outside of a fecal mass, making it easier for the patient to pass. Some are oral, some are enemas, and still others are suppositories. Be sure the suppositories are inserted past the rectal sphincter or the patient will have a continuous urge to defecate.

Glycerin Suppositories

Glycerin suppositories are intended for young children. One trade name is Fleet Babylax. A parent should administer a suppository to a child 2 years old or younger only when ordered by a physician.

Mineral Oil

Mineral oil is a readily available over-the-counter laxative. As such, it easily lends itself to overuse. In addition to the usual problems that overuse of a laxative can cause, mineral oil can also cause a decrease in the absorption of the fat-soluble vitamins. Be alert to possible deficiencies in such patients.

Stool Softeners

Stool softeners actually cause liquid to enter a fecal mass. They may be prescribed to treat constipation or to prevent straining in the cardiac patient or others for whom straining is detrimental.

Docusate Sodium

Docusate sodium (Colace, Dialose) is available as capsules, liquid drops, or a syrup. It is not habit forming and has no contraindications. The reported few adverse reactions tend to be mild, including nausea, throat irritation, or a bitter taste.

The usual dose of docusate sodium is 50 to 200 mg daily, given with at least a half-glass of fluid if the liquid drops are used.

Casanthranol and Docusate Sodium

Peri-Colace combines a stool softener, docusate sodium, with the stimulant laxative casanthranol. Because of this addition, this medication can be habit forming.

The most common adverse reactions are nausea, diarrhea, cramping, and rash. The usual dose is 1 to 2 capsules or 1 to 2 tablespoons at bedtime.

ANTIDIARRHEAL DRUGS

The antidiarrheal drugs differ drastically within the classification in mode of action. They are prescribed to stop diarrhea. Some are local acting, used for their ability to adsorb excess liquid from the bowel and to soothe the bowel wall. Common examples of these are kaolin, pectin, and the combination of these two, Kaopectate.

Other antidiarrheals have systemic actions to decrease the peristaltic action of the bowel.

NURSING ALERT

Some antidiarrheal drugs are opiates or contain an opiate, such as paregoric or parepectolin (a combination of paregoric, kaolin, and pectin). These are habit forming and addictive.

The most commonly prescribed systemic antidiarrheals are not opiates.

Diphenoxylate Hydrochloride with Atropine Sulfate

ACTIONS AND USES Diphenoxylate hydrochloride with atropine sulfate is a Schedule V controlled substance. Diphenoxylate hydrochloride is chemically related to meperidine (a narcotic analgesic) and is habit forming. Atropine sulfate is an anticholinergic added to the medication to discourage abuse.

This combined drug (Lomotil) is used for diarrhea. In addition to the dangers of addiction, it can cause respiratory depression.

Other adverse reactions can include drowsiness and dizziness, depression and confusion, urticaria and pruritus, nausea and vomiting, headache, flushing, and dry skin.

ASSESSMENT Assess the patient's stools. Note the color, amount, and consistency. Assess the patient's hydration status. Be sure to take baseline vital signs, especially respiration rate.

Check the patient's history for allergy to either ingredient of the drug. This drug is also contraindicated in patients with diarrhea caused by an enterotoxin-producing bacterium or pseudomembranous enterocolitis. It should not be given to a patient with obstructive jaundice.

PLANNING AND IMPLEMENTATION The usual dose of Lomotil is 20 mg a day in four divided doses. Teach your patient the safety precautions necessary because of drowsiness and dizziness. Institute these precautions if the patient is in a health care facility.

Teach the patient to avoid alcohol while taking this medication.

EVALUATION Determine the effectiveness of this drug by continuing to note color, amount, and consistency of stools. Evaluate also for any adverse reactions the patient may experience.

NURSING ALERT

▼▼▼▼▼▼▼▼▼▼▼▼▼▼▼▼▼▼▼▼▼▼▼▼▼

Look for signs of an overdose, which can be serious. An overdose can cause respiratory depression and coma and lead to possible brain damage and even death.

▲▲▲▲▲▲▲▲▲▲▲▲▲▲▲▲▲▲▲▲▲▲▲▲▲

Evaluate for any interactions with other medications. This drug should not be given with monoamine oxidase (MAO) inhibitor because it can lead to hypertensive crisis. The effects of barbiturates, tranquilizers, or alcohol are potentiated by Lomotil.

Loperamide Hydrochloride

ACTIONS AND USES Loperamide hydrochloride (Imodium) is not habit forming. It is given for nonspecific diarrhea or for conditions that may cause chronic diarrhea. The drug slows the motility of the bowel and affects the flow of water and electrolytes through the bowel.

Adverse reactions from this drug tend to be fairly mild, although allergy is a possibility. The patient may experience nausea and vomiting, drowsiness or dizziness, or a dry mouth.

ASSESSMENT The assessments for and contraindications to this drug are the same as for diphenoxylate hydrochloride with atropine sulfate.

PLANNING AND IMPLEMENTATION Loperamide is available in capsule form. The usual dose is 4 mg initially followed by 2 mg after each diarrheal stool. The total dose for a 24-hour period should not exceed 16 mg.

Take safety precautions essential for drowsiness and dizziness. Be sure the patient understands the need to continue these after discharge. Driving and operating hazardous machinery are dangerous.

EVALUATION Determine effectiveness by noting amount, color, and consistency of stools as well as the presence or absence of adverse reactions. Continue to monitor the patient for hydration level while diarrhea continues.

EXERCISES

CASE STUDIES

1. Your patient is a 12-year-old boy. He was admitted for severe abdominal pain in the right lower quadrant. He is to go for diagnostic testing today and has an order for a Fleet Enema. What is your best action?

2. Ms. S.J., age 37 years, has been diagnosed with irriable bowel syndrome. Her physician has prescribed methylcellulose daily. What teaching should you perform? How should you instruct the patient to take the medication?

3. Mr. B.F., age 61 years, is to receive castor oil to empty the bowel before diagnostic testing. What dose would you expect the physician to order? What could you do to improve the taste of the medication for Mr. B.F.? At what time of the day should the medication be administered? For what should Mr. B.F. be assessed?

4. Mr. B.F. was diagnosed with temporary constipation due to inappropriate daily habits. What teaching could you do to help him establish good bowel habits? If Mr. B.F. is prescribed a laxative, how long would you expect the order to last? When should Mr. B.F. seek medical attention?

5. Ms. A.M., age 45 years, was diagnosed with severe diarrhea and prescribed diphenoxylate hydrochloride with atropine sulfate. What is the purpose of the atropine sulfate in this medication? What teaching should be done for Ms. A.M.? What assessments are essential for this patient? What nursing interventions are needed?

MENTAL AEROBICS

1. Keep a log of your patients for a specific period (a week or two). Keep track of those prescribed either a laxative or an antidiarrheal agent. Note why the drug was being used.

2. Observe at the office of a gastroenterologist or a clinic that deals with gastrointestinal problems. What medications were prescribed? Which ones were laxatives or antidiarrheal agents? What conditions were they prescribed for? What teaching was done for each of the patients?

3. Observe diagnostic testing of the gastrointestinal system, including upper and lower tract x-rays, sigmoidoscopy, or esophagogastroduodenoscopy. Why was it necessary to have the bowel completely clear for these tests? Are there other tests that would have the same requirement?

DIGESTANTS AND NUTRITIONAL SUPPLEMENTS

LEARNING OBJECTIVES

After studying this chapter, you should be able to:

1. Describe the action and uses of digestants.

2. Describe adverse reactions and appropriate nursing responsibilities relating to the use of digestants.

3. State the appropriate method of administration of digestants.

4. Determine appropriate nursing assessment and interventions relating to the use of the nursing process in the care of patients receiving nutritional supplements.

5. State adverse reactions to nutritional supplements.

6. Select appropriate patient teaching for a patient receiving a nutritional supplement.

7. Define vitamin, supplement, precursor, intrinsic factor, and extrinsic factor.

8. Classify vitamins as fat-soluble or water-soluble.

9. State the chemical name of each vitamin.

10. Identify the rationale for supplementation of common vitamins.

11. Demonstrate how to administer vitamin supplements to a patient by use of the nursing process.

12. Define mineral.

13. List common sources and uses of and adverse reactions to iron.

14. State the rationale for supplementation of iron.

15. State appropriate nursing implications for the patient receiving a mineral supplement.

16. Demonstrate how to administer minerals to a patient by use of the nursing process.

DRUGS YOU WILL LEARN ABOUT IN THIS CHAPTER

Digestants

pancrelipase (Cotazym, Entolase, Ku-Zyme, Pancrease, Viokase, Zymase)

pancreatin (Creon)

pancrelipase (amylase, protease, and lipase), cellulase, hyoscyamine sulfate, phenyltoloxamine citrate (Kutrase)

pancreatin, pepsin, bile salts (Entozyme)

pancreatin, pepsin, bile salts, hyoscyamine sulfate, atropine sulfate, scopolamine hydrobromide, phenobarbital (Donnazyme)

lactase

Vitamins

Fat-soluble vitamins

vitamin A, retinol (Aquasol A)

vitamin D, calciferol

vitamin E, tocopherol (Aquasol E)

vitamin K, menadiol

vitamin K_1, phytonadione (Mephyton, Aqua-MEPHYTON)

Water-soluble vitamins

vitamin C, ascorbic acid

vitamin B_1, thiamine

vitamin B_2, riboflavin

vitamin B_3, niacin (nicotinic acid, niacina-mide, Nicobid, Nicolar)

vitamin B_6, pyridoxine

vitamin B_{12}, cyanocobalamin

folic acid (folate, Folvite)

folinic acid (leucovorin)

Minerals

calcium carbonate

calcium chloride

calcium gluceptate

calcium gluconate

calcium lactate

phosphorus (K-Phos, Neutra-Phos)

magnesium (Beelith, Mag-Ox 400, Uro-Mag)

ferrous sulfate (Feosol)

iron dextran (Imferon)

DIGESTANTS

Digestants are digestive enzymes (many of them pancreatic enzymes) that our bodies normally produce (Fig. 56–1). In some persons, the enzymes are not produced or cannot reach the site of action because of a disease or disorder. The enzyme must then be replaced with a supplement. Without the enzyme, the

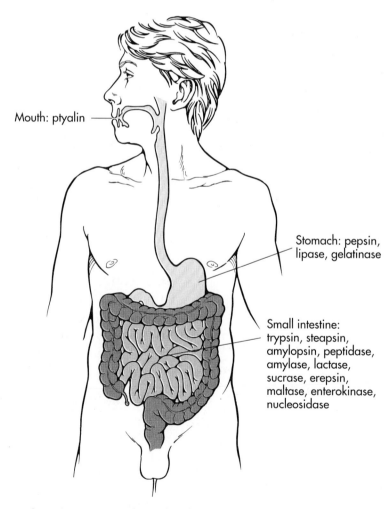

Mouth: ptyalin

Stomach: pepsin, lipase, gelatinase

Small intestine: trypsin, steapsin, amylopsin, peptidase, amylase, lactase, sucrase, erepsin, maltase, enterokinase, nucleosidase

Figure 56–1. Our bodies produce many enzymes that aid in digestion. Among them are ptyalin (mouth); pepsin, lipase, and gelatinase (stomach); trypsin, steapsin, amylopsin, peptidase, amylase, lactase, sucrase, erepsin, maltase, enterokinase, and nucleosidase (small intestine).

patient normally experiences gastrointestinal symptoms, such as nausea, vomiting, diarrhea, bloating, cramping, and flatulence. The food the patient eats is not fully metabolized, so there may also be signs of malnutrition. The patient may also experience a lack of appetite, which further complicates the nutritional picture.

Pancrelipase

ACTIONS AND USES Pancrelipase (Cotazym, Entolase, Ku-Zyme, Pancrease, Viokase, Zymase) contains three enzymes: lipase, protease, and amylase. These enzymes are responsible for hydrolyzing fats into fatty acids and glycerol, breaking down protein into amino acids, and converting carbohydrates into dextrins and other short-chain sugars. These then become available to the body as nutrients (bioavailable). The enzymes become active in the duodenum after they have passed through the stomach.

Pancrelipase is given to those with inadequate pancreatic enzymes who cannot digest fats. Disorders that may cause this include cystic fibrosis, chronic pancreatitis, and cancer of the pancreas. Replacement of pancreatic enzymes is also necessary after gastrectomy or pancreatectomy.

The enzymes of pancrelipase are obtained from the pancreas of a hog. Therefore, persons who are allergic to pork may also be allergic to pancrelipase. Adverse reactions are unusual and normally associated only with large doses. The patient may experience nausea and diarrhea, hyperuricemia, and hyperuricosuria.

ASSESSMENT To best determine need and establish a baseline for comparison, perform a thorough nutritional status assessment, including normal daily intake. Determine the patient's normal bowel routine and the presence of diarrhea or other symptoms. Assess the stools for the five F's—frequency, foul, fatty, foamy, and they float. This indicates inadequate digestion.

In addition to pork allergies, check the patient's history for other allergies. Some preparations contain povidone-iodine or benzyl alcohol.

Because of the increased bioavailability of dextrin and sugars, it is potentially possible for diabetics to experience difficulty with the normally well controlled serum glucose level. Warn your diabetic patient of this so the patient can inform the physician of any changes in the condition.

PLANNING AND IMPLEMENTATION Pancrelipase is available as pow-

der, capsules containing enteric coated spheres, and tablets or enteric coated tablets. The powders or the spheres can be sprinkled onto a small amount of cold food.

N U R S I N G   A L E R T
▼▼▼▼▼▼▼▼▼▼▼▼▼▼▼▼▼▼▼▼▼▼▼▼▼▼▼▼▼▼▼▼▼▼

Caution the patient not to hold the product in the mouth long, not to chew the spheres, and to eat all of the food onto which the medication is sprinkled. Do not use alkaline foods. Use soft foods such as applesauce, pudding, or gelatins. If the powder or melted spheres contact skin or mucous membranes, irritation results. Inhalation of the powder causes irritation of the nasal mucosa and respiratory congestion. Inhalation of the powder can also precipitate an asthma attack.

▲▲▲▲▲▲▲▲▲▲▲▲▲▲▲▲▲▲▲▲▲▲▲▲▲▲▲▲▲▲▲▲▲▲▲

The dose of pancrelipase depends on the formula used, but it should be administered just before a meal or snack so the enzymes are available to help digest the food. Caution the patient to omit a missed dose. It will not accomplish any action if it is taken on an empty stomach and may cause irritation of the gastrointestinal tract lining.

Because the product must remain dry, caution the patient not to store the product in the refrigerator because this can draw moisture.

EVALUATION To evaluate the effectiveness of the enzyme supplementation, reassess nutritional status, nutritional intake, frequency of diarrhea and other symptoms, and the stools for the five F's.

If a patient takes an overdose of the enzymes, diarrhea or other gastrointestinal upset may develop. No toxic effect has been reported.

Pancrelipase interacts with some common over-the-counter medications. Certain antacids decrease the effects of pancrelipase, and pancrelipase decreases the absorption of iron preparations. Caution the patient not to take any other drugs, even over-the-counter preparations, without consulting the physician first.

Pancreatin

Pancreatin (Creon) is similar to pancrelipase and contains the same three enzymes. Information about the two preparations is essentially the same.

Combination Pancreatic Enzymes

Kutrase

Kutrase capsules contain pancrelipase (amylase, protease, and lipase), cellulase, hyoscyamine sulfate (Donnatal, an anticholinergic and antispasmodic), and phenyltoloxamine citrate (a nonbarbiturate sedative). The antispasmodic and sedative are added to further treat gastrointestinal spasms and cramping associated with a lack of pancreatic enzymes.

Entozyme

Entozyme is a tablet of pancreatin, pepsin, and bile salts. The pepsin is released in the stomach. Pancreatin and the bile salts are released in the small intestine, their site of action.

Donnazyme

Donnazyme tablets contain pancreatin, pepsin, bile salts, hyoscyamine sulfate, atropine sulfate, scopolamine hydrobromide, and phenobarbital. The pepsin, hyoscyamine, atropine, and scopolamine dissolve and begin to work in the stomach. The pancreatic enzymes are released in the small intestine. Hyoscyamine, atropine, and scopolamine are antispasmodics. Phenobarbital acts as a sedative.

Lactase

ACTIONS AND USES To fully understand the actions of ▲▲▲▲▲▲▲▲▲▲▲▲▲▲ lactase, you must understand the normal digestive process involving lactose and lactase. Lactose is a nonabsorbable disaccharide that is normally hydrolyzed by lactase. Lactase is an enzyme made by the villi of the intestines.

If lactose is not hydrolyzed because of a lack of lactase, it stays in the intestine and gathers an increased amount of intestinal fluid. This excess fluid causes bloating, cramps, and diarrhea. Lactose is eventually broken apart by the normal intestinal flora, but the process produces increased carbon dioxide and hydrogen. This causes flatulence and abdominal pain. The hydrogen can also be detected in the person's breath.

This abnormal metabolism of lactose is called lactose intolerance. It is more commonly seen after the age of 4 or 5 years; peak occurrence is in the teens and early 20s. Lactose intolerance is more likely in adult blacks, Asians, Native Americans, and eastern European Jews. The signs and symptoms of lactose intolerance occur after ingestion of a large volume of milk or dairy products.

Lactase supplementation is therefore used for persons suffering from symptoms of lactose intolerance.

ASSESSMENT Assess the patient's normal nutritional ▲▲▲▲▲▲▲▲▲▲ intake and nutritional status. Assess for the symptoms of lactose intolerance and the frequency of their occurrence.

If the patient is diabetic, the milk sugar will now become bioavailable. Galactosemics should not have milk, regardless of lactase supplementation.

Take note of any allergies the patient may have. Those with penicillin or mold allergies are more likely to be allergic to lactase.

PLANNING AND IMPLEMENTATION Lactase is available ▲▲▲▲▲▲▲▲▲▲▲▲▲▲▲▲▲▲▲▲▲▲▲▲▲▲ as drops or capsules. The normal dose is to swallow 1 to 2 capsules with a normal serving of milk or dairy product. The contents of the capsule or the drops can also be sprinkled over the dairy product. This does not alter the taste if it is done immediately before eating or drinking.

The patient may also choose to pretreat milk by adding 5 to 15 drops or 1 to 2 capsules per quart of milk. Because this is done in advance, the milk may taste sweeter than normal, although the appearance remains unchanged. Patients can also buy pretreated milk, cottage cheese, and processed American cheese in some stores or order it through a catalogue.

EVALUATION To determine the effectiveness of the en- ▲▲▲▲▲▲▲▲▲▲▲ zyme, look for improvement in the signs or symptoms the patient was experiencing. The patient is the best judge of many of these, although the nurse can make some nonsubjective observations about the frequency of diarrhea.

VITAMINS

ACTIONS AND USES Vitamins, organic compounds nor- ▲▲▲▲▲▲▲▲▲▲▲▲▲▲▲▲ mally found in our daily diets, help regulate the metabolism and promote the efficient use of other nutrients. Vitamins can be divided into two subclasses: fat-soluble and water-soluble.

Fat-soluble vitamins can be stored in the body in the muscle, fat, or other tissues. Because they are stored, the body does not need to have a new supply of these vitamins every day. If no supply is furnished day after day, however, these stores become depleted. Therefore, a recommended daily allowance has been established for each fat-soluble vitamin to prevent depletion of these stores.

Certain diseases, conditions, and substances interfere with the absorption of fat-soluble vitamins from our diet. If the diet is deficient in fat, then it will be deficient in fat-soluble vitamins. If the patient has a condition that makes it difficult to digest fat and absorb it from the diet, such as gallbladder, pancreatic, or other gastrointestinal (GI) diseases, then the body will have difficulty absorbing fat-soluble vitamins. If the patient overuses mineral oil as a laxative, fat and fat-soluble vitamins will be flushed from the body. Fat-soluble vitamins include vitamins A, D, E, and K.

Water-soluble vitamins are not stored by the body, so a new supply of these vitamins must be obtained each day. These vitamins can easily be destroyed or washed away by cooking techniques, such as using too much water. Water-soluble vitamins include vitamin C and the B-complex vitamins.

The body uses minerals to make vitamins. Much of the information about vitamins and minerals is intertwined. Minerals are also needed to maintain the fluid balance in the body, both intracellular and extracellular.

ASSESSMENT When a patient is prescribed a vitamin or mineral supplement, it is often because of a faulty diet. The nurse can promote wellness best by determining what the patient's usual diet is like. Ask the patient to recall what was eaten and the amounts eaten in the previous 24 hours. Also assess the patient for signs and symptoms of deficiency of the affected vitamin or mineral.

Some vitamins and minerals contain additives, preservatives, or colors. Be sure to assess the patient's history for and ask the patient about any allergic reactions to these substances.

PLANNING AND IMPLEMENTATION Vitamins and minerals are often prescribed to the patient in multivitamin and multimineral compounds. Be sure the patient is aware of how to take the medication. Some patients do not take vitamins and minerals seriously. Caution the patient not to exceed the recommended daily allowance or prescribed amount of these medications.

Encourage a well-balanced diet. Teach the recommended guidelines by use of the food pyramid. Determine which foods in each group the patient likes. Ask the patient to select meals that follow the guidelines. Correct these choices as necessary.

Keep all vitamins and minerals in airtight containers. Keep the containers in a dark, cool place. Be sure moisture does not accumulate inside the container.

The refrigerator is not an appropriate place for tablets or capsules.

EVALUATION A few days or even weeks after therapy has been initiated, ask the patient to recall intake from the previous 24 hours to determine whether your diet teaching has been effective. Make suggestions as necessary.

Evaluate the patient for any signs or symptoms of vitamin or mineral deficiencies. A decrease in or the prevention of the deficiency indicates effectiveness of the medication.

Table 56–1 lists substances that interact with vitamins and minerals.

Fat-Soluble Vitamins

Vitamin A, Retinol

ACTIONS AND USES The physician prescribes vitamin A (Aquasol A) to treat a deficiency of the vitamin. It may also be used as a supplement to prevent deficiency.

Overuse of vitamin A, because it is stored by the body, may lead to hypervitaminosis A. Patients experiencing this reaction may complain of a headache, nausea and vomiting, and joint and bone pain. The patient may be irritable and have a yellow-orange discoloration to the skin, dry skin that may desquamate, alopecia, and even an enlarged liver. Infants may have bulging fontanelles.

ASSESSMENT Before beginning therapy, assess the patient for signs or symptoms of vitamin A deficiency. These may include an increased frequency of infection, decreased vision in dim light (night blindness), and dry, itchy skin.

Check the patient's history carefully. The use of vitamin A is contraindicated in malabsorption syndromes, severe renal impairment, and hypervitaminosis A.

PLANNING AND IMPLEMENTATION The dose prescribed depends on the level of deficiency. In general, the physician attempts to determine what the patient's normal intake of vitamin A is and then to "make up the difference" between the intake and the recommended daily allowance. The patient may receive 4000 to 50,000 International units (IU) orally each day. When vitamin A is given intramuscularly (IM), the patient may receive up to 100,000 IU each day for 3 days and then 50,000 IU for the next 2 weeks.

Table 56–1. Interactions with Vitamins and Minerals

VITAMIN/ MINERAL	DECREASED EFFECTS OF VITAMIN/ MINERAL	INCREASED EFFECTS OF VITAMIN/ MINERAL	DECREASED EFFECTS OF OTHER DRUG	INCREASED EFFECTS OF OTHER DRUG	OTHER INTERACTION
Vitamin A	Antilipemics, laxatives, mineral oil	Oral contraceptives			
Vitamin D	Antilipemics, glucocorticoids		Cardiac glycosides, antacids with magnesium, thiazide diuretics, glucocorticoids		
Vitamin E	Antilipemics, mineral oil		Iron supplements		
Vitamin K	Antilipemics, mineral oil, anticonvulsants, salicylates, antiinfectives, antibiotics		Oral anticoagulants		
Vitamin C	Salicylates, primidone	Iron supplements, folic acid supplements	Anticoagulants, cyanocobalamin		
Thiamine				Neuromuscular blockers	
Riboflavin	Phenothiazines, tricyclic antidepressants, probenecid, alcohol				
Niacin			Probenecid, sulfinpyrazone		Lovastatin
Pyridoxine	Isoniazid, hydralazine, penicillamine, chloramphenicol, estrogens, immunosuppressants, oral contraceptives, alcohol				

Table 56–1. Interactions with Vitamins and Minerals *Continued*

VITAMIN/ MINERAL	DECREASED EFFECTS OF VITAMIN/MINERAL	INCREASED EFFECTS OF VITAMIN/ MINERAL	DECREASED EFFECTS OF OTHER DRUG	INCREASED EFFECTS OF OTHER DRUG	OTHER INTERACTION
Vitamin B$_{12}$	Chloramphenicol, antineoplastics, aminoglycosides, colchicine, some potassium supplements, vitamin C supplements, cimetidine, alcohol				
Folic acid	Sulfonamides, triamterene, methotrexate, estrogen, steroids, oral contraceptives, phenytoin, alcohol				
Folinic acid		Fluorouracil	Anticonvulsants		
Calcium	Dairy products, cereals, spinach, rhubarb		Tetracyclines		
Phosphorus	Antacids with magnesium, aluminum, or calcium		Antacids with magnesium, aluminum, or calcium	Salicylates	Antihypertensives, corticosteroids, potassium supplements, potassium-sparing diuretics
Magnesium			Tetracyclines		
Iron			Tetracyclines		

When administering an oral liquid, you may offer the solution to the patient straight or mixed with food or juice. The IM route is normally used only if the oral route is impossible. Caution the patient not to double the dose if one dose is missed. This is true for all fat-soluble vitamins.

Encourage the patient to increase dietary intake of vitamin A. All of the following are good sources of vitamin A: liver, egg yolk, deep yellow or dark green fruits and vegetables, whole milk, and margarine or butter. Other foods may be fortified with vitamin A.

EVALUATION To determine whether the medication has been effective, look for decreased signs of deficiency. If a large dose is prescribed, also look for any decreases in red or white blood cells or an increase of the sedimentation rate or prothrombin time. Report these to the physician.

N U R S I N G   A L E R T
▼▼▼▼▼▼▼▼▼▼▼▼▼▼▼▼▼▼▼▼▼▼▼▼▼▼▼▼▼▼

Also look for any signs of vitamin A toxicity. These are the same reactions as described for hypervitaminosis A. Vitamin A toxicity may also cause increased blood glucose, blood urea nitrogen (BUN), serum calcium, cholesterol, and triglyceride levels.

▲▲▲▲▲▲▲▲▲▲▲▲▲▲▲▲▲▲▲▲▲▲▲▲▲▲▲▲▲▲

Vitamin A may interact with some medications. Look for any signs of interactions. Antilipemics, laxatives, and mineral oil decrease the absorption of vitamin A. Oral contraceptives can increase the effects of vitamin A and lead to toxic effects.

Vitamin D, Calciferol

ACTIONS AND USES Vitamin D supplements are often given to patients with renal failure to treat hypocalcemia. For the same reason, the supplement may be ordered for the patient with hypoparathyroidism.

Vitamin D supplement is associated with side effects. These are the signs or symptoms of hypercalcemia, such as GI upset, metallic taste, dry mouth, weight loss, polydipsia, polyuria, possibly kidney stones, photophobia, conjunctivitis, watery nose, fatigue or sleepiness, decreased libido, pruritus, hypertension, irregular pulse, increased systemic temperature, headache, or muscle or bone pain.

ASSESSMENT Assess the patient to be given a vitamin D supplement for signs or symptoms of hypocalcemia or a deficit of this vitamin. This may include rickets or osteomalacia.

Check the patient's history for any evidence of hypercalcemia or vitamin D toxicity. These contraindicate the use of a vitamin D supplement. Look also for any history of sarcoidosis or hyperparathyroidism. In these patients, use extra caution in administering this drug.

PLANNING AND IMPLEMENTATION Vitamin D supplement is given either orally or intravenously (IV). The dose and the route depend on the degree of deficiency. The oral dose is usually started at 0.25 µg per day and gradually increased upward to 2.0 µg per day. Vitamin D may also be measured in International units.

If the patient is being given an oral dose and will be going home with the medication, caution the patient not to double the dose if one dose is missed. This can cause hypervitaminosis. Teach the patient the signs of hypervitaminosis D, which are the side effects described with actions and uses.

If the supplement is given IV, the usual dose is 0.5 to 3.0 µg administered three times a day.

When the patient is prescribed a vitamin D supplement, teach and encourage the proper diet to increase the intake of vitamin D, unless there is reason to contraindicate such a diet. The most common source in the American diet is fortified milk and other fortified products. Also encourage the patient to have regular exposure to sunlight if this source has been lacking, but caution against sunburn.

Establish safety precautions for patients who are experiencing muscle twitching from severe hypocalcemia. This twitching can proceed to convulsions.

Also monitor laboratory reports for possible effects. Watch the levels of serum calcium, BUN, and both serum and urine creatinine. Look for any increase in the serum alkaline phosphatase levels; this may signal the beginning of hypercalcemia. The serum cholesterol level may be falsely elevated when this supplement is being taken.

EVALUATION When evaluating for effectiveness of this drug, look for a decrease in or prevention of the signs and symptoms of vitamin D deficit. Watch also for improved serum calcium levels.

Be cautious with patients who use the product at home without medical advice.

N U R S I N G   A L E R T
▼▼▼▼▼▼▼▼▼▼▼▼▼▼▼▼▼▼▼▼▼▼▼▼▼▼▼▼▼▼

Overuse of vitamin D can lead to kidney stones and damage.

▲▲▲▲▲▲▲▲▲▲▲▲▲▲▲▲▲▲▲▲▲▲▲▲▲▲▲▲▲▲

Many drugs interact with this supplement. If the patient is using cardiac glycosides, antacids that contain magnesium, or a thiazide diuretic, contact the physician to report. The absorption of vitamin D supplements is decreased if the patient is taking an antilipemic. Glucocorticoids are antagonistic.

Continue to monitor the patient for any signs or symptoms of hypervitaminosis D throughout drug therapy.

Vitamin E, Tocopherol

ACTIONS AND USES Vitamin E (Aquasol E) may be ordered for low-birth-weight infants. Infants born prematurely or of low weight for another reason are at risk for hemolysis of the red blood cells. Vitamin E deficiency may be the cause, and if it is the cause, a supplement can help prevent or treat the problem.

Topical preparations of vitamin E are ordered for skin irritations, such as chapping. Many lotions and creams available over-the-counter contain vitamin E for this reason. Vitamin E is also used as an antioxidant in foods.

Use and overuse of vitamin E can lead to adverse reactions, such as fatigue, headache, rash, or blurred vision. Vitamin E can also cause GI upset or, in severe cases, necrotizing enterocolitis.

ASSESSMENT When assessing the patient who is to receive vitamin E supplements, look carefully for any signs or symptoms that indicate a deficiency of this vitamin. These include irritability, muscle weakness, edema, or even hemolytic anemia. Be sure a definitive diagnosis has been reached if the patient has anemia. If it is iron deficiency anemia, vitamin E is used only with extra caution.

N U R S I N G   A L E R T

Although low-birth-weight infants are one of the most likely groups to receive vitamin E supplements, they also warrant extreme caution. Vitamin E given to infants in this group has been associated with increased risk for necrotizing enterocolitis.

If the patient also has a vitamin D deficiency, the risk of bleeding is increased.

PLANNING AND IMPLEMENTATION Vitamin E supplements are given orally at a usual dose of 30 to 75 IU per day. Topical doses are generally prescribed as needed.

When the oral route is ordered, vitamin E should be given with or just after meals to decrease GI upset. Chewable tablets are not to be swallowed whole. Vitamin E oral solutions may be taken straight or mixed with food or juice at the patient's discretion.

If the patient is to go home with this supplement, caution against doubling the dose if one dose is missed. As with all fat-soluble vitamins, this can lead to hypervitaminosis. Encourage a diet high in vitamin E. Foods that contain high levels of vitamin E include green leafy vegetables, whole grains and especially wheat germ, vegetable oils, nuts, seeds, and liver. Teach the patient not to exceed the recommended daily allowance when taking vitamin E supplements without medical supervision.

Monitor the patient's serum cholesterol and serum triglyceride levels. Both of these may be increased if large doses of the supplement are prescribed.

EVALUATION When evaluating for the effectiveness of this drug, look for a decrease in or prevention of the signs and symptoms of vitamin E deficiency. Look for decreased skin irritation if the supplement is ordered topically.

Watch for drug interactions. Vitamin E is known to interact with antilipemics and mineral oil, with decreased absorption of the supplement. The effects of an iron supplement given concurrently with vitamin E are decreased.

Vitamin K, Menadiol

ACTIONS AND USES Vitamin K supplement is given for many reasons. It may be ordered to prevent hypoprothrombinemia and bleeding tendencies. These may be induced by anticoagulants or salicylates. It may be used to treat deficiencies caused by antibiotic interference with the normal intestinal flora that helps produce vitamin K. It may be given to those who lack bile. It is administered prophylactically to the newborn before the establishment of normal flora. It is used in vitamin K malabsorption syndromes.

Menadiol is converted by the body to vitamin K. It can produce adverse reactions in the patient. Some may be disturbing but not life-threatening, such as GI upset, rash, hives, and flushing. Other reactions may indicate a much more severe response to the drug, such as hemolysis, hemolytic anemia, kernicterus, or hyperbilirubinemia.

ASSESSMENT When the patient is prescribed a vitamin K supplement, assess for any signs of bleeding, whether overt or covert (occult). Look for obvious signs of hemorrhage or blood loss as well as for blood in the stool, urine, or mouth. Assess for bruising.

N U R S I N G   A L E R T

Check the patient's history and chart carefully for any report of allergy to sulfites if the injectable form is to be given. The injectable solutions contain bisulfite. These allergic reactions are more common in asthmatic patients.

Look for a history of liver disease because this warrants extra caution. Caution is also necessary in the premature infant. The use of this supplement is contraindicated during the last few weeks of pregnancy to help prevent hemorrhagic disease in the newborn.

PLANNING AND IMPLEMENTATION Menadiol may be administered orally, subcutaneously (SC), IM, or IV. The usual oral dose is 5 to 10 mg every day. The usual injectable dose is 5 to 15 mg one or two times a day.

For the patient prescribed an oral supplement, teach the importance of taking the drug as directed. If a dose is forgotten, advise the patient to take it as soon as remembered unless the next dose is also due. Caution the patient not to double the dose because this may lead to hypervitaminosis.

The parenteral route may cause redness, swelling, and pain at the site. Caution the patient in advance. Increase the pressure time for any injection site because of the increased risk for bleeding.

Regardless of the route prescribed, teach the patient to increase intake of vitamin K in the diet. Foods that contain a high level of vitamin K include green leafy vegetables, egg yolks, and liver.

If the patient is experiencing bleeding tendencies, caution against hazardous activities, such as shaving, flossing the teeth, or more obvious hazards like working around sharp materials. It may be necessary to use a soft toothbrush or even to use only mouthwash for a short time. Look for and report any nosebleeds or blood in the stool, urine, or emesis; any bruising or petechiae; black tarry stool; blood in the mouth; and excessive menses.

Caution the patient against taking any over-the-counter medications. It is especially important not to take any products containing salicylates. Teach the patient to inform all physicians or dentists that the medication is being taken and of the bleeding tendencies experienced. The patient should carry identification and wear medical alert jewelry at all times.

EVALUATION To evaluate the effectiveness of this drug, look for improvement of the prothrombin time and decreased bleeding occurrences.

Be aware of possible interactions. The effects of oral anticoagulants are decreased when they are taken with vitamin K supplements. The body's need for vitamin K is increased if the patient is prescribed an anticonvulsant, salicylates, anti-infectives, or antibiotics. Antilipemics and mineral oil interfere with the absorption of this supplement.

Vitamin K₁, Phytonadione

ACTIONS AND USES Phytonadione is another form of vitamin K supplement with actions and uses similar to those of menadiol. It does not counteract heparin but is effective against coumarin derivatives. The oral form will not be absorbed without bile salts present in the GI system.

PLANNING AND IMPLEMENTATION Phytonadione can be given orally (MEPHYTON) or SC, IM, or IV (AquaMEPHYTON). The IV route is generally used only if all other routes have not been tolerated because this route has caused deaths. The IM route is painful. If the sites are not rotated for repeated doses, induration may develop.

The injectable solution must be protected from the light to maintain full potency.

The dose is individualized to the disorder and the age of the patient.

EVALUATION Evaluation for this form of the supplement is the same as that described for menadiol. When the oral dose is administered, expect an improvement in the prothrombin time in 6 to 10 hours. When the injectable form is used, improvement is usually seen in 1 to 2 hours.

Water-Soluble Vitamins

Vitamin C, Ascorbic Acid

ACTIONS AND USES Vitamin C has been shown to be useful for many conditions. Supplements of this vitamin are prescribed to treat and prevent scurvy, which may appear in some patients as a result of special circumstances, such as hemodialysis. An increased amount of vitamin C is required during pregnancy, after trauma, during any healing process, or during infection because it is necessary for the formation of collagen used for tissue repair. An increased amount is also needed during times of increased stress, if the patient has suffered a burn, or if the patient is a smoker. Vitamin C helps keep the gums healthy and strengthens the blood vessels. Vitamin C supplements may be used to facilitate iron absorption, to acidify the urine, and to treat folic acid deficits because it helps metabolize the folic acid. Some practitioners believe vitamin C can prevent the common cold.

Vitamin C supplements are also associated with some adverse reactions. Although vitamin C is not a stored vitamin, large doses of the supplement can cause GI upset, headache, drowsiness, fatigue, and flushing of the skin. It can also lead to kidney stones and deep venous thrombosis. Large doses of vitamin C may even precipitate a sickle cell crisis.

ASSESSMENT Assess the patient for signs or symptoms ▲▲▲▲▲▲▲▲▲▲ of the disorder being treated. If scurvy is the rationale for use, look for malaise, fatigue, pain in the legs or joints, petechiae, and bleeding gums.

Look for an increased occurrence of infection or slow wound healing in the patient's history if either of these is the rationale for use.

Check the patient's history for recurrent kidney stones. This patient will have an increased risk for additional recurrences, and caution should be used.

PLANNING AND IMPLEMENTATION The prescribed dose ▲▲▲▲▲▲▲▲▲▲▲▲▲▲▲▲▲▲▲▲▲▲▲▲▲▲▲▲▲▲▲ of vitamin C depends on the rationale for use and can range from 45 to 500 mg per day. Large doses can give the patient diarrhea and burning on urination. Vitamin C supplements can be administered orally, SC, IM, or IV. The SC and IM routes are painful. Rapid IV administration can cause the patient to become dizzy and faint.

If the oral route is used, be sure the physician specifies which form of the drug to use. Capsules and tablets are to be swallowed whole. Chewable vitamin C is also available and should be chewed. Effervescent tablets are to be dissolved completely just before drinking the solution. Other oral solutions may be mixed with food or juice at the patient's request.

Regardless of the route chosen by the physician, teach the patient to increase dietary intake of vitamin C. Foods high in vitamin C include all citrus fruits, strawberries, pineapple, cabbage, green peppers, cantaloupe, green leafy vegetables, broccoli, Brussels sprouts, and tomatoes. Encourage the patient to cook the fruit or vegetable as little as possible, to cook in small amounts of water, and never to add baking soda to cooking vegetables. Teach the patient to store fresh produce in airtight containers. These practices help preserve the vitamin C content of the food.

Caution the patient not to double the dose for missed doses. The excess vitamin C will simply be washed from the body and not be effective. If the patient is taking megadoses of vitamin C at home, report this to the physician. Do not encourage the patient to stop taking the drug all at once. Sudden withdrawal from these large doses of the vitamin may cause a rebound deficiency because the body has become used to the higher level. Megadoses have also been associated with false-positive results of testing for occult blood in the stool, false-positive response to urine glucose with use of the Clinitest, and false-negative response to urine glucose with use of Tes-Tape.

EVALUATION Effectiveness of the drug is determined ▲▲▲▲▲▲▲▲▲▲ by a decrease in the signs or symptoms that prompted the prescription. The nurse can also test the pH of the urine.

Some drug interactions have been noted with vitamin C. The effects of anticoagulants are decreased when they are given with vitamin C. The effects of the vitamin C supplement are decreased if it is given with salicylates or primidone (Mysoline, an anticonvulsant).

Vitamin B$_1$, Thiamine

ACTIONS AND USES Thiamine supplements are pre- ▲▲▲▲▲▲▲▲▲▲▲▲▲▲▲▲ scribed to treat beriberi, the disorder caused by thiamine deficiency. Thiamine may also prevent Wernicke's encephalopathy. If the patient suffers from a GI disease, alcoholism, or liver cirrhosis, thiamine supplementation may prevent a potential thiamine deficit.

Adverse reactions to this water-soluble, nonstored vitamin are rare. Those that have been reported include pruritus, weakness, restlessness, GI upset, respiratory distress, and even vascular collapse.

ASSESSMENT Assess the patient prescribed a thiamine ▲▲▲▲▲▲▲▲▲▲ supplement for any signs or symptoms of a thiamine deficit. These may include GI upset, irritability, hypersensitivity to noise, fatigue, neuritis, paresthesia (especially of the toes or feet), muscle weakness or pain, paralysis of the legs, atrophy of the muscles, depression, confusion psychoses, visual disturbances, ataxia, edema, cardiac arrhythmias, and even heart failure.

PLANNING AND IMPLEMENTATION Thiamine can be administered orally, generally at doses from 1 to 30 mg per day, or IM or IV at doses of 50 to 100 mg three times a day. The dose and route chosen by the physician depend on the condition being treated. Adverse effects are especially rare with the oral route. IM injection of thiamine may be painful. You may use a cool compress over the site to ease the pain.

The IV route for thiamine can be dangerous. It is associated with a feeling of warmth, nausea, pruritus, hives, pulmonary edema, or cyanosis and can even cause death. Perform an intradermal test before the administration of the full dose to check for hypersensitivity.

Encourage the patient to increase thiamine intake in the diet. Encourage foods such as whole grains (especially wheat germ), meats (especially pork or liver), raw vegetables, peas, beans, nuts, fish, peanuts, eggs, and items made with brewers' yeast.

EVALUATION Evaluate the patient often for any signs or symptoms of a deficit. Look for improvement or worsening of these symptoms.

If the patient is to go to surgery, be sure the anesthesiologist is aware of the order for thiamine. The effects of neuromuscular blockers are increased by the concurrent use of thiamine.

Vitamin B₂, Riboflavin

ACTIONS AND USES Riboflavin supplements are used to treat or prevent a deficit. The most common adverse reaction is bright yellow urine.

ASSESSMENT Assess the patient for dermatitis, stomatitis, fatigue, eye inflammation or irritation, photophobia, and cracks at the corners of the mouth. These are signs and symptoms of riboflavin deficit.

Because this is a water-soluble vitamin and excess amounts are washed from the body, there are no generally accepted contraindications or precautions.

PLANNING AND IMPLEMENTATION The dose of this oral drug is between 1 and 30 mg every day given in divided doses. Teach the patient to omit any missed doses because excess will be excreted from the body unused. Encourage a diet high in riboflavin, including such foods as milk and dairy products, whole grains, enriched flour and products made with enriched flour, meats (especially organ meats or chicken), nuts and legumes, and green leafy vegetables. Teach the patient to store milk in a lightproof container. Plastic see-through cartons allow the riboflavin to be destroyed. Also teach the patient to avoid alcohol because this depletes the body of riboflavin and impairs its absorption.

Warn the patient about the possibility of bright yellow urine. The patient could become alarmed without this precaution.

EVALUATION Effectiveness of this drug is determined by a decrease in the signs or symptoms of the deficit. If the supplement is given for prevention, the lack of these symptoms on a continuing basis is the tool used for evaluation.

Riboflavin interacts with some drugs. The patient will require larger doses or dietary intake of riboflavin with use of phenothiazines, tricyclic antidepressants, and probenecid or if alcohol is abused.

Vitamin B₃, Niacin

ACTIONS AND USES Niacin (nicotinic acid, niacinamide, Nicobid, Nicolar) is classed as a lipid-lowering agent as well as a vitamin. It is used to prevent or treat pellagra and hyperlipidemia because it helps metabolize lipids.

Adverse reactions are usually seen only with the higher dosage range or the IV route. These may include GI upset, flushing, pruritus, and headache. Much rarer reactions can include metallic taste, peptic ulcer, liver damage, increased blood sugar level, symptoms of gout, rash, blurred vision, and orthostatic hypotension.

ASSESSMENT The physician should order baseline laboratory tests, including uric acid level, liver profile, and serum glucose level. If the drug is being used as a lipid-lowering agent, laboratory tests should also include serum cholesterol and triglyceride levels.

Assess the patient before the first dose of the medication for any symptoms of pellagra. These symptoms include dermatitis, stomatitis, glossitis, weakness, fatigue, confusion, memory loss and delirium, GI upset, and anemia.

N U R S I N G   A L E R T

▼▼▼▼▼▼▼▼▼▼▼▼▼▼▼▼▼▼▼▼▼▼▼▼▼▼▼▼▼▼▼▼▼▼▼▼

Check the history carefully for an allergy to aspirin. Some of the niacin preparations contain yellow dye No. 5, tartrazine, which is closely related to aspirin.

▲▲▲▲▲▲▲▲▲▲▲▲▲▲▲▲▲▲▲▲▲▲▲▲▲▲▲▲▲▲▲▲▲▲▲▲

Look also for a history of liver disease, peptic ulcer, gout, glaucoma, or diabetes mellitus. Patients with these conditions need careful observation of the disorder.

PLANNING AND IMPLEMENTATION Niacin can be given ▲▲▲▲▲▲▲▲▲▲▲▲▲▲▲▲▲▲▲▲▲▲▲▲▲▲▲▲ orally, IM, SC, or IV. If the form is niacinamide, the same routes apply except SC.

The usual oral dose of niacin is 10 to 20 mg per day, or up to 1 to 2 g for lipid-lowering effects. The oral dose of niacinamide is 150 to 500 mg in divided doses. Doses for parenteral administration of niacin and niacinamide are the same: up to 3 g per day in divided doses IM (also SC for niacin), and 50 to 300 mg per day in divided doses IV. Do not give IV solutions stronger than 2 mg per milliliter and not faster than 1 mL per minute.

When either form of vitamin B_3 is given orally, it should be given with food or milk to decrease GI upset. The oral form is to be swallowed whole unless it is a liquid.

If large doses of the medication are prescribed, warn the patient that flushing and a headache are commonly experienced. Large doses can also cause GI upset, warmth, itching, and tingling of the skin.

Encourage a diet high in niacin content. Niacin-rich foods include meats, fish, eggs, milk and dairy products, green leafy vegetables, peanut butter, sesame seeds and soybeans, whole grains, and enriched flour. Also encourage a fat-reduced diet as prescribed by the physician if the agent is given for its lipid-lowering properties.

EVALUATION Look for a decrease in symptoms of the ▲▲▲▲▲▲▲▲▲▲ conditions for which the drug was prescribed. If it is used as a supplement, evaluate for prevention of or decrease in symptoms of a deficit. If it is used as a lipid-lowering agent, evaluate the serum cholesterol and triglyceride levels often.

Evaluate for interactions with lovastatin. Lovastatin (Mevacor) is another lipid-lowering agent. When niacin and lovastatin are used together, the patient may experience myopathy. The effects of probenecid (Benemid) and sulfinpyrazone (Anturane), both antigout agents, are decreased when they are used concurrently with niacin.

Vitamin B₆, Pyridoxine

ACTIONS AND USES Pyridoxine supplementation is ▲▲▲▲▲▲▲▲▲▲▲▲▲▲▲▲ used to prevent or treat pyridoxine deficits. It may also help treat niacin deficits because pyridoxine is involved in the metabolism of niacin.

Pyridoxine may be prescribed to prevent or treat neuropathy. It is often prescribed in conjunction with isoniazid (an antitubercular agent), penicillamine (an antirheumatic), or hydralazine (an antihypertensive) to prevent the neuropathy that can be associated with these drugs.

Adverse reactions are rare and are usually associated only with an overdose. It is possible that the patient could experience sensory neuropathy.

ASSESSMENT Signs and symptoms of pyridoxine deficit ▲▲▲▲▲▲▲▲▲▲ include dermatitis, irritability and possibly seizures, GI upset, increased susceptibility to infection, and anemia. Note these symptoms before the first dose of the medication.

There are no commonly accepted contraindications to the use of pyridoxine. Check the patient's history for Parkinson's disease that is being treated with levodopa.

PLANNING AND IMPLEMENTATION Pyridoxine may be ▲▲▲▲▲▲▲▲▲▲▲▲▲▲▲▲▲▲▲▲▲▲▲▲▲▲▲▲▲▲▲ ordered as an oral, SC, IM, or IV drug. The usual dose is 2.5 to 10 mg per day. If the rationale for use is to counteract the neuropathy associated with isoniazid, penicillamine, or hydralazine, the dose is increased to 10 to 300 mg per day depending on the drug involved.

Pyridoxine is almost always given orally. The exception is if the oral dose is contraindicated or not tolerated. Be sure the patient knows to swallow capsules and tablets whole if they are extended-release versions. Regular capsules can be emptied and mixed with jam or a similar foodstuff at the patient's request.

SC and IM administration of pyridoxine stings or burns. As always, rotate the sites of injection. These routes can also cause numbness, drowsiness, and decreased serum folic acid levels.

Teach the patient not to double the dose if a dose is forgotten after going home. Encourage a diet high in pyridoxine. You can encourage bananas, green leafy vegetables, potatoes, lima beans, whole grains (especially wheat germ), meats (especially organ meats), fish, eggs, and legumes.

Caution the patient against overmedicating. Many patients consider vitamin supplements harmless. Megadoses of pyridoxine can cause numbness of the feet, incoordination, and an unsteady gait.

EVALUATION Evaluate the effectiveness of this drug by ▲▲▲▲▲▲▲▲▲▲ checking for improvement of deficit signs or symptoms. If the drug is given to treat or prevent neuropathy, look for an improvement in sensation and decreased pain.

If the patient has Parkinson's disease that is treated with levodopa, the effects of the levodopa may be decreased. Check for increased symptoms of the disorder.

All of the following drugs or substances require increased doses or dietary intake of pyridoxine when they are being taken: isoniazid, hydralazine, penicillamine, chloramphenicol, estrogens, immunosuppressants, oral contraceptives, and alcohol.

Vitamin B₁₂, Cyanocobalamin

ACTIONS AND USES Vitamin B_{12} requires two parts to be a whole. The body must take in a substance known as the extrinsic factor, and the body must make a substance known as the intrinsic factor.

The extrinsic factor is found only in animal product sources. These include meats (especially organ meats), seafood, egg yolk, cheeses, milk, oysters, and yogurt. Therefore, persons who are strict vegetarians (those who eat no meat, milk, or eggs) may need a supplement of the extrinsic factor or vitamin B_{12}.

The intrinsic factor is produced by cells in the GI tract. At times, diseases or surgeries of these structures may cause a depletion of the intrinsic factor and therefore of vitamin B_{12}. A supplement may be ordered for those persons who have had gastric cancer, gastrectomies, or other GI diseases to treat or prevent a deficiency.

Another disorder that can require supplementation of vitamin B_{12} is pernicious anemia. This disorder leads to a lack of the intrinsic factor for an unknown reason.

When vitamin B_{12} supplement is given, it is to prevent or treat GI lesions, neurological damage, or a blood disorder that may result from a deficiency. If oral cyanocobalamin is given, the patient must be producing the intrinsic factor and must have a sufficient intake of calcium.

When cyanocobalamin is given, the patient can experience adverse reactions. Watch for complaints of itching, urticaria, or diarrhea. Note any generalized edema, signs or symptoms of peripheral vascular thrombosis, or low potassium levels.

ASSESSMENT Before the first dose of cyanocobalamin, assess the patient for any symptoms of pernicious anemia, such as pallor, neuropathies, red or inflamed tongue, or signs of psychosis. The physician should order a baseline laboratory work-up, including serum potassium and serum folic acid levels and a reticulocyte count.

Because a history of optic nerve atrophy is a contraindication to the use of cyanocobalamin, check the chart for and ask the patient about any history of eye conditions. Also test the visual acuity. Report abnormalities to the physician immediately.

N U R S I N G   A L E R T
▼▼▼▼▼▼▼▼▼▼▼▼▼▼▼▼▼▼▼▼▼▼▼▼▼▼▼▼▼▼▼▼▼

If a preparation containing benzyl alcohol is to be used, the patient cannot be a premature infant. Benzyl alcohol has been associated with fatalities in this group.

▲▲▲▲▲▲▲▲▲▲▲▲▲▲▲▲▲▲▲▲▲▲▲▲▲▲▲▲▲▲▲▲▲

Extra caution should be exercised with patients who have any history of cardiac disease, uremia, or folic acid or iron deficiencies. Check the chart for and ask the patient about these disorders.

PLANNING AND IMPLEMENTATION Cyanocobalamin can be given orally, SC, or IM. The usual oral dose is 1 to 25 µg per day. The oral route is ineffective if the patient has any GI diseases or malabsorption syndromes due to the lack of the intrinsic factor.

Oral cyanocobalamin may be mixed with food and should be given at mealtimes to decrease GI upset. Teach the patient about dietary sources that increase cyanocobalamin intake if there is no philosophical objection.

The dose for the SC and IM routes is 30 µg per day for 5 to 10 days, then 100 to 200 µg once a month. The IM route is painful. Rotate sites for both SC and IM injections.

EVALUATION Check your reassessments of the patient frequently for signs and symptoms of a deficiency of vitamin B_{12}. Look also for improvement of laboratory values.

Evaluate for any drug interactions. There can be decreased absorption or effects of cyanocobalamin if the patient is using chloramphenicol, antineoplastics, aminoglycosides, colchicine, certain potassium supplements, vitamin C supplements, cimetidine, and alcohol. Be sure to teach the patient to warn any physician who prescribes a new medication that cyanocobalamin is being taken.

Folic Acid

ACTIONS AND USES Folic acid (folate, Folvite) is ordered to treat macrocytic anemias and prevent certain birth defects. It helps the body to produce red and white blood cells. This process is called hematopoiesis. The patient may experience a rash or fever, bright yellow urine, and a decrease of serum vitamin B_{12} levels.

ASSESSMENT Assess the patient for any signs or symptoms of anemia, such as weakness and fatigue, irritability, feeling cold more readily than others do, and a low red or white blood cell count. The physician should order a baseline hemoglobin level, hematocrit, and reticulocyte count.

Some of the preparations may contain benzyl alcohol. Do not give these to premature infants. Pernicious anemia is also a contraindication for the use of folic acid.

Be especially cautious with the patient whose anemia has not yet been diagnosed. Some types of anemia (such as pernicious anemia) do not benefit from folic acid supplementation and may even be worsened.

PLANNING AND IMPLEMENTATION Folic acid can be administered orally, SC, IM, or IV. The usual dose is 0.1 to 1.0 mg per day. IM doses must be given deeply into a large muscle, such as the gluteus medius. If the IV push route is chosen by the physician, do not give the medication any faster than 5 mg per minute.

Regardless of the route, be sure to warn the patient about the possibility of bright yellow urine. This could be cause for alarm if it is unexpected.

Encourage the patient to eat a diet high in folic acid. Foods high in content include raw fruits and vegetables (especially broccoli, green leafy vegetables, asparagus, and corn), organ meats, foods made with yeast, whole grains, and legumes.

EVALUATION Monitor the laboratory results of the hemoglobin level, hematocrit, and reticulocyte count. Improvement is usually seen at its peak in 5 to 10 days.

Effectiveness of the folic acid may be altered by other drugs. These effects are decreased if the patient is taking a sulfonamide, triamterene, or methotrexate. An increased dose is often ordered if the patient is receiving estrogen, steroids, oral contraceptives, or phenytoin or drinks alcohol.

Folinic Acid

Folinic acid (leucovorin, a derivative of folic acid) is most often used after large doses of methotrexate when the patient has osteosarcoma. It may also be used to counteract the effects of an overdose of folic acid antagonists. However, it is not useful in treating anemias or pernicious anemia.

Folinic acid may be given orally, IM, or IV. The injectable route may be preferred if the patient is expected to vomit. The dose to be given is determined by the physician and dictated by the serum methotrexate levels.

Two common drug interactions exist. If folinic acid is given with fluorouracil (another antineoplastic), there is an increased chance of toxic effects and of death. Folinic acid counteracts the effectiveness of anticonvulsants. Assess these patients frequently for increased occurrence of seizures.

MINERALS

Minerals are essential to our bodies. They account for approximately 4% of our body weight. Minerals are present in all foods but have no caloric value. They are present in all body tissues and fluids. Our bodies use minerals to make vitamins and to maintain fluid balance, both intracellular and extracellular.

Minerals can be divided into two subclasses: macronutrients and micronutrients. Placement in these classes depends on the amount needed by the body. Macronutrients are needed in much greater quantities than micronutrients are. This does not imply, however, that either is less important. Macronutrients include calcium, magnesium, and phosphorus. Micronutrients include iron, fluoride, iodine, and sulfur.

Calcium

ACTIONS AND USES Calcium is the mineral most likely to be deficient, especially in women. Our bodies need calcium for bone and tooth formation, blood clotting, stimulation of muscle contraction and nerve transmission (especially the heart), absorption of vitamin B_{12}, activation of the pancreatic enzymes, and secretion of insulin.

If our body does not receive enough calcium, signs and symptoms of a deficit appear. This deficit is called rickets. It is associated with bone deformities such as knock-knees, bowlegs, pigeon breast (pectus carinatum), thickened wrists and ankles, tingling or even paresthesia in the fingers or toes, tetany, and cardiac arrhythmias.

Calcium supplements (calcium carbonate, calcium chloride, calcium gluceptate, calcium gluconate, calcium lactate) can be ordered to treat or prevent this deficiency. Disorders that may lead to calcium deficiency are hypoparathyroidism, achlorhydria, and pancreatitis. Calcium supplements may also be ordered after menopause to help prevent osteoporosis.

Calcium supplements can cause adverse reactions. The patient may experience constipation, hypotension, nausea and vomiting, and even kidney stones. If the product is delivered intravenously (IV), adverse reactions may also include phlebitis, cardiac arrhythmias, and even cardiac arrest.

ASSESSMENT Before beginning calcium therapy, assess the patient for any signs or symptoms of calcium deficit. You will need to know the degree to which the patient experiences these symptoms so they can be compared with assessments during and after therapy.

Check the patient's laboratory result of the serum calcium level. Hypercalcemia is a contraindication to the use of calcium. If the test result or assessment of the patient indicates possible hypercalcemia, report this to the physician immediately.

Check the patient's history for and ask the patient about any past kidney stones or ventricular fibrillation. Both of these are contraindications to the use of calcium supplement.

N U R S I N G   A L E R T

Extra caution must be exercised for the patient receiving calcium supplements who is also receiving digitoxin or suffering respiratory insufficiency, renal disease, or cardiac disease. Check for signs of digitoxin toxicity or worsening of the condition.

PLANNING AND IMPLEMENTATION Because calcium supplementation can be accomplished by many different forms and routes, be sure the physician specifies exactly the calcium salt to be used, the route to be used, and the schedule.

Given orally, calcium is usually prescribed at a level of 1 to 2 g per day. The usual IV dose is 4.5 to 14 mEq.

Adults need 800 mg of calcium per day. The physician attempts to "make up" for the deficit with the dose prescribed. Encourage the patient to increase dietary intake of calcium by eating more milk and dairy products, egg yolks, green leafy vegetables, whole grains, legumes, and nuts. A diet high in vitamin D is also desirable. See the evaluation section for exceptions to this.

Give oral calcium supplements 1 hour after meals and at bedtime. It is possible that an order for vitamin D supplementation is to be given concurrently. Do not give calcium supplements with other medications that are enteric coated. These should be separated by at least 1 hour, or the enteric coating is likely to dissolve in the patient's stomach.

Because oral calcium supplements are associated with constipation, teach the patient methods to prevent the constipation. Instruct the patient to increase fluid intake, eat a high-fiber diet, and increase physical activity.

Two common calcium products that you may see ordered are Caltrate and Citracal. Caltrate is an oral supplement available as tablets. Citracal, also an oral supplement, is available as tablets or effervescent tablets. Oral forms of calcium supplementation are calcium lactate, calcium gluconate, and calcium carbonate.

If the supplement is ordered IV, be sure to warm the solution to body temperature, then place the IV into a large vein. This prevents vein irritation and phlebitis.

Monitor the IV site frequently. Infiltration can cause tissue sloughing. An infiltrated site may need to be treated with hyaluronidase, 1% procaine, or heat. The physician will order the treatment desired.

Do not allow the patient to sit up immediately after an IV dose of calcium. Ask the patient to remain lying down for 15 to 30 minutes to prevent postural hypotension.

IV forms of supplementation include calcium gluconate, calcium glucceptate, and calcium chloride.

EVALUATION Monitor the serum calcium level and report improvements or worsening to the physician. Reassess for signs and symptoms of the deficit.

Monitor the patient for any signs or symptoms of overdose. This may include gastrointestinal (GI) upset, colic, paralytic ileus, constipation, thirst, laryngospasms, or cardiac arrhythmias.

Be aware of many different interactions. Some of the same foods that are normally encouraged when a calcium deficit exists are capable of interfering with the absorption of oral calcium supplements. Foods that interfere include dairy products, cereals, spinach, and rhubarb. Two drug interactions are also common. The use of calcium supplements decreases the absorption of tetracyclines from the GI system. Aluminum-containing antacids may be used as a calcium supplement, but be sure not to use these for patients with impaired renal function.

Phosphorus

ACTIONS AND USES Phosphorus is needed by our body for bone and tooth formation, formation of soft tissue, metabolism of other nutrients, storage of fat, and maintenance of acid-base balance (it acts as a buffer).

Phosphorus supplements (K-Phos, Neutra-Phos) also contain potassium, calcium, and sodium.

Phosphorus supplements are classified as phosphate urinary acidifiers or as phosphorus supplements, depending on the formula. They may be used with methenamine mandelate (Mandelamine) to increase antibacterial activity.

Phosphorus supplements can cause GI upset, electrolyte imbalance, and bone or joint pain.

ASSESSMENT Assessments to be performed depend on the rationale for use of the drug. If it is being given as a supplement, assess for the signs and symptoms of a deficit. If it is being given as a urinary acidifier, assess the urine pH.

Check the patient's history for any phosphate kidney stones, hyperphosphatemia, or loss of renal function below 30%. These are contraindications to the use of phosphorus supplements.

Extra caution is needed for patients with cardiac disease or hypertension, fluid or electrolyte imbalances, liver cirrhosis, or Addison's disease.

The physician should order baseline laboratory tests of serum phosphate, serum potassium, serum calcium, and serum sodium levels.

PLANNING AND IMPLEMENTATION Adults need 800 mg of phosphorus a day. The dose of supplementation depends on the degree of deficit, the normal intake for this patient, and the formula being ordered. Supplements are available as tablets, powder, or capsules.

It is possible that the patient may experience a mild laxative effect during the first few days of therapy. Warn the patient of this possibility and teach the patient to report prolonged diarrhea. The physician may need to alter the dose or discontinue the drug.

Monitor all laboratory results carefully, especially serum electrolyte values.

Encourage the patient to eat high-protein foods that are good dietary sources of phosphorus.

EVALUATION Effectiveness of the drug is determined by decreased signs of a deficit or by effectiveness of methenamine mandelate therapy.

Evaluate for antagonistic effects of concurrent use of antacids containing magnesium, aluminum, or calcium. Check for possible hypernatremia if phosphorus supplements are used with antihypertensives or corticosteroids. Look for signs of hyperkalemia if the patient is receiving potassium supplements or potassium-sparing diuretics. The effects of salicylates are increased if they are used with phosphorus supplements.

Magnesium

ACTIONS AND USES Magnesium is used to help synthesize protein, stimulate muscle contraction and nerve transmission, and regulate thyroxine secretion. If the body lacks a sufficient intake of magnesium, tetany results.

Magnesium supplements (Beelith, Mag-Ox 400, Uro-Mag) may be used as supplements or as antacids. They may also be ordered to be taken concurrently with pyridoxine.

ASSESSMENT Do a dietary assessment of the patient's intake of magnesium. Look for any signs or symptoms of magnesium deficit.

Check the patient's history for any kidney disease. This patient will require extra caution during therapy because the kidney is the primary site of excretion of magnesium.

PLANNING AND IMPLEMENTATION Adult requirements for magnesium differ by sex. Women require 300 mg per day; men need 350 mg. The physician orders a dose on the basis of the level of deficit, the patient's usual intake of magnesium, and the formula used.

Encourage the patient to increase intake of foods high in magnesium. Dietary sources include vegetables, cereals, dairy products, and seafood.

EVALUATION Watch serum levels of magnesium for improvements. Reassess the patient frequently for decreased occurrence of tetany.

Caution the patient that magnesium supplements may result in a laxative effect. Teach the patient to report prolonged diarrhea.

Magnesium-containing antacids interfere with tetracycline absorption, and they should not be used together.

Ferrous Sulfate

ACTIONS AND USES The body needs iron for the synthesis of hemoglobin and for glucose metabolism. Without sufficient intake of iron, the patient can experience anemia.

Iron supplements can cause GI upset. This includes nausea, vomiting, diarrhea, or constipation. The stool may become black.

ASSESSMENT Assess the patient for signs or symptoms of anemia, including weakness and fatigue, irritability, feeling cold when others do not, and feeling cold to the touch. The physician should order a baseline hemoglobin level and hematocrit.

PLANNING AND IMPLEMENTATION Ferrous sulfate (Fe-osol) is available as an elixir, tablets, or capsules. Be sure to mix the elixir with water or fruit juice if the patient cannot tolerate it "straight." Never mix it with milk products or those containing alcohol. Instruct the patient to drink the solution through a straw and not to swish the solution around in the mouth before swallowing. The iron elixir will stain the teeth a dark yellow-brown. Although the staining is not permanent, it is distressing to the patient while it lasts.

Instruct the patient to take all iron preparations with meals if it causes GI upset. The physician may choose to decrease the dose and then slowly increase it again until the desired level is achieved. Also warn the patient about the possibility of black stool to prevent alarm.

Adult requirements vary by sex. Men need 10 mg per day. Women need nearly double at a level of 18 mg per day. The dose of supplementation is determined by the patient's level of deficit, the formula used, the patient's usual intake, and the patient's ability to tolerate the supplement.

Encourage the patient to increase intake of iron through foods such as meats (especially organ meats), egg yolks, green leafy vegetables, legumes, and nuts.

Iron products should not be taken with tetracyclines. The absorption of the tetracycline will be altered. The two drugs should be separated by at least 2 hours if they must be taken concurrently.

EVALUATION Reassess the patient's baseline symptoms and laboratory results to determine effectiveness of the medication. Evaluate for compliance because GI upset may have caused the patient to stop taking the medication.

N U R S I N G   A L E R T

Iron supplements can produce toxicity. If an overdose of the supplement is taken (or a child accidentally ingests someone else's medication), be advised that this is poisonous. Contact the poison control center nearest to you immediately.

Iron Dextran

ACTIONS AND USES Iron dextran (Imferon) is an injectable iron preparation. It is given only if oral supplementation is not possible.

Iron dextran is considered a dangerous medication because of the possibility of anaphylaxis and death. This injectable can also lead to a headache, faintness, bronchospasms, and hematuria. It can cause birth defects if it is given during pregnancy. Given IV, iron dextran can cause low blood pressure, chest pain, tachycardia, flushing, and phlebitis. Intramuscular (IM) iron dextran can cause arthralgia, myalgia, a sterile abscess, staining of the tissue, cellulitis, or even necrosis. Either route can cause GI upset and rash or itching.

Laboratory values can be altered by injectable iron dextran. There may be falsely elevated serum bilirubin levels and falsely lowered serum calcium levels. Serum iron levels will not be accurate for several days after the medication.

ASSESSMENT Assessments are the same as for the oral iron preparation, plus some extra contraindications and precautions. Anemia not associated with iron deficiency is considered a contraindication to the use of this drug.

N U R S I N G   A L E R T

Use extra caution with patients who have liver dysfunction, an acute kidney infection, or rheumatoid arthritis (may cause an exacerbation). Also be aware that iron dextran is possibly carcinogenic.

PLANNING AND IMPLEMENTATION The dose of iron dextran is highly individualized. All oral iron preparations should be discontinued before the beginning of iron dextran therapy. A test dose should be administered before full IM or IV iron dextran doses are given.

If the IM route is to be used, it is best if the patient is lying down on the side. Give the medication by the Z-track method to avoid tissue staining. Never mix this medication with other medications or solutions. Give the IM injection into the gluteus medius muscle only. Never use a smaller muscle like the arm. Inject deeply using a 2- to 3-inch, 19- or 20-gauge needle. This injection is painful. The IM dose should not be more than 2.0 mL per day, which is 100 mg of iron.

If the IV route is to be used, be sure to give the medication slowly and undiluted at a rate of 1 mL per minute or slower.

EVALUATION
▲▲▲▲▲▲▲▲▲▲ Evaluation is the same as for the oral iron preparation.

E X E R C I S E S

CASE STUDIES

1. Ms. E.J., age 72 years, complains of diarrhea. She has been taking megadoses of vitamins. What questions do you need to ask her? What vitamin is most likely responsible for her diarrhea if she is taking it?

2. Your patient is to have an IM injection of iron supplement. What are your responsibilities before administering this drug? What method would you use to administer the drug?

3. B.W., a 6-year-old boy, must have pancreatic enzymes because of cystic fibrosis. When should he receive this medication? What are your responsibilities?

LEARNING ACTIVITIES

Perform a survey of laypersons. Ask questions to determine the layperson's basic understanding of vitamins and minerals. Examples of questions you may wish to ask include the following:

What is the best way to ensure that you have all the vitamins and minerals your body requires?

What problems, if any, can vitamins produce if they are taken in excess?

What vitamins, if any, should be taken in large doses?

What minerals, if any, should be taken in large doses?

Write some questions of your own. When the survey is over, look at the answers you received. What do the answers have in common? Are there misconceptions that many laypersons hold about vitamins and minerals? Share your results with other nursing students and health care personnel.

UNIT TWELVE

DRUGS THAT AFFECT THE ENDOCRINE SYSTEM

In your study of anatomy and physiology, you learned of the concept of homeostasis, the mechanisms whereby the systems of the body are kept in a state of balance. The endocrine system is no exception to this. As you recall, endocrine glands are internal and have no ducts (Fig. XII–1). Secretions from the endocrine glands are called hormones, which are carried by blood or lymph to other glands or tissues. Each hormone is specialized and delivers a specific message to a particular target organ or gland.

The hypothalamus, which is located in the brain (Fig. XII–2), acts like a thermostat to regulate hormone levels. The hypothalamus produces substances called neurohormones or hypothalamic releasing factors.

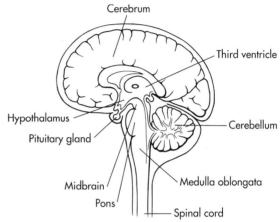

Figure XII–2. The hypothalamus, located in the brain, regulates hormone levels to keep the body in a state of homeostasis.

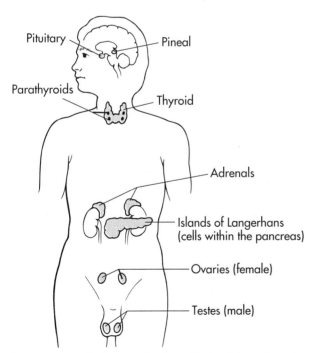

Figure XII–1. Endocrine glands are located throughout the body. Because they have no ducts, their secretions (called hormones) are carried by the blood or lymph to various areas of the body.

The hormones of the body affect homeostasis (the balance of the body's systems). They do this by a process called negative feedback, which involves a stimulating gland, a target gland, and hypothalamic releasing factors (neurohormones). The stimulating gland secretes a hormone (often called a tropic hormone), which is carried by the bloodstream to a specific target. The target gland receives the message of the hormone and responds, often by secreting another hormone.

The level of hormone circulating in the bloodstream is regulated by the hypothalamus through the release of neurohormones. (The term neurohormones is sometimes used because the nervous and circulatory systems are used to transmit the messages to the glands.)

The hypothalamus secretes the hypothalamic releasing factors, and these neurohormones transmit the message to the stimulating gland to increase its secretions.

As the stimulating gland responds, so does the target gland. Thus, the level of hormone secreted by the target gland increases. As the level of hormone secreted by the target gland increases, the amount of hypothalamic releasing factor decreases. This process is called negative feedback.

As the blood level of the hypothalamic releasing factor decreases, the stimulating gland decreases secretion of its hormone. In response, the target gland also decreases secretion of its hormone.

As the hormone from the target gland decreases, the hypothalamus releases the hypothalamic releasing factor. The whole process repeats, with the stimulating gland increasing the secretion of hormone until the target gland responds with the appropriate action. In this way, homeostasis is maintained.

PITUITARY HORMONES

LEARNING OBJECTIVES

After studying this chapter, you should be able to:

1. Discuss the concept of the feedback mechanism as it relates to the anterior pituitary gland and the thyroid and adrenal glands, appropriately describing the function of the stimulating gland, the target gland, and the hypothalamus.

2. Prepare a care plan for a patient receiving thyrotropin, corticotropin, or vasopressin.

DRUGS YOU WILL LEARN ABOUT IN THIS CHAPTER

Anterior Pituitary Hormones

Thyroid-stimulating hormone (TSH) or thyrotropic hormone

thyrotropin (Thytropar)

Adrenocorticotropic hormone (ACTH)

corticotropin (ACTH)

Acthar

Acthar gel

Somatotropin (STH) or human growth hormone (hGH)

somatotropin (Asellacrin, Humatrope, Nutropin) somatrem (Protropin)

Gonadotropic hormones

follicle-stimulating hormone (FSH)

luteinizing hormone (LH)

interstitial cell-stimulating hormone (ICSH)

lactogenic hormone or prolactin (PRL)

Posterior Pituitary Hormones

Antidiuretic hormone (ADH) or vasopressin

vasopressin (Pitressin Synthetic)

vasopressin tannate (Pitressin Tannate)

desmopressin (DDAVP)

lypressin (Diapid)

Oxytocin

The pituitary gland is considered the master gland because it controls many of the other glands of the body. The pituitary gland is the size of a pea and is located in the brain in a depression of the sphenoid bone. It has two distinct parts that function as separate glands called the anterior pituitary and the posterior pituitary. Each part produces different hormones (Table 57–1).

The diagnostic and therapeutic uses of the pituitary hormones are listed with their dosages in Table 57–2.

ANTERIOR PITUITARY HORMONES

Thyroid-Stimulating Hormone or Thyrotropic Hormone

The anterior pituitary gland secretes the thyroid-stimulating hormone (TSH), which stimulates the thyroid gland to produce the hormones thyroxine (T_4), triiodothyronine (T_3), and calcitonin. As the blood level of T_3 and T_4 increases, negative feedback occurs, and the hypothalamus decreases secretion of the

Table 57–1. Pituitary Gland Hormones

HORMONE	FUNCTION
Anterior Pituitary	
Thyroid-stimulating hormone (TSH) or thyrotropic hormone	Stimulates thyroid gland to secrete thyroxine (T_4), triiodothyronine (T_3), and calcitonin
Adrenocorticotropic hormone (ACTH)	Stimulates adrenal cortex to produce cortical hormones (glucocorticoids, mineralocorticoids, sex hormones) Aids in protecting the body during stress
Somatotropin (STH) or human growth hormone (hGH)	Promotes growth of all body tissues
Follicle-stimulating hormone (FSH)	In females: Regulates growth of ovarian follicles and estrogen secretion In males: Regulates growth of testes and development of sperm
Luteinizing hormone (LH) Interstitial cell-stimulating hormone (ICSH)	In females: Stimulates the development of the corpus luteum and secretion of progesterone In males: Stimulates the interstitial cells of the testes to increase production and secretion of testosterone
Lactogenic hormone or prolactin (PRL)	Stimulates the breasts to secrete breast milk
Melanocyte-stimulating hormone	Increases synthesis and dispersion of melanin
Posterior Pituitary	
Antidiuretic hormone (ADH) or vasopressin	Promotes reabsorption of water in the kidney tubules and stimulates smooth muscle tissue of blood vessels to constrict
Oxytocin	Stimulates contraction of the pregnant uterus and stimulates let-down and ejection of breast milk

hypothalamic releasing factors. As this stimulation of the anterior pituitary gland decreases, so does the secretion of TSH decrease.

When TSH secretion decreases, the thyroid gland decreases secretion of T_3 and T_4. As the level of these hormones decreases, the process repeats. The hypothalamus releases neurohormones that stimulate the anterior pituitary to increase TSH secretion. TSH stimulates the thyroid to increase T_3 and T_4 secretion.

If there is an anterior pituitary deficiency of TSH, the symptoms of hypothyroidism develop.

ACTIONS AND USES There is little use for TSH (thyrotropin) in medicine because T_3 and T_4 are both available as animal extracts or synthetics, which are much less expensive. TSH is sometimes used to differentiate whether hypothyroid

Readonly.

Table 57-2. Pituitary Medications

DRUG	DOSAGE
Thyroid-stimulating hormone (TSH) or thyrotropic hormone thyrotropin (Thytropar)	Diagnostic dose to differentiate primary from secondary hypothyroidism: 10 units IM or SC for 1–3 days
Adrenocorticotropic hormone (ACTH) corticotropin (ACTH, ATHAR, ATHAR gel)	Diagnostic dose to differentiate primary from secondary adrenocortical hypofunction: up to 80 units IM or SC in divided doses Therapeutic dose: aqueous, 40 units IM or SC in 4 divided doses; gel, 40 units q12–24 h
Somatotropin (STH) or human growth hormone (hGH) somatotropin (Asellacrin, Humatrope, Nutropin) Somatrem (Protropin)	Asellacrin: therapeutic dose in growth failure due to STH deficiency: 2 units (1.0 mL) IM 3 times a week with a minimum of 48 h between injections Dosage is doubled if growth does not exceed 1 inch in 6 months Humatrope 0.06 mg/kg (0.16 IU/kg) SC or IM 3 x wk Nutropin 0.3 mg/kg (approx. 0.78 IU/kg) per wk. SC or IM Somatrem (Protropin) up to 0.1 mg/kg (0.26 IU/kg) 3 x wk
Gonadotropic hormones Follicle-stimulating hormone (FSH) Luteinizing hormone (LH) Interstitial cell-stimulating hormone (ICSH) Lactogenic hormone or prolactin (PRL)	See chapter 62
Posterior Pituitary Hormones	
Antidiuretic hormone (ADH) or vasopressin (Pitressin Synthetic)	Therapeutic dose Child: 2.5–10 units IM or SC bid–qid prn or intranasal individualized dosage Adult: 5–10 units IM or SC bid–qid prn or intranasal individualized dosage
vasopressin tannate (Pitressin Tannate)	Therapeutic dose Child: 1.25–2.5 units IM q 2–3 days Adult: 2.5–5 units IM q 2–3 days
desmopressin (DDAVP)	Therapeutic dose: intranasal, 0.1 mL bid; SC or IV, 0.25–0.5 mL bid
lypressin (Diapid)	Therapeutic dose: intranasal, 1–2 sprays each nostril qid
oxytocin (Pitocin)	See chapter 64

symptoms are due to anterior pituitary hypofunction or thyroid hypofunction.

An example of a pharmaceutical preparation of this hormone is thyrotropin (Thytropar).

Adverse actions include headache, tachycardia, atrial fibrillation, congestive heart failure, nausea, menstrual irregularities, and anaphylactic reactions.

ASSESSMENT Perform cephalocaudal assessment and
▲▲▲▲▲▲▲▲▲▲ document findings as baseline data. Assess laboratory values for serum TSH, T$_3$, and T$_4$ levels.

PLANNING AND IMPLEMENTATION The dose of TSH is
▲▲▲▲▲▲▲▲▲▲▲▲▲▲▲▲▲▲▲▲▲▲▲▲▲ administered intramuscularly (IM) or subcutaneously (SC). Monitor the injection sites for irritation. Monitor the patient for signs and symptoms of anaphylaxis.

TSH administration may cause thyroid enlargement (hyperplasia). Enlargement may not be apparent externally, but an enlarged gland may be pressing on the esophagus. Caution the patient to report choking and difficulty in swallowing (dysphagia) or hoarseness and difficulty with speech (dysphasia).

EVALUATION Assess the patient and compare findings
▲▲▲▲▲▲▲▲▲▲ with baseline data. Monitor laboratory values for changes in TSH, T$_3$, and T$_4$ levels.

Adrenocorticotropic Hormone

The anterior pituitary secretes the adrenocorticotropic hormone (ACTH). As the blood level of ACTH increases, the cortex of the adrenal gland is stimulated to produce the adrenocortical hormones, primarily the glucocorticoids.

As the blood level of the glucocorticoids increases, negative feedback occurs. The hypothalamus decreases secretion of the hypothalamic releasing factors. The anterior pituitary decreases secretion of ACTH. As the level of ACTH decreases in the blood, the adrenal cortex decreases secretion of the glucocorticoid hormones.

When the blood level of the glucocorticoids decreases, the hypothalamus secretes more hypothalamic releasing factor. The anterior pituitary secretes more ACTH, and the adrenal cortex responds by secreting the glucocorticoids.

A deficiency of ACTH causes symptoms of adrenal insufficiency. This life-threatening condition is referred to as Addison's disease.

Examples of pharmaceutical preparations of ACTH include corticotropin (ACTH), Acthar, and Acthar gel.

ACTIONS AND USES There is little use for ACTH (ad-
▲▲▲▲▲▲▲▲▲▲▲▲▲▲▲▲▲ renocorticotropin or corticotropin) in medicine because the pharmaceutical preparations are widely available and less expensive. ACTH is sometimes used to evaluate adrenocortical function and to manage acute exacerbations (flare-ups) of multiple sclerosis.

Adverse actions include rash, urticaria, hypotension, tachycardia, dyspnea, dizziness, convulsions, personality changes, psychoses, edema, fragile skin, bruising, impaired wound healing, hyperpigmentation, muscle weakness, hypokalemia, and many others.

ASSESSMENT Perform a cephalocaudal assessment and
▲▲▲▲▲▲▲▲▲▲ document the findings as baseline data. Assess the patient's laboratory values for serum ACTH levels.

PLANNING AND IMPLEMENTATION These preparations
▲▲▲▲▲▲▲▲▲▲▲▲▲▲▲▲▲▲▲▲▲▲▲▲▲ are given SC and IM. Be alert for hypersensitivity reactions.

N U R S I N G   A L E R T
▼▼▼▼▼▼▼▼▼▼▼▼▼▼▼▼▼▼▼▼▼▼▼▼▼▼▼▼▼▼▼▼

If used for a time, ACTH causes negative feedback to the anterior pituitary. ACTH levels will decrease, as will stimulation to the adrenal gland. The secretion of adrenocortical hormones will decrease. This could have life-threatening consequences if the ACTH therapy is suddenly stopped.

▲▲▲▲▲▲▲▲▲▲▲▲▲▲▲▲▲▲▲▲▲▲▲▲▲▲▲▲▲▲▲▲▲▲▲▲▲▲

Advise patients to take their medication exactly as prescribed and to notify the physician if they discontinue it for any reason (see Chapter 58 for more information).

Contraindications to the use of ACTH include congestive heart failure, allergies to pork, pregnancy, tuberculosis, cirrhosis, renal insufficiency, diabetes, and psychotic tendencies.

EVALUATION Review daily cephalocaudal assessments
▲▲▲▲▲▲▲▲▲▲ and compare with baseline data to evaluate for improvement in symptoms. Review laboratory reports of serum ACTH levels.

Somatotropin or Human Growth Hormone

Somatotropin (STH), or human growth hormone (hGH), regulates growth of bones and tissues. The growth function is also influenced by the thyroid hormones and insulin. When a body is deficient in the amount of STH/hGH produced, a condition called dwarfism results. In this condition, the child fails to develop normally.

Natural sources of somatotropin, such as Asellacrin, are limited and difficult to obtain. As a result, they are extremely expensive and often cost the family thousands of dollars per month. Recent technology has made available synthetic products (Humatrope, Nutropin, Protropin) that are identical to natural somatotropin. These are manufactured by recombinant DNA technology from a strain of *E. coli* that has been modified by the addition of the gene for the human growth hormone. As synthetic products become more widely available, the cost of treatment is expected to be much less than with the natural sources.

ACTIONS AND USES Somatotropin acts to alter intracellular transport of amino acids, calcium absorption and excretion, reabsorption of phosphorus, intracellular glucose metabolism, and formation of cartilage. It may be used when the condition of dwarfism exists.

Adverse actions include excess calcium in the urine, renal calculi, hyperglycemia, and irritation at the injection site.

ASSESSMENT Assess the child's height, weight, and head circumference. Plot the measurements on the appropriate boy's or girl's growth chart. Review family history and genetic background to assess for individual family differences. Assess laboratory tests for serum STH/hGH, ACTH, and TSH levels.

PLANNING AND IMPLEMENTATION Synthetic products are available as a vial of white powder that must be reconstituted with the 5 mL of diluent included in the package. Aim the stream of diluent against the wall of the vial. Roll the vial gently to mix it. DO NOT SHAKE THE SOLUTION. If the solution is cloudy or contains particles that do not dissolve, it must be discarded. Use only clear solution.

Store powder under refrigeration at 36° to 46°F (2° to 8°C). Do not freeze. After reconstitution, solutions are stable up to 14 days if refrigerated at these same temperatures.

Treatment must begin before closure of the epiphyseal plate in the long bones and continue for many years until puberty, when closure of the epiphyses occurs. After epiphyseal closure, there is no further growth in height.

Use of somatotropin is contraindicated in any patient with evidence of active tumor. Those with intracranial lesions must be inactive and treatment must be completed before therapy with somatotropin is begun. Patients must be examined frequently for recurrence of tumor growth.

Somatotropin is administered IM or SC several times a week, so the family is often instructed in injection technique to decrease the number of clinic visits. Encourage families to keep all clinic appointments because dose must be individualized.

Emotional care should include methods of improving self-esteem because children are often sensitive to differences in their size compared with that of their peers. Emphasize development of interests and hobbies for which size is not important. If the child is interested in sports, emphasize those in which small size can be used to advantage. Swimming, tennis, golf, track, and sailing are a few of those sports.

Teach the patient and family the signs and symptoms of hyperglycemia and encourage them to report these promptly to the physician. The physician may order periodic monitoring of fingerstick blood glucose levels. Teach the patient and family to perform this test.

Thyroid and adrenocortical function may also be affected. Monitor for signs and symptoms of hypofunction or hyperfunction of these glands. Document and report symptoms to the physican.

Slipped epiphyses occur more frequently in children receiving somatotropin therapy because of the growth spurts that occur. Teach patients and their parents to report to the physician if hip pain or a limp occurs.

EVALUATION Patients occasionally have antibodies against the medication and fail to respond to therapy. Therefore, ongoing evaluations of height, weight, and head circumference must be made. Review laboratory results of serum STH/hGH levels and serum ACTH, TSH, calcium, phosphorus, and glucose levels.

Gonadotropic Hormones

The gonadotropic hormones derive their name from the fact that they stimulate the gonads. They include

- Follicle-stimulating hormone (FSH)
- Luteinizing hormone (LH)
- Interstitial cell-stimulating hormone (ICSH)
- Prolactin (PRL), which is also called the lactogenic hormone

Follicle-Stimulating Hormone

FSH regulates growth of the ovarian follicles in females and growth of the testes and development of sperm in males.

Luteinizing Hormone

After ovulation, LH stimulates the development of the corpus luteum at the site of the ruptured follicle on the ovary.

Interstitial Cell-Stimulating Hormone

In males, ICSH stimulates the interstitial cells of the testes to increase their production of testosterone.

Prolactin or the Lactogenic Hormone

PRL stimulates the breasts to produce or secrete breast milk.

For further discussion of FSH, LH, ICSH, and PRL, see Unit Thirteen.

Melanocyte-Stimulating Hormone

This hormone increases synthesis and dispersion of melanin. It produces a patient's natural skin color. Pharmaceutical products are not available.

POSTERIOR PITUITARY HORMONES

Antidiuretic Hormone/Vasopressin

Antidiuretic hormone (ADH) promotes the reabsorption of water in the proximal convoluted tubules of the kidney. It also stimulates constriction of the smooth muscle tissue of blood vessels, which increases blood pressure.

Hypofunction of the posterior pituitary gland results in a deficiency of ADH. This condition is called diabetes insipidus. Diabetes insipidus causes a person to void profuse amounts of dilute urine, which results in dehydration.

Some examples of pharmaceutical preparations of the ADH hormone are vasopressin (Pitressin Synthetic) and vasopressin tannate (Pitressin Tannate), desmopressin (DDAVP), and lypressin (Diapid).

ACTIONS AND USES ADH affects the distal convoluted ▲▲▲▲▲▲▲▲▲▲▲▲▲▲▲▲ tubules of the kidney nephron to regulate the reabsorption of water. This helps the body to conserve fluids and to maintain a normal fluid balance. It also constricts peripheral blood vessels, which raises blood pressure. Therefore, ADH is said to have vasopressor activity, and that is why it is also called vasopressin.

Vasopressin (Pitressin) is used to treat diabetes insipidus to prevent dehydration.

Symptoms of excessive dose include blanching skin, nausea, and abdominal cramps. Other possible adverse effects are tremors, sweating, vomiting, vertigo, drowsiness, convulsions, and coma.

ASSESSMENT Assess the patient for signs and symp- ▲▲▲▲▲▲▲▲▲▲▲ toms of dehydration. Also assess the patient's intake and output for a 24-hour period and the vital signs. Document data as baseline information.

Assess the chart for laboratory values of serum electrolytes and specific gravity of the urine.

PLANNING AND IMPLEMENTATION Monitor the intake ▲▲▲▲▲▲▲▲▲▲▲▲▲▲▲▲▲▲▲▲▲▲▲▲▲▲▲▲▲ and output, the vital signs, and the weight each day.

Preparations of vasopressin can be given subcutaneously (SC), intramuscularly (IM), or by nasal spray. Dose is individualized. Observe patients for 10 to 15 minutes after administration of medication.

If symptoms of excessive dose occur, the patient should consume one to two glasses of water. Reassure the patient that symptoms last only a few minutes. Notify the physician of these symptoms before another dose so that the dose may be reduced if necessary.

Patients should be knowledgeable about appropriate methods of administration. Instruct them in the possible adverse effects and the appropriate interventions. Remind them to keep all appointments and to take their medication consistently.

If traveling, the patient should keep the medication at all times and not put it in the luggage. ADH may not be readily available at all pharmacies and may be difficult to replace.

Nasal spray is used most frequently because of the ease of self-administration. If administered SC or IM, sites should be rotated. Teach patients to evaluate intake and output. They may be taught to do specific gravity tests at home.

EVALUATION Review laboratory values, especially spe- ▲▲▲▲▲▲▲▲▲▲ cific gravity and electrolytes. Evaluate intake records to determine whether they are approximate to the amounts listed for output. Compare vital signs and weight with baseline assessments to observe for dehydration or water retention.

Oxytocin

Oxytocin is used in women as part of the oxytocin challenge test during pregnancy, to stimulate labor, to control postpartum hemorrhage, or to cause ejection of milk (see Chapter 64).

E X E R C I S E S

CASE STUDIES

1. Ms. M.C.'s 4-year-old daughter has been under treatment with Asellacrin for a deficiency of STH. What must Ms. M.C. be taught about techniques of administration for this medication? Why was this medication started at such an early age? How long can this medication be used? What assessments are important for the nurse to make at each clinic visit?

2. Mr. J.H. has a condition called diabetes insipidus. His treatment consists of intranasal administration of vasopressin. What side effects should be reviewed with him? What is the appropriate intervention if these side effects should occur? What laboratory values should be evaluated?

LEARNING ACTIVITIES

Role play the concept of negative feedback. Be sure to include the role of the hypothalamic releasing factors.

STEROID HORMONES

LEARNING OBJECTIVES

After studying this chapter, you should be able to:

1. Discuss the actions of the adrenocortico-steroid drugs.

2. List some of the conditions for which they are used.

3. State the source of these hormones.

4. List the major adverse effects of these drugs.

5. State appropriate nursing interventions to prevent or control these adverse effects.

6. Write a teaching plan for a patient receiving one of these hormones.

DRUGS YOU WILL LEARN ABOUT IN THIS CHAPTER

Glucocorticoids

cortisone acetate (Cortistan, Cortone)

hydrocortisone (Cortisol, Cortef)

prednisolone (Cortalone)

betamethasone (Celestone)

methylprednisolone (Medrol)

dexamethasone sodium phosphate (Decadron)

hydrocortisone sodium succinate (Solu-Cortef)

methylprednisolone sodium succinate (Solu-Medrol)

methylprednisolone acetate (Depo-Medrol)

prednisone (Deltasone, Colisone)

triamcinolone (Aristocort, Kenacort)

Mineralocorticoids

desoxycorticosterone acetate (DOCA, Percoten Acetate)

desoxycorticosterone pivalate (Percorten Pivalate)

fludrocortisone acetate (Florinef Acetate)

Humans have two adrenal glands, one above each kidney. Each gland has two parts: the outside or cortex, and the inside or medulla. Each part produces hormones but acts on different tissues and in a different manner. This chapter focuses on the hormones produced by the cortex, which are often referred to as steroids.

The cortex produces three main groups of hormones: the glucocorticoids, the mineralocorticoids, and the sex hormones.

Glucocorticoids aid in the metabolism of carbohydrates, proteins, and fats. They help maintain a "carbohydrate reserve" in the body for use in times of stress when we need extra energy. They suppress inflammatory responses in the body and also help maintain a normal blood pressure.

Mineralocorticoids aid in the regulation of electrolytes by controlling the reabsorption of sodium and the secretion of potassium by the kidney tubules. Table 58–1 lists dosages of glucocorticoids and mineralocorticoids.

Sex hormones may influence some secondary sex characteristics of males and females. They are produced here in small amounts. These are primarily androgens, but some estrogens are also produced. (Androgens and estrogens are discussed in Chapters 61 and 62.)

Table 58-1. Steroids	
DRUG	**DOSAGE**
Glucocorticoids	
cortisone acetate (Cortistan, Cortone)	25–300 mg PO or IM qd or alternate days (individualized)
hydrocortisone (Cortisol, Cortef)	5–30 mg PO bid–qid, increased to 80 mg PO qid in acute situations
hydrocortisone sodium succinate (Solu-Cortef)	Initial dose: 100–250 mg IV or IM Maintenance dose: decrease to 50–100 mg IM as indicated
prednisolone (Cortalone)	2.5–15 mg PO bid–qid
methylprednisolone (Medrol)	2–60 mg PO in 4 divided doses
methylprednisolone acetate (Depo-Medrol)	40–80 mg IM qd
methylprednisolone sodium succinate (Solu-Medrol)	10–250 mg IV or IM q4h
betamethasone (Celestone)	0.6 to 7.2 mg PO qd
dexamethasone sodium phosphate (Decadron)	Cerebral edema: 10 mg IV, then 4–6 mg IM q6h for 2–4 days, then taper for 5–7 days Shock: 1–6 mg/kg IV single dose or 40 mg IV q2–6h prn Inflammation/allergy: 0.25–4 mg PO bid–qid
prednisone (Deltasone, Colisone)	2.5–15 mg PO bid–qid each day or qod

Table 58-1. Steroids *Continued*	
DRUG	**DOSAGE**
triamcinolone (Aristocort, Kenacort)	4–48 mg PO qd divided bid–qid
Mineralocorticoids	
desoxycorticosterone acetate (DOCA Acetate, Percoten Acetate)	2–5 mg IM qd
desoxycorticosterone pivalate (Percorten Pivalate)	25–100 mg IM q 4 wk
fludrocortisone acetate (Florinef Acetate)	0.1–0.2 mg PO qd

Adrenocorticosteroids, corticosteroids, and steroids all refer to the same thing. They can occur naturally or be manufactured synthetically. They are often labeled as glucocorticoids, mineralocorticoids, or mixed steroids. For our purposes, it is not important for the student to *memorize* to which of these specific groups the many drugs belong, but simply to understand the main differences in the actions of each group, to recognize the individual drugs as steroids, and to check appropriate resources when necessary.

In Chapter 57, we discussed that the anterior pituitary secretion of adrenocorticotropic hormone (ACTH) stimulates the adrenal cortex to produce its hormones. When there is enough of these hormones circulating in the bloodstream, the hypothalamus signals the anterior pituitary to decrease its secretion of ACTH (negative feedback). When steroids are taken as medications, they initiate the process of negative feedback.

Our hypothalamus is unable to distinguish between hormones produced in our own bodies and those we take as medications. Therefore, taking steroids also initiates the negative feedback message to the anterior pituitary to decrease secretion of ACTH. The problem with this is that when we stop taking the steroids, it takes a while for the anterior pituitary to stimulate the adrenal cortex to get its hormone secretions back up to normal levels. This produces a life-threatening condition known as addisonian crisis, which must be treated immediately.

Addisonian crisis may begin with cyanosis, temperature elevation, and symptoms of shock (such as rapid pulse and respirations and dropping blood pressure). The patient may complain of headache, nausea and vomiting, abdominal pain, diarrhea, confusion, and restlessness.

GLUCOCORTICOIDS

There are numerous examples of steroids. Some of the most commonly used glucocorticoids are cortisone acetate (Cortistan, Cortone), hydrocortisone (cortisol, Cortef), prednisolone (Cortalone), betamethasone (Celestone), methylprednisolone (Medrol), dexamethasone sodium phosphate (Decadron), hydrocortisone sodium succinate (Solu-Cortef), methylprednisolone sodium succinate (Solu-Medrol), methylprednisolone acetate (Depo-Medrol), prednisone (Deltasone, Colisone), and triamcinolone (Aristocort, Kenacort).

Glucocorticoids are administered by many different routes, including intravenous, intramuscular, and oral. They can be injected into joints (intra-articular), applied topically to the skin, and onto the mucous membranes, or instilled rectally. Ophthalmic and otic preparations are available.

ACTIONS AND USES There are many physiological effects of steroids. Metabolism is altered as more glucose is formed or released from the liver, protein is broken down, and cell division is inhibited. Fluid and electrolyte balance is altered as sodium and water are retained and potassium is excreted. Red blood cell production increases, coagulation factors increase, and capillaries become more fragile. These effects are sometimes beneficial and at other times are side effects, depending on the reason for use.

Steroids are capable of relieving the symptoms of numerous painful and disabling illnesses. Their anti-inflammatory action benefits many with collagen diseases, connective tissue injuries, rheumatic conditions, ocular and otic conditions, colitis, emphysema, allergies, blood diseases, and many other disorders. They often help produce remission of symptoms in malignant neoplasms. In patients receiving organ transplants, they suppress immune system responses that cause organ rejection. In emergency situations such as anaphylaxis, addisonian crisis, cerebral edema, increased intracranial pressure, septic shock, and other types of shock, they are used for their general overall effects of maintaining blood pressure and helping stabilize the patient. The mechanism of action is often unknown.

ASSESSMENT Assessments include baseline vital signs, weight, and any others pertinent to the condition being treated. Determination of serum glucose and electrolyte levels may be ordered before long-term therapy. Assess for a history of gastric ulcer, diabetes mellitus, glaucoma, cataracts, and emotional depression or other disturbances.

PLANNING AND IMPLEMENTATION Whenever steroids are used for purposes other than replacement therapy, the potential benefits must be weighed against the risk of harmful and toxic effects. The risk of complications depends on the dose ordered and the length of the therapy.

Monitor patients for signs and symptoms of fluid and electrolyte disturbances, such as edema, hypertension, hypokalemia, congestive heart failure, and pulmonary edema. Dietary considerations may be low-sodium and high-potassium foods. Monitor intake, output, and daily or weekly weights; the frequency of monitoring is determined by the severity of the symptoms.

Peptic ulcers, perforation, and hemorrhage can occur. Symptoms of gastrointestinal problems include abdominal distention, nausea, gastritis, hematemesis, and tarry stools. Teach patients to observe the color of their stools. Administer oral medications with meals or antacids. Report repeated gastrointestinal complaints to the physician.

Skin may become thin and fragile. Wounds may heal more slowly. Infection may occur more easily. Petechiae and ecchymosis indicate capillary fragility. Handle patients gently to avoid trauma. Apply tape carefully and remove it gently because tears occur easily. Instruct patients in good hygiene practices.

Potassium losses cause decreased muscle mass and weakness. Calcium losses predispose patients to osteoporosis and pathological fractures. Encourage patients to be as active as possible and emphasize safety precautions. Adequate amounts of calcium should be included in the diet.

Central nervous system stimulation occurs in some patients and may cause convulsions, headache, vertigo, neuritis, paresthesias, and mental changes (anxiety, depression, or euphoria). Teach family members to observe for symptoms of these and for changes in mood. Encourage patients to discuss their feelings with significant others and their physician. Suicide precautions may be necessary, especially in patients with pre-existing emotional conditions.

Red blood cell production and coagulation factors increase, which predisposes patients to thrombi and emboli. Instruct patients to avoid trauma. Encourage activity and discourage rubbing of the legs. Report chest or leg pain to the physician.

Children taking steroids for prolonged periods sometimes experience stunted physical growth. Emotional support and esteem-building measures may be necessary.

Women sometimes experience menstrual irregularities, which makes accidental pregnancies possible. Offer birth control information.

Release of glycogen from the liver is increased and insulin action is antagonized, which causes elevations in serum glucose levels or diabetes mellitus in susceptible persons. Monitor serum glucose levels in those patients or advise the patients to monitor fingerstick blood glucose levels. Teach patients and families the signs and symptoms of diabetes mellitus and the need to report the occurrence of symptoms to the physician as soon as they are noted.

Long-term use of steroids may cause cataracts or glaucoma. Encourage routine eye examinations. Teach signs and symptoms to patients and families so they may be reported as early as possible.

Cushingoid (or Cushing's-like) appearance results with long-term use. Symptoms include a rounded face (moon face), rounded protuberance at the back of the neck (buffalo hump), increased facial and body hair in women (hirsutism), potbelly, weight gain, stretch marks (striae) on the abdomen and hips, increased skin pigmentation, oily skin, and acne. Emotional support may be necessary.

The adrenal gland atrophies with long-term steroid use because of negative feedback. Therefore, this medication may not be withdrawn suddenly or symptoms of Addison's disease may occur suddenly. This is referred to as Addisonian crisis and is a life-threatening condition. Carefully monitor patients who are NPO and discuss the situation with the physician. Parenteral replacement will be necessary.

The choice of drug, dose, and route varies with the condition being treated. The drug is usually administered to mimic the pattern of normal hormone secretion. Doses are given once or twice a day, in early morning and repeated in approximately 6 hours if necessary. The usual dose is designed to meet the patient's needs under normal conditions of stress. In situations of increased physical or emotional stress, the dose may be doubled or tripled to compensate for the increased need. The physician aims to create a balance between deficiency and side effects.

It is not unusual for the patient to be on alternate-day regimens. This means that the dose changes every other day. For example, the patient takes the medication twice a day on Monday, Wednesday, Friday, and Sunday but only once a day on Tuesday, Thursday, and Saturday. Some other patients are on intermittent schedules; they take the steroids daily for a prescribed number of weeks and then, after tapering the dose, omit the steroids for a prescribed number of weeks.

The nurse and patient must be aware of the patient's normal regimen.

Patient teaching should include all of the preceding information. Be sure to emphasize that these medications may cause a life-threatening emergency if they are withdrawn suddenly. Patients must understand the seriousness of this and consult the physician about any problems with the drug and proposed changes in their regimen before initiation. If the steroids are to be discontinued for any reason, the dose is tapered and the patient is gradually weaned from the medication. This is to permit the hypothalamus to recognize the lower level of hormone in the bloodstream and to stimulate the anterior pituitary to increase secretion of ACTH. The increased stimulation of the adrenal cortex permits it to increase production of its hormones.

Encourage frequent medical and ophthalmic examinations.

To minimize the occurrence of systemic effects, apply topical skin preparations sparingly and only onto the affected areas. Do not apply occlusive dressings without a physician's order.

Because of interactions with a wide variety of medications, the patient should not take non-prescription medications without consulting the physician. Teach the patient to be certain to inform all practitioners who may be prescribing medications of the entire drug regimen. Barbiturates, phenytoin, and rifampin decrease the effects of glucocorticoids, and the physician may wish to increase the dose. Aspirin and other medications that increase bleeding tendencies and gastrointestinal distress must be used with caution if they are taken with glucocorticoids.

Before medical and dental procedures, physicians and dentists should be informed that steroids are being taken because bleeding, response to infection, and healing processes may be altered.

An identification card and Medic-Alert device should be carried at all times.

EVALUATION Compare vital signs and weight with ▲▲▲▲▲▲▲▲▲▲ baseline assessments. Monitor intake and output. Assess wounds for signs of healing or infection. Monitor serum glucose and electrolyte values. Monitor stools for occult blood at intervals. Question patients about gastrointestinal disturbances. Monitor symptoms of medical conditions being treated for improvement or deterioration.

MINERALOCORTICOIDS

Some examples of mineralocorticoids are desoxycorticosterone acetate (DOCA, Percoten Acetate), desoxycorticosterone pivalate (Percoten Pivalate), and fludrocortisone acetate (Florinef Acetate).

Desoxycorticosterone is available for intramuscular injection or in implantable pellet form. Fludrocortisone is an oral preparation.

ACTIONS AND USES Aldosterone is the most important
▲▲▲▲▲▲▲▲▲▲▲▲▲▲▲▲ of the mineralocorticoids. This hormone increases sodium reabsorption and potassium excretion at the distal convoluted tubules in the nephrons of the kidneys. This is known to increase the extracellular fluid volume and increase blood pressure.

Adverse actions include hypokalemia, edema, hypertension, and cardiac enlargement.

Mineralocorticoids are used to replace hormones that are lacking because of hypofunction of the adrenal cortex.

ASSESSMENT Assess the patient for objective signs and
▲▲▲▲▲▲▲▲▲▲ subjective symptoms, weight, and vital signs. Document data as baseline information. Assess for a history of hypertension, congestive heart failure, or cardiac disease. Assess serum electrolyte levels.

PLANNING AND IMPLEMENTATION Monitor intake, out-
▲▲▲▲▲▲▲▲▲▲▲▲▲▲▲▲▲▲▲▲▲▲▲▲▲▲▲▲▲▲▲ put, and weight daily. Monitor vital signs frequently, as ordered by the physician. Be alert for signs and symptoms of adverse effects and report them to the physician as soon as possible.

If treatment is for adrenal insufficiency, glucocorticoids must also be administered.

Teach patients about sodium-rich foods and encourage them to reduce their intake of them. Teach dietary sources of potassium to include in the daily diet. Potassium supplements may also be ordered by the physician.

Intramuscular forms of the drug are oil-based medications that must be administered by use of a large-gauge needle, deep into the gluteus medius muscle. Rotate the injection sites and monitor for localized irritation.

Pellets are implanted subcutaneously into loose tissues on the inner aspects of the thighs or the upper arms. They provide effects for 8 to 12 months. Monitor sites for localized irritation.

Patients with adrenal insufficiency are susceptible to hypoglycemia. Teach patients to avoid concentrated sugars, to eat meals at regular times, and to choose protein or complex carbohydrates for snacks. Be sure they understand the signs and symptoms and the need to report their occurrence to the physician.

EVALUATION Monitor serum electrolyte levels, vital
▲▲▲▲▲▲▲▲▲▲ signs, and weight. Compare findings with baseline data.

E X E R C I S E S

CASE STUDIES

1. Mr. J.K. has been taking steroids for several years for Addison's disease. If he were to suddenly stop taking his medication, what would happen? Why would this occur?

2. Ms. A.D. has taken prednisone for about 5 years for a chronic obstructive pulmonary disease. Lately, she noticed that she has many ecchymotic areas on her arms and legs. Today, when you are administering her medication, she asks you about these. How should you reply?

3. When Mr. D.P. had postoperative renal shock, the physician ordered methylprednisolone sodium succinate (Solu-Medrol) IV. What assessments will you make as you observe for the effectiveness of the drug?

LEARNING ACTIVITIES

1. Role play the interaction of the anterior pituitary gland, the hypothalamus gland, and the adrenal gland.

2. Role play the patient teaching what should be initiated between the nurse and the patient who is beginning cortisone therapy for Addison's disease.

CHAPTER 59

THYROID HORMONES AND ANTITHYROID DRUGS

LEARNING OBJECTIVES

After studying this chapter, you should be able to:

1. Discuss the actions of the thyroid replacement hormones and the antithyroid medications.

2. List the conditions for which each is used.

3. State the source of each of these medications.

4. List the adverse effects of each.

5. Prepare an appropriate care plan for a patient receiving any one of these drugs.

DRUGS YOU WILL LEARN ABOUT IN THIS CHAPTER

Thyroid Medications

thyroglobulin (Proloid)

levothyroxine sodium (Synthroid, Levothroid)

liothyronine sodium (Cytomel)

liotrix (Thyrolar)

Calcitonin (Calcimar)

Antithyroid Medications

propylthiouracil (PTU)

methimazole (Tapazole)

Iodine Preparations

Lugol's solution

saturated solution of potassium iodide (SSKI)

Radioactive Iodine

sodium iodide (I 131)

The thyroid gland, located in the neck, is the largest of the endocrine glands. It is composed of two lateral lobes on either side of the larynx, connected by a narrow strip of thyroid tissue called the isthmus. The thyroid is often said to resemble a butterfly or bow tie. The three hormones produced and secreted by the gland are thyroxine (T_4), triiodothyronine (T_3), and calcitonin.

T_4, the principal hormone of the gland, and T_3 affect all body cells by increasing metabolism for production of heat and energy. Normal mental development and normal growth depend on adequate secretion of these two hormones.

For these hormones to be produced, there must be adequate iodine in the blood. Natural sources of iodine are seafoods or vegetables grown in iodine-rich soil. However, because many people live in areas of the country where these sources are not available, use of iodized salt in cooking and food preparation is the major source of iodine.

The thyroid gland is stimulated or controlled by the anterior pituitary gland with the hypothalamus gland acting as the regulator. The hypothalamus secretes the hypothalamic releasing factor (a neurohormone), which stimulates the anterior pituitary gland to secrete the thyrotropic hormone or thyroid-stimulating hormone (TSH). As the blood level of TSH increases, the thyroid gland is stimulated to increase the secretion of its hormones (T_4 and T_3) into the bloodstream. When the blood level of the thyroid hormones increases, the hypothalamus (again acting like a thermostat) decreases secretion of the hypothalamic releasing factors. In response, the anterior pituitary decreases the secretion of TSH (negative feedback). As the level of TSH decreases, the thyroid gland decreases the secretion of its hormones, thus maintaining homeostasis.

The normal thyroid state is said to be euthyroid. Too much thyroid secretion produces a hyperthyroid state, and too little thyroid secretion produces a hypothyroid state.

The third thyroid hormone is calcitonin, which assists in the regulation of blood calcium levels. It inhibits the resorption (breakdown) of bone, thereby preventing the release of calcium from the bone into the blood. High serum calcium levels cause increased secretion of calcitonin until the serum calcium levels fall back into normal ranges.

Table 59–1 lists the drugs and dosages that pertain to the thyroid.

THYROID MEDICATIONS

Thyroid extract for pharmaceutical preparations can be obtained from cows and pigs. However, it is usually produced synthetically because it is more uniform in its potency.

Thyroid hormones can be administered orally or parenterally by the intramuscular, subcutaneous, or intravenous route. The most common route is oral. The hormone is absorbed in the intestine, but a significant amount is lost in the feces. Therefore, normal gastrointestinal function is significant in determining the oral dose required to produce therapeutic effects.

Regardless of the route of administration, the drugs have a latent period before their effects are seen. Onset of action may be days, with peak action occurring after weeks or months of treatment. The effects tend to be cumulative and to persist for some time after the drug is discontinued. Doses are individualized and are determined by monitoring serum TSH, T_3, and T_4 levels.

Certain factors, such as estrogen therapy and pregnancy, can alter the circulation of the drug and its availability for use in the body. They may sometimes cause enlargement of the thyroid gland.

Some examples of thyroid hormone drug preparations are thyroglobulin (Proloid), levothyroxine sodium (Synthroid, Levothroid), liothyronine sodium (Cytomel), and liotrix (Euthroid, Thyrolar). Notice that some of the trade names are similar to terms we have just discussed. For example, Synthroid sounds like synthetic thyroid, and Euthroid sounds like euthyroid.

Table 59–1. Thyroid Hormone and Antithyroid Medications

DRUG	DOSAGE
Thyroid Medications	
thyroglobulin	Child 　1–4 mo: initial dose: 　　15–30 mg PO qd, 　　increased q 2 wk; 　　maintenance dose: 　　30–45 mg PO qd 　4–12 mo: 60–80 mg 　　PO qd 　Older than 12 mo: 60– 　　180 mg PO qd Adult 　Initial dose: 15–30 mg 　　PO qd, increased by 　　15–30 mg q 2 wk Maintenance dose: 60– 　　180 mg PO qd
levothyroxine sodium (Synthroid, Levothroid)	Child (younger than 　12 mo): initial dose: 　0.025–0.05 mg PO qd, 　increased by 0.05 mg 　PO q 2–3 wk to total 　dose of 0.1–0.4 mg PO Adult 　**Myxedema:** initial 　　dose: 0.2–0.5 mg IV; 　　if no response within 　　24 h, increase 0.1– 　　0.3 mg IV 　**Hypothyroidism:** 　　initial dose: 0.025– 　　0.1 mg PO, increased 　　by 0.05–0.1 mg q 1–4 　　wk; maintenance 　　dose: 0.1–0.4 mg 　　PO qd

ACTIONS AND USES Thyroid hormones influence the ▲▲▲▲▲▲▲▲▲▲▲▲▲▲▲▲ metabolism of every tissue and organ in the body. They increase the metabolic rate that elevates the temperature, pulse, respirations, oxygen consumption, and cardiac output. They increase the metabolism of carbohydrates, proteins, and fats.

Thyroid hormones are used to maintain the euthyroid state when a patient is experiencing a condition known as hypothyroidism. In adults, this condition is

Table 59–1. Thyroid Hormone and Antithyroid Medications *Continued*

DRUG	DOSAGE
liothyronine sodium (Cytomel)	**Child** younger than 3 y: initial dose: 5 mcg PO qd, increased by 5 mcg q 3–4 days older than 3 y: 50–100 mcg PO qd **Adult** Initial dose: 5 mcg PO qd, increased by 12.5–25 mcg qd q 1–2 wk Maintenance dose: 25–75 mcg PO qd
liotrix (Thyrolar)	Initial dose: 15–30 mg PO qd, increased by 15–30 mg q 1–2 wk
Calcitonin (Calcimar)	100 IU per day IM or SC
Antithyroid Medications	
propylthiouracil (PTU)	**Adult** Initial dose: 100 mg PO tid; increased to 300 mg q8h until euthyroid Maintenance dose: 100 mg PO qd to tid
methimazole (Tapazole)	**Adult** Initial dose: mild, 5 mg PO tid; moderately severe, 10–15 mg PO tid; severe, 20 mg PO tid, continue until euthyroid Maintenance dose: 5 mg PO qd to tid

Table 59–1. Thyroid Hormone and Antithyroid Medications *Continued*

DRUG	DOSAGE
Iodine Preparations	
Lugol's solution	0.1–0.3 mL tid in water; after meals; for 2–3 wk before surgery
saturated solution of potassium iodide (SSKI)	5 gtt in water tid; after meals; for 2–3 wk before surgery
Radioactive Iodine	
sodium iodide I 131	4–10 millicuries PO; may repeat after 6 wk according to serum thyroxine levels

sometimes called myxedema; in children, it is often referred to as cretinism. Thyroid hormones are also used as replacement therapy after surgical removal of all or part of the gland (thyroidectomy) or after destruction of the gland by radiation therapy.

Adverse actions include symptoms of the hyperthyroid state, such as increased appetite, weight loss, temperature elevation, tachycardia, mild hypertension, and intolerance to heat. The skin is flushed, warm, and moist. Other symptoms include nervousness, anxiety, insomnia, tremors, diarrhea, and protruding eyeballs (exophthalmos). In women, there may be scant or irregular menses.

ASSESSMENT Document the subjective symptoms of ▲▲▲▲▲▲▲▲▲▲ hypothyroidism, such as lethargy, forgetfulness, and intolerance to cold. Assess for a history of thyroidectomy or radiation to the head or neck area. Assess for a history of hypertension or heart disease. Note evidence of mental slowness. Assess for dry skin and dry or brittle hair. Assess height, weight, and vital signs.

Assess laboratory test results of TSH, T_4, and T_3 levels. In hypothyroidism, the TSH levels are increased, whereas the T_4 and T_3 levels are decreased. Other tests are sometimes ordered, such as tests of thyroid uptake and thyroid excretion, thyroid scans, and radioactive iodine tests. These may indicate the cause of the abnormal TSH, T_4, and T_3 levels.

An additional assessment for the child with cretinism includes observation for retarded mental and physical development. Assess for eye contact and alertness to surroundings. It is important to note the time of onset of symptoms, especially if the infant is being breast-fed. Some of the mother's hormones pass through the breast milk to the infant, so symptoms may increase as frequency of breast-feeding decreases or weaning takes place. Assess height, weight, and head circumference and plot the measurements on growth charts appropriate for the sex and chronological or adjusted age of the child. Use standardized screening tools, such as the Denver II Developmental Screening Tool, to document achievement of developmental milestones.

Document all findings as baseline data.

PLANNING AND IMPLEMENTATION Thyroid hormones ▲▲▲▲▲▲▲▲▲▲▲▲▲▲▲▲▲▲▲▲▲▲▲▲▲▲▲▲▲ are usually administered orally, except in emergencies. They should be taken at the same time each day, early in the day and on an empty stomach. In severe deficiencies, the initial dose is usually small. This is done to prevent a sudden rise in metabolism that could cause serious cardiovascular complications, such as congestive heart failure and pulmonary edema. The dose is progressively increased in a period of 2 to 4 weeks. During that time, the patient should be monitored for adverse effects, such as a pulse rate above 80 beats per minute, increased blood pressure, edema, or complaints of chest pressure or pain. If possible, teach the patient or caregivers to monitor these values at home and report changes to the physician.

Monitoring and documentation of symptoms helps the physician to determine whether the individualized dose is appropriate to obtain and maintain the euthyroid state. There must always be monitoring for signs of hyperthyroidism. Monitor vital signs, weight, skin color, and temperature. Question the patient about increased appetite, tolerance to heat, nervousness, anxiety, insomnia, or tremors. Monitor bowel patterns and menstrual cycles. Note the appearance of the eyes. Report changes in symptoms to the physician because the dose may need to be altered.

Persons receiving warfarin derivatives as anticoagulation therapy or aspirin therapy may experience increased bleeding tendencies, and the dose of the anticoagulant may need to be reduced. Teach the patient to report increased bruising, bleeding gums, epistaxis, or hematuria.

Because thyroid hormones increase metabolism, people with a tendency toward diabetes mellitus may have symptoms of the disease after thyroid hormone therapy is begun. Teach patients to report increased thirst, urination, appetite, and weight loss. Diabetic patients have an increased need for insulin or oral hypoglycemic agents; advise them to monitor their serum glucose levels more closely until metabolism stabilizes.

Persons with a cortisone deficiency, such as in hypoadrenalism or Addison's disease, may experience the life-threatening symptoms of addisonian crisis after thyroid therapy is begun. Instruct patients to maintain their follow-up visits with the physician and to report symptoms of dizziness, irritability, weakness, or increased pigmentation.

Estrogens may decrease the level of circulating thyroid hormones.

Communication with physicians about all medications being taken is imperative. Doses of thyroid hormones may have to be increased in hypothyroid patients.

Nonprescription medications should be taken with caution because many of them may cause adverse reactions. For example, many cold and allergy preparations contain ephedrine, which also increases metabolism. Patients may experience tachycardia and an elevation in blood pressure.

Instruct patients to maintain follow-up visits with their physician because the need for thyroid hormones fluctuates with age and with stressful events in life. The dose may need to be increased or decreased at intervals.

N U R S I N G   A L E R T
▼▼▼▼▼▼▼▼▼▼▼▼▼▼▼▼▼▼▼▼▼▼▼▼▼▼▼▼▼▼▼▼

Children with cretinism should be referred to community resources for early intervention services. Parents may need to be taught play activities that will promote achievement of developmental milestones and readiness to learn.

▲▲▲▲▲▲▲▲▲▲▲▲▲▲▲▲▲▲▲▲▲▲▲▲▲▲▲▲▲▲▲▲▲

EVALUATION Compare vital signs and weight with ▲▲▲▲▲▲▲▲▲▲ baseline assessment findings. Monitor serum TSH, T_4, and T_3 levels. Monitor patients for improvement in symptoms of hypothyroidism. Many of the symptoms of hypothyroidism and hyperthyroidism are subjective, so encourage the patient to describe them and communicate clearly to the physician.

In addition, children with cretinism must have height, weight, and head circumference documented on the appropriate growth charts. Developmental assessments must be repeated at regular intervals to be certain that developmental milestones are being achieved.

CALCITONIN

Calcitonin is available as a synthetic preparation (Calcimar Synthetic) or as an extract from salmon (calcitonin-salmon). It is available for intramuscular or subcutaneous administration. The subcutaneous route is preferred for patients who must self-administer the drug. Solutions are available in 2-mL vials that contain 200 International units (IU) per milliliter. Average dosage is 100 IU per day. Research is being conducted to determine the effectiveness of a reduced dosage of 50 IU per day, but these data are not yet available.

ACTIONS AND USES Calcitonin acts with hormones from the parathyroid glands to maintain homeostasis of serum calcium levels. The primary action of calcitonin is on the bone, but some effect is also noted on the kidney. Calcitonin inhibits bone resorption by decreasing the number of cells responsible for bone breakdown (osteoclasts). It is also believed to increase the number of cells that are responsible for the building of new bone (osteoblasts). The excretion of phosphate, calcium, and sodium are increased because the reabsorption of these elements by the renal tubules is inhibited.

Calcitonin is used to treat Paget's disease (also called osteitis deformans), a disorder characterized by abnormal and accelerated bone formation and resorption. It is also used to treat hypercalcemia in patients with carcinoma, multiple myeloma, or hyperparathyroidism. Hypercalcemic emergencies can be treated with calcitonin and other agents that lower the serum calcium levels. Once the specific cause of the emergency has been determined, other treatments may be more appropriate.

Postmenopausal osteoporosis may be treated with calcitonin, calcium, and vitamin D to prevent the progressive loss of bone mass.

Adverse actions may include allergic reactions ranging in severity from localized inflammation at the injection site to bronchospasm, swelling of the tongue and throat, and anaphylaxis.

Other reported adverse actions are nausea and vomiting (which tend to disappear as treatment is continued), flushing of the face or hands, and skin rashes.

ASSESSMENT Question the patient about and review the chart for a history of allergies. Estrogen may delay the process of osteoporosis, so the physician may assess serum estrogen levels. Assess menstrual history to determine whether menopause is beginning, in progress, or past and review the chart for a history of surgical removal of the ovaries. Assess the patient's entire medication regimen because estrogen is often ordered as adjunctive therapy. Assess subjective complaints of muscle and bone pain. Assess serum calcium levels. X-rays and bone density studies may also be ordered as assessments.

PLANNING AND IMPLEMENTATION Physicians may order skin testing before treatment, especially in those with a history of other allergies. Observe patients carefully for at least 20 to 30 minutes the first few times injections are given to determine initial response to the hormone.

Calcitonin is stored in the refrigerator at 36° to 46° F (2° to 8°C). The solution should be discarded if it is not clear and colorless.

If patients or caregivers are to administer calcitonin at home, they must be taught procedures for appropriate preparation and injection of the drug. Be sure to include information on asepsis, rotation of sites, injection technique, disposal of equipment, and storage of the medication. Allow ample time for practice and supervision of the first few injections.

Patients with postmenopausal osteoporosis may need calcium and vitamin D supplements ordered by the physician. Provide nutritional information on dietary sources of these elements, recipes, and assistance with menu planning as needed.

Teach patients appropriate weight-bearing activities and exercises that will assist in the prevention of bone loss.

Dosages for hypercalcemia are often higher than the average dose. The intramuscular route must be used if the ordered dose exceeds 2-mL volume. Doses may need to be divided and given in alternative sites.

EVALUATION Monitor serum calcium levels and compare them with baseline data and normal values. Monitor urine samples at intervals for the presence of sedimentation. Coarse granular casts and casts containing renal tubule epithelial cells have been reported but disappeared after the drug was discontinued.

Compare periodic x-rays and bone density studies with baseline data. Monitor the patient's complaints of bone and muscle pain and compare with the baseline data.

People with Paget's disease must be monitored carefully and evaluated at intervals. There is an increased risk that the disease will progress to osteogenic sarcoma.

ANTITHYROID PREPARATIONS

Substances that inhibit the thyroid gland from producing its hormones are considered to be antithyroid. Some of these work at the level of the anterior pituitary gland by decreasing secretion of thyroid-stimulating hormone (TSH). Others interfere with the way the body synthesizes or produces triiodothyronine (T_3) and thyroxine (T_4). Some block the release of T_3 and T_4 into the circulation or reduce the ability of the peripheral tissues to use the thyroid hormones. Regardless of the manner of action, all of these substances reduce the physiological effects of the thyroid hormones and therefore reduce the signs and symptoms that accompany increased blood levels of the hormones.

Antithyroid medications are absorbed from the gastrointestinal tract and concentrated in the thyroid gland, where they perform their action. Just like the thyroid hormones, the antithyroid drugs have a latent period of days or weeks until their effect is evident because the body must first use up any thyroid hormones stored in peripheral tissues. The antithyroid drugs are excreted by the kidneys.

Medications that inhibit the production or use of the thyroid hormones include propylthiouracil and its related compounds. Propylthiouracil (PTU) and methimazole (Tapazole) are the chief antithyroid drugs used in the United States. Both are oral preparations. Doses are individualized, depending on the age of the patient and the severity of the condition.

ACTIONS AND USES Antithyroid medications are used ▲▲▲▲▲▲▲▲▲▲▲▲▲▲▲▲ in the treatment of hyperthyroidism, a condition also referred to as Graves' disease, exophthalmic goiter, thyrotoxicosis, or thyroid crisis. Hyperplasia (enlargement) of the thyroid gland sometimes occurs and becomes disfiguring or exerts pressure on the esophagus and trachea. Pressure causes symptoms of difficult speech (dysphasia) or difficulty in swallowing (dysphagia) and dyspnea. The antithyroid medications are used to block the production of thyroid hormones or their use by the peripheral tissues and thereby relieve the symptoms. Surgery sometimes follows the use of the antithyroid medications.

Hyperthyroidism may also occur as a side effect of therapy for hypothyroidism. When it results from therapy, treatment is usually limited to decreasing the dose of thyroid hormones.

The aim of antithyroid therapy is to produce the euthyroid state and put the disease in remission. If therapy precedes thyroidectomy, it is also intended to reduce the surgical risks produced by the toxic state.

Adverse actions of the antithyroid medications include symptoms of hypothyroidism, nausea, vomiting, diarrhea, jaundice, headache, drowsiness, rashes, and blood dyscrasias (such as agranulocytosis, leukopenia, granulocytopenia, and thrombocytopenia).

ASSESSMENT Document baseline descriptions of symp-
▲▲▲▲▲▲▲▲▲▲ toms, vital signs, and weight. Laboratory tests may include serum T_3 and T_4 levels, thyroid scans, and radioactive iodine uptake and excretion tests. Obtain a complete blood count with differential and record as baseline data.

PLANNING AND IMPLEMENTATION Antithyroid medica-
▲▲▲▲▲▲▲▲▲▲▲▲▲▲▲▲▲▲▲▲▲▲▲▲▲▲▲▲▲ tions have a relatively low frequency of adverse effects, but caregivers and patients must always be aware of their potential occurrence. The most common adverse effect is a skin rash with purpura and urticaria. In most cases, this is mild; but if it does not subside in a few days, the medication is changed to a different drug. Patients occasionally have a severe rash called exfoliative dermatitis, which requires immediate treatment. Teach patients and caregivers to report adverse effects to the physician.

Because of the possibility of blood dyscrasias and lowered resistance to infection, teach patients to protect themselves from communicable diseases until their blood counts return to normal. They should be taught to report fever, sore throat, cold symptoms, malaise, or jaundice. These symptoms often require that the drug be discontinued. Antibiotics may be needed to combat the infection. Recovery is generally spontaneous if the drug is discontinued immediately.

Antithyroid medications increase the vascularity of the thyroid gland. This is particularly undesirable in patients who will undergo thyroidectomy after the drug therapy. To counteract this effect, these patients are also given iodine for 10 days to 2 weeks before surgery.

Thrombocytopenia (a decrease in thrombocytes) and hypoprothrombinemia (decreased prothrombin levels) may also result. Teach patients about the increased tendency to bleed and warn them to avoid aspirin and products containing aspirin. If the patient is currently taking warfarin derivative anticoagulants, the dose must often be reduced below normal therapeutic levels to avoid the adverse effect of hemorrhage.

Because hyperthyroidism causes irritability, restlessness, and sleeplessness, encourage patients to get adequate rest. This will be difficult for them, so the environment should be quiet and as free of stress as possible. Caregivers should attempt to complete their care in a calm, organized, and efficient manner.

Because of the hypermetabolism with its weight loss, encourage the patient to consume a well-balanced, nutritious diet. Vitamins and minerals are sometimes added as supplements. Frequent feedings are usually needed. Stimulants such as coffee, tea, chocolate, colas, and other caffeine-containing beverages and foods should be avoided. Foods that stimulate peristalsis should be avoided until symptoms of a thyroid toxic state subside. Foods that are simple and easy to eat are often consumed more readily because the patient may be too restless to tolerate foods that require more time to eat. As the symptoms of hyperthyroidism decrease, calorie intake should be gradually reduced or the patient will begin to gain weight. If some weight gain is desired, it should be carefully monitored so obesity does not result.

Teach patients to avoid nonprescription drugs such as decongestants, which often contain stimulants.

Remind young women not to become pregnant while taking antithyroid therapy. Offer to review birth control methods. Thyroid hormones are vital to normal physical and mental development of the fetus. The antithyroid drugs can cross the placental barrier and can cause congenital cretinism in infants. Failure to recognize and treat this results in mental retardation. These drugs can also cross through to the infant through breast milk, so lactation is discouraged.

Some medications increase the thyroid-inhibiting properties of the antithyroid drugs, so good communications are important if the patient is being treated by more than one physician. It is especially important to notify the physician if phenylbutazone (Butazolidin), lithium, sulfonamides, or salicylates are being taken regularly.

While the physician is aiming to obtain the euthyroid state, the thyroid hormones are sometimes suppressed to the extent that hypothyroidism results. Remind patients to report lethargy, mental slowness, rapid weight gain, slow pulse, and any other changes in symptoms.

Some patients discontinue their treatment as symptoms improve. This will cause recurrence of symptoms, so they must be reminded to continue treatment.

Warn patients to store medications in their original containers. Methimazole should be stored away from heat and light.

EVALUATION At intervals, compare weight and vital signs with baseline data. Compare symptoms with those documented in the baseline data and note improvement. As symptoms improve, the dose of antithyroid medication is decreased.

Remember that hypothyroidism may result from treatment and that patients may subsequently need replacement of thyroid hormones. Serum T_3 and T_4 determinations may be ordered at intervals; compare these levels with previous values. Compare results of periodic blood counts with baseline data.

IODINE PREPARATIONS

Examples of concentrated iodine preparations are Lugol's solution in 5% and 10% concentrations and saturated solution of potassium iodide (SSKI).

ACTIONS AND USES People normally ingest adequate amounts of iodine in the foods they eat. The body concentrates the iodine in the thyroid gland and uses it in the manufacture of thyroid hormones. When a person is producing excessive thyroid hormones, iodine is sometimes administered in large doses. As the iodine saturates the thyroid gland, the activities of the gland decrease or cease. The level of thyroid hormones will then decrease and so will the toxic symptoms being experienced by the patient.

Iodine is often used in conjunction with the other antithyroid drugs and surgery. By combining these different modes of treatment, a nearly euthyroid state can be achieved before surgery. This dramatically decreases the frequency of operative and postoperative complications.

Iodine also decreases the vascularity of the thyroid gland, so it is often used as a preoperative preparation to avoid the complication of hemorrhage. This effect lasts 10 days to 2 weeks. At this time, the symptoms of toxicity and the vascularity of the gland are at their lowest. If surgery is delayed more than 2 weeks beyond the initiation of therapy, the effects of the iodine decrease and the advantage is lost.

ASSESSMENT Assessments include baseline descriptions of symptoms, vital signs, and weight. Assess serum thyroid-stimulating hormone (TSH), thyroxine (T_4), and triiodothyronine (T_3) levels. Thyroid scans and radioactive iodine uptake and excretion tests may also be ordered.

PLANNING AND IMPLEMENTATION Before administration of an iodine preparation, it is vital to determine whether the patient has an allergy to iodine. Be sure to question the patient about allergy to shellfish. Many people know they are allergic to these foods but do not understand that it is the iodine in the animal that causes the allergic reaction.

Even if the patient has not previously experienced an allergic reaction to iodine, the patient and caregivers should be taught that a reaction can occur at any time. Reactions can begin immediately after ingestion of the drug or hours later. Symptoms can be severe and life-threatening. Be alert for complaints of swelling or tightness in the throat, swelling of the face or other body parts, temperature elevation, joint pains, and dyspnea. Notify the physician immediately if these symptoms are noted. If treatment is not begun immediately, severe respiratory distress and death may result.

Iodine solutions have a metallic taste and are irritating to the gastric mucosa. To minimize this, they should be diluted in milk or juice and administered with a straw. Taking them with meals is also helpful.

Other adverse reactions include burning of the mouth and throat, sore teeth and gums, rash, temperature elevation, and symptoms of a head cold. Patients should know to report these to the caregivers.

Decongestants that contain stimulants are contraindicated in hyperthyroidism. Instead, humidifiers can be used to relieve nasal stuffiness.

Iodine solutions are sensitive to light. They should be kept in their original dark containers and stored away from heat and light.

N U R S I N G   A L E R T

▼▼▼▼▼▼▼▼▼▼▼▼▼▼▼▼▼▼▼▼▼▼▼▼▼▼▼▼▼▼▼▼▼▼

Iodines are poisons. Doses are often ordered in drops.

▲▲▲▲▲▲▲▲▲▲▲▲▲▲▲▲▲▲▲▲▲▲▲▲▲▲▲▲▲▲▲▲▲▲

Accuracy of measurement is important. Iodines should also be stored out of reach of youngsters or confused individuals.

A slow intravenous infusion of sodium iodide is sometimes ordered to be administered in doses ranging from 250 mg to 2 g per day. The intravenous route is usually used only if the patient is vomiting or is ordered NPO by the physician.

Patients will still be experiencing symptoms of hyperthyroidism, so all of the implications listed with the antithyroid preparations are relevant. Preoperative education and preparation may be initiated while the patient is awaiting the time for surgery.

EVALUATION Observe for improvement in symptoms ▲▲▲▲▲▲▲▲▲▲ as compared with baseline assessments. Monitor TSH, T_3, and T_4 levels and results of any other laboratory work ordered by the physician. Be constantly alert for symptoms of toxic effects or allergic reactions.

RADIOACTIVE IODINE

The most common form of radioactive iodine used therapeutically is the isotope called sodium iodide (I 131).

ACTIONS AND USES A radioactive form of iodine is ▲▲▲▲▲▲▲▲▲▲▲▲▲ sometimes prescribed for treatment of thyrotoxicosis or malignant neoplasms of the thyroid gland. It may be ordered before or instead of surgery. Because the thyroid gland concentrates iodine, the effects of the radioactivity are primarily confined to the thyroid gland, where it destroys the hyperactive tissue. Radioactive iodine destroys both normal and malignant cells.

ASSESSMENT Review diagnostic test results. Assess ▲▲▲▲▲▲▲▲▲▲ thyroid-stimulating hormone (TSH), triiodothyronine (T_3), and thyroxine (T_4) levels. Assess results of thyroid scans or uptake and excretion tests. Record symptoms and vital signs as baseline data.

PLANNING AND IMPLEMENTATION I^{131} can be given ▲▲▲▲▲▲▲▲▲▲▲▲▲▲▲▲▲▲▲▲▲▲▲▲▲▲▲▲ intravenously but is most often administered as an oral liquid or capsule. It is absorbed more effectively if it is taken after an 8- to 12-hour fast.

Radioactive isotopes are teratogenic and can cause defects in the fetus if they are administered during pregnancy. It is important to question women of childbearing age about the possibility of pregnancy and to administer the isotope during menses or within 7 days after menses. Birth control measures should be discussed. The isotope can also pass through breast milk to the infant, so lactation is contraindicated during the course of treatment. Because of the risk to the fetus or newborn infant, this mode of treatment is more prevalent in women and men older than 50 years.

Personnel in nuclear medicine must follow standard procedures to protect themselves during preparation and administration of the isotope. Protection includes the use of special gloves, lead aprons, monitoring badges to measure the amount of exposure, and special procedures to clean up spills.

After administration of the isotope, the patient's urine, saliva, perspiration, and vomitus are radioactive. The amount of radioactivity and the length of time that the radioactivity lasts are relevant to the dose administered. The dose for thyrotoxicosis is smaller than that administered for cancer of the thyroid gland; therefore, the amount of radioactivity is less.

Caregivers should be informed of institutional procedures for caring for patients with radioactive isotopes, and patients should be instructed in proper procedures for disposal of excretions. Patients should increase fluid intake for 48 hours to facilitate excretion of the isotope.

Caregivers should protect themselves according to institutional procedures, remembering that they are protected by three factors: time, distance, and shielding. They should limit the amount of time in contact with the patient, keep as much distance as possible between themselves and the patient, and use protective devices such as lead aprons or screens whenever possible. Proper procedures for handling excreta must be observed. Monitoring badges are worn to measure the amount of exposure received. Badges are assigned to individual employees and should never be shared. Pregnant women should not care for these patients.

Assess patients for complaints of fullness in the throat, swelling of the parotid glands, and metallic taste. These are usually minor, but the occurrence should be reported.

On discharge, instruct patients to avoid prolonged contact with children, such as holding them or sleeping with them, for approximately 1 week. Patients should also sleep in a room alone for 1 week. No special precautions are necessary with excreta.

Patients receiving therapeutic doses of radioactive iodine for treatment of malignant disease should be informed of the increased risk for development of leukemia later in life.

Therapeutic effects of the isotope will not be noted for 6 to 10 weeks after treatment. Radiation destroys both healthy and malignant cells, so patients frequently become hypothyroid after treatment. They will later need to receive replacement thyroid hormones.

Instruct patients about the symptoms of hypothyroidism and encourage them to report the occurrence so treatment can be initiated.

Provide emotional support because many patients experience anxieties about the illness and fear the effects of radiation.

EVALUATION Continue to monitor serum TSH, T_3, and ▲▲▲▲▲▲▲▲▲▲ T_4 levels. At intervals, compare vital signs and symptoms with the baseline data. Question patients about the possible occurrence of symptoms of hypothyroidism.

E X E R C I S E S

CASE STUDIES

1. Ms. S.E., age 45 years, presented to her physician complaining of coldness, fatigue, 20-pound weight gain in the past year, mental slowness, and other symptoms. Laboratory tests verified moderate to severe hypothyroidism (myxedema). The physician initially ordered levothyroxine sodium (Synthroid), 0.1 mg PO, and explained that he planned to increase the dose by 0.1 mg the following week and by 0.05 mg each week for several weeks thereafter. Explain the rationale for this dosage schedule. What symptoms will indicate effectiveness of therapy? What symptoms would indicate that the dose is too high for Ms. S.E.?

2. Four years ago, Ms. M.K. was diagnosed as having hypothyroidism. She has followed her treatment regimen faithfully and has maintained the euthyroid state. Recently, Ms. M.K. has been diagnosed as having diabetes mellitus. How will her hypothyroidism affect the diabetes?

3. Mr. J.G. is scheduled to have a subtotal thyroidectomy in 2 weeks. The physician has ordered Lugol's solution three times a day until surgery. What is the rationale for ordering this medication? What are the expected effects? What should Mr. J.G. be taught concerning administration of this medication? Of which side effects should he be aware? What should he do if side effects occur?

LEARNING ACTIVITIES

1. Fold a sheet of notebook paper into three lengthwise columns. Label the first column "hypothyroidism," the middle column "hyperthyroidism," and the third column "side effects of thyroid medications." List the appropriate symptoms in the first two columns. Use a medical-surgical textbook for reference if necessary. Then, in the third column, list the side effects. Compare your work with a classmate's.

2. Role play the interaction between the anterior pituitary gland, the hypothalamus gland, and the thyroid gland. Have one student represent each gland. Be sure to include the negative feedback concept. Role play the interaction when the thyroid gland is unable to respond to the stimulation from the anterior pituitary gland. Have another student role play a patient with hypothyroid symptoms. How does administration of thyroid medications affect this interaction? Have another student represent a thyroid medication. Have another student role play a patient with hyperthyroid symptoms.

HYPOGLYCEMIC DRUGS AND INSULIN ANTAGONISTS

LEARNING OBJECTIVES

After studying this chapter, you should be able to:

1. Discuss the action of the oral hypoglycemic agents, the insulins, and the antagonist glucagon.

2. List the use of the hypoglycemic agents and their antagonist.

3. State the source of these medications.

4. List the side effects of these medications.

5. State appropriate nursing interventions related to the adverse effects.

6. Prepare a plan of care for a patient receiving one or more of these medications.

DRUGS YOU WILL LEARN ABOUT IN THIS CHAPTER

Oral Hypoglycemics

  acetohexamide (Dymelor)

  chlorpropamide (Diabinese)

  tolazamide (Tolinase)

  tolbutamide (Orinase)

  glipizide (Glucotrol)

  glyburide (Micronase, DiaBeta)

Insulins

  Rapid-acting

  Regular

  Semilente

  Humulin R

  Novolin R

  Intermediate-acting

  NPH (neutral protamine Hagedorn)

  Lente

  Humulin N

  Novolin N

  Long-acting

  PZI (protamine zinc insulin)

  Ultralente

  Humulin U

  Novolin L

Insulin Antagonists

  glucagon

The pancreas is a fish-shaped organ located slightly to the left and behind the stomach. It is an organ that contains both exocrine and endocrine glands. The exocrine glands have ducts to carry secretions to another organ or outside of the body. The pancreatic enzymes amylase, lipase, and trypsin are produced by exocrine glands and are secreted into the duodenum.

Endocrine glands have no ducts. They release their secretions directly into the circulatory system. In the pancreas, the endocrine glands are called the islands (or islets) of Langerhans. These specialized cells are scattered throughout the pancreas. Their secretions are two hormones called insulin and glucagon, which antagonize each other.

The main hormone, insulin, is secreted by the beta cells of the islands of Langerhans. Insulin lowers blood glucose levels by assisting in the metabolism of glucose and the transport of glucose across the cell membrane. Once inside the cell, glucose can be used for energy or stored as glycogen for later use.

The other hormone is glucagon, which is secreted by the alpha cells of the islands of Langerhans. Glucagon raises blood glucose levels by stimulating the liver to metabolize glycogen into glucose for release into the bloodstream.

If insulin and glucagon are in balance, glucose is being used properly and a state of homeostasis exists. Serum glucose levels are normal. "Normal ranges" vary with each laboratory, so they must be stated on the laboratory report. In general, values of 80 to 120 mg per 100 mL blood are considered normal for fasting serum glucose levels.

Diabetes mellitus is a condition in which there is inadequate insulin secretion. When this occurs, there is not enough glucose available for cell metabolism even though there is glucose in the bloodstream. This causes an abnormal breakdown of proteins and fats. Incomplete fat metabolism produces acetone and leads to a condition called ketoacidosis. Serum glucose levels rise, and a condition known as hyperglycemia results.

If there is not enough glucagon secreted or if too much insulin is secreted, the body cells may use up the available glucose. A condition called hypoglycemia results when the serum glucose levels fall.

If the serum glucose levels fall below 70 mg per 100 mL, signs of sympathetic nervous system activity occur. Perspiration, tachycardia, weakness, trembling, and anxiety may be noted. This release of catecholamines is a compensatory mechanism to antagonize the effect of the insulin. Hyperglycemia and glycosuria (glucose in the urine) can result. This is referred to as the Somogyi effect.

Drugs used to lower the serum glucose levels are referred to as hypoglycemic agents or hypoglycemics. The oldest of the hypoglycemics is insulin, which was discovered in 1921 by Doctors Banting and Best of Toronto, Canada. The hormone insulin was originally obtained from the pancreas of pigs and cows. In recent years, however, advances in DNA technology have allowed scientists to duplicate insulin molecules from a harmless strain of *Escherichia coli*. The products are chemically, physically, and biologically equivalent to pancreatic human insulin. Humulin and Novolin are trade names of synthetic human insulin. When injected into the body, insulin lowers the serum glucose level just as the human insulin does. Insulin is always administered by parenteral methods because it is destroyed by the digestive enzymes if the enteral route is used.

Insulin-dependent diabetes mellitus (IDDM) requires insulin for control of the serum glucose levels because the pancreas is unable to produce adequate amounts of insulin. The people with IDDM are also said to have type I diabetes. Type I diabetes may occur at any age.

Oral hypoglycemics have been available for use since 1955. They are derivatives of the group of drugs called sulfonamides and are called sulfonylureas. These drugs are *not* oral insulin, although patients often mistakenly call them that.

Sulfonylureas act in the islands of Langerhans to increase insulin secretion by the beta cells. They cannot be used by everyone because they are not effective if the beta cells are nonfunctional.

Non–insulin-dependent diabetes mellitus (NIDDM) does not require insulin for control of the serum glucose levels. People with NIDDM are said to have type II diabetes. This is usually a maturity-onset disease, that is to say, it usually occurs later in life (around age 40 years or later). The majority of people with diabetes have this type.

Examples of oral hypoglycemics are acetohexamide (Dymelor), chlorpropamide (Diabinese), tolazamide (Tolinase), tolbutamide (Orinase), glipizide (Glucotrol), and glyburide (Micronase, DiaBeta).

Insulin and the oral hypoglycemics are discussed separately.

stimulate body to produce insulin

ORAL HYPOGLYCEMICS

ACTIONS AND USES Oral hypoglycemics act to lower
▲▲▲▲▲▲▲▲▲▲▲▲▲▲▲▲ the serum glucose levels by stimulating the beta cells of the pancreas to secrete more insulin. Use of these agents is limited to those people who have some functioning beta cells. Persons with type II diabetes are adults. As the aging process continues, sometimes all of the beta cells cease to function, and the person becomes insulin dependent.

Adverse actions include nausea, epigastric distress, rash, pruritus, increased sensitivity to the sun, jaundice, and vague neurological symptoms (such as weakness and numbness of the extremities). Hypoglycemic reactions may also occur. Anemia, thrombocytopenia, and leukopenia are possible.

ASSESSMENT Question patients about or observe for
▲▲▲▲▲▲▲▲▲▲ symptoms of hyperglycemia. These include increased urine output (polyuria), increased thirst (polydipsia), increased hunger (polyphagia), unexplained weight loss, weakness, dim or blurred

vision, increased number of infections, or delay in wound healing. Also note whether the breath, perspiration, or urine has a sweet or fruity odor.

Assess serum glucose levels by venipuncture or fingerstick for an increase (hyperglycemia) or decrease (hypoglycemia). Assess urine for the presence of glucose (glycosuria) and ketones (ketonuria).

PLANNING AND IMPLEMENTATION One error that many
▲▲▲▲▲▲▲▲▲▲▲▲▲▲▲▲▲▲▲▲▲▲▲▲▲▲ persons with type II diabetes make is to believe that their illness is not as serious as that of other diabetics. This may lead them to be careless and inconsistent with their treatment, which may result in more rapid progression of their disease and eventual complications. A major point of patient teaching is to impress people that proper attention to all aspects of treatment allows *control* of their disease and decrease in or delay of the onset of complications. Treatment does not cure the disease.

Allergic reactions to sulfonylureas are not common, but exercise caution in people with allergy to sulfonamides.

Take care with patients who have renal, hepatic, thyroid, or other endocrine disorders. Monitor patients for renal insufficiency and cumulative effects of the hypoglycemics. Report these to the physician immediately.

Include information about the condition of diabetes mellitus and the medication in patient teaching. Patients who understand their illness are more likely to follow the plan of care. Important aspects to be included are diet, weight management, exercise, personal hygiene, avoidance of infection, wound care, and foot care. Teach the patient how to test serum glucose levels or glucose levels in the urine. Teach symptoms of hyperglycemia and hypoglycemia and the appropriate interventions for each. Emphasize the importance of reporting symptoms to the physician and the need to follow medical advice. People who attempt to alter their medication dosage to control symptoms without consulting the physician are risking serious complications or death.

Advise patients to avoid consumption of alcohol. Headache, flushed face, dizziness, and shortness of breath may result from alcohol intake.

Teach patients to note and report symptoms of adverse effects. The physician may wish to change them to a different oral hypoglycemic.

Increased sensitivity to the sun may occur. Teach methods of protecting the skin from the harmful rays of the sun by avoiding bright midday sun and covering exposed areas with clothing or sunscreen. Sunglasses and large brimmed hats are also helpful.

Increased bleeding or bruising tendencies may

indicate thrombocytopenia. Leukopenia may cause an increased tendency toward infections. Anemia is possible. All changes in condition should be reported to the physician.

Increased stress caused by emotions, infection, surgery, or trauma may cause the body to release more glycogen into the bloodstream and increase the need for hypoglycemics. Instruct patients to monitor their glucose levels or urine more frequently at these times. Elevations should be reported to the physician. Discourage self-adjustment of medication unless it is specifically approved by the physician.

Oral hypoglycemics should be taken 30 minutes before meals. This allows the medication to stimulate the beta cells to increase the secretion of insulin.

Teach patients to notify the physician if pregnancy is suspected. Oral hypoglycemics may cause birth defects.

EVALUATION Monitor serum glucose levels for devia-
▲▲▲▲▲▲▲▲▲▲ tions from normal values and monitor urine for the presence of ketones. Monitor patients for symptoms of hypoglycemia and hyperglycemia.

Encourage the elderly and those with renal problems to maintain adequate fluid intake. Evaluate intake and output for adequacy.

INSULINS

ACTIONS AND USES Insulin is manufactured by the
▲▲▲▲▲▲▲▲▲▲▲▲▲▲▲▲ beta cells of the pancreas. Its action is to lower blood glucose levels by enabling the glucose to cross the cell membrane for use by the cell in energy production or storage. It functions on a negative feedback system: insulin is secreted when the serum glucose levels go up, and insulin secretion is reduced when the serum glucose levels decrease. Inadequate production of insulin or a poor response to secreted insulin results in the condition of diabetes mellitus. People who are insulin dependent are said to have type I diabetes.

Adverse effects include hypoglycemic reactions, insulin resistance, and tissue atrophy or hypertrophy at injection sites.

ASSESSMENT Question all patients with diabetes about
▲▲▲▲▲▲▲▲▲▲ or observe for symptoms of hyperglycemia. These include increased urine output (polyuria), increased thirst (polydipsia), increased hunger (polyphagia), unexplained weight loss, weakness, dim or blurred vision, increased number of infections, or delay in wound healing. Also note whether the breath,

perspiration, or urine has a sweet or fruity odor. Also assess patients for symptoms of hypoglycemia.

Assess serum glucose levels by venipuncture or fingerstick for abnormal values. Assess urine for glycosuria and ketonuria.

PLANNING AND IMPLEMENTATION Caregivers must be
▲▲▲▲▲▲▲▲▲▲▲▲▲▲▲▲▲▲▲▲▲▲▲▲▲▲ aware of three basic properties of all insulins, regardless of whether they are animal products or synthetically manufactured products. These properties are the *onset,* the *peak,* and the *duration.* The onset is when the dose of insulin begins to act in the body. The peak is when insulin exerts its maximal action (i.e., when the blood glucose is the lowest). The duration is the length of time the dose of insulin is acting in the body (Fig. 60–1).

The properties are sometimes modified or altered by the manufacturer by the addition of zinc or protamine (a protein). These modifiers slow the absorption of insulin from the injection site, thereby prolonging the onset and duration of action.

Insulins are divided into three categories or types on the basis of their properties (Table 60–1).

Unmodified regular insulin is the only type suitable for intravenous administration and therefore is the type required in emergency situations.

Regular insulin can also be administered by subcutaneous (SC) injection. When the SC method is used, the dose is usually administered 20 to 30 minutes before a meal. Onset of action averages 20 minutes to 1 hour after SC injection. Average peak action is 2 to 5 hours after injection. Average duration of action is 6 to 8 hours. Some examples of rapid-acting insulins are Regular insulin, Semilente insulin, Novolin R, and Humulin R.

Those insulins categorized as having an intermediate action have an average onset of action at 1 to 2 hours after injection, peak 8 to 12 hours later, and average 18 to 24 hours in duration. Some examples of intermediate-acting insulins are NPH insulin, Lente insulin, Novolin N, and Humulin N. All of these insulins contain modifiers.

Long-acting insulins have an average onset of action at 4 to 8 hours after injection, peak 14 to 20 hours later, and average 36 or more hours in duration. Some examples of long-acting insulins are PZI insulin, Ultralente insulin, Humulin U, and Novolin L. These also contain modifiers.

Because the serum glucose levels are lowest during the peak action time, hypoglycemic symptoms are most likely to occur then. These symptoms are also referred to as insulin shock, insulin reaction, or hypoglycemic episodes. Instruct patients about these symptoms (Table 60–2) and make them aware of the time of day or night that these are most likely to occur with the type of insulin they are taking. For example, if a patient takes regular insulin at 8 AM, hypoglycemia is most likely to occur between 10 AM and 1 PM (2 to 3 hours later).

Teach patients that ingesting a rapidly absorbed form of glucose, such as orange juice or candy, will quickly alleviate the symptoms of hypoglycemia. Items such as these should be kept on hand at all times for emergency use. Some people find that small tubes of cake icing are a convenient form of glucose to carry in their pocket or purse. As soon as possible, the person should consume a more complex form of carbohydrate, such as a sandwich, skim milk, or fruit, to prevent a return to the hypoglycemic state after the rapidly absorbed glucose is used by the cells.

N U R S I N G   A L E R T
▼▼▼▼▼▼▼▼▼▼▼▼▼▼▼▼▼▼▼▼▼▼▼▼▼▼▼▼▼▼

If hypoglycemic episodes occur regularly, the physician should be notified. The diet, the insulin, or the exercise regimen will need to be altered.

▲▲▲▲▲▲▲▲▲▲▲▲▲▲▲▲▲▲▲▲▲▲▲▲▲▲▲▲▲▲▲

Insulin is measured in units. Insulin is most commonly available in U-100 concentrations. This means that each milliliter contains 100 units. The label on the vial states the concentration.

The syringe used for administration must be an insulin syringe calibrated in units.

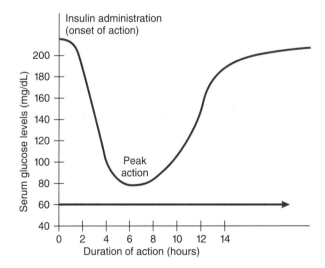

Figure 60–1. All insulins have three basic properties: onset (when the dose begins to act in the body), peak (when the insulin exerts its maximal action), and duration (the length of time the dose of insulin is acting in the body).

Table 60–1. Insulins

NAME	ACTION	PROPERTIES		
		Onset (h)	Peak (h)	Duration (h)
Regular	Rapid	1/2–1	2–3	5–7
Semilente	Rapid	1/2–1	4–7	12–16
Humulin R	Rapid	1/2–1	2–5	5–16
Novolin R	Rapid	1/2–1	2–5	5–16
NPH	Intermediate	1–2	8–12	24–28
Lente	Intermediate	1–2	8–12	18–24
Humulin N	Intermediate	1–2	4–12	16–18
Novolin N	Intermediate	1–2	4–12	16–18
PZI	Long	4–8	14–20	36+
Ultralente	Long	4–8	10–18	36+
Humulin U	Long	4–8	12–18	24–28
Novolin L	Long	4–8	7–15	16–28

(handwritten margin note: Know — How many hrs after to take place)

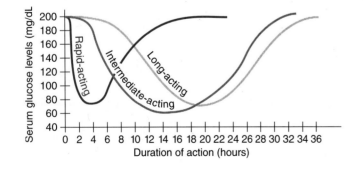

NURSING ALERT

▼▼▼▼▼▼▼▼▼▼▼▼▼▼▼▼▼▼▼▼▼▼▼▼▼▼▼▼▼▼▼▼

Insulin is always ordered and administered in units.

▲▲▲▲▲▲▲▲▲▲▲▲▲▲▲▲▲▲▲▲▲▲▲▲▲▲▲▲▲▲▲▲

It should also be stated on the syringe that it is to be used with U-100 insulin. Always compare the label on the vial with the marking on the syringe. Use of an

Table 60–2. Diabetes Mellitus

DEFINITION The inability to properly metabolize carbohydrates, resulting in incomplete metabolism of fats and production of ketones.

	IMPORTANT DISTINGUISHING FACTORS	
TERMS	**Hyperglycemia** Diabetic coma Ketoacidosis	**Hypoglycemia** Insulin shock Insulin reaction Hyperinsulinism
CAUSES	Insufficient insulin Excessive food Too little exercise Other medications Illness	Excessive insulin Too little food (meals delayed, omitted, vomited) Excessive exercise Other medications Illness
ONSET	Slow (may be days)	Sudden (minutes)
LABORATORY FINDINGS	Hyperglycemia (above 120 mg/100 mL) Glycosuria Ketonuria	Hypoglycemia (below 80 mg/100 mL)
SYMPTOMS	Flushed face Skin dry Skin warm Acetone odor Polydipsia Polyuria Polyphagia Full, bounding pulse Kussmaul respirations (air hunger; rapid, deep breaths) Behavioral changes (euphoric, irritable) Weakness Sleepiness Seizures Coma	Pallor Diaphoresis Skin cool, clammy Rapid, thready pulse Rapid respirations Behavioral changes (irritable) Weakness Sleepiness Tremors Seizures Coma

Table 60–2. Diabetes Mellitus *Continued*

TREATMENT	Fluids Insulin	Rapidly absorbed carbohydrates (orange juice, candy, tube of cake icing) Glucagon, IV dextrose
RESPONSE TO TREATMENT	Slow	Rapid

Treatment emphasis is on patient education concerning *diet, insulin* (or oral hypoglycemic medication), *exercise,* and *maintenance of health.*

inappropriate syringe would result in an error in dose. Insulin dose is individualized and based on the serum glucose levels.

Insulin resistance sometimes develops and the physician orders larger doses of insulin. To minimize the volume of insulin to be injected with each dose, the physician may prescribe insulin in higher concentrations, such as U-500. The syringe must then be marked for use with U-500 insulin. Serious consequences would result if the wrong concentration of insulin were used.

Check the expiration date on the vial before using the contents. Discard outdated insulin.

Do not use insulin that has changed color. Modified insulins appear cloudy or milky white. Other insulins are clear. If they are any other color, they should be discarded.

Modified insulins are suspensions and precipitate when at rest. Rotate them to mix the solute evenly into the solution. Roll the vial between the palms of the hands. Do not shake the vial because this causes formation of bubbles and may result in an error in dose.

Insulin needles are a very fine 25 to 28 gauge and ½ to ⅝ inch in length. Administration into subcutaneous tissue can be obtained with a 45- or 90-degree angle, depending on whether the patient is thin or obese.

Serum glucose levels of some people are difficult to regulate and require a specific type of insulin. Physicians sometimes order two types of insulin mixed into one dose (Fig. 60–2). Review the Drug Administration Guidelines for mixing two insulin preparations for injection in Chapter 9.

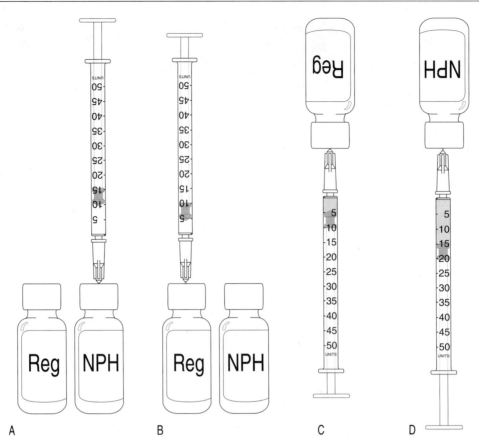

Figure 60–2. *A.* Inject into the vial of modified (cloudy) insulin the volume of air that is equal to the ordered dose of modified insulin (example: 10 units of NPH insulin). Withdraw the needle. *B.* Inject into the vial of unmodified (clear) insulin the volume of air that is equal to the ordered dose of unmodified insulin (example: 5 units of regular insulin). *C.* Withdraw the ordered dose of unmodified insulin. Remove all air bubbles in the usual manner. *D.* Insert the needle into the vial of modified insulin and withdraw the ordered dose of modified insulin. *Be careful not to aspirate any air into the syringe during this step.*

Lipodystrophy sometimes occurs at the injection sites. This can be manifested as either atrophy or hypertrophy. Tissue atrophy displays itself as a pitted appearance to the site. Lipohypertrophy at the site appears as a swelling. Either of these symptoms is more likely to occur if injections are frequently given in the same site. Systematic rotation of sites is an important preventive measure to teach. Appropriate sites include the upper arms, abdomen, thighs, scapula area, and buttocks (Fig. 60–3). For self-administration, patients often find the abdomen and thighs easiest to reach. Family members are often taught to give injections to allow use of the sites that are harder to reach. Some form of record keeping will help the patient remember which site was last used.

Administration of cold insulin may increase the frequency of lipodystrophy. Insulin may be kept refrigerated for long-term storage (as in the pharmacy), but for daily use it should just be kept in a cool place. Avoid excessive heat and strong light.

After injection, press the site but do not rub. Rubbing the site may increase skin irritation or increase the rate of absorption of the insulin.

As with all injections, aseptic technique should be maintained. Patients with diabetes are particularly susceptible to infection.

Because insulin is a protein substance, allergic reactions can occur to the beef, pork, or modifiers. Localized reactions are pruritus, redness, stinging, urticaria, warmth, and edema. These sometimes subside with continued use. Careful monitoring for further symptoms should continue during therapy. Often, the physician will change the prescription to the other type (i.e., beef or pork) or may order human insulin.

Other medications affect control of diabetes. Hyperglycemic effects occur with alcohol, steroids, estrogen, lithium, some diuretics, epinephrine, and other drugs. Hypoglycemic effects occur with monoamine oxidase (MAO) inhibitors, salicylates, sulfonamides, oral anticoagulants, and other drugs. Physicians should be informed of all medications being taken so that dietary requirements and medication doses can be altered appropriately.

Smoking delays absorption of insulin because nicotine constricts blood vessels. Instruct patients to delay smoking for at least 30 minutes after injection.

Pregnancy often increases insulin requirements dramatically, and a condition called gestational diabetes mellitus may occur. Pregnant patients are often under the care of a specialist.

Patients should not skip meals. Hypoglycemia may result.

Exercise should be done consistently and not sporadically. Sudden increases in activity level may cause hypoglycemic episodes.

Serum glucose levels and urine assessments should be performed at home as directed by the physician. Serum glucose monitoring is thought to be more accurate than urine glucose assessments because renal function affects the amount of glucose excreted in the urine. Urine may also be assessed for the presence of ketones. Instruct patients in the method ordered by their physician and give them ample opportunity to demonstrate their skill in performing these assessments.

Some physicians order specific doses of rapid-acting insulin to be given on the basis of the results of serum glucose levels or urine assessments. This is referred to as *insulin coverage.* Self-adjustment of the insulin dose should not be done unless it is approved by the physician.

Advise patients to always wear medical identification. Behavioral changes resulting from hypoglycemic or hyperglycemic episodes can be misinterpreted and may delay the patient's obtaining prompt treatment.

Advise patients to always carry a rapidly absorbed form of carbohydrate for emergency use.

Remember that control of diabetes mellitus depends on a balance of diet, medication, and exercise. Long-term complications of the disease are more likely in people who do not maintain normal serum glucose levels. Therefore, remind patients to notify the physician if symptoms of hypoglycemia or hyperglycemia occur more than just occasionally. Serum glucose levels are influenced by many factors, such as stress, infection, dietary intake, and exercise. If glucose levels are frequently abnormal, overall health, lifestyle, and treatment need to be reviewed by the physician.

EVALUATION Monitor serum glucose levels and urine ▲▲▲▲▲▲▲▲▲▲ assessments. Monitor patients for symptoms of hypoglycemia and hyperglycemia episodes.

INSULIN ANTAGONISTS

Glucagon

Medications that act to elevate the blood sugar level are antagonists of insulin and are often called hyperglycemics. In some instances, this is a side effect of a

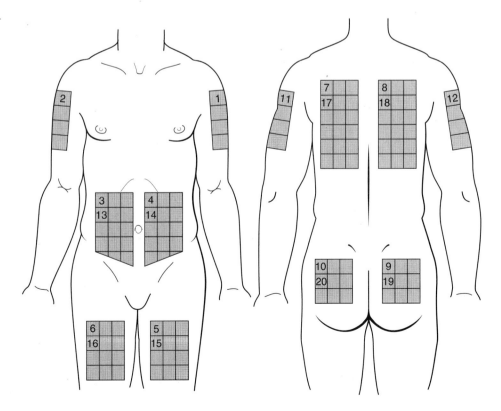

Figure 60–3. Appropriate sites for insulin injections include the upper arms, abdomen, thighs, scapula area, and buttocks.

medication that has been ordered for another purpose. At other times, it is a desirable effect used to treat hypoglycemic reactions. The drug most commonly ordered for treatment of a hypoglycemic reaction is glucagon.

Glucagon is a hormone secreted by the alpha cells of the islets of Langerhans of the pancreas. It works on the negative feedback principle to help maintain homeostasis of the blood sugar by stimulating the release of glycogen from the liver. Insulin lowers the blood sugar, glucagon elevates it.

For glucagon to be effective, one must have normal hepatic function and adequate glycogen reserves. Therefore, it is not effective in starvation, adrenal insufficiency, chronic hypoglycemia, and many of those with juvenile-onset diabetes.

Glucagon cannot be administered orally because it is destroyed by the enzymes in the digestive tract. It is administered by the subcutaneous (SC), intramuscular (IM), or intravenous (IV) route.

ACTIONS AND USES Glucagon antagonizes the effect of
▲▲▲▲▲▲▲▲▲▲▲▲▲▲▲▲ insulin. It is used to treat severe insulin-induced hypoglycemic reactions when the patient is unable to ingest glucose or IV glucose therapy is not readily available. Those who lapse suddenly into coma or who have combative behaviors that make it difficult to encourage glucose consumption are candidates for use of glucagon. In these cases, the physician may choose to order glucagon for the patient to have on hand for emergency use.

Adverse effects include nausea and vomiting.

ASSESSMENT Assess the person for consciousness and
▲▲▲▲▲▲▲▲▲▲ the ability to swallow and to cooperate. Assess the serum glucose levels.

PLANNING AND IMPLEMENTATION Teach family or sig-
▲▲▲▲▲▲▲▲▲▲▲▲▲▲▲▲▲▲▲▲▲▲▲▲▲▲▲▲▲▲ nificant others the symptoms of hypoglycemia and the importance of notifying the physician in emergency situations. Also teach the methods of preparing and injecting glucagon.

Glucagon is available in kits that contain the dry, white powder in a vial or ampule and sterile diluent in another vial. The solution must be prepared before use and the remainder kept refrigerated. It may be stored in the refrigerator up to 3 months after reconstitution.

The usual dose of glucagon is 0.5 to 1 mg injected SC or IM. Improvement of the condition should be evident within 5 to 20 minutes. If necessary, the dose may be repeated after 20 minutes. No more than two doses (total) are given. Further doses are usually not

effective. (IV use is limited to practitioners who are licensed to administer IV medications.)

It is important to arouse the patient from coma as soon as possible. The hyperglycemic effect of glucagon lasts only about an hour, and it is then often followed by secondary hypoglycemia. If possible, the person should consume a feeding that includes rapid-acting carbohydrates for immediate effect and complex carbohydrates for a more prolonged effect.

If the patient does not regain consciousness or cooperativeness within 30 minutes, IV glucose administration is usually necessary.

Teach family or caregivers the importance of maintaining an airway and preventing aspiration in the unconscious patient.

Patients often have no memory of events preceding the hypoglycemic episode. Review the diabetic teaching regimen and emphasize preventive measures.

EVALUATION Continue monitoring the patient after
▲▲▲▲▲▲▲▲▲▲ the episode to be certain that the condition has stabilized. Monitor serum glucose levels and monitor for symptoms of hypoglycemia and hyperglycemia.

E X E R C I S E S

CASE STUDIES

1. Your patient, a 12-year-old girl, is a new diabetic. While you are teaching her to administer her insulin, she asks why she cannot just take a pill like her grandmother does. How will you explain this to her?

2. Mr. N.R., age 35 years, likes to go out with his friends and drink a few beers and enjoy a pizza. When he comes home, he tests his serum glucose with his home monitoring device. If his glucose level is elevated, he then gives himself an injection of 5 or 10 units of insulin. He has not told his physician of this practice because he does not think it is necessary. Explain why this is a dangerous practice.

3. Mr. E.V. works as an accountant. He is careful about maintaining his diabetic regimen and is a conscientious person. He recognizes the importance of avoiding excess weight gain, so on weekends he likes to get additional exercise. He often plays several hard games of racquet ball with his friends. Lately, he has had hypoglycemic reactions after playing and has needed to consume his emergency glucose supply to alleviate his symptoms. What teaching is it important to review with Mr. E.V.?

LEARNING ACTIVITIES

1. Role play the part of a nurse teaching her newly diagnosed patient about hyperglycemia. Have a classmate role play the patient who is having some difficulty comprehending.

2. Role play the part of the patient in case study 2. Have a classmate role play the nurse.

3. Demonstrate to your classmates the appropriate techniques for mixing 10 units of Regular insulin and 20 units of NPH insulin. Explain the rationale for your steps as you would explain to a patient.

DRUGS THAT AFFECT THE REPRODUCTIVE SYSTEM

This unit includes many of the drugs that affect the reproductive system. Some of the classifications are hormones, others are not. Among the anterior pituitary hormones are those called *gonadotropic* because they stimulate the gonads to develop and to secrete other hormones. Some drugs block secretion of or antagonize the actions of hormones, so they have been included in the same chapter to offer the contrast and comparisons of their actions.

ANDROGENS

LEARNING OBJECTIVES

After studying this chapter, you should be able to:

1. Discuss the action of androgens in men and women.

2. List conditions for which androgens may be used in men and women.

3. Name examples of androgens.

4. Prepare an appropriate plan of care for patients receiving androgens.

DRUGS YOU WILL LEARN ABOUT IN THIS CHAPTER

Natural Androgens

testosterone (Andro 100, T pellets)

testosterone cypionate (DEPO-Testosterone)

testosterone enanthate (Andro L.A., Delatest)

testosterone propionate (Testex)

Synthetic Androgens

danazol (Danocrine)

fluoxymesterone (Halotestin)

methyltestosterone (Android, Testred)

nandrolone phenpropionate (Durabolin)

stanozolol (Winstrol)

Negative feedback affects the reproductive system as well as the endocrine system because the endocrine system controls the reproductive hormones. In this situation, the stimulating gland is once again the anterior pituitary gland. Remember, we called it the master gland. The target glands in the male reproductive system are the testes.

The interstitial cell-stimulating hormone (ICSH) is produced by the anterior pituitary gland. This hormone is the male equivalent of the luteinizing hormone (LH) secreted in females. ICSH stimulates the interstitial cells in the male gonads, or testes, to produce testosterone (Fig. 61–1). Testosterone is the hormone responsible for producing the primary and secondary male sexual characteristics (Box 61–1).

The follicle-stimulating hormone (FSH) is also produced by the anterior pituitary to stimulate the seminiferous tubules in the testes to produce sperm.

Testosterone is necessary for sperm production. Therefore, there is an interrelationship between the actions of ICSH, FSH, and testosterone. Beginning at puberty, the hypothalamus influences this process by secreting hypothalamic releasing factors. These regulate the blood levels of all of the gonadotropic hormones (negative feedback mechanism) and thus maintain homeostasis of the male hormones (Box 61–2).

Aging gradually decreases this process. As early as age 20 years, the hormones peak and begin to decrease, but they continue to be secreted for many years. Some men may continue producing significant amounts of these hormones even past the age of 80 years.

The male hormones, testosterone and its derivatives, are called *androgens*. Androgens are also produced in small amounts by the adrenal cortex.

For pharmaceutical use, natural forms of testosterone are obtained from the testes of bulls. Synthetically produced androgens are called *anabolic steroids*. Anabolism refers to the "building up" phase of metabolism. Anabolic agents promote the building of new body tissues.

Androgens may be administered to men or women for various conditions. Our hypothalamus is unable to distinguish between hormones produced in our own bodies and those we take as medications. Therefore,

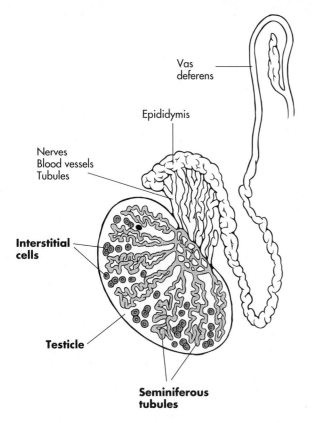

Figure 61–1. The interstitial cell-stimulating hormone, produced by the anterior pituitary gland, stimulates the interstitial cells in the testes to produce testosterone.

in the woman. As a result, infertility and changes in secondary sex characteristics may occur.

Table 61–1 lists the dosages of natural and synthetic androgens.

ACTIONS AND USES The main actions of androgens are
▲▲▲▲▲▲▲▲▲▲▲▲▲▲▲▲▲ the production of male secondary sex characteristics and the maintenance of male reproductive structures, including sperm production. Therefore, they are used as a replacement for testosterone deficiency caused by hypogonadism or cryptorchidism. Sometimes they are used in cases of infertility due to a low sperm count (oligospermia).

The androgens are taken for several weeks, causing suppression of the anterior pituitary hormones ICSH and FSH (negative feedback). The theory is that when the androgens are discontinued, a rebound phenomenon occurs, and the anterior pituitary will surge out an increase in FSH and ICSH. This should then cause an increase in testosterone and sperm production.

Some types of cancers are treated with hormones. In discussing the use of hormones for cancer therapy, it is important to understand the difference in the terms therapeutic and palliative. With *therapeutic* treatments, the patient's general condition and prognosis should improve. With *palliative* treatments, some aspects of the patient's condition may improve, but in general, the prognosis is not improved. In fact, the

---

Box 61–1. Male Sexual Characteristics

Primary
Development of reproductive structures
Function of reproductive structures
Sperm production

Secondary
Body/facial hair
Deep voice
Broad shoulders
Narrow hips
Large muscle mass

Box 61–2. Anterior Pituitary–Testosterone Negative Feedback Cycle

Anterior pituitary secretes interstitial cell-stimulating hormone (ICSH).
ICSH stimulates the interstitial cells of the testes.
Interstitial cells increase production of testosterone.
Testosterone levels increase in the bloodstream. (When testosterone levels are adequate, the anterior pituitary secretes follicle-stimulating hormone (FSH), which stimulates the gonads to produce sperm.)
Hypothalamus decreases secretion of hypothalamic releasing factors, which signals the anterior pituitary to decrease ICSH.
ICSH levels decrease in the bloodstream.
Interstitial cells decrease production of testosterone.
Testosterone levels decrease in the bloodstream. (When testosterone levels are inadequate, FSH levels are also low, and the sperm production decreases.)
Hypothalamus increases secretion of hypothalamic releasing factors, which signals the anterior pituitary to increase ICSH.

Thus the cycle repeats. In this manner, homeostasis of the male hormones is maintained.

---

taking androgens initiates the negative feedback message to the anterior pituitary to decrease secretion of the gonadotropic hormones ICSH and FSH in the man and FSH and LH in the woman. The problem with this is that when the person stops taking androgens, it takes a while for the anterior pituitary to stimulate the gonads to produce testosterone and sperm in the man and estrogen, progesterone, and ova

Table 61-1. Androgens

DRUG	DOSAGE
Natural Androgens	
testosterone (Andro 100, T pellets)	Male hypogonadism: 10–25 mg 2–3 times/wk IM; 2–6 pellets (75 mg each) SC q 3–6 mo
testosterone cypionate (DEPO-Testosterone) and testosterone enanthate (Andro L.A., Delatest)	Male hypogonadism: 50–400 mg q 2–4 wk IM Female: Palliation inoperable breast cancer: 50–400 mg q 2–4 wk IM
testosterone propionate (Testex)	Male: Replacement therapy 25–50 mg IM 2–3 × wk
Synthetic Androgens	
danazol (Danocrine)	Female endometriosis: 400 mg PO bid for 3–9 mo Female fibrocystic breast disease: 100–400 mg qd PO in 2 divided doses for 2–6 mo
fluoxymesterone (Halotestin)	Male hypogonadism: 2–10 mg PO qd Female breast cancer: 15–30 mg PO qd in divided doses
methyltestosterone (Android, Testred)	Male hypogonadism: 10–50 mg PO qd; buccal: 5–25 mg qd
nandrolone phenpropionate (Durabolin)	Severe debility, some anemias: 50–100 mg/wk IM
stanozolol (Winstrol)	To increase hemoglobin in some cases of aplastic anemia: 2 mg PO tid

expected life span may be lessened. However, the patient may feel better and therefore be more active. The question is one of quality of life versus quantity of life. It is a personal decision. For example, some people want to live as long as they possibly can, regardless of their condition (quantity of life). Other people want to live as long as they are physically and emotionally able to participate in and enjoy life (quality of life).

Androgens are sometimes used for palliative treatment of male reproductive tumors. Reproductive tumors often grow faster in the presence of reproductive hormones, and that is what makes this a palliative treatment. However, androgens increase protein building and increase density of bone. This serves to increase lean body mass and strength. Anabolic hormones also increase one's feeling of well-being (libido). Those with an increased libido are more alert, report a decrease in pain levels, tend to have an increased appetite, and are more willing participants in activities.

Female reproductive tumors, such as breast tumors, grow faster when female hormones (primarily estrogen) are present in the body. Androgens are sometimes used as therapeutic treatment in women because they suppress or override the effects of estrogen in the body. The tumor does not thrive in this environment, so it will grow more slowly or even atrophy.

Because of their anabolic effects, androgens are used to reverse the tissue wasting (catabolism) that often accompanies debilitating diseases or the long-term use of corticosteroids. They are also used for prevention or management of postmenopausal osteoporosis in men.

In women, androgens are sometimes used to suppress postpartum breast engorgement and lactation. In women with endometriosis, anabolic steroids may be used to suppress the estrogen levels. This causes atrophy of normal endometrium as well as the ectopic endometrial implants. Menstrual periods cease until approximately 3 months after the medication is discontinued. If the patient has been infertile because of the endometriosis, it is hoped that fertility will be restored after the therapy is completed.

Anabolic steroids are also used to treat women with fibrocystic breast disease. Suppression of the estrogen levels causes atrophy of the breasts and relief from the cysts.

Androgens increase bone marrow function, especially red blood cell production. Because of this, they are used to treat some anemias, such as aplastic anemia and those present in chronic renal failure.

There are numerous examples of androgens. Some of the most commonly used natural hormones are testosterone (Andro 100, T pellets), testosterone cypionate (DEPO-Testosterone), testosterone enanthate (Andro L.A., Delatest), and testosterone propionate (Testex).

Some commonly used synthetic androgens are danazol (Danocrine), fluoxymesterone (Halotestin), methyltestosterone (Android, Testred), nandrolone phenpropionate (Durabolin), and stanozolol (Winstrol).

Adverse actions include nausea, vomiting, and diarrhea. Serum sodium, calcium, phosphorus, cholesterol, and potassium levels are elevated. Clotting factors are decreased. Other adverse actions are hypoglycemia, pruritus, jaundice of skin or sclera, and alteration in libido.

Men may experience breast enlargement (gynecomastia) and persistent, painful erections (priapism). These sometimes occur early in therapy but may disappear when the dose is decreased. Inability to have an erection (impotence) may also occur. Long-term use in men may increase male pattern baldness and acne.

Women receiving androgens for an extended time will usually experience an absence of menstrual periods (amenorrhea) or other menstrual irregularities. Hot flashes, headaches, sleep disorders, decreased libido, vaginitis, and other symptoms of estrogen lack may appear. Symptoms of virilization may occur, such as an increase in facial and body hair (hirsutism), lowered voice, breast atrophy, clitoral enlargement, and increase in muscle mass. Voice changes are usually permanent. Other changes are usually reversed when medication is discontinued. These symptoms do not occur with short-term use, such as for prevention of postpartum engorgement and lactation.

ASSESSMENT Assess vital signs and weight and assess ▲▲▲▲▲▲▲▲▲▲ for any symptoms pertinent to the condition being treated. When relevant, ask the patient about pain levels and menstrual cycle information. Document assessment findings as baseline data. The physician sometimes orders determination of serum electrolyte and fasting serum glucose levels and liver function tests to establish baseline data. Sodium and glucose levels may be altered.

PLANNING AND IMPLEMENTATION Androgens have ▲▲▲▲▲▲▲▲▲▲▲▲▲▲▲▲▲▲▲▲▲▲▲▲▲▲▲▲ limited use in prepubescent patients because they stimulate premature closure of the epiphyses and will stunt growth.

Androgens are commonly administered by intramuscular (IM) and oral routes. They may occasionally be administered by the buccal route. They may also be implanted as pellets into the subcutaneous layers of the skin.

Forms used for IM injection are often prepared as oil-based preparations because the oil delays absorption and therefore prolongs the action of the medication. Oil-based medications to be stored a long time are kept in the refrigerator. If retrieved directly from the refrigerator, they will have to be warmed before use. This may be done by placing the vial or ampule in a shallow container of warm water for a few minutes. The container may also be rolled rapidly between the palms for a few minutes. Warming makes the solution flow more easily so it can be aspirated without difficulty. Use a larger gauge (20 to 22 gauge) IM needle, 1 1/2 to 2 inches in length. Inject into a large muscle mass, such as the gluteus medius muscle. Rotate injection sites and check sites for signs of inflammation or abscess because the oil delays absorption and often causes irritation of the tissues.

Weight gain and headaches may result from the hypernatremia. Teach patients to monitor weights weekly or daily if necessary. Weight gain of 2 pounds or more per week often indicates fluid retention. Advise patients about foods high in sodium and teach them to avoid these. Intake and output may need to be monitored. Teach patients to report headaches.

Administering the medications with food or milk may relieve gastrointestinal symptoms. Teach patients to report symptoms that do not improve because they could indicate elevated calcium levels in the blood (hypercalcemia).

If hypercalcemia occurs, teach patients to consume 2000 to 3000 cc of fluid per day (unless other conditions contraindicate this) to help flush the kidneys and prevent formation of kidney stones. Teach that weight-bearing activities, such as walking, help decrease calcium loss from bones. This loss of calcium may lead to osteoporosis and the possibility of pathological fractures.

Itching of the skin (pruritus) and jaundice of skin or sclera may indicate a hepatotoxic effect and should be reported to the physician.

Teach patients to report any increase in bleeding or bruising tendencies. Patients receiving anticoagulants may need doses decreased.

Diabetics should monitor carefully for symptoms of hypoglycemia. Doses of oral hypoglycemics and insulin may need to be decreased.

Monitor emotional status for symptoms of anxiety or depression. Encourage patients to verbalize feelings and to seek support if they are aware of these feelings.

As mentioned previously, therapy with androgens produces negative feedback to the anterior pituitary to decrease the gonadotropic hormones. In men, the decreased FSH and ICSH result in decreased sperm count (oligospermia) and possible inability to have an erection (impotence). Report changes in sexual function to the physician. Offer emotional support.

In women, therapy with androgens also produces negative feedback to the anterior pituitary to decrease the gonadotropic hormones FSH and LH. This results in anovulation and amenorrhea. Reassure the patient that these are temporary symptoms and that her periods and potential for conception will return 2 to 3 months after therapy is discontinued.

Muscle spasms in the back, neck, and legs also bother many women. Teach relaxation techniques and reassure them that these are also temporary symptoms. Increasing dietary intake of calcium may provide some relief.

In recent years, there has been an increase in the abuse of anabolic steroids by athletes. This practice has many serious consequences for both men and women. Health care workers should always counsel against this practice by informing abusers of the hazards.

EVALUATION Monitor patients for changes from baseline assessments. Monitor laboratory reports for abnormal results, especially electrolyte and blood glucose levels and results of liver function tests. Document improvement in symptoms or occurrence of adverse effects.

E X E R C I S E S

CASE STUDIES

1. A 55-year-old man has had carcinoma of the prostate for several years. At this point, he is weak and has great difficulty getting out of bed. He has a poor appetite, sleeps a lot, and cries often. The physician has discussed the possibility of testosterone therapy to alleviate his symptoms. Would this be considered therapeutic or palliative treatment? How do you think this treatment will affect his prognosis?

2. A 43-year-old woman has recently been diagnosed with breast carcinoma. The physician recommends treatment with testosterone. What is the anticipated effect of using this hormone? What patient teaching would you include in her plan of care?

LEARNING ACTIVITIES

1. Prepare a patient teaching sheet, to be distributed to adolescents, discussing the use and abuse of anabolic steroids in sports. With the approval of your instructor, distribute the sheets in local schools, pediatric units of hospitals, or pediatricians' offices.

2. Review the medication lists of patients in a geriatric unit. Prepare a list of those receiving androgens. Include their age, gender, and diagnoses. Share the information with a group of your classmates. Have each classmate prepare a plan of care specific for the assigned patient.

ESTROGENS AND ANTIESTROGENS

LEARNING OBJECTIVES

After studying this chapter, you should be able to:

1. Discuss the action of estrogens in men and women.

2. Discuss the action of antiestrogens in women.

3. List conditions for which estrogens and antiestrogens may be used.

4. Name examples of estrogens and antiestrogens.

5. Prepare an appropriate plan of care for patients receiving estrogens or antiestrogens.

DRUGS YOU WILL LEARN ABOUT IN THIS CHAPTER

Estrogens

  estradiol (Estrace)

  conjugated estrogens (Premarin)

  esterified estrogens (Estratab, Menest)

  chlorotrianisene (TACE)

  estradiol cypionate (Depo-Estradiol Cypionate, Depogen, Dura-Estrin)

  estradiol valerate (Delestrogen, Gynogen L.A.)

  estropipate (Ogen)

  diethylstilbestrol (stilbestrol, DES)

Antiestrogens

  tamoxifen citrate (Nolvadex)

  clomiphene citrate (Clomid)

In the female reproductive system, the feedback mechanism is the regulator of the hormones. The anterior pituitary gland (master gland) is the stimulating gland, and the target glands are the ovaries.

The follicle-stimulating hormone (FSH) is produced by the anterior pituitary gland. FSH stimulates a follicle in the ovary to mature. This maturing follicle is referred to as a graafian follicle (Fig. 62–1). The graafian follicle produces the hormone estrogen, which is responsible for the primary and secondary female sexual characteristics (Box 62–1).

The anterior pituitary also produces the luteinizing hormone (LH). This hormone stimulates the rupture of the graafian follicle, thus releasing the ovum in a process called ovulation. The area of the ruptured follicle on the ovary is now referred to as the corpus luteum. LH stimulates the corpus luteum to produce a hormone called progesterone.

Beginning at puberty, the hypothalamus regulates the blood levels of these hormones by secreting hypothalamic releasing factors, which signal the anterior pituitary to secrete FSH and LH. As the levels of FSH and LH increase, the hypothalamus decreases its secretion of hypothalamic releasing factors. As a result, the anterior pituitary decreases secretion of FSH and LH (negative feedback mechanism). Through this process, homeostasis of the female hormones is maintained and the female menstrual cycle is regulated (Box 62–2).

Aging gradually causes atrophy of the ovary, which decreases the secretion of estrogen and progesterone. Sometime around 45 to 55 years of age, the woman experiences the process of menopause, and the menstrual cycle ceases. This marks the end of her childbearing years. The ovaries continue secreting estrogen in gradually decreasing amounts.

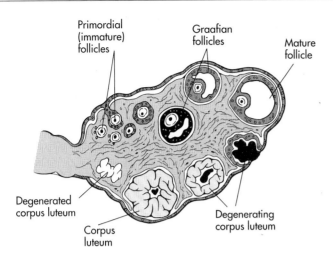

Figure 62–1. The follicle-stimulating hormone causes an immature follicle in the ovary to mature. The maturing follicle is called the graafian follicle. After the mature follicle ruptures, the area is called the corpus luteum.

Box 62–1. Female Sexual Characteristics

Primary
Development of reproductive structures
Function of reproductive structures
Production of ova

Secondary
Breast development
Higher pitched voice
Broad hips
Less muscle mass and more fat deposits

The adrenal cortex also produces small amounts of estrogen in both men and women. During pregnancy, the placenta produces estrogen and other hormones, so it is often referred to as a temporary endocrine gland.

Estrogens used for pharmaceutical preparations are obtained by extraction from natural sources such as placentas. Large animals, such as horses, produce large amounts of urine. Hormones are excreted in the urine. Therefore, some people breed mares and retrieve the urine for use by the pharmaceutical companies.

All naturally occurring estrogens, such as estrone, estradiol, and estriol, are steroids that are converted to estriol by the body. Estradiol, the most potent of these, is produced by the ovaries. Estradiol is metabolized to the chemical compound of estrone, which is half as potent. Estrone is further metabolized to estriol, which is considerably less potent. Estrogens

are also frequently produced synthetically. Some of these products are steroidal and some are nonsteroidal.

Several forms of estrogen are available commercially. Oral preparations, which may be tablets or capsules, are absorbed rapidly by the mucous membranes of the gastrointestinal tract and carried to the liver by the portal circulation. Vaginal creams and suppositories are also absorbed by the mucous membranes and are usually used for their localized effects on vaginal tissues. Estrogen may be absorbed through the skin, so there are circumstances when skin patches are an effective means of hormone administration. Pellets are effective for long-term use because when they are inserted into the subcutaneous tissues,

---

Box 62–2. Anterior Pituitary-Estrogen-Progesterone Negative Feedback Cycle

Days 1–10
The anterior pituitary secretes follicle-stimulating hormone (FSH).
FSH stimulates a follicle in the ovary to mature and produce estrogen.
Estrogen levels increase in the bloodstream.
Estrogen stimulates the *proliferation* (development) of the endometrium of the uterus.
Hypothalamus decreases secretion of hypothalamic releasing factors, resulting in decreased anterior pituitary secretion of FSH.
Anterior pituitary secretion of luteinizing hormone (LH) increases.

Days 10–14
Ovarian follicle ruptures (ovulation).

Days 14–28
LH stimulates the corpus luteum to develop and produce progesterone.
Progesterone levels increase in the bloodstream.
Progesterone stimulates the *secretory phase* of the endometrium. (Uterine glands begin to secrete a viscid fluid.)
After 8 to 10 days (unless pregnancy has occurred), the hypothalamus decreases secretion of hypothalamic releasing factors, resulting in decreased secretion of LH.
The corpus luteum degenerates, and progesterone levels in the blood decrease.
The endometrium regresses, and menstruation starts (day 1 of a new cycle).
The hypothalamus increases secretion of the hypothalamic releasing factors, and the anterior pituitary increases FSH secretion.

Thus the cycle repeats. In this manner, homeostasis of the female hormones is maintained.

Table 62–1. Estrogens and Antiestrogens

DRUG	DOSAGE
Estrogens	
estradiol (Estrace)	Menopausal symptoms, hypogonadism, primary ovarian failure: 1–2 mg qd PO (cycle 3 wk on, 1 wk off)
estradiol cypionate (Depo-Estradiol Cypionate, Depogen, Dura-Estrin)	Menopausal symptoms: 1–5 mg IM q 3–4 wk
estradiol valerate (Delestrogen, Gynogen L.A.)	Menopausal symptoms: 5–20 mg IM; repeat after 2–3 wk Inoperable prostate cancer: 30 mg IM q 1–2 wk or 1–2 mg PO tid
conjugated estrogens (Premarin)	Menopausal symptoms: 0.3–1.25 mg PO qd in cycles Abnormal uterine bleeding: 25 mg IM/IV; repeat in 6–12 h Osteoporosis: 1.25 mg PO qd in cycles Female hypogonadism: 2.5 mg PO bid–tid in cycles
esterified estrogens (Estratab, Menest)	Prostate cancer: 1.25–2.5 mg PO tid Female hypogonadism: 2.5 mg qd–tid PO in cycles Menopausal symptoms: 0.3–3.75 mg PO qd in cycles

Table 62–1. Estrogens and Antiestrogens
Continued

DRUG	DOSAGE
estropipate (Ogen)	Atrophic vaginitis: 0.2 mg vaginal suppository qd or cream q hs Female hypogonadism: 1.25–7.5 mg PO qd in cycles or 0.1–2 mg/wk IM Menopausal symptoms: 0.625–5 mg PO qd in cycles
chlorotrianisene (TACE)	Prostate cancer: 12–25 mg PO qd Female menopausal symptoms: 12–25 mg PO qd in cycles
diethylstilbestrol (stilbestrol, DES)	Female hypogonadism: 0.2–0.5 mg PO qd Male breast cancer: 15 mg qd PO
Antiestrogens	
tamoxifen citrate (Nolvadex)	Female breast cancer: 10–20 mg PO bid
clomiphene citrate (Clomid)	Female infertility to induce ovulation: 50–100 mg PO qd × 5 days, starting on fifth day of cycle; repeat until conception occurs or three courses of therapy are completed

they are stored in fatty tissues and are released slowly. Solutions for injection are commonly prepared as oil-based solutions to prolong their action. Intravenous solutions are an aqueous base. The choice of preparation depends on the reason for use, cost, convenience, and reliability of the patient. Table 62–1 lists estrogens and antiestrogens and their dosages.

ESTROGENS

ACTIONS AND USES The primary action of estrogen is
▲▲▲▲▲▲▲▲▲▲▲▲▲▲▲▲ the maintenance of the reproductive structures, including ova production. Secondary actions are related to the secondary sex characteristics or those characteristics that give the feminine appearance (higher pitched voice, broad hips, increase in subcutaneous fat, breast development).

Estrogens affect metabolism in several other ways. Calcium and phosphorus are retained and used in the formation of bone. Fatty tissues and general metabolism are increased. The kidneys retain more sodium, so the body retains more water. Glucose metabolism is decreased, cholesterol and lipids are decreased, and coagulation factors are increased.

Estrogens are sometimes used with progesterone to prevent pregnancy from occurring. Because of the cyclic interaction of estrogens and the gonadotropic hormones, administration of estrogens causes negative feedback to occur. The anterior pituitary gland then decreases the production of FSH and LH, which in premenopausal women prevents the ovary from developing and releasing ova.

There are numerous other uses for estrogens in both women and men. In women, they are used to treat hypogonadism, prevent postpartum engorgement or lactation, relieve symptoms of surgical menopause, treat the symptoms of naturally occurring menopause, treat atrophic vaginitis, and prevent postmenopausal osteoporosis. Estrogens are used to relieve symptoms of dysmenorrhea, endometriosis, and dysfunctional uterine bleeding. They are sometimes used for palliative treatment of postmenopausal patients with inoperable breast cancer. (Remember that palliative treatments improve the quality of life but may decrease the quantity of life.)

In men, estrogens may be used therapeutically to antagonize the hormone testosterone in the treatment of inoperable prostatic and testicular carcinomas. (Remember that therapeutic treatments are expected to slow the growth of the tumor and increase both the quantity and quality of life.)

Some examples of estrogen preparations are estradiol (Estrace), conjugated estrogens (Premarin), esterified estrogens (Estratab, Menest), chlorotrianisene (TACE), estradiol cypionate (Depo-Estradiol Cypionate, Depogen, Dura-Estrin), estradiol valerate (Delestrogen, Gynogen L.A.), estropipate (Ogen), and diethylstilbestrol (stilbestrol, DES).

All estrogen products have similar adverse effects when they are prescribed at similar dosages. Because estrogens affect so many body functions, there are many potential adverse effects. Of course, as with all medications, there is a great variance in individual response to the different products based on the person's body chemistry, the reason for use, and the length of therapy.

Adverse effects occur in men because estrogen antagonizes the androgenic hormones and causes symptoms of feminization to occur. Symptoms include higher pitched voice, breast enlargement (gynecomastia), increase in fat deposits on the hips, loss of facial and body hair, testicular and penile atrophy, and impotence. A decrease in libido includes a decline in sexual interest, moodiness, and possibly depression.

If estrogens are used before the onset of puberty, closure of the epiphyseal line occurs prematurely and causes stunted growth.

Other adverse effects in women are as follows:

Genitourinary system: changes in menstrual flow, amenorrhea, dysmenorrhea, breakthrough bleeding, increase in the size of fibroid tumors, and infertility.

Breasts: tenderness, enlargement, and sometimes secretions.

Cardiovascular system: hypertension and increased coagulability of the blood, which may lead to thrombophlebitis, cerebrovascular accident (CVA), and myocardial infarction, particularly in women older than 30 years who smoke cigarettes.

Gastrointestinal system: nausea, vomiting, abdominal cramps, bloating, and jaundice. Estrogen seems to increase the concentration of cholesterol in bile, which often leads to cholelithiasis (formation of gallstones). Risk of gallbladder disease in postmenopausal women is two to three times higher than that in premenopausal women. Jaundice may occur as a symptom of blockage of the biliary tree or because of altered liver function.

Skin: chloasma (mask of pregnancy) and linea nigra (pigmented line down the center of the abdomen from sternum to pubis) may occur but are not harmful. Photosensitivity, dermatitis, and hives may also occur.

Even though estrogens induce a feeling of well-being in women who have an estrogen deficiency, high levels tend to produce depression. This can progress to psychosis in some women, particularly if there is a history of depressive illness.

Some adverse effects are prevalent in both male and female patients. Many of these relate to the tendency of estrogen to increase levels of renin and angiotensin. This favors retention of sodium and water with resultant edema, hypertension, and weight gain. Edema may also aggravate certain other conditions, such as asthma, epilepsy, migraines, heart disease, and renal disease.

People who wear contacts often note intolerance to their lenses. Edema changes the shape of the eye somewhat, so the lens may not fit properly. Corneal irritation and ulceration may occur.

Glucose tolerance is decreased during estrogen therapy. This may lead to symptoms of diabetes mellitus.

ASSESSMENT The reason for use of the hormone determines which assessments are appropriate. Assess weight and vital signs along with symptoms relevant to the condition being treated. Record menstrual history in women. Document all of this as baseline data. Determination of serum glucose and cholesterol levels may be ordered before long-term therapy.

PLANNING AND IMPLEMENTATION Since estrogen use
▲▲▲▲▲▲▲▲▲▲▲▲▲▲▲▲▲▲▲▲▲▲▲▲▲▲▲▲▲▲▲▲▲ in men is for treatment of reproductive malignant neoplasms, symptoms of feminization are not reasons to stop therapy unless the patient requests it. Caregivers must explain to the patient and significant others that these are expected effects and offer emotional support as necessary.

Use in prepubescent girls with hypogonadism usually induces development of the female reproductive tract and feminization. Because estrogen administration also speeds closure of the epiphyseal line in long bones, normal growth of long bones may not occur. Be prepared to explain this to patients and their parents and to offer emotional support as needed.

Changes in menstrual flow, amenorrhea, dysmenorrhea, and breakthrough bleeding sometimes disappear after a few weeks or months of therapy. They should be reported to the physician. Sometimes, depending on the reason for therapy, progesterone is added to the therapy to decrease these symptoms. Increase in the size of fibroid tumors and infertility should be reported to the physician and *may* be reason to discontinue therapy.

Breast enlargement, tenderness, and secretions should be reported to the physician so they can be monitored. Often these will decrease or disappear within a few weeks.

Because smoking predisposes the patient to the adverse cardiovascular effects, encourage the patient to decrease the amount she smokes and to stop completely if possible. Teach her the signs and symptoms of hypertension, thrombophlebitis, CVA, and myocardial infarction so that she may monitor for them and report their occurrence to the physician.

Gastrointestinal symptoms may be relieved if oral medications are taken with meals. Teach patients to monitor for yellow discoloration of skin and sclera, dark urine, or light (clay-colored) stools and to report these immediately.

Encourage patients to use a sunblock and to cover exposed areas of skin if photosensitivity becomes a problem.

For a long time, there has been controversy about possible carcinogenic effects of estrogens. Prolonged or high levels of estrogens in postmenopausal women have been associated with 4.5 to 13.9 times greater incidence of endometrial cancer. Study results have been for and against the possibility of an increased risk of breast and cervical cancers in premenopausal women. Estrogen therapy is contraindicated in women who have had cancer of the reproductive tract or breast. Obviously, it would be wise for patients to share any concerns with the prescribing physician and to share any information of family history of these types of cancers, especially if they involved the patient's grandmother, mother, or sister. Also teach patients receiving estrogens the proper procedures for breast self-examinations. Emphasize the importance of monthly breast self-examinations, annual breast examinations by the physician, and annual pelvic examinations with Pap smears. The physician may order baseline and follow-up mammograms.

Estrogens are also known to be teratogenic, that is, capable of causing defects in the fetus. Diethylstilbestrol (DES) was formerly given to pregnant women to prevent abortion. The incidence of vaginal and cervical cancers in their female children and genital malformations (hermaphroditism or pseudohermaphroditism) in their male children is significantly greater than that in the nonexposed population. There are also studies indicating an increase in thyroid cancers in female children of mothers who took estrogen during pregnancy. Congenital limb deformities have also been known to occur. Certainly this indicates that estrogens should not be taken during pregnancy. Teach patients to report to their physicians immediately if they suspect they are pregnant.

Because of these known carcinogenic and teratogenic factors for offspring and because estrogen is secreted in breast milk, use of estrogens in lactating women is contraindicated.

Patients and their significant others should be aware of the possibility of depression. Encourage patients to discuss any symptoms with their physician as soon as they are noted. Caregivers should monitor for symptoms of mood alteration.

Patients with asthma, epilepsy, migraines, heart disease, and renal disease should discuss the condition with their physicians. Teach these patients to observe for and report any increase in symptoms.

Instruct patients to inform their ophthalmologist of the use of estrogens and of any eye symptoms that may occur.

Glucose tolerance is decreased during estrogen therapy. Teach patients who are predisposed to diabetes mellitus to monitor for the occurrence of symptoms or worsening of symptoms. Antidiabetic medications or other adjustments in treatment may be needed.

Caution women using estrogen vaginal creams against using them before intercourse because they can be absorbed by the skin of the penis and cause reduced potency and some degree of feminization of the partner. Teach that the use of condoms during intercourse and applying the cream *after* intercourse will avoid these effects.

Women taking estrogens orally must be taught the proper regimen for their treatment. Many times, estrogens are ordered on a cyclic regimen (for example: take 3 weeks then skip 1 week, or take day 1 through 25 of the cycle with progesterone added on days 16 through 25). Verify that patients are taking medications appropriately by requesting them to explain to you how they take them.

Estrogens may present significant interactions with some other medications. Certain antibiotics are known to decrease the effectiveness of estrogens. This may be of particular significance if the estrogens are being taken for contraception. Advise patients to use some other form of contraception in addition to their birth control pills until the antibiotic is discontinued and they have begun their next menstrual cycle.

Teach patients who take warfarin that estrogen decreases the anticoagulant effects. The physician should be advised of the use of estrogens so that the prothrombin times and warfarin dose may be monitored appropriately.

Estrogens may inhibit the metabolism of phenytoin, resulting in phenytoin toxicity. Teach patients to monitor for the adverse effects of nystagmus, sedation, and lethargy. Physicians may order determination of serum phenytoin levels, and a decreased dose may be required.

Estrogens also reduce the level of circulating thyroid hormones. Communication with physicians about all medications being taken is imperative. The physician may order periodic analysis of triiodothyronine and thyroxine levels. Doses of thyroid hormones may have to be increased in hypothyroid patients.

EVALUATION Estrogens were the first drugs considered under the federal Food and Drug Administration rule that patients be provided with information about the adverse effects and risks of use. Frequently evaluate whether patients are taking the medications as prescribed and if they understand which adverse effects should be reported.

Physicians may wish to order tests of serum glucose levels and glucose tolerance, determination of liver enzyme activities, or studies of renal function for those who take estrogens for long periods or those who exhibit symptoms of renal or hepatic malfunction.

ANTIESTROGENS

Tamoxifen

Tamoxifen citrate (Nolvadex) is a drug with potent antiestrogen effects. It acts to block estradiol at estrogen receptor sites on target tissues such as the breast.

ACTIONS AND USES Tamoxifen is used for treatment of breast cancer and sometimes advanced ovarian cancer in women. With blocking of estradiol, the cancer cells grow more slowly or atrophy.

Because this drug blocks the effects of estrogen, symptoms of menopause will occur. Patients should expect headaches, menstrual changes, hirsutism, thinning of hair on the head, hot flashes, dizziness, and decrease in libido. Some patients experience photosensitivity, rashes, and dryness of the skin. Nausea, vomiting, anorexia, edema, blurred vision, leukopenia, thrombocytopenia, and bone pain may occur.

ASSESSMENT Document the patient's menstrual history and weight as baseline data. Assess the chart for white blood cell and platelet counts.

PLANNING AND IMPLEMENTATION Encourage patients to protect skin from ultraviolet light with sunblocks and protective clothing. Advise them to avoid direct sunlight when possible.

Nausea, vomiting, and anorexia may be relieved by taking medications with food.

Discourage the addition of salt to foods and encourage avoidance of high-sodium foods to minimize the edema. Monitor and record weights and symptoms of edema.

Reassure the patient who is experiencing bone pain. Bone pain usually indicates that the drug will produce a good response. Analgesics are usually ordered to relieve pain.

Leukopenia lowers resistance to infection. Teach patients to avoid persons with colds, flu, or other contagious illnesses. Encourage good nutrition and hygiene to increase resistance to infection. Thrombocytopenia increases bleeding tendencies. Teach patients to avoid trauma because bruising may occur from mild trauma.

Pregnancy should be avoided during antiestrogen therapy. Remind patients that menstrual irregularities and other symptoms make it difficult to determine whether ovulation is occurring. Condoms, diaphragms, or spermicidal preparations should be used on all occasions of intercourse.

Encourage patients to keep all scheduled appointments with physicians.

EVALUATION Menopausal symptoms indicate antiestrogen effects. Physicians may order white blood cell and platelet counts to monitor effects.

Clomiphene

Clomiphene is a synthetic drug that binds to estrogen receptor sites on target tissues to prevent or block the action of estrogen on those tissues. This prevents the normal negative feedback from inhibiting the follicle-stimulating hormone (FSH) and luteinizing hormone (LH) secretion by the anterior pituitary. Therefore, increased amounts of the gonadotropic hormones are secreted, the ovaries are stimulated to produce and release ova, and the corpus luteum is stimulated to produce progesterone.

ACTIONS AND USES Clomiphene is used to treat infer-
▲▲▲▲▲▲▲▲▲▲▲▲▲▲▲ tility resulting from anovulatory cycles. As the ovaries receive increased stimulation, one or more ova are released at ovulation. Pregnancy occurs in 25% to 30% of the women who take this drug, and 8% to 10% of those pregnancies result in multiple births. Most of these multiple births are twins.

Adverse actions such as ovarian enlargement or cysts may occur from the overstimulation of the ovaries. Fluid retention may occur and cause dizziness, hypertension, edema, bloating, blurred vision, photophobia, and headaches. Hot flashes and breast tenderness may occur.

ASSESSMENT Assessments include detailed discussion
▲▲▲▲▲▲▲▲▲▲ of the menstrual cycle to determine whether a pregnancy exists. Assess the chart to determine whether the physician ordered a pregnancy test, and verify the results. Document vital signs and weight as baseline data.

PLANNING AND IMPLEMENTATION Clomiphene is usu-
▲▲▲▲▲▲▲▲▲▲▲▲▲▲▲▲▲▲▲▲▲▲▲▲▲▲▲ ally started on the fifth day of the menstrual cycle in an effort to increase the gonadotropic hormones and cause ovulation. Patients must be taught to take basal body temperatures immediately on awakening and while still in bed. This is to minimize the effects of activity on metabolism and body temperature. They must be instructed in the proper way to graph the temperatures on a chart and taught to recognize when ovulation has occurred. There is a drop in basal body temperature a day or two before ovulation and a sharp increase (0.6° to 1.0°F) in temperature immediately after ovulation. Patients should plan to have intercourse during the 3 days after ovulation to maximize the chance of conception.

Teach patients to report pelvic or abdominal pain. This may signify the presence of ovarian enlargement or cysts.

Teach safety factors, such as to always rise slowly from a sitting or lying position. Driving or hazardous activities should be avoided until response to the drug can be determined. Remind patients to weigh themselves two or three times a week and to report sudden gains of 2 pounds or more per week. Headaches, blurred vision, and photophobia should be reported to the physician.

Reassure patients that hot flashes and breast tenderness will be relieved when the drug is discontinued.

Teratogenic effects are possible. Teach patients to notify the physician immediately if pregnancy is suspected. If pregnancy is verified, the drug is discontinued.

If pregnancy does not occur, the therapy can be repeated for two more cycles.

EVALUATION Compare vital signs, weight, and symp-
▲▲▲▲▲▲▲▲▲▲ toms with pretherapy findings. Review the patient's graph of basal body temperature. Pelvic examination or pregnancy tests are used to verify conception.

E X E R C I S E S

CASE STUDIES

1. Ms. L.S., age 52 years, is taking estrogen for relief of severe menopausal symptoms. What points of patient teaching should be emphasized to her because of her age?

2. Mr. J.F. has been taking estrogen for 6 months for treatment of testicular cancer. Lately, his wife has noted that he is much more emotional than he was previously, often to the point of being tearful. She has called the office and asks you why this is happening. What would you reply?

3. Ms. M.C., age 61 years, is using estrogen vaginal cream to treat symptoms of atrophic vaginitis. What would you include in her teaching plan?

4. The physician has scheduled Ms. K.E., age 25 years, to take tamoxifen for a right breast cancer. She asks you what to expect from this drug. What will you tell her?

LEARNING ACTIVITIES

1. Review the charts of four patients who are taking estrogens. List their age, gender, reason for therapy, and any other medications they are currently taking that may interact with the estrogen. Have a classmate prepare a teaching plan for each patient that indicates the type of interaction to expect and any relevant interventions. Present your information to the class.

2. Prepare a care plan for a 35-year-old woman who is taking estrogen to prevent symptoms of menopause after a hysterectomy and bilateral oophorectomy for treatment of endometriosis. Be sure to include points of patient teaching. Have a classmate prepare a care plan for a 35-year-old man who is taking estrogen for treatment of testicular cancer after bilateral orchiectomy. Be sure to include points of patient teaching. Compare the two plans for the class.

PROGESTERONE

LEARNING OBJECTIVES

After studying this chapter, you should be able to:

1. Discuss the actions of progesterone.

2. List conditions for which progesterone and the synthetic preparations may be used.

3. Name examples of progesterone and the synthetic preparations.

4. Prepare an appropriate plan of care for patients receiving progesterone or the synthetic preparations.

DRUGS YOU WILL LEARN ABOUT IN THIS CHAPTER

hydroxyprogesterone caproate (Delalutin, Hylutin, Duralutin)

medroxyprogesterone acetate (Provera, Depo-Provera)

norethindrone (Norlutin)

levonorgestrel implants (Norplant system)

Previous chapters describe the anterior pituitary gland's production of the gonadotropic hormones, which include the luteinizing hormone (LH). This hormone stimulates the rupture of the graafian follicle and the release of the ovum. The hormone progesterone is then produced from the corpus luteum, which forms at the site of the ruptured follicle.

During days 14 to 28 of the menstrual cycle, progesterone increases in the bloodstream, stimulating the secretory phase of the endometrium. Progesterone raises the basal body temperature about 1°F. Detecting this temperature change confirms ovulation. At this time, the uterine glands secrete a viscid fluid that will sustain the zygote if pregnancy occurs. Progesterone also changes the cervical secretions to a scanty viscid material that forms the mucous plug if pregnancy occurs. The corpus luteum maintains the progesterone levels until the placenta is developed enough to produce adequate amounts. Progesterone suppresses uterine contractility, which would precipitate an abortion. It also suppresses T lymphocytes in the immunological response, which would cause rejection and abortion of the fetus. It stimulates further development of the ducts and glands of the breasts to prepare for lactation.

If fertilization of the ovum does not occur, the hypothalamus decreases secretion of hypothalamic releasing factors after 8 to 10 days. As a result, the anterior pituitary gland decreases secretion of LH. The falling LH levels cause the corpus luteum to degenerate, and serum progesterone levels decrease. The endometrium degenerates, and menstruation begins. This is day 1 of a new menstrual cycle.

For pharmaceutical purposes, progesterone is obtained from natural sources, such as placentas. It is not administered orally because oral doses are rapidly metabolized by the liver. Injections are often prepared in oil-based solutions to delay the absorption and prolong the effects. Progesterone is excreted primarily in the urine, and a small amount is excreted in feces.

Synthetic preparations are somewhat different chemically and are called progestins or progestogens. These products are more effective when they are administered orally.

Progesterone intrauterine devices (IUDs) are no longer popular in the United States because of the many adverse effects attributed to IUDs.

The implanting of progesterone capsules or pellets into subcutaneous tissues is gaining in popularity because they may remain in place up to 5 years. With use of a local anesthetic, the capsules are inserted just under the skin on the inner surface of the upper arm through a small incision. The procedure usually takes 5 to 10 minutes.

The choice of preparation depends on the reason for use, cost, convenience, and reliability of the patient.

Some examples of preparations are hydroxyprogesterone caproate (Delalutin, Hylutin, Duralutin), medroxyprogesterone acetate (Provera, Depo-Provera), norethindrone (Norlutin), and levonorgestrel implants (Norplant system). Progesterone preparations and their dosages are listed in Table 63–1.

ACTIONS AND USES The primary action of progesterone is to preserve the pregnancy. Progesterone is necessary for placental development, for increase in development of uterine muscle during pregnancy, for further breast development in pregnancy, and for inhibition of uterine contractions during pregnancy. Progesterone also inhibits anterior pituitary production of gonadotropic hormones. Therefore, development of other ova and ovulation are prevented.

Progesterone and its derivatives are used to treat amenorrhea, functional uterine bleeding, endometriosis, and uterine carcinoma. Progestins and progestogens are often used in combination with estrogen to inhibit ovulation and prevent conception. The progesterone injections and implants are also used for contraception.

Progesterone can also be used in some cases of infertility. Because of the cyclic interaction of progesterone and the gonadotropic hormones, administration of progestogen will cause negative feedback to occur. The anterior pituitary gland will decrease the production of follicle-stimulating hormone (FSH) and LH, which in premenopausal women will prevent the ovary from developing and releasing ova. The theory is that when the progesterone is stopped, the anterior pituitary will rebound with a surge of FSH. This will stimulate the development of ova, and ovulation will follow.

Adverse effects include acne, rashes, nausea, vomiting, breast tenderness and secretions, menstrual changes, liver dysfunction, and phlebitis. Sodium retention with resultant edema, weight gain, hypertension, and headaches may occur. Glucose tolerance is decreased. Localized irritation may occur at sites of injection or insertion of implants. Cervical erosions and uterine fibromas as well as teratogenic effects on the fetus have sometimes occurred.

ASSESSMENT Assess weight and vital signs. Document assessment findings along with symptoms relevant to the condition being treated. Record menstrual history. The physician may order tests to assess liver function and serum glucose levels before long-term use.

PLANNING AND IMPLEMENTATION Progesterone and its derivatives are known to be teratogenic and therefore should not be used during pregnancy or lactation. Heart and limb defects are known to occur, as is masculinization of the female fetus. Advise women of possible side effects before the initiation of therapy. Therapy should be initiated immediately after the last normal menstrual period or abortion. If for any reason a woman suspects she is pregnant after therapy has been initiated, she should immediately report this to her physician.

N U R S I N G   A L E R T

Patients with a history of breast or genital cancer should be advised not to use progesterone therapy.

Teach patients to report to the physician if acne and rashes occur. Nausea and vomiting may be prevented

Table 63–1. Progesterone Preparations and Dosages	
hydroxyprogesterone caproate (Delalutin, Hylutin, Duralutin)	*Menstrual disorders:* 125–375 mg IM q 4 wk; stop after 4 cycles *Uterine cancer:* 1–5 g wk IM
medroxyprogesterone acetate (Provera, Depo-Provera)	*Abnormal uterine bleeding:* 5–10 mg PO qd 5–10 days, beginning on the 16th day of the cycle *Secondary amenorrhea:* 5–10 mg PO qd for 5–10 days *Endometrial cancer:* 400–1000 mg/wk IM
norethindrone (Norlutin)	*Amenorrhea, abnormal uterine bleeding:* 5–20 mg PO qd days 5–25 of menstrual cycle
levonorgestrel implants (Norplant system)	*Contraception:* see Chapter 66 for details

by taking oral preparations with meals. Symptoms tend to subside after a few months.

Instruct patients in techniques of breast self-examination and remind them to have annual breast examinations by a physician.

Menstrual changes, such as prolonged menstrual bleeding, spotting between periods, or no bleeding for several months, should be discussed with the physician. Also remind the patient of the importance of annual pelvic examinations and Pap smears.

Sodium retention may aggravate other conditions, such as asthma, migraines, and epilepsy. Teach patients to always discuss all other conditions and all medications being taken with any physicians providing them with medical care. Also remind them to weigh themselves weekly, to report sudden increases in weight, and to observe for edema. Dietary sodium may have to be restricted.

Progesterone sometimes causes androgenic effects and may result in hirsutism and thinning of the hair on the head. Tell patients to discuss these with the physician.

Teach patients to observe for and report jaundice of skin or sclera, dark urine, or clay-colored stools. These may indicate liver dysfunction.

N U R S I N G   A L E R T

▼▼▼▼▼▼▼▼▼▼▼▼▼▼▼▼▼▼▼▼▼▼▼▼▼▼▼▼▼

Injection of oil-based solutions may cause irritation of the tissues and abscess formation. Use large muscle masses for injections and rotate sites.

▲▲▲▲▲▲▲▲▲▲▲▲▲▲▲▲▲▲▲▲▲▲▲▲▲▲▲▲▲

Capsules and pellets may also cause temporary redness and inflammation at insertion sites. Patients should report to the physician if these do not disappear in a short time. Discoloration of the skin at the insertion site often remains until the implant is removed.

Teach patients to assess for signs and symptoms of phlebitis and to report these immediately.

Warn persons with diabetes that progesterone can decrease glucose tolerance. Teach them to monitor serum glucose levels or urine checks more frequently and to report abnormal results or symptoms to the physician. Dosages of antidiabetic medications may need to be adjusted. Teach the signs and symptoms to people with a tendency toward the development of diabetes.

Physicians should be aware that the antitubercular drug rifampin may enhance the metabolism of progestins. This necessitates an increased dose of progestins to maintain therapeutic levels.

EVALUATION Frequently evaluate whether patients
▲▲▲▲▲▲▲▲▲▲ are taking the medications as prescribed and if they understand which side effects to report.

Physicians may order determination of serum glucose levels, glucose tolerance tests, and liver enzyme tests at intervals for those who take progesterone for a prolonged time.

E X E R C I S E S

CASE STUDY

Ms. M.K. has been having intermittent uterine bleeding for several weeks. Her physician is contemplating the use of progesterone injections for a diagnosis of dysfunctional uterine bleeding. What questions will you include when taking Ms. M.K.'s history in the physician's office?

LEARNING ACTIVITIES

Prepare a care plan for Ms. M.K., who is taking progesterone injections for dysfunctional bleeding. Be sure to include points of patient teaching.

OXYTOCICS AND OXYTOCIN ANTAGONISTS

L E A R N I N G   O B J E C T I V E S

After studying this chapter, you should be able to:

1. Discuss the actions of oxytocin, oxytocic medications, and drugs that antagonize oxytocin.

2. State the uses of these medications.

3. List adverse effects of each medication.

4. Prepare an appropriate plan of care for a patient receiving each of these medications.

DRUGS YOU WILL LEARN ABOUT IN THIS CHAPTER

Oxytocic Drugs

   oxytocin (Pitocin, Syntocinon)

   Syntocinon nasal spray

Ergot Derivatives

   ergonovine maleate (Ergotrate Maleate)

   methylergonovine maleate (Methergine)

Abortifacients

   dinoprostone (Prostin E2, prostaglandin E_2)

   hypertonic (20%) sodium chloride

Antagonists, Uterine Relaxants, and Tocolytics

   ritodrine HCl (Yutopar)

   terbutaline sulfate (Brethine, Bricanyl)

   magnesium sulfate

The posterior pituitary gland produces two main hormones. Antidiuretic hormone is discussed in Chapter 57. Oxytocin is a hormone secreted in progressively increasing amounts during pregnancy. As the blood level of oxytocin increases, the uterus becomes more irritable and the contractions of labor begin. The contractions of labor normally become progressively stronger and result in dilatation and effacement of the cervix and expulsion of the infant through the birth canal. After delivery, the oxytocin level in the blood progressively decreases. During this time, it continues to cause uterine contractions that help control bleeding and hemorrhage from the placental site.

Oxytocin also stimulates the glandular cells of the breast to contract and release milk into the lactiferous ducts of the breasts. As the lactating mother puts the infant to breast, the infant's sucking stimulates the posterior pituitary gland to secrete more oxytocin. The increasing blood level of oxytocin triggers the anterior pituitary gland to secrete the hormone prolactin, which is responsible for milk production by the secretory cells of the breasts.

The increased oxytocin level in the lactating mother also continues to keep the uterus firm. Thereby, it offers increased protection from uterine hemorrhage and a more rapid involution of the uterus.

Several types of synthetic preparations have an oxytocic effect. The three main groups are the oxytocics, the ergot derivatives, and the abortifacients. Although the general effect is similar, they act somewhat differently and are used for different purposes (Table 64–1). Therefore, they are discussed separately.

Table 64–1. Oxytocics and Oxytocin Antagonists

DRUG	DOSAGE
Oxytocic Drugs	
oxytocin (Pitocin, Syntocinon)	Dilute 1 ampule/10 units per 1000 mL D5W or 0.9% NaCl; administer by infusion pump as a secondary IV Initial rate: 1–2 milliunits/min; may be increased at 15- to 30-min intervals until a normal labor pattern is established; maximal rate: 1–2 mL/min (20 milliunits/min) After normal contractions are well established, the dose is often decreased
Syntocinon nasal spray	1–2 sprays in each nostril 2–3 min before breastfeeding or pumping of the breasts
Ergot Derivatives	
ergonovine maleate (Ergotrate Maleate)	Postpartum bleeding: 0.2 mg IM initially; repeat in 2–4 h if needed for maximum of 5 doses; or 0.2–0.4 mg PO q6–12 h for 2 days
methylergonovine maleate (Methergine)	Control of uterine hemorrhage: 0.2 mg IV infused for 60 sec or more; may dilute with 5 mL 0.9% NaCl
Abortifacients	
dinoprostone (Prostin E2, prostaglandin E$_2$)	Second-trimester pregnancy, intrauterine fetal death up to 28 wk: 20-mg suppository high in the posterior vaginal fornix; repeat q3–5h until abortion is complete

Table 64–1. Oxytocics and Oxytocin Antagonists *Continued*

DRUG	DOSAGE
hypertonic (20%) sodium chloride	Abortion after 16 wk gestation: up to 250 mL slowly instilled by amniocentesis at approximately 1 mL/min (after aspiration of an equal amount of amniotic fluid)
Oxytocin Antagonists, Uterine Relaxants, and Tocolytics	
ritodrine hydrochloride (Yutopar)	IV infusion: 0.1 mg/min until contractions stop or until the maximal infusion rate of 0.35 mg/min is reached; continue for 12 h after labor is stopped; PO therapy is begun 30 min before termination of IV therapy PO: 10 mg q2h for 24 h, then 10–20 mg q4–6h to maximal dose of 120 mg qd; continued as long as suppression of preterm labor is desired; if contractions recur, IV treatment is reinstated
terbutaline sulfate (Brethine, Bricanyl)	IV: initiated at 10 mcg/min; gradually increased to 80 mcg/min PO: 2.5 mg q4–6h as long as suppression of labor is desired
magnesium sulfate	Initial dose: 2–4 g (4–8 mL of 50% solution) by slow IV bolus in 5 min Maintenance dose: 1–2 g hourly as an infusion of 8 mL 50% solution to 230 mL D5W; arrest of labor is achieved at magnesium plasma levels of 4–7 mEq/L; higher levels may inhibit cardiac and neurological function

OXYTOCIN

ACTIONS AND USES Oxytocin (Pitocin, Syntocinon) ▲▲▲▲▲▲▲▲▲▲▲▲▲▲▲ may be used in many different situations. There are times when the physician decides to induce (or initiate) labor artificially. Some reasons for doing this may be prolonged rupture of fetal membranes, post-term pregnancy, placental insufficiency, pregnancy-induced hypertension, induction of a therapeutic abortion, or abortion for a fetal demise (an infant that has died in the uterus). Also, there are times when labor begins spontaneously but the contractions do not develop the normal pattern of frequency, intensity, or duration. The physician may then decide to augment (stimulate or intensify) the contractions. After delivery, if the uterus does not contract sufficiently to control bleeding from the placental site, the physician must initiate measures to prevent or control postpartum hemorrhage.

N U R S I N G   A L E R T
▼▼▼▼▼▼▼▼▼▼▼▼▼▼▼▼▼▼▼▼▼▼▼▼▼▼▼▼▼▼▼▼

Because medications given to the pregnant woman cross the placental barrier and often affect the fetus, situations involving a live, term pregnancy require more assessments and precautionary measures.

▲▲▲▲▲▲▲▲▲▲▲▲▲▲▲▲▲▲▲▲▲▲▲▲▲▲▲▲▲▲▲▲

Adverse effects include nausea, vomiting, hypertension, tachycardia, and arrhythmias with hypotension. Tetanic uterine contractions may also occur and may result in fetal distress, abruptio placentae, or ruptured uterus. Edema, oliguria, or anuria indicates water intoxication and may lead to convulsions and coma. Allergic reactions are possible. Infants may experience bradycardia, tachycardia, hypoxia, and anoxia during the labor. Hyperbilirubinemia may occur in the infant after delivery.

Induction and Augmentation

ASSESSMENT Before induction or augmentation, the ▲▲▲▲▲▲▲▲▲ physician must determine lie, presentation, and position of the infant and adequacy of the maternal pelvis. The cervix must be assessed to see whether it is "ripe" or ready for induction. Be aware of the physician's findings.

Assess the chart or ask the patient for a history of previous uterine or cervical surgery because this may predispose to uterine rupture. Assess the number of previous pregnancies. Mothers who are considered grand multiparas are also at risk for the complication of uterine rupture.

Assess the history and the mother's abdomen for size of the baby and presence of twin pregnancy (or other multiples). Assess for the presence of polyhydramnios (excessive amniotic fluid), which will also predispose her to uterine rupture.

Assess baseline vital signs of the mother, including the temperature, pulse, respirations, and blood pressure. Assess the fetal heart rate and the frequency, intensity, and duration of any contractions. Also be aware of the reason for induction to anticipate and plan appropriate nursing interventions.

PLANNING AND IMPLEMENTATION Be aware of appro-
▲▲▲▲▲▲▲▲▲▲▲▲▲▲▲▲▲▲▲▲▲▲▲▲▲▲ priate dosages and
precautions.

N U R S I N G   A L E R T
▼▼▼▼▼▼▼▼▼▼▼▼▼▼▼▼▼▼▼▼▼▼▼▼▼▼▼▼▼▼▼▼

Be aware of the physician's whereabouts in case of a problem with mother or baby.

▲▲▲▲▲▲▲▲▲▲▲▲▲▲▲▲▲▲▲▲▲▲▲▲▲▲▲▲▲▲▲▲

Monitor vital signs, fetal heart rate, and uterine contractions every 15 minutes (or more frequently if necessary) during the time of incremental increases in the rate of infusion. Report variances in vital signs from baseline data. In the event of changes in maternal or fetal vital signs, turn the mother to her left side to increase blood flow to the placenta. Oxygen may be necessary.

N U R S I N G   A L E R T
▼▼▼▼▼▼▼▼▼▼▼▼▼▼▼▼▼▼▼▼▼▼▼▼▼▼▼▼▼▼▼▼

Blood pressures should not be taken during a uterine contraction. They may vary by as much as 20 mm Hg. Take blood pressures during the relaxation phase of the uterine contraction.

▲▲▲▲▲▲▲▲▲▲▲▲▲▲▲▲▲▲▲▲▲▲▲▲▲▲▲▲▲▲▲▲

If the duration of contractions becomes longer than 90 seconds, turn the mother on her left side to increase blood flow to the placenta. Report this symptom immediately. Oxygen may be necessary. Oxytocin infusion will be stopped until normal uterine activity resumes and then slowly increased again.

N U R S I N G   A L E R T

▼▼▼▼▼▼▼▼▼▼▼▼▼▼▼▼▼▼▼▼▼▼▼▼▼▼▼▼▼▼▼▼

Magnesium sulfate should be available as the antidote for tetanic contractions.

▲▲▲▲▲▲▲▲▲▲▲▲▲▲▲▲▲▲▲▲▲▲▲▲▲▲▲▲▲▲▲▲

If nausea and vomiting occur, turn the mother's head to the side or elevate the head of the bed. Stay with her to prevent aspiration.

Monitor intake, output, and edema. Report edema, oliguria, or anuria immediately.

Electronic fetal monitors should be used to assist in the monitoring of the fetus and the uterine activity.

If the mother's and baby's conditions are stable, frequency of assessments may be decreased after normal labor is established if institutional policy allows this.

After delivery, monitor the infant for hyperbilirubinemia. Report jaundice of the skin and sclera to the pediatrician.

EVALUATION Compare maternal blood pressure, pulse, ▲▲▲▲▲▲▲▲▲▲ and respirations and fetal heart rates with baseline assessments. Monitor uterine contractions for frequency, intensity, and duration. Monitor intake, output, and edema.

Postpartum Hemorrhage

Intravenous or intramuscular oxytocin may be used after delivery to cause a firm uterine contraction for control of bleeding from the placental site.

ASSESSMENT Postpartum assessments are primarily ▲▲▲▲▲▲▲▲▲▲ for shock and hemorrhage. Assess vital signs, fundus, and lochia at least every 15 minutes for the first hour or two, hourly for 1 to 2 hours, then every 4 hours or according to institutional policy. Also assess color and warmth of skin.

PLANNING AND IMPLEMENTATION Because the uterus ▲▲▲▲▲▲▲▲▲▲▲▲▲▲▲▲▲▲▲▲▲▲▲ is empty, there is no risk of rupture. Monitor the fundus for level, firmness, and position. The fundus should be firm, at the umbilicus or below, and in the midline. If it is not, massage it and manipulate it until it is. Report variances.

N U R S I N G   A L E R T

▼▼▼▼▼▼▼▼▼▼▼▼▼▼▼▼▼▼▼▼▼▼▼▼▼▼▼▼▼▼▼▼

A full or distended urinary bladder raises and displaces the uterus from midline position. Encourage the patient to keep the bladder empty.

▲▲▲▲▲▲▲▲▲▲▲▲▲▲▲▲▲▲▲▲▲▲▲▲▲▲▲▲▲▲▲▲

Lochia is monitored for amount and color. Saturation of more than one perineal pad per hour during the first 2 hours after delivery is abnormal and must be reported. Report bright red blood and clots as well as a constant trickle of bright lochia when the fundus is firm.

EVALUATION Compare vital signs with baseline find-▲▲▲▲▲▲▲▲▲▲ ings. Skin should be pink, warm, and dry. The fundus should be firm and in the midline, at or below the umbilicus. Lochia should be moderate and without clots.

N U R S I N G   A L E R T

▼▼▼▼▼▼▼▼▼▼▼▼▼▼▼▼▼▼▼▼▼▼▼▼▼▼▼▼▼▼▼▼

Oxytocin may be used in the first, second, third, and fourth (recovery) stages of labor.

▲▲▲▲▲▲▲▲▲▲▲▲▲▲▲▲▲▲▲▲▲▲▲▲▲▲▲▲▲▲▲▲

Syntocinon Nasal Spray

ACTIONS AND USES Syntocinon nasal spray is used to ▲▲▲▲▲▲▲▲▲▲▲▲▲▲ stimulate "let-down" or ejection of milk in lactating patients.

Adverse effects are rare. Hypertension may possibly occur if the patient is susceptible to this problem and if she uses the spray frequently.

ASSESSMENT Assess for the presence of milk, proper ▲▲▲▲▲▲▲▲▲▲ positioning of the infant, and proper breast-feeding techniques. Assess blood pressure and document baseline data.

PLANNING AND IMPLEMENTATION The patient should ▲▲▲▲▲▲▲▲▲▲▲▲▲▲▲▲▲▲▲▲▲▲▲▲▲▲▲▲▲▲ be in an upright position. She should blow the nose to clear the nasal passages before use. One to two sprays are used in each nostril, 2 to 3 minutes before breast-feeding or pumping of the breasts.

EVALUATION Ask the mother if she felt let-down. Ask ▲▲▲▲▲▲▲▲▲▲ whether milk was seen dripping from the breasts. Monitor the infant for signs of contentment after feeding. Breasts will feel softer after feeding or pumping.

ERGOT DERIVATIVES

The ergot derivatives are obtained from a fungus that infects the seed of the rye grain. The ergot alkaloids ergonovine maleate (Ergotrate Maleate) and methylergonovine maleate (Methergine) are potent uterine muscle stimulants.

ACTIONS AND USES Ergot derivatives are used to control or prevent postpartum hemorrhage in cases of uterine atony. They act rapidly and efficiently. Within 1 minute after intravenous administration, 2 to 3 minutes after intramuscular administration, and a few minutes after oral administration, firm tetanic contractions of the uterus will occur.

Because of the rapidity and force of action, these drugs would cause adverse effects on the fetus, so they are contraindicated during labor. Adverse effects on the mother may include headaches, palpitations, chest pain, dizziness, nausea, and numbness or tingling of the extremities.

NURSING ALERT

Ergot derivatives are to be used only during the third or fourth stage of labor after the delivery of the infant.

ASSESSMENT Assess vital signs, height and firmness of the uterus, amount and color of lochia, and color and condition of the skin. Document these as baseline data. Because ergot derivatives also cause constriction of blood vessels, review the chart for a history of hypertension or vascular diseases, such as Raynaud's or Buerger's diseases.

PLANNING AND IMPLEMENTATION Intravenous solutions are stored in the refrigerator, but daily supplies may be kept at cool room temperature for 60 to 90 days. Store in tightly closed, light-resistant containers. Discard the solution if it is discolored.

Monitor, report, and chart uterine level and firmness and amount and color of lochia.

Remember that caudal and spinal anesthesias potentiate hypertensive and cardiovascular effects.

Tell patients to report the subjective symptoms of headaches, palpitations, chest pain, dizziness, nausea, and numbness or tingling of extremities. Report these to the physician.

Monitor for nausea and vomiting. Take measures as necessary to prevent aspiration.

Monitor extremities for color, temperature, and capillary refill. Report symptoms of vascular impairment immediately.

Tell patients to expect uterine cramping but to report if it is severe. Severe cramps indicate that the dose should be reduced.

EVALUATION A firm fundus located at or below the umbilicus, a decrease in lochia and clots, and fewer complaints of uterine cramping indicate that the drug is being effective.

ABORTIFACIENTS

Drugs used to cause abortions are called abortifacients. Abortions are performed in cases of intrauterine fetal death, benign hydatidiform mole, missed or incomplete spontaneous abortions, and personal choice. The uterus is usually not responsive to oxytocin or the ergot derivatives until several weeks into the second or even the third trimester of pregnancy. Other drugs that may be effective earlier are the prostaglandins and hypertonic (20%) sodium chloride.

Prostaglandins are hormone-like substances produced by various tissues of the body. Some of these have actions resembling those of the hormone oxytocin.

Dinoprostone

ACTIONS AND USES Dinoprostone (Prostin E2, prostaglandin E_2) is a synthetic prostaglandin used for abortions up to 28 weeks of gestation. It causes the uterus to contract in a manner similar to spontaneous labor.

Dinoprostone vaginal gel is sometimes used in term pregnancy to produce cervical softening and dilatation before induction or augmentation of labor with oxytocin.

Adverse effects include nausea, vomiting, diarrhea, fever, diaphoresis, headache, hypertension or hypotension, dizziness, flushing, tachycardia, dyspnea, joint pain, bronchospasm, and rash.

ASSESSMENT Assess the chart for the reason for use and assess the patient's emotional state. Knowledge of the diagnosis is necessary to give appropriate emotional care to the patient.

Assess the chart for a history of glaucoma, epilepsy,

allergies or asthma, and migraines that might be aggravated by this medication.

Assess the chart for a history of previous uterine surgery because the scar may rupture.

Assess baseline vital signs of the mother and assess the fetal heart rate if this is a live pregnancy. Assess vaginal drainage if this is a missed or incomplete spontaneous abortion or hydatidiform mole. Document your findings as baseline data.

PLANNING AND IMPLEMENTATION Knowledge of the ▲▲▲▲▲▲▲▲▲▲▲▲▲▲▲▲▲▲▲▲▲▲▲▲▲▲▲▲ diagnosis helps the nurse to anticipate the appearance of the products of conception and prepare the patient for this if necessary. Those with an unexpected fetal demise need assistance with stages of grief; those with an elective abortion may need support in their decision. Monitor the patient's emotional state to determine appropriate therapeutic communication.

Suppositories are stored in the freezer and must be removed and warmed at room temperature in their foil wrapping. Suppositories are inserted high in the posterior fornix of the vagina. Nurses must be knowledgeable about licensure restrictions and institutional restrictions concerning who may administer these medications. Instruct the patient to remain supine for at least 10 minutes to allow the suppository to melt.

Warn patients that stimulation of the gastrointestinal tract usually occurs. Institute supportive measures if nausea, vomiting, and diarrhea occur. The physician sometimes orders premedication with antiemetics and antidiarrheal agents.

Fever occurs in approximately 50% of the patients. This may be accompanied by diaphoresis. Fluids should be increased, and sponging may be necessary.

Monitor for adverse effects and report these to the physician.

Observe for onset of labor. Suppositories may be repeated every 2 to 4 hours with a physician's order.

Monitor progress of labor. Be aware that products of conception will be delivered as soon as there is adequate dilatation and effacement of the cervix, not necessarily after 10 cm as with a term pregnancy.

EVALUATION Compare vital signs with baseline assess-▲▲▲▲▲▲▲▲▲▲ ments. Evaluate effectiveness of uterine contractions. Evaluate emotional status of the patient to determine effectiveness of support measures.

Hypertonic (20%) Sodium Chloride

ACTIONS AND USES Hypertonic saline solution is used ▲▲▲▲▲▲▲▲▲▲▲▲▲▲ to abort live pregnancies or intrauterine fetal deaths after 16 weeks' gestation.

The physician aspirates up to 250 mL of amniotic fluid by amniocentesis and slowly instills an equal amount of sodium chloride solution (approximately 1 mL per minute). The solution acts as an oxytocic, and labor usually begins within several hours or days. The dose may be repeated in 48 hours if labor has not begun. Patients who fail to respond to the second dose may be given oxytocin, but the two drugs are not given together.

Adverse effects occur if the solution is accidentally injected into a blood vessel. Hypernatremia with severe dehydration and increased intravascular volume could occur.

ASSESSMENT Before the procedure, assess the chart for ▲▲▲▲▲▲▲▲▲▲ any history of blood disorders, cardiac disease, hypertension, epilepsy, renal impairment, or uterine surgery. These may be contraindications for the procedure. Assess vital signs and document them as baseline data.

PLANNING AND IMPLEMENTATION Direct the patient to ▲▲▲▲▲▲▲▲▲▲▲▲▲▲▲▲▲▲▲▲▲▲▲▲▲▲ drink at least 2 liters of water on the day of the procedure to improve salt excretion.

If intravascular injection occurs, symptoms are usually evident within 1 minute. Tell the patient to report any sudden sensation of heat, pain, burning, thirst, ringing in the ears, or headache during instillation of solution. Monitor for tachycardia, hypotension, flushed face, mental confusion, or vomiting. Instillation should be stopped immediately to prevent cerebral dehydration and death.

Some hospitals or clinics may allow the patient to leave the facility and return when labor begins.

Physicians usually allow pain medications to be administered liberally during labor because there is no concern for fetal injury.

Monitor labor as with any other patient. Continue to observe for complications of pulmonary edema, pulmonary embolism, and coagulation disorders. Offer emotional support as indicated by the situation.

EVALUATION Compare vital signs with baseline as-▲▲▲▲▲▲▲▲▲▲ sessments. Monitor intake and output. Evaluate the emotional status of the patient.

ANTAGONISTS, UTERINE RELAXANTS, AND TOCOLYTICS

During pregnancy, there is a progressive increase of the blood level of natural oxytocin. This normally prompts labor to begin about 38 to 40 weeks after conception. Sometimes, however, labor begins early and poses a risk to the fetus. Any labor after 20 weeks but before the beginning of the 38th week is called premature labor. The risk to the fetus depends on its gestation. Obviously, the infant who is closer to term is usually more developed and therefore has a better chance of survival. Most infant deaths that are not related to birth defects are due to prematurity. Since the 1980s, it has become possible to stop many of these premature labors, allowing the pregnancy to progress to term and thus decreasing the fetal mortality rate.

Several drugs are currently used to inhibit uterine activity and stop preterm labor. These drugs are often referred to as uterine relaxants or tocolytics. Commonly used drugs are ritodrine hydrochloride (Yutopar) and terbutaline sulfate (Brethine, Bricanyl).

ACTIONS AND USES The main drugs being used are classified as beta-adrenergic receptor stimulants. They act primarily on the beta$_2$-receptors to relax the uterine, bronchial, and vascular smooth muscle. The effect on the uterus is to decrease the frequency, intensity, and duration of the contractions. These drugs are used when there is no underlying cause for the premature labor that might cause further problems for the fetus if the labor is stopped.

Sometimes, especially in large doses, the beta$_1$-receptors are stimulated, causing maternal and fetal tachycardia and arrhythmias as adverse effects. Serum glucose and insulin levels may also increase. Tremors and feelings of inner tremulousness or anxiety are fairly common. Nausea, vomiting, diaphoresis, tinnitus, drowsiness, or restlessness may occur.

ASSESSMENT Assess the history to determine the gestation of the pregnancy. These drugs are contraindicated before the 20th week. Review the patient's history for any indication of cardiovascular disease, hypertension, hyperthyroidism, diabetes mellitus, asthma, or allergies. These disease processes may be potentiated by these medications.

Assess vital signs and the fetal heart rate. Assess the frequency, intensity, and duration of uterine contractions. Document these as baseline data.

Assess the chart for significant laboratory results, such as serum glucose levels, electrolyte values, and hematocrit.

PLANNING AND IMPLEMENTATION An intravenous (IV) infusion is started, and the patient is given approximately 500 mL in 15 to 20 minutes. The medication is then diluted in another IV solution and administered per infusion pump as a secondary IV line according to the physi-

cian's order. If there are no serious adverse effects, the dose is usually increased every 10 minutes until the desired effect is achieved or the maximal dose is reached. Monitor the IV flow carefully. Monitor vital signs frequently during this time.

The mother should be positioned on her left side with pillows placed for support and comfort. Teach the patient and her support person to use relaxation techniques, such as breathing and massage, but *not* uterine massage because it may increase uterine contractions.

Uterine contractions and fetal heart rate should be monitored continuously by electronic fetal monitor.

Monitor maternal vital signs frequently and as ordered by the physician.

Physicians may order patients to be NPO or to receive ice chips only in case the medication does not work and the labor progresses.

Monitor patients with diabetes carefully for symptoms of hyperglycemia or hypoglycemia.

Report tremors and feelings of inner tremulousness or anxiety. The physician may order that the dose be decreased.

After labor has ceased, the physician may order oral medication. Oral medications are given with food or milk to decrease the frequency of nausea and vomiting. The oral doses are initiated *before* the discontinuation of the IV infusion to allow time for the oral medication to take effect. Follow orders carefully.

After the infusion is discontinued, monitor for recurrence •of labor. Teach patients to report any uterine cramping.

The patient's activity is progressively increased. Dizziness and hypotension may occur with position changes, so teach patients to dangle before rising. Assist with ambulation as necessary. Monitor laboratory values for evidence of hypokalemia or other electrolyte imbalances. Teach patients to report symptoms of muscle cramps, weakness, tremors, and nausea. Monitor for confusion, lethargy, or anxiety. Monitor intake, output, and daily weights. Monitor for edema and teach patients to report symptoms of edema, such as tight rings and swollen feet.

Pulmonary edema may occur if the patient is also receiving corticosteroids. Monitor as before and assess lung sounds. Teach patients to report if a cough develops.

After delivery, infants are monitored for hypoglycemia and electrolyte imbalance.

EVALUATION Compare maternal vital signs and fetal heart rate with baseline assessments. Monitor uterine contractions for decrease or increase in frequency, intensity, and duration. Compare laboratory values with baseline values. Compare weights with baseline findings.

Magnesium Sulfate

Magnesium sulfate, which is classified as a central nervous system depressant and anticonvulsant, is also classed with the tocolytic drugs. It may be administered by the intramuscular (IM) or intravenous (IV) routes.

ACTIONS AND USES In obstetrics, magnesium sulfate is
▲▲▲▲▲▲▲▲▲▲▲▲▲▲▲ sometimes used to control the complications of pregnancy-induced hypertension, preeclampsia and eclampsia, and preterm labor after 20 weeks. It is also used as an antidote for oxytocin when the side effect of tetanic contractions occurs.

By depressing the central nervous system, there is a relaxation effect on the smooth muscles of the body. This can be effective in lowering blood pressure and in relaxing uterine musculature.

Adverse effects include depression of the central nervous system and oliguria or anuria of mother and infant. Cardiopulmonary arrest may result. An intense feeling of heat and flushed skin are often experienced when initial IV doses are administered. IM doses cause pain and irritation of the tissues.

ASSESSMENT Assessments vary somewhat, depending
▲▲▲▲▲▲▲▲▲▲ on the use and the expected effect of the drug. In all cases, assess the mother's vital signs to establish baseline data. Use of an electronic fetal monitor is strongly recommended to monitor the fetal heart rate and variability. The frequency, intensity, and duration of uterine contractions should be monitored by the electronic fetal monitor or by palpation. The monitor should be in place before initial administration of the magnesium sulfate to establish a baseline for comparison.

If the drug is being used to treat pregnancy-induced hypertension or preeclampsia, obtain a baseline weight and assess for peripheral edema.

Assess level of consciousness and reflexes. Document findings as baseline data.

Assess the chart for serum magnesium, calcium, and electrolyte levels.

PLANNING AND IMPLEMENTATION Initiate safety pre-
▲▲▲▲▲▲▲▲▲▲▲▲▲▲▲▲▲▲▲▲▲▲▲▲▲▲▲ cautions. Because this drug depresses the central nervous system, reflexes, judgment, and responses may be slowed. Keep side rails up at all times. Assist patients if they are permitted to ambulate. If magnesium sulfate is being used for pregnancy-induced hypertension, preeclampsia, or eclampsia, seizure precautions should already have been initiated.

Monitor level of consciousness, reflexes, maternal vital signs, uterine contractions, and fetal heart rate and variability. Anticipate a decrease in all of these. Check the physician's order or institutional protocols for guidelines about the frequency of assessments and minimal levels to be maintained.

Monitor intake and output. Check the physician's order or institutional protocols for minimal amounts of urine output per hour. Expect minimal outputs to average 30 mL per hour or 100 mL in 3 hours. If hourly outputs are ordered, request an order for a Foley catheter.

The IV route is the usual route of administration. The magnesium is usually run as a secondary line, so the infusion can be slowed or stopped while the primary line is maintained for administration of emergency drugs should side effects or other complications occur. An infusion pump should be used to safely monitor the infusion rate. Sometimes an initial bolus of the drug is administered by IV push. Follow legal and institutional restrictions for IV push procedures. Reassure the patient that an intense feeling of heat and flushed skin are often experienced initially.

Magnesium sulfate is occasionally administered by the IM route. Follow standard procedures for drugs that are irritating to tissues. A 2 1/2- to 3-inch needle length may be necessary to administer the medication deep into the tissues. The dose is often ordered as 4 to 5 g of 50% solution given in divided doses into each buttock.

Severe depression of the central nervous system may cause cardiopulmonary arrest. Cardiopulmonary resuscitation procedures may be necessary. Be knowledgeable of the antidote calcium gluconate, which may be ordered if toxic effects of magnesium occur.

Notify the nursery when magnesium sulfate therapy is initiated because the drug will affect the fetus. At delivery, the infant may need resuscitation because of the depressant effects on the central nervous system.

If labor progresses or if complications occur, anticipate the possibility of a cesarean delivery.

EVALUATION Compare level of consciousness, reflexes,
▲▲▲▲▲▲▲▲▲▲ maternal vital signs, and fetal heart rate and variability with baseline assessments. Check the physician's orders and institutional protocols for frequency of evaluations. Monitor uterine contractions for changes in frequency, intensity, and duration. Compare laboratory values with baseline values. Monitor outputs and report diminished amounts according to the physician's orders and institutional protocols. Compare weights and presence of edema with baseline findings.

After delivery, monitor infants for central nervous system depression and the need for resuscitation. Evaluate magnesium and calcium levels and compare them with normal newborn levels. The physician will determine whether IV calcium gluconate is necessary.

E X E R C I S E S

LEARNING ACTIVITIES

1. Write a nursing care plan for a 16-year-old primigravida who is to have labor induced with IV Pitocin because of a 43-week post-term pregnancy.

2. Ask a classmate to role play a multigravida labor patient. You portray the labor nurse. The physician has ordered Pitocin augmentation because of her irregular pattern of contractions. Mom feels that continued ambulation will stimulate her labor contractions and is willing to do so with her IV on a mobile pole. Explain why you want her to return to bed to have continuous fetal monitoring.

3. Explain why the ergot derivatives are not used during first and second stages of labor.

4. Why should a patient be assessed for nausea and vomiting during induction of labor with dinoprostone (Prostin E2, prostaglandin E_2 suppositories)?

5. The patient is receiving magnesium sulfate intravenously for treatment of her pregnancy-induced hypertension. Prepare a nursing care plan that reflects knowledge of the drug as it relates to the condition.

MISCELLANEOUS DRUGS USED IN OBSTETRICS

LEARNING OBJECTIVES

After studying this chapter, you should be able to:

1. Discuss the actions of each of the listed drugs.

2. State the uses of each of these drugs for mothers and newborns.

3. List the adverse effects of each of these drugs.

4. Prepare an appropriate plan of care for a patient receiving any of these drugs.

DRUGS YOU WILL LEARN ABOUT IN THIS CHAPTER

calcium (calcium lactate, calcium gluconate)

vitamin K, phytonadione (AquaMEPHYTON, Konakion)

RhoGAM

naloxone HCl (Narcan)

Drugs belonging to several different classifications are frequently used during pregnancy, during labor and delivery, and in the admission nursery. These drugs and their dosages are listed in Table 65–1.

CALCIUM

Calcium is a mineral that is important to homeostasis of many of the body systems. Calcium deficiencies during pregnancy may result in osteoporosis and periodontal disease in the pregnant woman and rickets in the infant. When serum levels decline, tetany or convulsions may occur.

There is a narrow margin of safety between the amount of this element necessary to maintain therapeutic blood levels and the amount that may cause toxic effects. The body has limited ability to excrete excess chemicals, and harmful levels may occur within a short time.

ACTIONS AND USES In pregnancy, calcium lactate is ▲▲▲▲▲▲▲▲▲▲▲▲▲▲▲▲ often ordered as part of a multivitamin and mineral supplement to replace maternal nutrients depleted by the developing infant. When it is taken as directed, there should not be any adverse effects except possibly nausea, indigestion, constipation, or gastrointestinal hemorrhage.

Calcium gluconate may be ordered intravenously (IV) as the antidote for toxic effects of magnesium in pregnant women being treated for pregnancy-induced hypertension, preeclampsia, or eclampsia and in their newborn infants. Calcium is a necessary element for proper muscle response to nerve stimulation. In this situation, its desired effect is to increase the contractility of cardiac muscles and increase cardiac output.

Emergency treatment in adults requires the use of 500 mg to 1 g IV calcium, but there can be serious side effects during its administration. Hypotension, syncope, bradycardia, arrhythmias, and cardiac arrest may result. Patients may complain of heat waves during IV administration. If the IV solution infiltrates, necrosis and sloughing of tissues often result.

The intramuscular (IM) route is used only if the patient's condition has deteriorated to circulatory collapse and no IV site is accessible. In adults, the site should be the gluteus medius muscle; in infants, the lateral thigh muscle is used. Burning, necrosis, and sloughing of tissues may result from IM injection. Cellulitis and soft tissue calcification may also occur.

Table 65-1. Obstetric Drugs

DRUG	DOSAGE
calcium (calcium lactate, calcium gluconate)	500 mg to 1 g IV; repeat q 1–3 days prn as determined by serum calcium levels
vitamin K, phytonadione (AquaMEPHYTON, Konakion)	0.5–1 mg SC or IM immediately after birth; repeat in 6–8 h if needed
RhoGAM	1 vial IM up to 72 h after delivery or abortion
naloxone hydrochloride (Narcan)	Adults: 0.4–2 mg IV, SC, or IM; may repeat q 2–3 min as needed, up to a total of 10 mg; if no response is noted, other causes for the respiratory depression should be investigated Neonates: 0.01 mg/kg into the umbilical vein, SC, or IM; repeat in 2–3 min for a total of 3 doses

ASSESSMENT Assess the maternal vital signs and the ▲▲▲▲▲▲▲▲▲▲ fetal heart rate. Assess Chvostek's sign in the mother. Tap the cheek near the ear over the facial nerve. Twitching of the nose, mouth, and eye on the side tapped is a sign of calcium deficiency. (Chvostek's sign is normally present in newborns, so this test is not significant until about 2 months of age.) Document findings as baseline data.

PLANNING AND IMPLEMENTATION During administra-▲▲▲▲▲▲▲▲▲▲▲▲▲▲▲▲▲▲▲▲▲▲▲▲▲▲▲▲▲ tion, cardiac arrhythmias and bradycardia may occur and lead to cardiac arrest. The drug is administered slowly, and the physician may order cardiac monitoring during administration. Personnel should be prepared to begin cardiopulmonary resuscitation if necessary. Continue to monitor maternal vital signs and fetal heart rate throughout administration. Reassure the patient that feelings of flushing and heat waves are normal occurrences.

The patient should remain recumbent for a short while after administration. Further dosage is based on serum calcium levels.

Frequently monitor the IV site for infiltration because necrosis and sloughing of tissues may result. If the IV solution infiltrates, stop the infusion immediately and notify the supervisor.

After birth, monitor the infant's serum calcium levels because they may be low also. IV calcium gluconate may be needed.

Teach patients who are taking oral calcium to monitor stools. Dark stools may indicate bleeding. Instruct patients to report this to the physician.

EVALUATION Compare serum calcium levels with nor-▲▲▲▲▲▲▲▲▲▲▲ mal values. Compare vital signs with baseline assessments. Monitor Chvostek's sign. Observe for tetany or convulsions if calcium levels are low.

VITAMIN K

Vitamin K is a fat-soluble vitamin used by the liver to manufacture prothrombin and other clotting factors. It is ingested in foods but requires digestible fat and bile salts in the digestive tract for absorption to occur in the small intestine. Newborns have immature intestines and also do not ingest the appropriate food sources. One pharmaceutical preparation of vitamin K is phytonadione (AquaMEPHYTON, Konakion).

ACTIONS AND USES Because of the trauma that the ▲▲▲▲▲▲▲▲▲▲▲▲▲▲▲▲ infant incurs during the delivery process, many physicians order vitamin K as a prophylactic measure to prevent neonatal hemorrhage. An injection of phytonadione is administered to the infant shortly after birth to assist with clotting.

In newborns, the most commonly occurring adverse effects are a nodule at the injection site, flushed appearance, and tachycardia.

ASSESSMENT Obtain vital signs in the delivery room to ▲▲▲▲▲▲▲▲▲▲ establish the baseline for comparison. Assess the infant for signs of hemorrhage. The most likely sites in the newborn are the umbilical cord, the head, and the skin. Check the cord clamp or tie as soon as the infant arrives in the nursery and assess for bruising or petechiae. The head circumference is usually obtained in the delivery room or on admission to the nursery. Assess the fontanelles for tension. The initial cephalocaudal assessment provides the baseline data for later comparisons.

PLANNING AND IMPLEMENTATION In the nursery, in-
▲▲▲▲▲▲▲▲▲▲▲▲▲▲▲▲▲▲▲▲▲▲▲▲▲▲▲ itially take vital
signs at frequent intervals and compare them with the
baseline assessments. Check the cord frequently for
bleeding. Assess skin every shift and compare with
baseline findings. If new bruises or petechiae are
noted, report them. Assess fontanelles every shift for
signs of tension. If the infant shows irritability or
other signs of increasing cerebral pressure, the head
circumference may be checked and compared with the
baseline measurement. Neuro checks are then indicated. If a circumcision is performed, monitor the site
for bleeding. Document all abnormal observations and
report them to the physician.

EVALUATION Compare assessments with baseline as-
▲▲▲▲▲▲▲▲▲▲ sessments. Monitor any laboratory values, such as blood counts, hemoglobin levels, or
platelet counts, and compare with normal values.

RHOGAM

RhoGAM is classified as an immune globulin. Immune globulins are prepared from serum of people
who have immunity to a particular antigen. They are
expected to confer passive immunity to persons exposed to a particular antigen. Passive immunity
confers immediate protection, but it is short-acting.
RhoGAM confers passive immunity to pregnant
women experiencing Rh incompatibility.

The Rh factor is a protein attached to the red blood
cells of some people. These persons are said to be
Rh-positive. Those who do not have this protein are
said to be Rh-negative. If Rh-positive blood is introduced into the bloodstream of an Rh-negative person,
the Rh factor is a foreign protein or antigen to that
person. The antigen stimulates the production of
antibodies, which attempt to defend the body against
this foreign invader. When this antibody production
occurs, the person is said to be sensitized.

When the placenta separates from the uterus after
delivery of the infant, it is possible for a small amount
of the fetal blood to enter the maternal blood vessels
at the placental site. If the mother is Rh-negative and
the infant is Rh-positive, these Rh-positive red blood
cells will stimulate the production of antibodies
against the Rh factor. These antibodies do not harm
the red blood cells of the Rh-negative mother.

However, if this sensitized Rh-negative mother
becomes pregnant with an Rh-positive infant, these
antibodies can cross the placenta and hemolyze
(destroy) the infant's red blood cells. This can cause
erythroblastosis fetalis or newborn hemolytic disease,
which may be fatal for the infant.

ACTIONS AND USES RhoGAM confers passive immu-
▲▲▲▲▲▲▲▲▲▲▲▲▲ nity to an Rh-negative mother who
is pregnant with an Rh-positive infant. The drug is
used to prevent sensitization of the Rh-negative
mother to the Rh factor on her Rh-positive infant's
blood cells.

RhoGAM is administered intramuscularly. The
most common adverse effects are irritation at the
injection site and a slight temperature elevation.
However, remember that this immunization is prepared from a serum, and anaphylaxis is possible.

ASSESSMENT Be aware of the patient's history. Assess
▲▲▲▲▲▲▲▲▲▲ the chart for her blood type. During
history taking, ask whether she has had any previous
Rh-positive pregnancies or any abortions that could
have caused her to build antibodies against the Rh
factor. Ask her if she has ever received a blood
transfusion because she may also have been sensitized
during a transfusion accident if Rh-positive blood was
infused. Assess for a history of allergies or serum
reactions.

PLANNING AND IMPLEMENTATION Many obstetricians
▲▲▲▲▲▲▲▲▲▲▲▲▲▲▲▲▲▲▲▲▲▲▲▲▲▲▲▲▲▲ order administration of a prophylactic dose to the woman at 28 weeks'
gestation. This is usually half the normal postpartum dose.

When a woman is admitted to the obstetric unit,
note her Rh factor on the chart. Communicate her
status to the delivering physician and the nursery
personnel.

At delivery, a blood sample is often obtained from
the blood of the infant's cord. The baby's Rh factor is
determined, and a test called a Coombs' test is
performed. This test indicates whether antibodies
against the Rh factor are present in the infant's
circulation.

If the infant is Rh-positive and the Coombs' test
result is positive for antibodies, then the mother is
already sensitized and RhoGAM will not be useful.
Notify the pediatrician of the results and monitor
the infant for complications. Offer emotional support
to the mother during the infant's treatment, which
may include exchange blood transfusions and photo-
therapy.

If the infant is Rh-positive and the Coombs' test
result is negative, then the mother has not been
previously sensitized. RhoGAM is indicated to prevent
any sensitization that may have occurred during this
pregnancy. Report results of the cord blood samples to
the obstetrician. If RhoGAM is ordered, it is to be
given to the mother within 72 hours of delivery.

Check the chart for known allergies. Ask the patient
whether she has ever had a reaction from an immunization or blood product.

Note that people of some religious persuasions, such as Jehovah's Witnesses, Christian Scientists, and others, may object to receiving serum and may refuse this treatment on the basis of their religious beliefs. Be certain that this is discussed with the patient to her satisfaction and that she understands the implications for future pregnancies so she may make an informed choice. Offer to contact her religious advisor if she desires.

Check institutional policies about administration of a serum. Often, two nurses check the serial number on the vial and record the serial number when the injection is charted. The empty vial is often required to be returned to the laboratory and kept until it is determined whether a reaction has taken place.

RhoGAM is to be given intramuscularly, deep into the large muscle mass of the gluteus medius. Observe for side effects.

EVALUATION Verify documentation of physician's order ▲▲▲▲▲▲▲▲▲▲ and documentation that the patient received RhoGAM (or refused it) within 72 hours of delivery.

NALOXONE

Narcotic antagonists are sometimes used to counteract the effects of narcotics. Different drugs act in different ways. Naloxone hydrochloride (Narcan) is particularly useful in known or suspected narcotic-induced respiratory depression in both mothers and infants.

ACTIONS AND USES As you know, many drugs taken by ▲▲▲▲▲▲▲▲▲▲▲▲▲▲▲▲ a pregnant patient have the ability to cross the placental barrier and affect the infant. Unfortunately, some pregnant women do not consider the infant when they are gratifying their own cravings for illegal drugs. Therefore, a patient may be admitted to a labor unit while already being under the influence of an illegal drug or a legal drug that she is abusing. Sometimes a patient experiences an adverse reaction to a narcotic that was administered to help control labor pain or pain after a cesarean birth. Depending on the drug received, the time of its peak action, and the time of delivery, the infant may be born sedated (a condition called asphyxia neonatorum) and need to be resuscitated.

The exact mechanism of the action of naloxone is not known, but it seems to compete for and displace narcotic analgesics from their receptor sites. There appears to be no pharmacological activity if naloxone is administered to a patient who has not taken a narcotic before its administration. This drug is considered the safest of the narcotic antagonists to be administered when the cause of respiratory depression has not been determined.

Adverse effects that may be observed are nausea and vomiting, perspiration, tachypnea, tachycardia, and hypertension. Those patients who are addicted to narcotics may proceed into withdrawal symptoms.

ASSESSMENT Assess vital signs and level of conscious-▲▲▲▲▲▲▲▲▲▲▲ ness in the laboring patient. In the newborn, assessing the Apgar scores gives valuable information about the vital signs, reflexes, and respiratory effort.

PLANNING AND IMPLEMENTATION Be prepared to ad-▲▲▲▲▲▲▲▲▲▲▲▲▲▲▲▲▲▲▲▲▲▲▲▲▲▲▲▲▲▲▲ minister oxygen or perform resuscitation as needed. Improvement should be noted in 1 to 2 minutes, and effects last up to 4 hours. If no response is noted after administration of naloxone, other causes for the respiratory depression should be investigated.

EVALUATION Observe the rate and depth of respira-▲▲▲▲▲▲▲▲▲▲▲ tions and the state of alertness. In the neonate, the Apgar score may be repeated.

E X E R C I S E S

LEARNING ACTIVITIES

1. Explain the rationale for such careful monitoring during IV calcium infusions.

2. The proud new father is observing nursery admission procedures on his first-born son. He becomes anxious when you mention that the physician has ordered the injection of vitamin K (AquaMEPHYTON, Konakion), which you are preparing to administer to the infant. Explain the rationale for this injection.

3. An Rh-negative mom has delivered an Rh-positive infant. She does not understand why you are giving the RhoGAM to her instead of the baby. Explain in a manner to be understood by this 15-year-old patient.

4. Explain to the parents why the pediatrician is giving naloxone (Narcan) to their infant in the delivery room. Apgar scores are 6 and 7, and there are no risk factors listed on the chart.

CONTRACEPTIVE DRUGS

LEARNING OBJECTIVES

After studying this chapter, you should be able to:

1. Discuss the action of the various contraceptive medications listed.

2. Name examples of each type of contraceptive medication.

3. List adverse effects of each type of contraceptive medication.

4. Prepare a teaching plan for a patient seeking counseling for contraceptive medications.

DRUGS YOU WILL LEARN ABOUT IN THIS CHAPTER

Ovulation Control Pill

  Combination type

    Enovid

    Norlestrin

    Ortho-Novum

  Fluctuating progestin levels

    Ortho-Novum 7/7/7

    Tri-Norinyl

medroxyprogesterone acetate suspension (Depo-Provera)

levonorgestrel (Norplant)

Family planning, or the process of determining when to have and when not to have a pregnancy, is an important issue. At present, there is a broad range of contraceptive methods from which to choose. *Personal acceptance* of the method influences the choice and the proper use of the method. Some factors that influence choices are medical problems, comfort in touching the genitalia, convenience in relation to the sexual activity, cost of the medication, and religious beliefs. Patient education should include information about convenience, cost, advantages and disadvantages, pregnancy rate, protection from sexually transmitted diseases, and dangers involved in the use of each method. If cost is a major factor, refer patients to their local health department or community family planning clinic, which are often lower cost. Encourage them to compare prices of products by phoning several local pharmacies.

There is no right or wrong method of birth control. The *best method* is the method accepted and correctly and consistently used.

The only *absolute* method of preventing pregnancy is abstinence. This method is free, has no side effects or dangers, and poses no risk of sexually transmitted diseases.

Other than by abstinence, pregnancy is prevented by methods that (1) prevent ovulation, (2) prevent fertilization of an ovum, or (3) prevent implantation of a fertilized ovum. Drugs that prevent ovulation are listed in Table 66–1.

METHODS THAT PREVENT OVULATION

Methods of contraception to prevent ovulation involve the use of hormones that alter the woman's menstrual cycle and prevent the release of ova from the ovary. The hormones used are estrogen and progesterone. The most commonly used form is the pill or tablet, which is taken orally. You may frequently see this form referred to as a birth control pill or ovulation control pill (OCP).

Table 66-1. Contraceptive Drugs

DRUG	DOSAGE
Combination Type	
Norlestrin 2.5/50	50 mcg ethinyl estradiol, 2.5 mg norethindrone acetate 1 qd × 21 days; off × 7 days or inert pill × 7 days
Ortho-Novum 1/35	35 mcg ethinyl estradiol, 1 mg norethindrone acetate 1 qd × 21 days; off 7 days or inert pill × 7 days
Fluctuating Progestin Levels	
Ortho-Novum 7/7/7	35 mcg ethinyl estradiol with 0.5 mg norethindrone acetate × 7 days; 35 mcg ethinyl estradiol with 0.75 mg norethindrone acetate × 7 days; 35 mcg ethinyl estradiol with 1 mg norethindrone acetate × 7 days; Off × 7 days
Tri-Norinyl	35 mcg ethinyl estradiol with 0.5 mg norethindrone acetate × 7 days; 35 mcg ethinyl estradiol with 1 mg norethindrone acetate × 9 days; 35 mcg ethinyl estradiol with 0.5 mg norethindrone acetate × 5 days; Off × 7 days
medroxyprogesterone acetate suspension (Depo-Provera)	150 mg IM q 3 mo; given within the first 5 days of a normal menstrual cycle or birth of an infant
levonorgestrel (Nor-plant)	6 silicone capsules; 36 mg levonorgestrel SC

Students may wish to review the concept of negative feedback, the normal female menstrual cycle, and the effects and adverse effects of estrogen and of progesterone.

ACTIONS AND USES The OCPs are generally composed of estrogen and one of the synthetic oral forms of progesterone, such as progestin or progestogen. Progesterone itself cannot be given by the oral route because it is inactivated by the digestive enzymes. The OCP acts to suppress or inhibit follicle-stimulating hormone and luteinizing hormone by increasing the blood levels of estrogen and the progestins. In this manner, they interfere with the negative feedback mechanism, which would normally allow release of an ovum from the ovary. Thus, OCPs are used as a method of contraception by inhibiting ovulation.

Other uses include regulation of the period in those women who tend to have no pattern to their menstrual cycle. For a heavy flow or painful periods, as when hypermenorrhea or endometriosis exists, the OCP controls how long the cramping and bleeding last and thus provides some relief for these women.

ASSESSMENT Before initiation of OCP use, assess the patient's menstrual history for regularity or irregularity, duration of flow, and occurrence of pain. Assess for possibility of pregnancy because taking OCPs during pregnancy can cause fetal defects or abortion. Ask the patient whether she smokes; if so, determine the amount smoked per day and the number of years smoked. Smoking predisposes to vascular disease, which may increase her risks of side effects and complications. Assess for the family's and patient's history of vascular disease, cardiac problems, diabetes mellitus, cancer of breast or reproductive organs, liver disease, hypertension, obesity, renal dysfunction, depression, migraines, and seizure disorders; all of these may increase risks of side effects and complications. Age is significant, because women older than 35 years have a greater chance of having these disorders. Some of the less serious adverse effects include those common to estrogen and progesterone, such as nausea, vomiting, uterine cramping, breakthrough bleeding, edema, chloasma, breast tenderness, and rashes.

PLANNING AND IMPLEMENTATION Teach patients that they should use an additional form of birth control during the first month of OCP therapy until the next period.

Teach patients that when the pills are stopped, there is no "carry-over protection" from pregnancy.

Manufacturers often package OCPs in attractive

cases with flowers or butterflies on them, which is enticing to children. Because the pills are small, children may think that they are candy, such as may be found in toy doctor or nurse kits. Also, to remember to take the OCP every day, women often leave the packages in their purse or on the bedside table where they are easily accessible. It is therefore important to teach women to keep OCPs in a place safe from children, as they would with any other medication.

Teach women with diabetes to monitor symptoms or fingerstick serum glucose levels often. OCPs decrease glucose tolerance (increase blood glucose levels).

Encourage women to decrease the number of cigarettes smoked per day to minimize the vasoconstrictive effects. Teach the symptoms of thrombophlebitis to be reported to the physician.

Women with hypertension should monitor their blood pressure frequently.

Caution patients with conditions influenced or aggravated by fluid retention (asthma, migraines, cardiac and renal dysfunction, seizure disorders, depression) to monitor for edema. Advise them to notify the physician of problems.

Fluid retention may alter the shape of the eyeball and cause contact lenses to fit improperly. The increased pressure may lead to corneal ulceration. Those who wear contact lenses should have eye examinations annually or more often. Tell these patients to notify their ophthalmologist or oculist that they are taking OCPs.

Omitting pills increases the likelihood of conception. If one pill is omitted, instruct the patient to take two the next day. If two or three pills are omitted in one cycle and there is a chance that pregnancy *could* occur, advise the use of another form of contraception *in addition* to the remaining OCPs.

If several pills are omitted in one cycle and it is possible that a pregnancy *could have occurred,* continuing the OCP may cause fetal abnormalities. Therefore, the pills should be stopped and another form of contraception should be used until pregnancy is confirmed or disaffirmed.

Some drugs, such as antibiotics, decrease the effectiveness of the pill. An additional form of contraception should be added during that cycle. Teach patients to remind their physician, dentist, or ophthalmologist that they are taking OCPs *every time* a new medication is prescribed.

Discuss the advantages and disadvantages of OCPs so that women can make an informed choice about the method of contraception.

Advantages OCPs are effective if they are taken as directed. They offer a convenient form of protection for those who wish to have spontaneous sexual inter-course and do not want to stop their activities to insert or apply their protection.

Disadvantages The burden is on the woman to remember to take her pill every day. There are a significant number of adverse effects and risks involved. OCPs cannot be used after delivery until involution has taken place and the menstrual cycle is re-established. They should not be used during lactation because the hormones may interfere with the establishment of an adequate milk supply. They also "cross through" in the breast milk and may cause adverse effects in the infant.

Effectiveness Rate If OCPs are taken as directed, they are 98% to 99% effective.

Encourage women to have regular physical examinations with pelvic examinations, Pap tests, and mammograms as recommended. Although it may seem like there are a lot of adverse effects with OCPs, remember that there are also adverse effects and complications from pregnancy! Women desiring long-term protection from conception (more than 5 years) may wish to consider other birth control options.

ADDITIONAL TEACHING OCPs are classified by the manner in which the hormones are distributed throughout the cycle. Teach patients additional information about the particular type of OCP ordered by the physician.

Combination Type Estrogen is most effective for suppression of ovulation. If it is given alone, however, it causes nausea, vomiting, edema, breakthrough bleeding, and prolonged menses. To decrease these problems, progestins are combined with the estrogens. Teach the patient to start the first pill on the fifth day of her cycle. Remember that the first day of the cycle is the first day of menstrual bleeding.

One hormone pill is taken per day for 20 days. Packages are often prepared with five to eight pills of a different color to be taken (one each day) until the "period" or menses begin. These pills may be placebos made of inert ingredients, or some manufacturers add iron as an added measure to prevent anemia. They do not contain hormones, however. The main reason for taking them is to help the woman remember the pill-taking habit. She should start a new packet of pills on day 5 of the menses. Examples of this type of OCP are Norlestrin and Ortho-Novum.

Sequential Type With this type of OCP, the woman also starts the packet on day 5 of her cycle. She takes one pill of estrogen for 15 days, followed by a pill containing both estrogen and progestins for 5 days. She stops all pills when menses start and begins a new packet on the fifth day of menses. There are fewer side effects with this type because the endometrium is not significantly altered from the normal cycle. However, pregnancy occurs more frequently with this type, especially if one or two pills are missed during the month. This type is still available in some European drug markets, but the Food and Drug Administration has ordered this type removed from the United States drug market until the problem of the high pregnancy rate is resolved.

Fluctuating Progestin Levels One type of OCP combines estrogen with fluctuating levels of progestins. The highest amount of progestins is contained in the pills taken at the time coinciding with the expected time of ovulation. This offers the greatest protection at the most likely time of conception. These pills have less frequency of adverse effects than the sequential type does, but they are somewhat less effective. Examples of this type are Ortho-Novum 7/7/7 and Tri-Norinyl.

Others Experimental work continues on other types of OCP and also on a male contraceptive pill. These are not currently available in the United States.

EVALUATION To evaluate the patient's learning, ask ▲▲▲▲▲▲▲▲▲▲ her to repeat the information you have given her or ask her to pretend to explain it to a friend.

Women with medical conditions that may be aggravated by the use of OCPs should have regular evaluations by their physicians for complications. Those with diabetes mellitus or a tendency toward it should have periodic monitoring of their serum glucose levels.

Medroxyprogesterone

Medroxyprogesterone acetate suspension (Depo-Provera) contains a chemical similar to the natural hormone progesterone.

ACTIONS AND USES Injections of medroxyprogesterone ▲▲▲▲▲▲▲▲▲▲▲▲▲▲▲ acetate act to prevent the maturation and release of ova from the ovary. The lining of the uterus is also altered to make it less likely for implantation of a zygote to occur.

Medroxyprogesterone is used as a longer acting but not permanent form of contraception. The action of this hormone provides 3 months of protection from pregnancy.

Adverse actions include headache, nervousness, nausea, dizziness, acne and dermatitis, change in appetite, weight gain, breast tenderness, hirsutism or alopecia, prolonged menstrual bleeding, spotting between periods, absence of periods, and demineralization of the bones.

ASSESSMENT Before use, assess the chart and the ▲▲▲▲▲▲▲▲▲▲ patient for pregnancy and history of breast cancer or fibrocystic disease. These are contraindications to the use of progesterone. Also ask the patient about and assess the chart for a history of diabetes mellitus, hypertension, thrombophlebitis, liver or gallbladder disease, and heart or kidney disease. The patient may need to be monitored more frequently for complications of these disorders.

PLANNING AND IMPLEMENTATION If the patient is ▲▲▲▲▲▲▲▲▲▲▲▲▲▲▲▲▲▲▲▲▲▲▲▲▲▲▲▲▲ breast-feeding, the injection is given 6 weeks after delivery. Medroxyprogesterone does pass through the breast milk, but there is no evidence of harm to the infant.

Assess injection sites for redness and irritation and teach patients to report these symptoms. Teach the importance of keeping scheduled appointments for injections to prevent ovulation.

Teach that menstrual bleeding often decreases, becomes irregular, and may even stop completely. When the injections are discontinued, the menstrual cycle will return to normal within a few months.

Weight-bearing activity and adequate calcium intake assist in preventing mineral loss from the bones. Instruct patients to report muscle and bone pain to the physician.

If there is any question that a pregnancy may have occurred while the woman is receiving medroxyprogesterone therapy, the physician should be notified.

Advantages Long-term reversible contraception is provided by this hormone. Sexual activity can be spontaneous.

Disadvantages Injections are uncomfortable. Patients must remember to keep appointments for injections.

Effectiveness Rate If injections are received at 3-month intervals, effectiveness is 99%.

EVALUATION At each visit, evaluate patients for the ▲▲▲▲▲▲▲▲▲▲ occurrence of adverse effects and for symptoms of pregnancy.

Levonorgestrel

The Norplant implant system consists of six thin silicone capsules that contain levonorgestrel, a synthetic progesterone. These are implanted under the skin of the inner aspect of a woman's upper arm with use of a local anesthetic (Fig. 66–1).

ACTIONS AND USES The implants release their hormones slowly, providing 5 years of protection from conception. They act by inhibiting ovulation and by thickening cervical mucus to interfere with sperm motility.

An additional adverse effect may be discoloration of skin on the arm over the placement site.

PLANNING AND IMPLEMENTATION Teach patients that the contraceptive effect begins within 24 hours if the capsules are inserted during the menstrual period. If they are inserted at any other time during the menstrual cycle, the woman must first be evaluated for possible pregnancy. Tell her to use some other form of contraception until her next period.

Some bruising and swelling may be present for a few days after the insertion procedure. She should avoid lifting heavy objects and protect the insertion area from trauma for a few days. The bandage may be removed after about 3 days. Teach her to observe for signs and symptoms of irritation. Encourage these same precautions when the implants are removed.

Teach her to report muscle and bone pain, abdominal discomfort, or the presence of vaginal or breast discharge.

Some women may miss periods while they are using the Norplant system. The physician should be consulted if there is possibility of pregnancy.

There are no known significant effects on the newborn infants of lactating mothers who have had the Norplant system inserted 6 weeks after delivery. (There are no data for use in lactating women before 6 weeks post partum.)

Patients should discuss with the physician any possible effects or interactions with other medications. For example, phenytoin (Dilantin) and other drugs used to prevent seizures may decrease the effectiveness of the implant. Monitor for adverse effects as listed previously.

Advantages Long-term reversible contraception is provided. Sexual activity can be spontaneous. No estrogen hormones are used.

Disadvantages Initial cost is high. Irritation of the insertion site is not common, but it is possible.

Effectiveness Rate Norplant is 99% effective at preventing pregnancy.

EVALUATION Because the implant is one of the newer methods of contraception, any possible adverse effects should be discussed with the physician. See OCPs for other evaluation.

METHODS THAT PREVENT FERTILIZATION

Fertilization or conception can be prevented in several different ways. There are natural methods that involve knowledge of the menstrual cycle, devices that act as barriers between sperm and ova, chemicals that kill sperm, and surgeries that prevent sperm and ova from being united.

Chemicals

Spermicidal preparations are composed of ingredients that immobilize and kill sperm. They are prepared as foams, creams, jellies, vaginal suppositories, and vaginal sponges that contain the chemicals. Those products that contain the chemical nonoxynol 9 are also believed to inhibit transmission of the human immunodeficiency virus (HIV).

ASSESSMENT Annual physical and pelvic examinations should be done to assess for infections or diseases.

PLANNING AND IMPLEMENTATION The woman must insert the chemicals

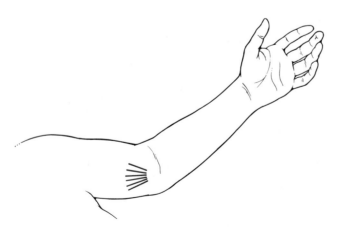

Figure 66–1. The Norplant contraceptive system consists of six silicone capsules that are implanted under the skin of the inner aspect of the woman's upper arm.

into her vagina while reclining on her back. Product directions should be read before use. Some products may be inserted up to 1 hour before intercourse. Other products are inserted immediately before intercourse. Suppositories must be in place long enough to melt and coat the vagina before intercourse. Sponges must be left in place 6 to 8 hours after intercourse. Douching must be avoided for 6 to 8 hours after intercourse with other forms.

Advantages These products are available without prescription and are relatively economical. These may be used with a condom or diaphragm to increase the effectiveness rate.

Disadvantages Chemicals are messy. They all become liquid at body temperature and drain out of the vagina. Those that must be inserted at the time of intercourse may interfere slightly with spontaneity. Some people experience contact dermatitis or allergies to the chemicals.

Effectiveness Rate Foams, jellies, and creams are 82% to 97% effective. Sponges are 80% to 91% effective. The rate of effectiveness depends on how carefully and consistently the product is used. Effectiveness rate is increased if the product is used in conjunction with a condom.

EVALUATION Ask the patient to verbalize the method ▲▲▲▲▲▲▲▲▲▲ of and the appropriate time for insertion. Have her explain how to evaluate for signs and symptoms of irritation.

E X E R C I S E S

CASE STUDY

A woman has just delivered an infant boy and is planning to breast-feed. Before discharge from the hospital, she tells you she plans to use the progesterone implants for birth control. How will you respond?

MENTAL AEROBICS

1. Explain how OCPs prevent conception.
2. Prepare a teaching plan for a 17-year-old high-school senior who comes to the clinic requesting a prescription for an OCP.
3. Your neighbor asks your advice. It seems she was ill with the flu and forgot to take her OCP for the past 4 days. What will you tell her?
4. How soon after receiving a Norplant implant can a woman safely engage in unprotected intercourse?

DRUGS USED TO PROMOTE FERTILITY

LEARNING OBJECTIVES

After studying this chapter, you should be able to:

1. Discuss the action of the various drugs used to promote fertility.

2. Name examples of each classification of fertility drug listed.

3. List the adverse effects of the listed fertility drugs.

4. Prepare an appropriate teaching plan for a couple taking one of the fertility drugs.

DRUGS YOU WILL LEARN ABOUT IN THIS CHAPTER

clomiphene citrate (Clomid)

bromocriptine mesylate (Parlodel)

menotropins USP (Pergonal)

progesterone

testosterone

DRUGS USED FOR FEMALE INFERTILITY

Fertility, or the ability to produce children, depends on many factors:

• The endocrine system must secrete the proper amounts of the hormones that influence the reproductive cycle.

• The circulatory system must be functioning to transport the hormones to the proper organs.

• The reproductive organs must be properly developed and functioning.

• The central nervous system must be functioning properly to transmit impulses to the proper glands and organs.

There are various causes of infertility in both men and women. There can be deficiencies of the pituitary hormones that regulate the production of ova or sperm. There can be cysts, infections, or tumors of the ovaries or testes and obstructions of any of the tubal structures that transport the ova or sperm. There may be defects in the structure of the ova and the sperm. A couple experiencing difficulty with conception should have careful examination by specialists to determine the specific cause of their infertility. Several drugs may be prescribed for those women and men experiencing infertility. Table 67–1 lists these drugs and their dosages.

Clomid

ACTIONS AND USES Clomiphene citrate (Clomid) is an
▲▲▲▲▲▲▲▲▲▲▲▲▲▲▲▲ "uncategorized drug" that acts on the anterior pituitary gland to increase secretion of follicle-stimulating hormone (FSH). It is used to stimulate ovulation in women experiencing anovulatory cycles. The increased FSH is intended to stimulate the ovary to release ova.

The ovaries are sometimes overstimulated and become enlarged or develop cysts. Several ova are often released and fertilized at once, resulting in multiple births.

Adverse actions include dizziness, edema, blurred vision, hot flashes, headaches, breast tenderness, or abdominal pain.

ASSESSMENT Because the patient has been trying to
▲▲▲▲▲▲▲▲▲▲ conceive, a pregnancy test and pelvic examination should be performed to assess for pregnancy before initiation of therapy. Use of the drug during pregnancy could cause teratogenic effects.

Table 67–1. Drugs Used to Promote Fertility	
DRUG	**DOSAGE**
clomiphene citrate (Clomid)	50–100 mg qd × 5 days; repeat until pregnancy occurs, up to 3 cycles
bromocriptine mesylate (Parlodel)	2.5 mg PO with a meal; gradually increase to 2 or 3 tablets qd with meals until pregnancy occurs
menotropins USP (Pergonal)	Women (dosage is individualized), initial dose: 1 ampule IM qd for up to 12 days, until blood and urine estrogen levels are equal to or greater than those of a woman with normal ovulatory activity; give 10,000 units hCG IM 1 day after last dose of menotropins; progesterone levels are then monitored and compared with those of women with normal ovulatory cycles. Men, pretreatment: 5000 IU hCG IM 3 times/wk × 4–6 mo or until secondary sexual characteristics develop and until serum testosterone levels are within normal range; follow with menotropins 1 ampule IM 3 times/wk with hCG 2000 IU IM twice/wk for at least 4 additional months; treatment continues until sperm counts are normal, which takes 74 ± 4 days
progesterone	Luteal phase defect: 12.5 mg IM qd or 25 mg bid intravaginally after ovulation; continue through 8–10 weeks of pregnancy (until placenta is developed enough to produce progesterone)

Table 67–1. Drugs Used to Promote Fertility *Continued*	
DRUG	**DOSAGE**
testosterone (Andro 100, T pellets)	Male hypogonadism: 10–25 mg 2–3 times/wk IM or 2–6 pellets (75 mg each) SC q 3–6 mo
testosterone cypionate (DEPO-Testosterone) testosterone enanthate (Andro L.A., Delatestryl Testate)	Male hypogonadism: 50–400 mg q 2–4 wk IM
testosterone propionate (Testex)	Male hypogonadism: 10–25 mg 2–4 times/wk IM

Assess baseline vital signs for later comparisons. Note skin color because jaundice may occur during therapy. Assess for a history of disorders that may be aggravated by fluid retention, such as migraines, seizure disorders, hypertension, and cardiac or renal conditions.

PLANNING AND IMPLEMENTATION Teach the patient
▲▲▲▲▲▲▲▲▲▲▲▲▲▲▲▲▲▲▲▲▲▲▲▲▲▲▲▲▲▲▲▲▲▲▲ to report adverse effects to the physician.

Teach the patient the methods of natural family planning listed in obstetrics textbooks. These methods can be used to determine the time of ovulation. The couple can then increase their sexual activity at that time to maximize their chances of conception.

Advise the patient to stop the drug immediately and report to the physician if she experiences abdominal pain. Ovarian cysts may enlarge and rupture, causing shock and bleeding. Caution the patient not to drive or work with hazardous equipment because dizziness or visual disturbances can occur.

For avoidance of teratogenic effects, the patient must stop the drug immediately and report to the physician if she believes she has conceived.

Provide emotional support for the couple as necessary. One or both partners are often feeling "guilty" because they are unable to perform a biological function that is so simple for others to accomplish. They frequently complain of the lack of spontaneity in their lovemaking because their activities are dictated by a calendar or hormone test. Encourage them to use imagination to keep their relationship fresh and relaxed.

EVALUATION Monitor vital signs and compare with baseline findings. Evaluate for jaundice. Pregnancy tests may be done to evaluate for conception. The physician will perform pelvic examinations to evaluate abdominal pain. Monitor for early signs of pregnancy.

Bromocriptine Mesylate

ACTIONS AND USES Bromocriptine mesylate (Parlodel) acts to suppress the production of prolactin by the anterior pituitary gland. It is used to inhibit lactation in postpartum women who do not desire to breast-feed. Bromocriptine decreases prolactin secretion in cases of infertility caused by amenorrhea related to hyperprolactinemia.

Adverse effects include nausea, vomiting, and nasal congestion. A "first-dose phenomenon" is dizziness or syncope on position change.

ASSESSMENT Assessments must be specific to the reason for use. If bromocriptine is being used to increase fertility, studies such as serum prolactin levels would have already been done to determine the possible cause of infertility. Establish baseline vital signs in all patients.

PLANNING AND IMPLEMENTATION Teach the patient to use nonhormonal contraceptive measures the first week to allow time to determine whether pregnancy has already taken place. This drug should not be taken during pregnancy. After it has been determined that the woman is not pregnant, advise her to discontinue all contraceptive measures.

A pregnancy test should be performed if menses are more than 3 days late. The medication is discontinued when pregnancy occurs.

Caution the patient to rise slowly from a lying or sitting position, especially when the drug is first begun, to avoid the first-dose phenomenon.

Instruct the patient to take the pills with meals or a snack to prevent nausea and vomiting.

EVALUATION Monitor blood pressure for hypotension. Monitor for and question the patient about dizziness or faintness. Monitor for nausea. Monitor for pregnancy if menses are late.

Menotropins USP

ACTIONS AND USES Menotropins USP (Pergonal) is a purified preparation of gonadotropins that have been extracted from the urine of postmenopausal women. It contains both follicle-stimulating hormone (FSH) and luteinizing hormone (LH). It is used to cause maturation of the ovarian follicle in women who have anovulatory cycles but *do not* have primary ovarian failure. It must be followed by a dose of human chorionic gonadotropin (hCG) to cause release of the mature ovum from the follicle.

Adverse effects include fever, nausea, vomiting, abdominal distention, flatulence, and diarrhea.

This therapy should be prescribed only by physicians thoroughly familiar with the regimen and its potentially serious complications. Hyperstimulation of the ovary, hemoperitoneum, arterial thromboembolism, and multiple births have been known to occur. Allergic responses are always a possibility with any drug.

ASSESSMENT Before institution of treatment, assess vital signs and weight. Various tests to determine the cause of infertility are performed, such as pelvic examination, endocrine examination, hysterosalpingogram, and cellular studies of the vaginal mucosa. A pregnancy test should be done to determine whether the patient has recently conceived.

PLANNING AND IMPLEMENTATION Administration is intramuscular (IM). Reconstitute the medication with 1 to 2 mL sterile saline before use and administer it immediately after preparation. Discard unused portions of the ampule. Dosage is individualized.

The gynecologist should examine the patient at least every other day to observe for the hyperstimulation syndrome. If estrogen levels are higher than normal cycles, the hCG is not given. This sometimes prevents development of the syndrome. Symptoms include mild to moderate ovarian enlargement, ascites, abdominal pain, and pleural effusion. The syndrome may develop rapidly in a 3- to 4-day period, usually within 2 weeks after the injections.

Couples are encouraged to engage in sexual intercourse daily, beginning the day before the hCG injection.

Teach patients to report nausea, vomiting, abdominal distention, flatulence, diarrhea, abdominal pain, edema, and difficulty breathing.

Monitor vital signs and the patient's complaints. Monitor intake, output, and weight. Collect urine specimens and blood samples as ordered.

EVALUATION Compare vital signs and weight with ▲▲▲▲▲▲▲▲▲▲ baseline assessments. Monitor results of blood or urine tests. If the physician determines the presence of ovulation but not conception, the dosage regimen may be repeated at least twice more before the dose is increased.

Progesterone

Progesterone can be used in some cases of infertility. Because of the cyclic interaction of progesterone and the gonadotropic hormones, administration of progestogen causes negative feedback to occur. The anterior pituitary gland decreases the production of FSH and LH, which in premenopausal women prevents the ovary from developing and releasing ova.

The theory is that when the progesterone is stopped, the anterior pituitary will rebound with a surge of FSH. This will stimulate the development of ova, and ovulation will follow. (See Chapter 63 for assessments, planning and implementation, and evaluation.)

DRUGS USED FOR MALE INFERTILITY

Menotropins USP

ACTIONS AND USES Menotropins USP (Pergonal) is ▲▲▲▲▲▲▲▲▲▲▲▲▲▲▲ sometimes used to treat men with infertility due to deficiency of the gonadotropins follicle-stimulating hormone (FSH) and interstitial cell–stimulating hormone (ICSH). Both are necessary for adequate sperm production.

Adverse actions include breast enlargement (gynecomastia) and tenderness.

ASSESSMENT Assessments include blood and urine ▲▲▲▲▲▲▲▲▲▲ tests to determine levels of testosterone and gonadotropins. Physical examination is performed to assess signs and symptoms of hypogonadism. Semen tests are performed to assess the number of sperm in the ejaculate, sperm motility, and numbers of abnormal sperm.

PLANNING AND IMPLEMENTATION Teach patients the ▲▲▲▲▲▲▲▲▲▲▲▲▲▲▲▲▲▲▲▲▲▲▲▲▲▲ importance of pro-

viding blood, urine, and semen samples to monitor therapy.

Inform patients that breast enlargement (gynecomastia) and tenderness will occur. Tell the patient that these will dissipate when the drug is discontinued. Provide emotional support as necessary.

EVALUATION Monitor results of blood and urine tests ▲▲▲▲▲▲▲▲▲▲ and semen analyses.

Testosterone

ACTIONS AND USES The main actions of androgens are ▲▲▲▲▲▲▲▲▲▲▲▲▲▲▲▲ the production of male secondary sex characteristics and the maintenance of male reproductive structures, including sperm production. Therefore, they are used as a replacement for testosterone deficiency caused by hypogonadism or cryptorchidism.

In cases of infertility due to a low sperm count (oligospermia), androgens are sometimes used to produce the negative feedback mechanism. The androgens are taken for several weeks, which causes suppression of the anterior pituitary hormones ICSH and FSH. The theory is that when the androgens are discontinued, a rebound phenomenon occurs, and the anterior pituitary will surge out an increase in FSH and ICSH. This should then cause an increase in testosterone and sperm production.

Adverse actions include breast enlargement (gynecomastia), persistent and painful erections (priapism), and acne.

ASSESSMENT Assessments include physical examina-▲▲▲▲▲▲▲▲▲▲ tion to determine the status of secondary sexual characteristics, blood and urine tests to determine hormone levels, and semen analyses.

PLANNING AND IMPLEMENTATION Encourage men re-▲▲▲▲▲▲▲▲▲▲▲▲▲▲▲▲▲▲▲▲▲▲▲▲▲▲▲▲▲ ceiving androgens to report side effects. Gynecomastia and priapism sometimes occur early in therapy but may disappear when the dose is decreased. Acne may occur or increase. Offer emotional support because patients are often embarrassed and frustrated.

EVALUATION Physical examination is necessary to ▲▲▲▲▲▲▲▲▲▲ determine the status of secondary sexual characteristics. Monitor results of blood and urine tests for hormone levels. Monitor reports of semen analyses.

E X E R C I S E S

LEARNING ACTIVITIES

1. Explain the risks of overstimulating the ovaries with Clomid.

2. Explain why hCG is used with Pergonal.

DRUGS THAT AFFECT THE EAR, EYE, AND SKIN

Have you ever considered what it would be like to be blind or deaf? For one thing, you would not be reading this text in the manner that you are, and you would not be sitting in a classroom listening to lecture unless you had special assistive devices. When a person has a condition of the ear or eye, however, it is frequently treated on an outpatient basis. This may lead some people to regard the problem as less than serious. Yet consider the alternatives: *deafness and blindness* are often the complications of untreated conditions of the ear and eye.

What of skin conditions? No big deal, right? Consider again the alternatives to an intact skin: *open portals* for entrance of bacteria and viruses into the body and its internal organs; *loss of sensation* due to damaged nerve endings in the skin; *amputation* due to damaged cells and infection. Shall we go on?

Although many of the medications included in these chapters are used for home treatment of various conditions, that does not imply that the conditions or their sequelae are to be taken lightly or that the medications are not as important to learn as any other. The importance of patient teaching cannot be over-emphasized, for when a patient is responsible for self-medication, he is also responsible for reporting signs and symptoms of complications of the condition or the medication.

DRUGS THAT AFFECT THE EAR

LEARNING OBJECTIVES

After studying this chapter, you should be able to:

1. Discuss the action of each of the listed classifications on the ear.

2. List the conditions of the ear for which each of the classifications is used.

3. Name examples of each of the classifications listed.

4. Discuss the adverse effects of drugs in the classifications listed.

5. Prepare an appropriate nursing care plan for a patient receiving one of the listed medications.

DRUGS YOU WILL LEARN ABOUT IN THIS CHAPTER

Anti-infectives

    acetic acid 2% to 5% solution

    boric acid solution (Ear-Dry, Swim Ear)

Antibiotics

    chloramphenicol (Chloromycetin Otic)

    neomycin sulfate

Corticosteroids

    dexamethasone sodium phosphate (Decadron)

    hydrocortisone acetate (Otall)

    methylprednisolone disodium phosphate (Medrol)

Combination Products

    colistin sulfate, neomycin, hydrocortisone acetate, thonzonium bromide (Coly-Mycin S Otic)

    oxytetracycline HCl (Terramycin with polymyxin B or polymyxin B sulfate with hydrocortisone)

    ceruminolytics

    carbamide peroxide (Debrox)

The ear is a sensory organ for hearing and equilibrium. It is composed of three sections: the external, middle, and internal ear (Fig. 68–1). The external ear has two main parts, the pinna (or auricle) and the external auditory canal. Bacterial and fungal infections of the canal are fairly common, especially in children, who have a shorter and straighter canal. The organisms can travel easily along the wall of the canal and hide in the dark, moist areas near the eardrum. The tympanic membrane, or eardrum, is at the end of this canal and is the division between the external and middle ear.

The middle ear is a space containing three bones or ossicles that vibrate, amplify sound waves, and transmit the sound waves through the oval window to the fluid of the inner ear. The eustachian tube connects the middle ear cavity with the pharynx. Its function is to equalize the air pressure on both sides of the eardrum, which allows the eardrum to vibrate when it is struck by sound waves. This tube is lined with mucous membrane, which often becomes a pathway for travel of organisms from the pharynx to the middle ear. Infection of the middle ear is called otitis media.

The most complicated part of the ear is the internal ear. It is also the most important part because it is here that the sound waves pass through the special fluid called perilymph, which is in the bony snail-shaped structure called the cochlea. Inside the cochlea

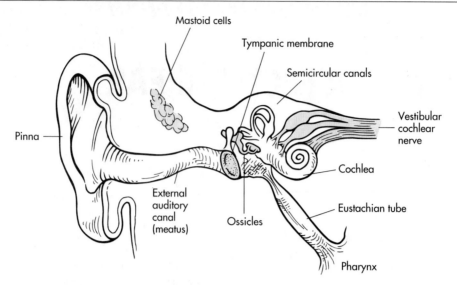

Figure 68-1. The human ear.

are the organs of Corti. These hair-like nerve receptors are connected to the nerve fibers in the cochlear nerve, a branch of the eighth cranial nerve that transmits the sensation of sound to the auditory area of the brain where it is interpreted. In the vestibule, or space around the cochlea, are three semicircular canals that contain fluids called perilymph and endolymph. The sensory receptors for equilibrium are located at the base of these canals. There are proprioceptors in the vestibule that obtain information on the position of the head and transmit the information by way of the vestibular branch of the eighth cranial nerve to the brain. Infections of the inner ear can damage the vestibulocochlear (auditory) nerve, causing impairment of hearing or balance.

Some ear conditions are treated with medications that are taken internally to achieve a systemic effect. These are usually antibiotics to treat infections, corticosteroids to decrease inflammation, or antihistamines to relieve the symptoms of dizziness and nausea that accompany inner ear conditions. These medications are discussed in previous chapters.

Other medications used to treat the ear are liquids. Liquid medications are instilled into the external auditory canal to treat bacterial and fungal infections, soften and remove cerumen, or suppress inflammation. Those medications instilled into the canal must be labeled *otic*.

Table 68–1 lists dosages of drugs for the ear. Before initiation of treatment of an ear infection or condition, the physician may order the ear canal to be irrigated for removal of any accumulated cerumen or drainage. Clean technique is used unless the eardrum is perforated, when aseptic technique is used.

Medications to be instilled into the external ear canal should be warmed to room temperature before instillation. Solutions that are too warm or too cold may cause the patient to experience nausea, vertigo, or pain. Avoid touching the ear with the dropper.

N U R S I N G   A L E R T
▼▼▼▼▼▼▼▼▼▼▼▼▼▼▼▼▼▼▼▼▼▼▼▼▼▼▼▼▼▼▼

To straighten the ear canal of an adult or older child, gently pull the pinna up and back.

To straighten the ear canal of a child 3 years old or younger, gently pull the pinna down and back.

▲▲▲▲▲▲▲▲▲▲▲▲▲▲▲▲▲▲▲▲▲▲▲▲▲▲▲▲▲▲▲

After instillation of medication into the ear canal, ask the patient to remain with the treated ear in a superior position for a few minutes to prevent the medication from draining out. Never occlude the external canal with a tight-fitting "plug" of any type. Occlusion increases the pressure on the tympanic membrane and may cause it to rupture. Gently wipe drainage away instead.

Sometimes, because of swelling in the external canal, the physician inserts a wick. Use of a wick facilitates drainage out of the ear or instillation of medications all the way to the tympanic membrane.

N U R S I N G   A L E R T
▼▼▼▼▼▼▼▼▼▼▼▼▼▼▼▼▼▼▼▼▼▼▼▼▼▼▼▼▼▼▼

Never treat a draining ear without a physician's order. The fluid may be the result of an infection that needs attention, or cerebrospinal fluid may be leaking from the brain.

▲▲▲▲▲▲▲▲▲▲▲▲▲▲▲▲▲▲▲▲▲▲▲▲▲▲▲▲▲▲▲

Table 68–1. Drugs that Affect the Ear

DRUG	DOSAGE
Anti-infectives	
acetic acid 2% to 5% solution	4–6 gtt tid–qid; insert saturated wick for first 24 h, then continue with instillations
boric acid solution (Ear-Dry, Swim Ear)	Fill canal with solution; repeat tid–qid
Antibiotics	
chloramphenicol (Chloromycetin Otic)	2–3 gtt into ear canal tid–qid
neomycin sulfate	2–5 gtt into ear canal tid–qid
Corticosteroids	
dexamethasone sodium phosphate (Decadron)	1–2 gtt into ear canal tid–qid
hydrocortisone acetate (Otall) (availability: 0.25%, 0.5%, 1%)	3–5 gtt into ear canal tid–qid
methylprednisolone disodium phosphate (Medrol)	2–3 gtt into ear canal tid–qid
Combination Products	
colistin sulfate, neomycin, hydrocortisone acetate, thonzonium bromide (Coly-Mycin S Otic)	3–5 gtt into ear canal tid–qid
oxytetracycline hydrochloride (Terramycin with polymyxin B or polymyxin B sulfate with hydrocortisone)	1/2-inch ointment into ear canal tid–qid

Table 68–1. Drugs that Affect the Ear *Continued*

DRUG	DOSAGE
Ceruminolytics	
carbamide peroxide (Debrox)	5-10gtts into ear canal bid for 3–4d

ANTI-INFECTIVES

Anti-infectives kill bacteria that may be present in the ear canal. Some are used as irrigations, others as instillations. Examples of those used as irrigations are acetic acid 2% to 5% solution and boric acid solution (Ear-Dry, Swim Ear).

ACTIONS AND USES Anti-infectives inhibit the growth of or kill bacteria. By decreasing bacterial growth, they reduce swelling and relieve the pruritus, erythema, and drainage associated with the infection. Common adverse effects are irritation, swelling, urticaria, and overgrowth of nonsusceptible organisms.

ASSESSMENT Assessments include visualization of the external ear canal and tympanic membrane with an otoscope to monitor redness and swelling. Assess the temperature. A temperature elevation may indicate the presence of systemic infection or inner ear infection.

PLANNING AND IMPLEMENTATION Teach the parents or significant others to make appropriate assessments. Demonstrate appropriate technique for instillation of medication into the external ear canal. Observe the caregiver doing the procedure so that you may reinforce appropriate actions.

EVALUATION Monitor vital signs and signs and symptoms of infection.

ANTIBIOTICS

Some anti-infectives are also classified as antibiotics. Examples are chloramphenicol (Chloromycetin Otic) and neomycin sulfate.

ACTIONS AND USES Antibiotics may be applied into the external auditory canal to be used for external ear infections. Adverse effects include burning and itching of the pinna or external auditory canal. Systemic effects can be burning and itching, urticaria, or rash. Sore throat can be an early sign of toxic effects.

ASSESSMENT Ask the patient or significant caregiver about the existence of allergies. Assess the external ear canal and tympanic membrane. Assess the vital signs.

PLANNING AND IMPLEMENTATION If the ear is draining, request an order for culture and sensitivity before initiation of therapy. Monitor for symptoms of conditions that result from overgrowth of nonsusceptible organisms, such as thrush, diarrhea, and vaginal infections.

EVALUATION Monitor the vital signs and signs and symptoms of infection and for adverse effects.

CORTICOSTEROIDS

Corticosteroid preparations, such as dexamethasone sodium phosphate (Decadron), hydrocortisone acetate (Otall), and methylprednisolone disodium phosphate (Medrol), are used to control inflammation, edema, and pruritus of the ear. Common adverse effects are suppression of the adrenal gland and masking of the symptoms of infection.

ACTIONS AND USES Corticosteroids are used to suppress the uncomfortable symptoms associated with an ear inflammation.

ASSESSMENT Assess the external ear canal and tympanic membrane. Assess the vital signs.

PLANNING AND IMPLEMENTATION Teach the caregiver the proper method of instillation. Teach the caregiver and the patient the side effects. Corticosteroids are contraindicated in viral infections, fungal infections, and perforated eardrum.

EVALUATION Monitor the vital signs and symptoms of infection and for adverse effects.

COMBINATION PRODUCTS

Two or more antibiotics, antibiotics and benzocaine, or antibiotics and corticosteroids are often combined to give the advantage of the effects of both types of drug in one prescription. Examples are colistin sulfate with neomycin, hydrocortisone acetate, and thonzonium bromide (Coly-Mycin S Otic) and oxytetracycline hydrochloride (Terramycin with polymyxin B or polymyxin B sulfate with hydrocortisone).

CERUMINOLYTICS

Cerumen sometimes hardens and blocks the external auditory canal. This can interfere with hearing and block the action of medications on the ear canal and tympanic membrane. When this occurs, a ceruminolytic such as carbamide peroxide (Debrox) may be ordered. The ear is then irrigated if necessary.

ACTIONS AND USES Drugs in this group are used to emulsify the cerumen. The cerumen then drains out of the canal spontaneously or with an irrigation.

ASSESSMENT Assess the hearing ability with an audiometer and assess the ear canal with an otoscope. The cerumen is visible in the canal. Assess for signs of inflammation and for drainage, which may indicate a perforated eardrum.

PLANNING AND IMPLEMENTATION A physician should examine the patient if there is a question of a perforated eardrum. Products of this type are contraindicated with perforation. It may be necessary to follow the treatment with irrigation of the canal to remove the emulsified cerumen. Be certain to instruct caregivers in appropriate ways of restraining young children and infants to prevent injury during the procedure.

EVALUATION Examine the ear canal with an otoscope to determine whether all the cerumen has been removed. Hearing may then be rechecked to accurately determine hearing levels.

E X E R C I S E S

LEARNING ACTIVITIES

A 2-year-old boy has bilateral otitis externa. The physician has prescribed 3 to 5 drops of colistin sulfate to be instilled in each ear qid. Prepare a teaching plan for his mother that includes facts about the medication, signs and symptoms to report to the physician, safety tips, and appropriate restraint techniques to use with the child.

DRUGS THAT AFFECT THE EYE

LEARNING OBJECTIVES

After studying this chapter, you should be able to:

1. Discuss the action of each of the listed classifications on the eye.

2. List the conditions of the eye for which each of the classifications is used.

3. Name examples of each of the classifications listed.

4. Discuss the adverse effects of drugs in the classifications listed.

5. Prepare an appropriate nursing care plan for a patient receiving one of the listed medications.

DRUGS YOU WILL LEARN ABOUT IN THIS CHAPTER

Cholinergics

    carbachol (Isopto Carbachol) 0.75%–3%

    pilocarpine HCl (Isopto Carpine)

    physostigmine sulfate (Eserine Sulfate ointment) 0.25%–0.5%

Anticholinergics

    atropine sulfate (Isopto Atropine) 0.125%–4% solution or 0.5%–1% ointment

    homatropine hydrobromide (Isopto Homatropine)

    scopolamine hydrobromide (Isopto Hyoscine)

Adrenergics

    epinephrine HCl (Adrenalin Chloride, Glaucon) 0.25%–2%

    tetrahydrozoline HCl (Visine, Murine) 0.05%

Adrenergic Blockers

    levobunolol HCl (Betagan) 0.25% to 0.5%

    timolol maleate (Timoptic) 0.25%–0.5%

    betaxolol (Betoptic) 0.25%–0.5%

Carbonic Anhydrase Inhibitors

    acetazolamide (Diamox)

    dichlorphenamide (Daranide)

Osmotic Diuretics

    glycerin (glycerol, Osmoglyn) 50% oral solution

    mannitol (Osmitrol) 15%–25% IV solutions

    glycerin, anhydrous (Ophthalgan) topical

Anesthetics

    tetracaine HCl (Pontocaine) 0.5%

    cocaine HCl 1%–4% solutions

Antiseptics

    benzalkonium chloride (Zephiran) 1:5000 solution

    boric acid (Blinx, Collyrium) 2% solution or 5%–10% ointment

    thimerosal 0.1% solution

    silver nitrate 1%

Antibiotics

bacitracin (Baciguent)

chloramphenicol (Chloromycetin)

erythromycin (Ilotycin) 0.5%

tobramycin (Tobrex)

polymyxin B sulfate

chloramphenicol and polymyxin B sulfate (Chlormyxin Ophthalmic)

Antifungals

natamycin (Natacyn)

Antivirals

idoxuridine (IDU, Dendrid, Herplex)

trifluridine (Viroptic)

vidarabine (Vira-A)

Corticosteroids

dexamethasone (Maxidex ophthalmic suspension)

dexamethasone sodium phosphate (Decadron Phosphate ophthalmic ointment)

polyvinyl alcohol (¼% Liquifilm tears, 3% Liquifilm Forte)

hydrocortisone acetate (Cortamed, Hydrocortone)

prednisolone sodium phosphate (Inflamase Mild 1/8% Ophthalmic, Inflamase Forte 1% Ophthalmic)

The eye is protected by the bones of the orbit, the eyelids and eyelashes, and tears. The epithelial sac, which separates the front of the eye from the eyeball, aids in the destruction of pathogens. The eyeball is composed of three layers (Fig. 69–1):

1. sclera, the white outer layer of tough connective tissue;
2. choroid, the second layer that contains a network of connective tissues and blood vessels; brown pigment prevents light rays from reflecting off the inner surface;
3. retina, the inner layer that contains ten layers of nerve cells, which include the rods and cones.

Rods function in dim light and are sensitive to light. They are necessary for general vision. Cones function in bright light and are sensitive to red, blue, and green color. Impulses received by the rods and cones are transmitted to the second cranial (optic) nerve and then to the occipital area of the brain, where they are interpreted.

When light rays enter the eye, they are refracted (bent) by different clear, colorless structures (refracting media) to be focused onto a small area of the retina. The refracting media are the

1. cornea, the clear part at the front of the eye;
2. aqueous humor, the fluid in the anterior chamber of the eye in front of the lens that helps maintain the outward curve of the cornea;

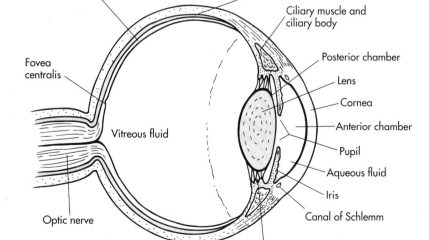

Figure 69–1. The human eyeball.

3. lens, the circular structure of jelly-like material with elastic properties so the shape can be changed to focus the light;

4. vitreous humor (body), a jelly-like substance that fills the space behind the lens.

The vitreous humor maintains the spherical shape of the eye and is not replaceable. The aqueous humor is constantly being reproduced from the vascular tissues of the ciliary body. It then flows into the posterior chamber, out through the pupil to the anterior chamber, and into the venous sinus called the canal of Schlemm in the corner where the cornea and the iris meet (Fig. 69–1).

Intrinsic muscles inside the eyeball are also part of the refractory process. The iris or pigmented part of the front of the eye controls the black opening in the center called the pupil. The iris is actually two sets of muscles, a circular set and a radial set arranged like the spokes of a wheel. They regulate the amount of light that enters the eye. Constriction of the circular muscles decreases the pupil size (miosis), and constriction of the radial muscles causes pupil dilation (mydriasis). The ciliary body is a flattened ring of muscles behind the iris that alters the shape of the lens to allow us to focus on objects close to us and then on those far away. This action is called accommodation.

Three pairs of extrinsic muscles surround each eye. These muscles must work in a coordinated fashion to permit smooth movement of the eyeball in various directions. In coordination with the muscles of the other eye, they permit proper vision.

Several different classifications of medications are used in the eye, but any medication instilled into the eye should be labeled *ophthalmic*. Eye medications are always dilute concentrations of medication, usually 1% to 2% strengths or fractions of 1%. Common ophthalmic drugs and their dosages are listed in Table 69–1.

Medications that constrict the pupil are referred to as miotics. Those that dilate the pupil are referred to as mydriatics.

Universal precautions and clean technique are maintained to prevent transmission of infection to the patient or the caregiver. You may wish at this time to review the Drug Administration Guidelines for administration of eye medications.

The following abbreviations are frequently used in medication orders:

OD = right eye
OS = left eye
OU = both eyes

Never touch the dropper to the eye. To prevent systemic absorption of the medication through the tear ducts into the nasal mucosa, hold pressure for 2 to

Table 69–1. Drugs that Affect the Eye

DRUG	DOSAGE
Cholinergics	
carbachol (Isopto Carbachol) 0.75%–3%	1 gtt bid–qid; ointment bid
pilocarpine hydrochloride (Isopto Carpine)	1–2 gtt bid–qid or as directed
physostigmine sulfate (Eserine Sulfate ointment) 0.25%–0.5%	1–2 gtt tid; ¼ inch of ointment into conjunctival sac
Anticholinergics	
atropine sulfate (Isopto Atropine)	0.125%–4% solution: 1–2 gtt bid–tid 0.5%–1% ointment: small amount bid–tid
homatropine hydrobromide (Isopto Homatropine)	Uveitis: 1–2 gtt 2%–5% q3–4h Cycloplegic refraction: 1–2 gtt 2%–5%; repeat in 5–10 min
scopolamine hydrobromide (Isopto Hyoscine)	1–2 gtt 0.1% bid–tid
Adrenergics	
epinephrine hydrochloride (Adrenalin Chloride, Glaucon) 0.25%–2%	1 gtt bid
tetrahydrozoline hydrochloride (Visine, Murine) 0.05%	1–2 gtt bid–tid
Adrenergic Blockers	
levobunolol hydrochloride (Betagan) 0.25%–0.5%	1 gtt bid

Table 69–1. Drugs that Affect the Eye *Continued*

DRUG	DOSAGE
timolol maleate (Timoptic) 0.25%–0.5%	1 gtt bid
betaxolol (Betoptic) 0.25%–0.5%	1 gtt bid; decrease to 1 gtt qd
Carbonic Anhydrase Inhibitors	
acetazolamide (Diamox)	250 mg qid or 500-mg sustained-release capsules bid Narrow-angle glaucoma: 250 mg q4h or bid PO, IM, or IV Open-angle glaucoma: 250 mg qd to 1 g PO, IM, or IV (divided into qid doses)
dichlorphenamide (Daranide)	Initial: 100–200 mg PO, followed by 100 mg q12h until desired response is achieved Maintenance: 25–50 mg qd–tid
Osmotic Diuretics	
glycerin (glycerol, Osmoglyn) 50% oral solution	0.5–2 g/kg
mannitol (Osmitrol) 15%–25% IV solutions	1.5–2 g/kg infused in 30–60 min
glycerin, anhydrous (Ophthalgan) topical	1–2 gtt after instillation of local anesthetic
Anesthetics	
tetracaine hydrochloride (Pontocaine) 0.5% solution	1–2 gtt immediately before procedure

Table 69–1. Drugs that Affect the Eye *Continued*

DRUG	DOSAGE
cocaine hydrochloride 1%–4% solutions	1–2 gtt immediately prior to procedure
Antiseptics	
benzalkonium chloride (Zephiran) 1:5000 solution	Used in some irrigating solutions
boric acid (Blinx, Collyrium)	2% solution to irrigate eye prn 5%–10% ointment to eye prn
thimerosal 0.1% solution	Used in some irrigating solutions
silver nitrate 1%	Neonates: 1 gtt into each eye shortly after birth
Antibiotics	
bacitracin (Baciguent)	Small amount into conjunctival sac several times qd or prn
chloramphenicol (Chloromycetin)	2 gtt solution q1h until improved or qid, depending on severity of infection
erythromycin (Ilotycin) 0.5%	Small amount 1 or more times qd
tobramycin (Tobrex)	1–2 gtt q4h Severe infection: 2 gtt q1h
polymyxin B sulfate	0.1%: 1–3 gtt 0.25%: q1h instillation

Table continued on following page

Table 69–1. Drugs that Affect the Eye *Continued*

DRUG	DOSAGE
Antifungals	
natamycin (Natacyn)	Individualized dose: 1 gtt q1–2h; after 3–4 days, reduce to 1 gtt 6–8 × qd
Antivirals	
idoxuridine (IDU, Dendrid, Herplex)	Solution: 1 gtt q1h in the day, q2h at nights Ointment: q4h or 5 times qd Discontinue if no response in 7 days, (maximal use, 21 days)
trifluridine (Viroptic)	1 gtt q2h while awake to a maximum of 9 gtt until re-epithelialization
vidarabine (Vira-A)	½ inch of ointment 5 times qd at 3-h intervals
Corticosteroids	
dexamethasone (Maxidex ophthalmic suspension)	1–2 gtt q1h; taper to 4–6 times qd as improvement occurs
dexamethasone sodium phosphate (Decadron Phosphate ophthalmic ointment)	1–2 gtt q1h; taper to 4–6 times qd as improvement occurs
polyvinyl alcohol (¼% Liquifilm tears, 3% Liquifilm Forte)	1–2 gtt as needed

Table 69–1. Drugs that Affect the Eye *Continued*

DRUG	DOSAGE
hydrocortisone acetate (Hydrocortone)	Solution: 1–3 gtt q1h while awake, q2h at night; decrease to 1 gtt tid–qid Ointment: tid–qid
prednisolone sodium phosphate (Inflamase Ophthalmic Mild ⅛%, Inflamase Forte 1% Ophthalmic)	1–2 gtt q1h; while awake, q2h at night as inflammation decreases Taper to 1gtt q4h, then 1 gtt 3–4 × d

3 minutes at the inner canthus of the eye with a clean cotton ball or tissue.

CHOLINERGICS

Cholinergic medications have actions that mimic those of acetylcholine from the parasympathetic nervous system. Therefore, cholinergics are also referred to as parasympathomimetic medications. To remember their actions, we need to recall those of the sympathetic and parasympathetic divisions of the autonomic nervous system. The autonomic nervous system makes "automatic" adjustments to various organs and systems of the body without conscious thought.

Examples of cholinergics used in the eye are carbachol (Isopto Carbachol) 0.75% to 3%, pilocarpine hydrochloride (Isopto Carpine), and physostigmine sulfate (Eserine Sulfate ointment) 0.25% to 0.5%.

ACTIONS AND USES The action of cholinergics on the ▲▲▲▲▲▲▲▲▲▲▲▲▲▲▲▲ eye is to produce contractions of the iris, which causes miosis, and to produce contractions of the muscles of the ciliary body, which affects accommodation. Cholinergics are used to decrease intraocular pressure in patients with closed-angle glaucoma. They widen the filtration angle where the cornea and iris meet. This permits the aqueous humor to flow out into the canal of Schlemm, where it is absorbed into the venous circulation.

Localized adverse effects are often transient and include burning and stinging of the eyes. If the medication is absorbed into the circulation, adverse systemic effects include increased perspiration and salivation, headache, abdominal cramping and diarrhea, hypotension, asthma attacks, and cardiac arrhythmias. These effects are less severe than those associated with drugs that block cholinesterase.

ASSESSMENT Assess baseline vital signs, visual acuity, ▲▲▲▲▲▲▲▲▲▲ and appearance of the eyes (i.e., bloodshot appearance, status of the pupils). Chart the location and description of the patient's headaches, and question the patient about bowel patterns. Assess also for a history of asthma and other respiratory conditions that may be aggravated by use of these drugs.

PLANNING AND IMPLEMENTATION Teach the patient ▲▲▲▲▲▲▲▲▲▲▲▲▲▲▲▲▲▲▲▲▲▲▲▲ or caregiver to wash hands before and after instillation of eye drops. Teach the proper technique of administration. Teach the patient to monitor for side effects and report to the physician if any occur. Caution patients that visual difficulty may occur in dim light or after dark. Advise the patient about safety factors, such as not to drive after dark and to light stairways and other dangerous areas of the home. These drops are contraindicated in conditions such as iritis, which would be worsened by constricted pupils. Monitor vital signs, cardiopulmonary status, gastrointestinal pain and spasm, urine output, and the physician's recordings of intraocular pressure.

EVALUATION Pupils will appear constricted. Symp-▲▲▲▲▲▲▲▲▲▲ toms such as reddened eyes and headaches will dissipate. Tonometer readings will indicate a decrease in intraocular pressure.

ANTICHOLINERGICS

Examples of anticholinergic medications that are used in the eye are atropine sulfate (Isopto Atropine) 0.125% to 4% solution or 0.5% to 1% ointment, homatropine hydrobromide (Isopto Homatropine), and scopolamine hydrobromide (Isopto Hyoscine).

ACTIONS AND USES Anticholinergic ophthalmic prep-▲▲▲▲▲▲▲▲▲▲▲▲▲▲▲ arations act to relax smooth muscles of the ciliary body and iris. They are used to produce mydriasis (dilation of the pupil) and cycloplegia (paralysis of the ciliary muscles). These effects are useful when the ophthalmic physician wishes to examine the interior of the eye or to measure refraction (the bending of light rays) when fitting a patient

for eyeglasses. Anticholinergics may be used to rest the eye when the uveal tract (iris, ciliary body, and choroid) is inflamed.

ASSESSMENT Assessments include those listed for cho-▲▲▲▲▲▲▲▲▲▲ linergics. Assess the chart for documentation of a history of glaucoma, hypertension, coronary artery disease, asthma, or pulmonary disease.

PLANNING AND IMPLEMENTATION Anticholinergics are ▲▲▲▲▲▲▲▲▲▲▲▲▲▲▲▲▲▲▲▲▲▲▲▲▲▲▲▲▲▲ contraindicated in patients with glaucoma. Warn patients to avoid driving and other hazardous activities because their ability to accommodate vision for close activities will be inhibited. Patients will be unable to read or perform activities that require close-up visual acuity. Eyes should be protected by dimming lights and wearing dark glasses in the sunshine. Be certain that patients know the possible adverse effects of atropine and know to report to their ophthalmic physician if these occur. Symptoms to report include flushing and dryness of the skin, blurred vision, rapid and irregular pulse, fever, delirium, and hallucinations. Coma may occur with hypotension, and respiratory depression and may lead to death, especially in the very young. Headache, eye pain, and other symptoms of glaucoma should be reported. Prolonged use may lead to conjunctivitis.

EVALUATION Compare vital signs and cardiovascular ▲▲▲▲▲▲▲▲▲▲ assessments with baseline assessments. Pupils will appear dilated.

ADRENERGICS

Adrenergic medications stimulate beta-receptor sites. Their actions mimic the sympathetic nervous system actions of epinephrine. Thus, they are sometimes referred to as sympathomimetics. Examples include epinephrine hydrochloride (Adrenalin Chloride, Glaucon) 0.25% to 2%, and tetrahydrozoline hydrochloride (Visine, Murine) 0.05%.

ACTIONS AND USES Adrenergics produce mydriasis (di-▲▲▲▲▲▲▲▲▲▲▲▲▲▲▲ lation of pupils), increase the outflow and decrease the production of aqueous humor, relax the ciliary muscle, and constrict the blood vessels of the eye. They are used to treat open-angle glaucoma, to produce mydriasis for examination of the eye, and to decrease congestion and hyperemia of the eye. Localized adverse effects include stinging, burning, and photophobia.

Systemic effects are not common. Tachycardia, palpitations and arrhythmias, hypertension, anxiety, trembling, and increased perspiration may result from the use of adrenergic medications.

ASSESSMENT Assess the chart for a history of hyper-
▲▲▲▲▲▲▲▲▲▲ tension, hyperthyroidism, heart disease, asthma, or diabetes mellitus. Symptoms of these illnesses may be aggravated by adrenergics. Assess the vital signs, cardiovascular status and, cardiopulmonary status. Document assessment findings.

PLANNING AND IMPLEMENTATION Caution patients to
▲▲▲▲▲▲▲▲▲▲▲▲▲▲▲▲▲▲▲▲▲▲▲ protect the eyes from bright lights.

Encourage patients with diabetes mellitus to monitor fingerstick blood glucose levels.

Caution patients who habitually use over-the-counter preparations containing tetrahydrozoline that intraocular pressure may increase. Teach them to discontinue use if headache or eye pain develops.

EVALUATION Monitor vital signs. Compare cardiovas-
▲▲▲▲▲▲▲▲▲▲ cular and cardiopulmonary assessments with the baseline data. Pupils will be dilated. Monitor the physician's records of intraocular pressure. Monitor for hyperglycemia.

ADRENERGIC BLOCKERS

Adrenergic blockers inhibit actions of the sympathetic nervous system, so they are sometimes also called sympatholytics. There are different types of adrenergic blockers. The ones discussed here block the beta-adrenergic receptors and prevent epinephrine and norepinephrine from stimulating them. Examples are levobunolol hydrochloride (Betagan) 0.5%, betaxolol (Betoptic) 0.25% to 0.5%, and timolol maleate (Timoptic) 0.25% to 0.5%.

ACTIONS AND USES The exact mechanism of action of
▲▲▲▲▲▲▲▲▲▲▲▲▲▲▲▲ the ophthalmic solutions is unknown, but they are thought to decrease the production of aqueous humor. They are used to reduce intraocular pressure in patients with chronic open-angle glaucoma. Adrenergic blockers do not affect pupil size and therefore have little or no effect on visual acuity.

Conjunctivitis, blepharitis, and keratitis are known to occur as localized adverse effects. Adverse systemic effects are not common but include bradycardia, arrhythmia, hypotension, and bronchospasm. These are more common in those with bronchial asthma, heart disease, or hypertension and in those using systemic beta-blockers for the same conditions.

ASSESSMENT Assess the chart for a history of bronchial
▲▲▲▲▲▲▲▲▲▲ asthma, heart disease, or systemic medication with other beta-blockers. Assess vital signs, cardiovascular status, and cardiopulmonary status.

PLANNING AND IMPLEMENTATION Warn patients that
▲▲▲▲▲▲▲▲▲▲▲▲▲▲▲▲▲▲▲▲▲▲▲▲▲▲▲▲▲▲ burning and stinging are common when drops are first instilled. Caution patients to report any symptoms of eye irritation that persist.

EVALUATION Compare vital signs and cardiovascular
▲▲▲▲▲▲▲▲▲▲ and cardiopulmonary assessment findings with baseline data. Symptoms of glaucoma will dissipate. Monitor the chart for the physician's records of intraocular pressure.

CARBONIC ANHYDRASE INHIBITORS

The enzyme carbonic anhydrase produces free hydrogen ions that are exchanged for sodium ions in the kidney tubules. The inhibitors interfere with this action, and therefore sodium, potassium, bicarbonate, and water are excreted. Examples of oral forms of carbonic anhydrase inhibitors are acetazolamide (Diamox) and dichlorphenamide (Daranide).

ACTIONS AND USES In the eye, bicarbonate is formed in
▲▲▲▲▲▲▲▲▲▲▲▲▲▲▲▲ the ciliary body and secreted into the aqueous humor. Water follows the bicarbonate and increases the intraocular pressure. The carbonic anhydrase inhibitors are used to interfere with this action and cause excretion of the bicarbonate, which in turn decreases secretion of the aqueous humor. Ophthalmic use of carbonic anhydrase inhibitors in conjunction with other medications decreases intraocular pressure in simple, open-angle glaucoma and sometimes in other types of glaucoma.

ASSESSMENT Review the patient's history for an al-
▲▲▲▲▲▲▲▲▲▲ lergy to sulfonamides because the inhibitors are sulfonamide derivatives. Also review for a history of chronic pulmonary, renal, or hepatic disease. Assess for symptoms of fluid and electrolyte imbalance and verify serum electrolyte results. Assess the chart for baseline intraocular pressures. Obtain baseline vital signs.

PLANNING AND IMPLEMENTATION Teach patients the
▲▲▲▲▲▲▲▲▲▲▲▲▲▲▲▲▲▲▲▲▲▲▲▲▲▲ following:

Store these medications in airtight, light-resistant containers.

Take the medication early in the day to obtain maximal benefit.

Drink 6 to 8 glasses of liquid a day unless contraindicated by other medical conditions.

Ingest food sources of potassium to prevent hypokalemia. Report to the physician the occurrence of signs or symptoms of hypokalemia, such as paresthesia, drowsiness, muscle weakness, respiratory distress, arrhythmias, headache, confusion, vomiting, and diarrhea.

Take the medication with meals if gastric distress occurs.

Caution patients not to drive or operate hazardous machinery until response to the medication has been determined.

EVALUATION Monitor vital signs and pulmonary, re-
▲▲▲▲▲▲▲▲▲▲ nal, and biliary status. Compare assessment findings with baseline data. Monitor for symptoms of fluid and electrolyte balance and serum electrolyte values. Monitor the physician's records of intraocular pressure.

OSMOTIC DIURETICS

Osmotic agents increase osmotic pressure of plasma. This causes extracellular fluid to be drawn into the blood and circulated to the kidney for excretion.

ACTIONS AND USES Osmotic agents decrease intraocu-
▲▲▲▲▲▲▲▲▲▲▲▲▲▲▲ lar fluid and pressure. They are used in patients with acute closed-angle glaucoma, preoperatively and postoperatively for patients undergoing iridectomy, in repair of retinal detachment, and for cataract extractions and keratoplasty.

Adverse actions include headache, nausea, vomiting, diarrhea, thirst, dehydration, and urinary retention. Congestive heart failure, circulatory overload with pulmonary edema, disorientation, agitation, and convulsions are possible.

Examples of osmotic diuretics used for eye conditions are glycerin (glycerol, Osmoglyn) 50% oral solution, mannitol (Osmitrol) 15% to 25% intravenous (IV) solutions, and anhydrous topical glycerin (Ophthalgan).

ASSESSMENT Assess vital signs and cardiopulmonary
▲▲▲▲▲▲▲▲▲▲ status. Document baseline findings. Assess for signs and symptoms of electrolyte imbalance or renal impairment. Assess the chart for reports of serum electrolyte levels and intraocular pressures. Review the patient's history for indications of cardiac, renal, or hepatic disease and diabetes mellitus. Obtain the patient's accurate weight because oral and IV doses are based on body weight. Assess the patient's mental status and level of consciousness and document as baseline information.

PLANNING AND IMPLEMENTATION Oral preparations
▲▲▲▲▲▲▲▲▲▲▲▲▲▲▲▲▲▲▲▲▲▲▲▲▲▲ are administered 60 to 90 minutes before surgery. Pour oral preparations over cracked ice and encourage patients to sip slowly. Excessive sweetness of these preparations causes nausea in some patients.

Before the instillation of some topical preparations, such as Ophthalgan, a topical anesthetic is to be instilled to prevent pain. Follow directions carefully.

IV infusion should be initiated 60 to 90 minutes before surgery and should take 30 to 60 minutes.

Monitor patients for symptoms of congestive heart failure and pulmonary edema, which may occur rapidly, especially with IV infusion. Monitor for urinary retention. When administration is to be by the IV route, insertion of an indwelling catheter may be ordered before the infusion.

Monitor for fluid and electrolyte imbalances, such as water intoxication or dehydration. Keep accurate measurements of intake and output.

Patients with diabetes mellitus may experience acidosis. Monitor for symptoms of hyperglycemia.

EVALUATION Compare vital signs, cardiopulmonary
▲▲▲▲▲▲▲▲▲▲ status, mental status, and level of consciousness with baseline assessment findings. Compare serum glucose and electrolyte levels with baseline values. Compare documented intraocular pres-sures with those documented before initiation of osmotic diuretic therapy.

ANESTHETICS

Examples of ophthalmic anesthetics are tetracaine hydrochloride (Pontocaine) 0.5% and cocaine hydrochloride 1% to 4% solutions.

ACTIONS AND USES Topical anesthetic drops are used
▲▲▲▲▲▲▲▲▲▲▲▲▲▲▲▲▲ to eliminate the blink reflex and to eliminate the pain associated with procedures per-

formed on the eye. Some diagnostic procedures, such as tonometry, may be performed after an anesthetic has been instilled into the eye. Other procedures, such as removal of a foreign body, suturing, suture removal, and radial keratotomy, also require an anesthetic. Adverse actions include rash and urticaria.

ASSESSMENT Assess the patient for allergies to medi-
▲▲▲▲▲▲▲▲▲▲ cations. Assess the eye for redness, ir-
ritation, and tearing. Stinging immediately after instillation is common. Assess vital signs and document them.

PLANNING AND IMPLEMENTATION Store the solution in
▲▲▲▲▲▲▲▲▲▲▲▲▲▲▲▲▲▲▲▲▲▲▲▲▲▲▲ a tightly closed container. Do not use the solution if it is discolored.

Protect the affected eye with a patch until the anesthetic has "worn off." The protective action of the blink reflex is inhibited.

EVALUATION Anesthetic is effective when pain is no
▲▲▲▲▲▲▲▲▲▲ longer felt and the blink reflex is inhib-
ited. The anesthetic has worn off when the blink reflex returns. Compare vital signs with baseline assessments.

ANTISEPTICS

Examples of ophthalmic antiseptics are benzalkonium chloride (Zephiran) 1:5000 solution, boric acid (Blinx, Collyrium) 2% solution or 5% to 10% ointment, thimerosal 0.1% solution, and silver nitrate 1%.

ACTIONS AND USES Some antiseptics retard the
▲▲▲▲▲▲▲▲▲▲▲▲▲▲ growth of organisms on a surface
through an unknown action. Antiseptics are used to irrigate and cleanse the eye of excess secretions. As a germicidal, they are used in cleansing solutions for contact lenses. Silver nitrate is sometimes used in the eyes of the neonate at delivery for preventive treatment of ophthalmia neonatorum. Adverse reactions include redness, irritation, drainage, and periorbital edema. Silver nitrate also stains the skin.

ASSESSMENT Assess for symptoms of redness, itching,
▲▲▲▲▲▲▲▲▲▲ or drainage. Document findings as baseline data.

PLANNING AND IMPLEMENTATION Do not use benzalko-
▲▲▲▲▲▲▲▲▲▲▲▲▲▲▲▲▲▲▲▲▲▲▲▲▲▲ nium chloride or thimerosal if abrasion is present in the eye. These

solutions may be toxic to the corneal cells. Do not use benzalkonium chloride with fluorescein dyes or sulfonamides. Do not use boric acid with polyvinyl alcohol (Liquifilm) because they are incompatible.

When irrigating an infected eye, turn the patient's head toward the affected side so drainage will not contaminate the unaffected eye.

Store silver nitrate wax ampules away from light. Liquid is clear and colorless. Discard solutions that are discolored. Bacitracin inactivates silver nitrate, so they should not be used together.

Silver nitrate stains the skin, so do not let drops fall onto the infant's face. It also stains clothing and bedding.

Wear dark glasses if bright light causes photophobia.

EVALUATION Compare symptoms with baseline as-
▲▲▲▲▲▲▲▲▲▲ sessments.

ANTIBIOTICS

Antibiotics are bactericidal (kill bacteria) or bacteriostatic (retard the growth of bacteria). There are many ophthalmic antibiotic solutions and ointments. Some products combine two or more antibiotics, which are sometimes combined with other drugs. Examples are bacitracin (Baciguent), chloramphenicol (Chloromycetin), erythromycin (Ilotycin) 0.5%, tobramycin (Tobrex), and polymyxin B sulfate.

ACTIONS AND USES Many ophthalmic antibiotics act to
▲▲▲▲▲▲▲▲▲▲▲▲▲▲▲▲ prevent protein synthesis in micro-
organisms, which prevents their reproduction and growth. They are used to treat superficial infections in the eye and sometimes to prevent ophthalmia neonatorum.

Adverse effects include worsening of symptoms, severe burning, and periorbital edema. Chloramphenicol may cause bone marrow hypoplasia and aplastic anemia with prolonged use.

ASSESSMENT Assess for allergies. Assess for redness,
▲▲▲▲▲▲▲▲▲▲ burning, itching, and drainage also.

PLANNING AND IMPLEMENTATION Some ointments may
▲▲▲▲▲▲▲▲▲▲▲▲▲▲▲▲▲▲▲▲▲▲▲▲▲▲▲▲▲▲ cause blurred vision.
Prolonged or intermittent use may cause hypersensitivity reactions and overgrowth of resistant organisms and fungi.

Notify the physician if adverse effects or worsening of symptoms occurs.

Chloramphenicol is not for long-term use. Report to

the physician if symptoms do not improve within 3 days.

Encourage the use of dark glasses if photophobia occurs.

EVALUATION Compare symptoms with baseline assessments.

ANTIFUNGALS

An example of an antifungal ophthalmic preparation is natamycin (Natacyn).

ACTIONS AND USES This drug acts to kill fungi or yeasts. It is used in blepharitis, conjunctivitis, and keratitis caused by fungi.

Adverse effects include blurred vision, photophobia, edema, hyperemia, and pain.

ASSESSMENT Assess for allergies, redness, burning, itching, and drainage.

PLANNING AND IMPLEMENTATION Prolonged or intermittent use may cause hypersensitivity reactions and overgrowth of resistant organisms and fungi. If no improvement is noted in 7 to 10 days, report to the physician. Therapy should normally continue for 14 to 21 days.

Notify the physician if severe burning, itching, periorbital edema, or worsening of symptoms occurs.

Encourage the use of dark glasses if photophobia occurs. If pain develops, notify the physician and discontinue use.

EVALUATION Compare symptoms with baseline assessments.

ANTIVIRALS

Examples of antiviral ophthalmic preparations are idoxuridine (IDU, Dendrid, Herplex), trifluridine (Viroptic), and vidarabine (Vira-A).

ACTIONS AND USES These medications act by interfering with DNA synthesis, which prevents reproduction of the virus. These products are effective for treating conjunctivitis and keratitis caused by herpes simplex virus types 1 and 2.

ASSESSMENT Assess for allergies, redness, burning, itching, and drainage.

PLANNING AND IMPLEMENTATION Idoxuridine is contraindicated in cases of deep ulcerations. Do not mix with other medications or boric acid eyewashes.

Herplex does not require refrigeration, but the other products do.

Treatment is continued for 3 to 5 days after healing has occurred to prevent recurrences.

Encourage the use of dark glasses if photophobia occurs. Discourage driving or operation of hazardous equipment if blurring occurs.

EVALUATION Compare symptoms with baseline assessments.

CORTICOSTEROIDS

Examples of ophthalmic preparations of corticosteroids are dexamethasone (Maxidex ophthalmic suspension), dexamethasone sodium phosphate (Decadron Phosphate ophthalmic ointment), polyvinyl alcohol (¼% Liquifilm Tears, 3% Liquifilm Forte) hydrocortisone acetate (Hydrocortone), and prednisolone sodium phosphate (Inflamase Mild ⅛% Ophthalmic, Inflamase Forte 1% Ophthalmic).

ACTIONS AND USES Steroids act to decrease inflammatory reactions and the invasion of leukocytes into an inflamed area. These medications are used to treat allergic reactions of the eye and all noninfectious inflammations of the eye.

Adverse actions are increased intraocular pressure, cataracts, blurred vision, and optic nerve damage. Decrease in leukocytes may cause interference with wound healing and exacerbation of bacterial, fungal, or viral infections.

ASSESSMENT Assess for a history of glaucoma, infection, diabetes mellitus, and increased intraocular pressure. Assess symptoms of redness, burning, and drainage. Assess visual acuity. Document assessment findings as baseline data.

PLANNING AND IMPLEMENTATION Steroids are used for a limited time only. Systemic effects and adrenal suppression may occur with long-term use.

Shake suspensions before use. Store suspensions in tightly closed containers.

Monitor intraocular pressures. Teach patients to report headache, eye pain, and blurred vision, which may indicate increased intraocular pressure.

Teach patients with diabetes mellitus to monitor fingerstick blood glucose levels and to report symptoms of hyperglycemia.

EVALUATION Compare symptoms with baseline assessment findings. Compare visual acuity and tonometry readings with baseline recordings.

E X E R C I S E S

LEARNING ACTIVITIES

1. Role play the following situations:

Mr. J.L. is using carbachol drops for his glaucoma. You note that his pupils are constricted. Mr. J.L. asks you to explain how that helps his glaucoma.

You are teaching a 55-year-old woman to instill homatropine drops. Include techniques of administration as well as side effects.

2. Prepare a nursing care plan for an 80-year-old man who is to receive IV Osmitrol tomorrow before his cataract extraction. Include the scientific rationale for your nursing interventions.

MENTAL AEROBICS

1. Discuss the advantages of the use of timolol maleate (Timoptic) drops over carbachol drops for treatment of glaucoma.

2. The patient is prescribed acetazolamide (Diamox) for treatment of his glaucoma. Why does the nurse ask him to discuss his allergies?

3. Explain to the patient how an osmotic diuretic works to decrease intraocular pressure.

DRUGS THAT AFFECT THE SKIN

LEARNING OBJECTIVES

After studying this chapter, you should be able to:

1. Discuss various classifications of drugs used to treat infections and wounds of the skin.

2. Name examples of each of the listed classifications.

3. Discuss adverse effects of drugs in each of the listed classifications.

4. Prepare a plan of care for a patient receiving one of these medications.

DRUGS YOU WILL LEARN ABOUT IN THIS CHAPTER

Anti-infectives

Antibiotics

aminoglycosides: gentamicin sulfate (Garamycin, Apogen), neomycin (Myciguent), neomycin B (Framycetin, Soframycin)

bacitracin (Baciguent, Bacitin)

nitrofurazone (Furacin)

Sulfonamides

silver sulfadiazine (Silvadene)

mafenide acetate (Sulfamylon)

Antivirals

acyclovir (Zovirax)

Antifungals

amphotericin B (Fungizone)

clotrimazole (Lotrimin, Mycelex)

nystatin (Mycostatin, Nilstat)

miconazole (Monistat)

tolnaftate (Tinactin)

Proteolytic Enzymes

collagenase (Santyl, Biozyme-C)

sutilaine (Travase)

trypsin (Granulex)

fibrinolysin and deoxyribonuclease (Elase, Elase-Chloromycetin)

Hydroactive or Hydrophilic Products

dextranomer (Debrisan)

Sorbsan rope or dressing

DuoDERM Hydroactive granules

Retinoids

tretinoin/retinoic acid (Retin-A, vitamin A acid)

Corticosteroids

hydrocortisone (Cort-Dome, Cortef, Hytone) 1%

methylprednisolone (Medrol) 0.25%

triamcinolone acetonide (Aristocort, Kenalog), 0.025%, 0.1%, 0.5%

betamethasone valerate (Betaderm, Valisone) 0.1%

Platelet-Derived Wound Healing Formula

  Procuren solution

Emollients

  aluminum paste

  glycerin (Corn Huskers Lotion)

  hydrophilic lotion or ointment

  liquid petroleum

  oatmeal (Aveeno Colloidal, Aveeno Oilated Bath)

  A & D ointment (Balmex, Desitin, Comfortine)

The skin or integumentary system is composed of two main layers:

1. the epidermis, which is composed of layers of epithelial cells; and

2. the dermis, which contains many blood vessels, nerve endings, and gland openings within a framework of connective tissue.

Below the dermis is the subcutaneous layer, which contains the sweat and oil glands and the nail beds. Elastic and fibrous connective tissue, along with a layer of fat, acts to insulate the body and connect the dermis to the muscles.

There are five functions of the skin:

1. *Protection.* The skin protects the deeper tissues from drying and acts as a mechanical barrier against pathogens. When the skin barrier is intact, there is no portal of entry for bacteria. The slightly acid secretions of the glands make the environment on the skin less conducive to the growth of microbes.

2. *Regulation of body temperature.* The skin regulates body temperature by providing a large radiating surface for dissipation of heat to the surrounding air. If blood vessels dilate and bring blood close to the surface, the temperature of the blood is lowered, and eventually the body temperature is lowered. Perspiration released onto the skin cools the body as the moisture is evaporated.

3. *Obtain information from the environment.* Through the profuse nerve endings, the person receives stimuli of sensations, such as pain, touch, pressure, and temperature. This permits the person to respond to factors in the environment that pose a threat to safety.

4. *Absorption.* This is a minimal function. Medicated creams and ointments are absorbed into the skin for a localized effect. Medicated dermal patches release medication that is slowly absorbed into the systemic circulation in sufficient quantities to affect the total body. Medications injected into *sub*cutaneous tissues are absorbed into the systemic circulation more rapidly than are those medications applied to the epidermis but more slowly than those injected into muscles and veins.

5. *Excretion.* This is also a minimal function. Small amounts of water and mineral salts are secreted onto the skin through the sweat glands. The amount excreted by the skin is usually negligible. In abnormal conditions, such as renal failure, amounts are often increased.

ACTIONS AND USES Several classifications of drugs, ▲▲▲▲▲▲▲▲▲▲▲▲▲▲▲ such as antibiotics, antivirals, antifungals, other anti-infectives, steroids, enzymes, and emollients, have effects on the body when they are applied to the skin. The amount of medication absorbed depends on the drug form. In general, smaller molecules are absorbed more readily than larger ones are, and water-based solutions are absorbed more readily than oil-based ointments are. The action and uses of each drug vary with the classification. Related chapters contain this specific information.

Hormones, antihistamines, antianginals, antihypertensives, and other medications may also be applied to the skin as pastes and patches, but systemic effects are expected from their use. Discussion in this chapter is limited to medications applied to the skin to treat conditions of the skin, nails, or hair.

ASSESSMENT Review the patient's history for allergies. ▲▲▲▲▲▲▲▲▲▲ Check to see whether specimens for culture and sensitivity studies have been obtained before initiation of therapy for skin infections.

Assess for any factors predisposing to the condition and document relevant information. Assess the patient's knowledge of the precipitating condition.

Measure and assess the appearance of the wound. Document exact measurements and descriptions as baseline data. If institutional policy allows and proper written consent is obtained from the patient, photographs of affected areas may be attached to the chart.

Obtain vital signs and document as baseline data. Document any signs and symptoms of systemic infection.

Assess the patient's complaints of itching, burning, or pain. Document findings as baseline data.

Also assess hearing ability, renal function, and hepatic function. Many of these preparations are ototoxic, nephrotoxic, or hepatotoxic. Review the chart for results of urinalysis and blood urea nitrogen (BUN) and creatinine levels. Review the patient's entire medication regimen to determine whether other ototoxic, hepatotoxic, or nephrotoxic drugs are being used. Such drugs may increase the chance for occurrence of toxic effects, especially when they are used on large, open wounds.

PLANNING AND IMPLEMENTATION If culture specimens ▲▲▲▲▲▲▲▲▲▲▲▲▲▲▲▲▲▲▲▲▲▲▲▲▲▲▲▲▲▲▲▲ have not been obtained, be sure to get a physician's order. Culture the wounds before initiation of therapy if skin infection is present.

Cleanse the area to remove accumulated debris before application of the ordered medication. Irrigations and whirlpool are particularly effective for large or deep wounds. Check the physician's orders carefully. Maintain universal precautions with all aspects of care. Always wash your hands before and after wound care procedures.

For the application of medications, wear sterile gloves or use a sterile tongue blade to avoid accidental absorption of the medication into your hands, to prevent contamination of your hands, and to maintain asepsis of the wounds. If the patient or significant other will be doing the wound care, teach aseptic procedures and explain the rationale.

Document wound appearance daily and compare with baseline data. Observe for irritation or symptoms of infection. Monitor the vital signs. Monitor the patient's complaints of discomfort. Notify the physician of any adverse reactions or changes in the patient's condition.

Monitor for signs and symptoms of the precipitating condition. Reinforce teaching related to the precipitating condition.

If the drug may be nephrotoxic, monitor intake, output, urinalysis results, and serum creatinine and BUN levels. If the drug may be ototoxic, monitor the patient's complaints of hearing changes and monitor hearing acuity.

When the patient is to be discharged, teach the importance of keeping follow-up appointments with the physician.

EVALUATION Compare the wound, rash, or lesion with ▲▲▲▲▲▲▲▲▲▲ baseline assessments. Compare daily assessments of any precipitating conditions with the baseline data.

When appropriate, compare measurements of intake and output and results of renal and hepatic function tests with baseline data. Compare hearing acuity with baseline results. Compare the patient's complaints of discomfort with those of preceding days.

Evaluate teaching. Ask the patient or significant other who is to do the wound care to explain or demonstrate procedures to you or to another family member.

ANTI-INFECTIVES

Antibiotics

Antibiotics for topical use are frequently prepared as creams. Apply them to the affected area two or three times a day as ordered by the physician.

Aminoglycosides

Aminoglycosides contain at least one sugar attached to an amino group. The first of these, streptomycin, was developed after penicillin and the sulfonamides and is often used in combined therapy with these drugs to give a broader spectrum of coverage. Examples of aminoglycosides commonly used as topical preparations include gentamicin sulfate (Garamycin, Apogen), neomycin (Myciguent), and neomycin B (Framycetin, Soframycin).

These bactericidal drugs act by interfering with protein synthesis. They are particularly effective against gram-negative bacteria and are frequently used to treat aerobic gram-negative infections. They have little effect against anaerobic organisms. Topical use of these drugs includes treatment of primary and secondary skin infections caused by sensitive strains of commonly occurring bacteria, such as streptococci, staphylococci, *Pseudomonas, Escherichia coli,* and *Klebsiella.* Topical preparations of these medications are usually creams or ointments, medicated gauze, and solutions for irrigation. Adverse actions include ototoxic and nephrotoxic effects, allergic reactions such as rash, urticaria, pruritus, fever, and stomatitis.

Remain alert for early signs of ototoxic effects, such as tinnitus and reduced perception of high-pitched sounds. Monitor intake and output (I & O) to detect early signs of nephrotoxic effects. Monitor for overgrowth of nonsusceptible organisms.

Solutions are unstable and must be used before the expiration date. Refrigerate unused portions.

Bacitracin

Bacitracin (Baciguent, Bacitin) is a local anti-infective agent produced by *Bacillus subtilis.*

Bacitracin may be bactericidal or bacteriostatic, depending on the organism and on the concentration of the drug. It acts by inhibiting cell wall synthesis. It is particularly useful against streptococci, staphylococci, and many other gram-positive organisms.

Nitrofurazone

Nitrofurazone (Furacin) has antibacterial activity against gram-positive and gram-negative bacteria. Its mode of action is unknown, but it is believed to inhibit carbohydrate metabolism within the organism. It is used to treat second- and third-degree burns, ulcers, superficial wounds, and infections.

Adverse reactions include nephrotoxic effects, erythema, burning, pruritus, edema, vesicle formation, or ulceration.

Generalized allergic reactions sometimes occur if nitrofurazone is applied continuously for 5 days or more. Discontinue use and notify the physician if symptoms occur.

If wet dressings are used, the surrounding skin must be protected with a barrier, such as zinc oxide.

Store the solution in light-resistant containers that are kept tightly closed. Discard discolored solutions.

Safe use during pregnancy or lactation has not been established.

Sulfonamides

Sulfonamides, or "sulfa drugs," were first developed in the 1930s and were the first effective systemic antimicrobials. Examples of topical preparations in use today are silver sulfadiazine (Silvadene) and mafenide acetate (Sulfamylon). (See Chapter 19 for more information.)

The sulfonamides are bacteriostatic, acting to inhibit the growth of bacteria by inhibiting the synthesis of folic acid, an essential enzyme. They do this by competing with p-aminobenzoic acid (PABA), which is essential for folic acid production. The bacteria cannot assimilate the sulfonamides. Topical uses are the treatment of leg ulcers, abrasions, second- and third-degree burns, and skin grafts. Applications are twice a day or as ordered by the physician.

Adverse actions include allergic reactions with symptoms of rash, pruritus, swelling, hives, blisters, and erythema. Mafenide acetate may also cause pain and burning at the site. Absorption through a large wound can cause eosinophilia, renal dysfunction, or hepatic dysfunction.

Monitor the patient's hygiene status and assist with personal care if necessary. Do not use cream that is discolored. Cleanse the area before application of the cream. Keep the area covered with cream continuously. Apply the cream only to affected areas.

Report to the physician if pain and burning persist because the drug may need to be discontinued. Monitor I & O. Monitor for signs and symptoms of electrolyte impairment.

Tell the patient to inform the physician if pregnancy is suspected. Use is contraindicated during pregnancy and lactation and in newborns.

Antivirals

Acyclovir

Acyclovir (Zovirax) effectively acts against the herpes virus by inhibiting DNA synthesis. Topical applications are used for herpes lesions on the lips (type I) and also for genital herpes (type II). Adverse actions from use of topical ointment include burning, rash, and pruritus.

Therapy should be initiated as soon as possible after onset of lesions. Apply sufficient amounts to cover the affected areas six times a day for 7 days.

Teach the patient to avoid contact with other body sites. Autoinoculation of other areas is possible. Wear a glove to apply acyclovir, and wash your hands frequently.

Newborns are especially vulnerable to this virus. Teach parents that herpes can cause death in newborns.

Pain and burning sensations from lesions should decrease after application of ointment.

Antifungals

Fungal infections may involve the hair, nails, and skin. They particularly affect areas that remain warm and moist, such as the feet, the axillary area, under the breasts, and the perineal area. Topical preparations may be in the form of creams, powders, solutions, or aerosol sprays applied two to three times a day as ordered by the physician. Topical preparations of antifungal medications include amphotericin B (Fungizone), clotrimazole (Lotrimin, Mycelex), nystatin (Mycostatin, Nilstat), miconazole (Monistat), and tolnaftate (Tinactin).

Most of the preparations act by affecting the integrity of the cell membrane of the fungus and thus permit loss of valuable elements from the cell. Antifungals can be fungistatic or fungicidal. They are used to treat conditions caused by *Candida* and *Tinea* organisms. Adverse reactions may include localized reactions, such as erythema, burning, blistering, and pruritus.

Salicylic acid and benzoic acid (Whitfield's ointment) and salicylanilide are keratolytic agents that promote softening and desquamation (shedding) of the outer layers of cells. This helps remove the fungi that tend to burrow down to the base of the keratin layer of the skin and also assists other drugs to penetrate the area. Keratolytic agents may cause such adverse reactions as swelling and softening of noninfected cells and open areas on the skin, which may act as portals for other organisms to enter the body.

Assess female patients to determine the presence of pregnancy. Safe use of clotrimazole in pregnancy (and in children younger than 3 years of age) has not been determined.

Note the presence of ulcerations or burns. These increase the absorption of medication and increase the likelihood of the occurrence of systemic side effects, such as nausea, vomiting, and diarrhea.

Take care to avoid inhalation of powders or aerosol sprays.

Teach patients to complete the full course of therapy as ordered by the physician, even if symptoms dissipate. This prevents recurrence of symptoms and the development of resistant strains of the organism.

PROTEOLYTIC ENZYMES

Proteolytic enzymes are proteins produced by microorganisms. They have been purified and otherwise prepared for medicinal use. Preparations include liquids, ointments, and aerosol sprays. Examples are collagenase (Santyl, Biozyme-C), sutilains (Travase), trypsin (Granulex), and a combination product called fibrinolysin and deoxyribonuclease (Elase). The last product is sometimes also combined with an antibiotic (chloramphenicol) and is called Elase-Chloromycetin.

These enzymes dissolve protein of tissue debris and wound exudate. They are used to clean and debride necrotic wounds, burns, and ulcers. Combining the antibiotic with the preparation adds a bactericidal action to the product. This is important because natural barriers to infection are inhibited. Proteolytic enzymes are used to liquefy fibrinous or purulent exudates.

Adverse actions include allergic responses, bleeding from the wound, and increased chance of infection in the wound.

Because these enzymes are a foreign protein (antigen) to the patient, the chance of allergic reaction is present. Monitor for increased inflammation in the tissues surrounding the wound and a rash. Teach patients to report symptoms of possible allergic reactions promptly.

Store ointments and solutions in cool areas. Do not shake or agitate solutions because the protein may be damaged.

Wounds must be cleansed at least daily and must be kept moist for enzymes to work. Avoid contact with healthy tissues because they may also be damaged. Coat surrounding wound edges with petroleum jelly. Avoid allowing the enzyme to contact the eyes. Be especially careful when using sprays.

Report to the physician if bleeding from the wound is increasing. The enzyme interferes with clot formation, and hemorrhage may result.

HYDROACTIVE OR HYDROPHILIC DRESSINGS

These preparations may be powders, granules, "rope," or topical wound dressings. The products are hydrophilic (capable of absorbing water). They are applied into shallow wounds or ulcers or are placed over them, where they cleanse by absorbing secretions from the wound. Examples are dextranomer (Debrisan), Sorbsan dressings and rope, and DuoDERM Hydroactive granules.

The absorption and capillary action remove microorganisms with the fluid and reduce edema and inflammation. They attract the secretions and form a gel that must be removed by irrigation before reapplication of the product. They do not appear to cause any irritation or side effects. Patients sometimes complain of some mild discomfort or "drawing" sensation due to the absorption action.

Hydroactive or hydrophilic dressings are used in the management of draining ulcerations or decubitus ulcers and some superficial draining skin lesions.

Assess the wound for the presence of secretions before initiation of therapy. Hydrophilic products should not be used in dry wounds because they have no effect. The wound must be irrigated before each use to remove as much loose debris and exudate as possible. The physician frequently orders normal saline for this purpose. Do not dry the wound.

Debrisan beads and DuoDERM granules are poured into the wound 1/8- to 1/4-inch thick. Sorbsan rope is packed loosely into the wound, allowing room for expansion as the exudate is absorbed. A loose gauze dressing is applied over the top and sealed on all four sides to prevent the loss of the product and exudate from the wound. Sorbsan dressings must also be covered with a gauze dressing. Treatments are usually ordered twice a day or more often until the amount of exudate diminishes.

Maintain aseptic technique throughout the procedure to prevent introduction of additional pathogens.

N U R S I N G   A L E R T

▼▼▼▼▼▼▼▼▼▼▼▼▼▼▼▼▼▼▼▼▼▼▼▼▼▼▼▼▼

Do not use petroleum jelly or other substance around the wound because it will inactivate the hydrophilic action of the product.

▲▲▲▲▲▲▲▲▲▲▲▲▲▲▲▲▲▲▲▲▲▲▲▲▲▲▲▲▲

When the wound is no longer moist, notify the physician so the procedure may be discontinued. Continued use may interfere with healing.

Store products tightly closed in their original package and in a dry place to prevent absorption of moisture before use.

These products are contraindicated in treatment of full-thickness wounds involving muscle, tendon, or bone and of ulcers resulting from infection, such as tuberculosis, syphilis, and deep fungal infections. Some vascular conditions and systemic lupus erythematosus may also be contraindications.

RETINOIDS

Tretinoin/retinoic acid (Retin-A, vitamin A acid) is a topical preparation of vitamin A used to treat mild to moderately severe cases of acne. Tretinoin acts to increase the growth of epithelial cells that line the comedones (blackheads) and loosens the cells. Within 6 to 8 weeks, the number of papules and pustules usually decreases, although the condition initially appears to worsen. Oral retinoid preparations, such as isotretinoin (Accutane), are used to treat severe cases of acne.

Adverse actions of tretinoin include sensations of warmth and stinging, erythema, blistering, peeling, and edema. Hyperpigmentation or hypopigmentation may also occur.

The area should be clean and dry. A light coat of lotion is applied once daily at bedtime. Inform the patient that some redness and scaling are expected. Teach the patient to avoid sunlight or ultraviolet light during therapy.

N U R S I N G   A L E R T

▼▼▼▼▼▼▼▼▼▼▼▼▼▼▼▼▼▼▼▼▼▼▼▼▼▼▼▼▼

Discontinue use if a sunburn occurs and do not resume until the burn is completely healed.

▲▲▲▲▲▲▲▲▲▲▲▲▲▲▲▲▲▲▲▲▲▲▲▲▲▲▲▲▲

Avoid use of other lotions, creams, medicated soaps, or cosmetics during therapy. They may interact with the tretinoin.

Do not use tretinoin if eczema is present. Avoid contact with mucous membranes. Do not take multivitamin tablets during therapy because most of these contain vitamin A and may contribute to toxicity.

CORTICOSTEROIDS

Topical corticosteroid preparations are available as lotions, creams, gels, and ointments. The site of application influences the choice of the form to be used. For example, gels stay in place better on hairy areas than other forms do, but they contain alcohol, which would irritate mucous membranes. Creams are better for wet, weepy tissues. To be effective, the medication must penetrate to the dermis. Occluding the area speeds this process. Ointments are more occlusive than other forms are, and lotions are least occlusive. To assist absorption, use a commercially prepared occlusive dressing or cover the area with plastic wrap.

Preparations are available in various concentrations. Different preparations have different potencies.

Recent changes in legislation have permitted over-the-counter sale of low-potency, topical corticosteroids. Examples of the numerous products available are hydrocortisone 1% (Cort-Dome, Cortef, Hytone), methylprednisolone 0.25% (Medrol), triamcinolone acetonide 0.025%, 0.1%, 0.5% (Aristocort, Kenalog), and betamethasone valerate 0.1% (Beta-derm, Valisone).

Topical forms of corticosteroids are used for their anti-inflammatory action. They act by constricting peripheral blood vessels, thereby decreasing blood flow to the inflamed area. They also interfere with localized prostaglandin production and alter neutrophil and lymphocyte response to stimuli. They are used for eczema, psoriasis, and rashes caused by a variety of conditions, such as discoid lupus erythematosus, poison ivy, and other allergens.

Adverse actions can be localized or systemic. Localized reactions include thinning of the epidermis, atrophy of the dermis, appearance of striae, and secondary infections. (See Chapter 58 for adverse systemic effects, which can be many and serious.)

N U R S I N G   A L E R T

▼▼▼▼▼▼▼▼▼▼▼▼▼▼▼▼▼▼▼▼▼▼▼▼▼▼▼▼▼

The steroids suppress normal body defense mechanisms. Antimicrobials are frequently ordered to be taken concurrently.

▲▲▲▲▲▲▲▲▲▲▲▲▲▲▲▲▲▲▲▲▲▲▲▲▲▲▲▲▲

If occlusive dressings are being used on large areas of skin surface, assess the temperature every 4 hours.

Notify the physician and remove dressings if the temperature rises.

Monitor patients for the occurrence of adverse systemic effects. Adverse systemic effects are likely to occur especially if potent forms of corticosteroids are being used, if large occlusive dressings are in place, or if an infant is being treated.

Teach patients all of this information. Caution against the indiscriminate use of steroids to treat conditions other than the one for which the medication was prescribed.

PLATELET-DERIVED WOUND HEALING FORMULA

Procuren Solution

Procuren is a solution prepared from the patient's own blood. A 60-mL sample of blood is withdrawn from the patient. The platelets are removed from that, and the growth factors are removed from the platelets.

Procuren contains five growth factors: platelet factor 4, platelet-derived growth factor, transforming growth factor-Beta, platelet-derived angiogenesis factor, and platelet-derived epidermal growth factor. The 60 mL of blood usually produces enough Procuren solution for daily applications for 10 weeks.

Topical application of Procuren solution promotes new granulation tissue, growth of new capillaries in the granulation tissue, and growth of new skin. Use of this product has begun a new era in wound healing. It acts to stimulate initial wound healing when it is used in treatment of chronic, nonhealing skin wounds, such as ulcers caused by diabetes, peripheral vascular disease, neuropathy, collagen disease, and pressure.

Assess the patient's chart for results of other diagnostic tests, such as x-rays, Doppler scans, transcutaneous oxygen measurements, and serum glucose tests.

The wound or ulcer must be cleaned or surgically debrided before Procuren use. Most wounds are infected, so antibiotic therapy must be maintained throughout the course of therapy. Monitor the patient for compliance with the medication regimen and for adverse effects of the antibiotic.

Procuren solution is kept frozen until needed. Each day, another tube should be moved to the refrigerator and permitted to thaw there for 24 hours.

N U R S I N G   A L E R T

▼▼▼▼▼▼▼▼▼▼▼▼▼▼▼▼▼▼▼▼▼▼▼▼▼▼▼▼▼▼▼▼▼▼▼

Be aware that Procuren is a blood product. Maintain appropriate blood and body fluid precautions.

▲▲▲▲▲▲▲▲▲▲▲▲▲▲▲▲▲▲▲▲▲▲▲▲▲▲▲▲▲▲▲▲▲▲▲

The treatment is usually done at night and left in place for 12 hours. Saturate gauze with the Procuren and pack it into the wound all the way to the edges. Cover the gauze with a petrolatum gauze to prevent evaporation, cover with gauze, and secure with a wrap dressing. Avoid taping directly onto the patient's skin to avoid further trauma to the skin. During the alternate 12 hours, the physician usually orders a gauze packing that is saturated with normal saline or an antibiotic solution.

To promote circulation, the patient is usually directed to assist weight bearing with crutches or a walker. Monitor safety or assist the patient as necessary. Teach the patient that elevation of the extremity is important. If a decompression pump is ordered for edema, teach the procedure to the patient. Teach the patient and caregivers principles of good skin care, foot care, prevention of skin breakdown, and skin assessment.

Also teach the patient to follow a balanced diet with adequate amounts of protein for tissue building and vitamin C for healing.

EMOLLIENTS

Emollients soften dry skin by preventing evaporation. They are used for protection of intact skin around draining wounds and ostomies, to heal cracked skin and nipples, and to soothe diaper rashes, sunburn, and abrasions. The area should be clean and dry before application.

Examples of emollient products are aluminum paste, glycerin (Corn Huskers Lotion), hydrophilic lotion or ointment, liquid petroleum, oatmeal (Aveeno Colloidal, Aveeno Oilated Bath), and A & D ointment (Balmex, Desitin, Comfortine).

E X E R C I S E S

MENTAL AEROBICS

1. List appropriate techniques for application of topical creams or ointments to the skin. Include the scientific rationale for your answer.

2. Discuss the actions and uses of proteolytic enzymes.

3. Compare and contrast the methods of application and the precautions for use during wound care between Debrisan and Elase.

4. Discuss the advantages of using a topical cream versus a gel and an ointment versus a liquid.

5. Discuss the actions and uses of Procuren.

USEFUL EQUIVALENCIES

Liquid

1 cc	= 1 mL
1000 mL	= 1 L
1000 L	= 1 kL
60 gtt	= 1 tsp
4 fl dr	= 1 tbsp
8 fl dr	= 1 fl oz
3 tsp	= 1 tbsp
2 tbsp	= 1 fl oz

8 fl oz	= 1 c
2 c	= 1 pt
16 fl oz	= 1 pt
2 pt	= 1 qt
4 qt	= 1 gal
1 mL	= 16 m
4 mL	= 1 fl dr
5 mL	= 1 tsp
30 mL	= 1 fl oz

500 mL	= 1 pt
1000 mL	= 1 qt
1 L	= 1 qt
4 L	= 1 gal
1 fl dr	= 4 mL
1 fl dr	= 1 tsp

Weight

1 g	= 1000 mg

1000 g	= 1 kg
1 kg	= 2.2 lb
16 oz	= 1 lb
1 oz	= 30 g
1 oz	= 16 dr
60 gr	= 1 dr
4 g	= 1 dr
1 g	= 15 gr
60 mg	= 1 gr

ABBREVIATIONS FOR UNITS OF MEASUREMENT

gram	g, G, or gm	kiloliter	kL	fluid dram	fl dr	quart	qt
		meter	M or m	ounce	oz	gallon	gal
milligram	mg	millimeter	mm	fluid ounce	fl oz	cup	c
kilogram	kg	kilometer	km	pound	lb	tablespoon	tbsp or T
liter	L or l	centimeter	cm	inch	in	teaspoon	tsp or t
milliliter	mL	grain	gr	foot	ft	minim	m
cubic centimeter	cc	dram	dr	pint	pt	drop, drops	gtt, gtts

CANADIAN TRADE NAMES OF DRUGS AVAILABLE IN THE UNITED STATES

The following list contains common trade names that are employed in Canada but not in the United States. In the list, trade names are in CAPITAL LETTERS, and generic names are in lowercase letters. Canadian trade names that are formed simply by affixing a manufacturer's prefix to a generic name (such as APO-FLURAZEPAM) are not included in the list. Drugs that are not available in the United States are not included in the list.

Generic Name	Trade Name	Generic Name	Trade Name
acetaminophen	ATASOL	clonazepam	RIVOTRIL
acetazolamide	ACETAZOLAM	clonidine	DIXARIT
acetohexamide	DIMELOR	clorazepate	NOVO-CLOPATE
acetylcysteine	AIRBRON	clotrimazole	CANESTEN, CLOTRIMADERM,
acetylsalicylic acid	ENTROPHEN		MYCLO, NEO-ZOL
albuterol, salbutamol	APO-SALVENT, NOVO-SALMOL	cyanocobalamin	RUBION
allopurinol	ALLOPRIN, PURINOL	cyclophosphamide	PROCYTOX
alprazolam	NOVO-ALPRAZOL	danazol	CYCLOMEN
aminophylline	COROPHYLLIN, PALARON	dexamethasone	SPERSADEX, DERONIL
amitriptyline	LEVATE	dextromethorphan	ROBIDEX, SUDATUSS
amoxicillin	APO-AMOXI, NOVAMOXIN,	diclofenac	NOVO-DIFENAC
	NU-AMOXI	dicyclomine	BENTYLOL, FORMULEX
amoxicillin-clavulanate	CLAVULIN	diethylstilbestrol	HONVOL
ampicillin	AMPICIN, APO-AMP, NU-AMPI	digitoxin	DIGITALINE
atropine	ATROPISOL	diltiazem	APO-DILTIAZ, NU-DILTIAZ
bacampicillin	PENGLOBE	dimenhydrinate	GRAVOL, NAUSEATOL,
bacitracin	BACITIN		TRAVEL AID
beclomethasone	BECLOFORTE	dinoprostone	PREPIDIL, PROSTIN
betamethasone	BETACORT, METADERM	diphenhydramine	ALLEDRYL
bretylium	BRETYLATE	dipyridamole	NOVO-DIPIRADOL
captopril	APO-CAPTO, NU-CAPTO	disopyramide	RYTHMODAN
carbamazepine	NOVO-CARBAMAZ, MAZEPINE	dopamine	REVIMINE
cephalexin	NOVO-LEXIN	doxepin	TRIADAPIN
chloramphenicol	SOPAMYCETIN, PENTAMYCETIN	doxycycline	APO-DOXY
chlordiazepoxide	SOLIUM	ergocalciferol	OSTOFORTE
chlorothiazide	SUPRES	ergotamine	GYNERGEN
chlorpheniramine	CHLOR-TRIPOLON	erythromycin	ERYTHROMID, APO-ERYTHRO
chlorpromazine	LARGACTIL	estrone	FEMOGEN
chlorpropamide	NOVO-PROPAMIDE	ethambutol	ETIBI
cimetidine	PEPTOL, NU-CIMET	flurazepam	NOVO-FLUPAM, SOMNOL
clidinium	APO-CHLORAX, CORIUM	flurbiprofen	FROBEN
clofibrate	NOVO-FIBRATE	folic acid	NOVO-FOLACID

Generic Name	Trade Name	Generic Name	Trade Name
furosemide	URITOL	phenylbutazone	NOVO-BUTAZONE
gentamicin	CIDOMYCIN, GENTAK, GENTRASUL	phytonadione	KONAKION
		pilocarpine	MIOCARPINE, SPERSACARPINE
glyburide	EUGLUCON, GEN-GLYBE	pindolol	NU-PINDOL
griseofulvin	GRISOVIN-FP	piroxicam	NOVO-PIROCAM, NU-PIROX
haloperidol	NOVO-PERIDOL	prazosin	APO-PRAZO, NOVO-PRAZIN, NU-PRAZO
heparin	HEPALEAN		
hydralazine	NOVO-HYLAZIN, NU-HYDRAL	prednisolone	INFLAMASE, NOVO-PRED, PRED
hydrochlorothiazide	APO-HYDRO	prednisone	WINPRED
hydrocodone	HYCODAN, ROBIDONE	primidone	SERTAN
hydrocortisone	CORTATE, HYCORT	prochlorperazine	STEMETIL
hydroxyzine	MULTIPAX	promethazine	HISTANTIL
ibuprofen	ACTIPROFEN, AMERSOL, NOVO-PROFEN	propantheline	BANLIN
		propranolol	NOVO-PRANOL
indomethacin	INDOCID, NOVO-METHACIN, NU-INDO	propylthiouracil	PROPYL-THYRACIL
		protriptyline	TRIPTIL
isoniazid	ISOTAMINE	pseudoephedrine	ELTOR
isosorbide	APO-ISDN, CEDOCARD	psyllium	FIBREPUR, NOVO-MUCILAX, PRODIEM
isosorbide dinitrate	CEDOCARD-SR, CORADUR, CORONEX		
		pyrazinamide	TEBRAZID
ketoprofen	APO-KETO, ORUVAIL, RHODIS	quinidine	BIQUIN
ketorolac	ACULAR	ranitidine	NU-RANIT
lactulose	ACILAC, RHODIALOSE	rifampin	ROFACT
levothyroxine	ELTROXIN	scopolamine	BUSCOPAN, TRANSDERM-V
lidocaine	XYLOGARD	secobarbital	NOVO-SECOBARB
lindane	HEXIT, KWELLADA	silver sulfadiazine	FLAMAZINE
lithium carbonate	CARBOLITH, DURALITH, LITHIZINE	simethicone	OVOL
		spironolactone	NOVO-SPIROTON
lorazepam	NOVO-LORAZEM, NU-LORAZ	sulfinpyrazone	ANTURAN, NOVO-PYRAZONE
methohexital	BRIETAL	sulindac	APO-SULIN, NOVO-SUNDAC
methylclothiazide	DURETIC	tamoxifen	APO-TAMOX, TAMOFEN, TAMONE
methyldopa	DOPAMET, NOVO-MEDOPA, NU-MEDOPA	testosterone	ANDRIOL
		testosterone-estradiol	NEO-PAUSE
methyltestosterone	METANDREN	tetracycline	APO-TETRA, NOVO-TETRA, NU-TETRA
metoclopramide	APO-METOCLOP, MAXERAN		
metoprolol	NOVO-METOPROL	tolbutamide	MOBENOL, NOVO-BUTAMIDE
metronidazole	NOVO-NIDAZOL, TRIKACIDE	tretinoin	STIEVAA, VITAMIN A ACID
nadolol	APO-NADOL	triamterene	APO-TRIAZIDE
naproxen	NAXEN, NEOPROX, NOVO-NAPROX, NU-NAPROX	triazolam	APO-TRIAZO, NOVO-TRIOLAM, NU-TRIAZO
nifedipine	APO-NIFED, NOVO-NIFEDIN, NU-NIFED	trihexyphenidyl	APARKANE, APO-TRIHEX
		vasopressin	PRESSYN
nitrofurantoin	NOVO-FURAN	verapamil	APO-VERAP, NOVO-VERAMIL, NU-VERAP
norethindrone	MICRONOR, NORLUTATE		
nystatin	NADOSTINE, NYADERM	vinblastine	VELBE
oxymetazoline	NAFRINE, OCUCLEAR	warfarin	WARFILONE
penicillin G	MEGACILLIN	zidovudine	NOVO-AZT
pentobarbital	NOVO-PENTOBARB, NOVA-RECTAL		
phenazopyridine	PHENAZO		
phenolphthalein	DOXIDAN		
phentolamine	ROGITINE		

Adapted from Lehne, R. A. (1994). *Pharmacology for nursing care* (2nd ed.). Philadelphia: W. B. Saunders.

GLOSSARY

AV (atrioventricular) term used in discussion of the conduction system of the heart.

Absorption the passage of a drug from the outside of the body to the bloodstream.

Accommodation alteration of the shape of the lens of the eye to allow us to focus on objects close to us and then on those far away.

Actions the physiological response elicited by a drug. The four major drug actions are depression, stimulation, irritation, and demulcence.

Addition when the effects of one drug are added to the effects of another drug, the combined effect of the drugs can be estimated by simply adding the separate effects; also called summative.

Adrenergic agonists drugs that mimic the sympathetic nervous system; also called sympathomimetics.

Adrenergic blockers a classification of drugs that prohibit the actions of the sympathetic nervous system; also called sympathomimetic blockers or sympatholytics.

Adverse reactions effects elicited by a drug that were not the desired effect and are unpleasant or even harmful.

Aerobes those microbes requiring oxygen for life or growth; *adj.* aerobic.

Aggregation agglutination or clumping.

Agonist a drug that stimulates a response from a receptor in the body.

Agranulocytosis an absence (decrease in the normal amounts) of granulocytes (a type of white blood cell).

Alcohol a colorless liquid obtained from fermentation or distillation, it acts as a sedative to the nervous system of the body.

Alcoholic one who drinks alcohol excessively and has either physical or psychological dependence on the substance.

Alkylating agents antineoplastic medications that interfere with cell division in rapidly growing tissues.

Allergen protein substance capable of producing an allergic reaction.

Allergic rhinitis allergic reaction that produces increased nasal mucus; sometimes called hay fever.

Amebiasis an infestation of the body by amebae.

Amebicides a group of drugs that work against amebae. amphetamines a classification of drugs that are central nervous system stimulants.

Anabolic steroids synthetically produced androgens.

Anabolism building-up phase of metabolism.

Anaerobes those microbes that do not require oxygen for life or growth and often survive best where it does not exist; *adj.* anaerobic.

Anaphylactic shock see anaphylaxis.

Anaphylaxis extreme hypersensitivity to a drug; an emergency situation; a severe allergic reaction that may result in death; often produces sudden and severe symptoms, including drop in blood pressure, pallor, cyanosis, respiratory distress, seizures, collapse, coma, and even death; also called anaphylactic shock.

Anesthesia a state of painlessness; a classification of drugs that are used to produce the state of painlessness for surgical purposes.

Ankylosis the permanent fusion of a joint.

Antagonism the counteraction of the effects of one drug by the effects of another drug.

Antagonist a drug that attaches to a receptor site without eliciting a response. It then prevents other chemicals from causing a response as well.

Anthelmintics a group of drugs used to treat an infestation by helminths or worms.

Antiarthropods a group of drugs used to treat an infestation by arthropods.

Antibiotics a classification of drugs used to fight infection by working against specific organisms.

Antibodies proteins made by the body to fight specific diseases when an antigen, such as a virus, bacterium, or toxin, enters the body.

Anticholinergics a classification of drugs that are antagonistic to the actions of the parasympathetic nervous system; also called cholinergic blockers, parasympathomimetic blockers, or parasympatholytics.

Anticonvulsants a classification of drugs used to treat seizures.

Antidiarrheals a classification of drugs given to stop diarrhea.

Antifungals a classification of drugs used to treat fungal or mycotic infections.

Antigens a foreign protein, such as a virus, bacterium, or toxin.

Antigout agents a classification of drugs that are given to treat gouty arthritis.

Antihistamine a classification of drugs that work against the actions of histamine.

Anti-inflammatory a group of drugs that are used to decrease the symptoms of inflammation.

Antimalarials a group of drugs used to treat malaria.

Antimetabolites antineoplastic medications that interfere with cell metabolism, function, or growth.

Antineoplastics drugs intended to destroy the cells of a neoplasm.

Antiprotozoals a group of drugs that work against a class of mostly unicellular animals; also called protozoacides.

Antipyretics a group of drugs that work to decrease the systemic temperature of the body.

Antiseptic an agent that can slow or stop the growth of microorganisms.

Antitoxin a serum containing a special type of antibody that fights the toxins, or poisons, from a specific antigen.

Antitussives a classification of drugs that are given to treat a cough.

Antiviral drugs a classification of drugs that work against viruses.

Anxiolytic a drug that relieves anxiety.

Apical-radial pulse a procedure for the assessment of patients with cardiac symptoms; one nurse listens to the apical pulse while another nurse palpates the radial pulse. A signal is given to start and stop the count so that it is done simultaneously. The counts are normally the same. If there is a difference greater than a few beats, it is called a pulse deficit.

Apothecary system the system of measurement that was once used widely by pharmacies to measure medications; units most often used include the grain, dram, fluid dram, and minim.

Arrhythmia irregular heart rhythm.

Arteriosclerosis a condition produced by unusually high levels of lipids in the blood, which hardens and increases the atherosclerotic plaque formation along the arterial walls.

Arthropods insects that include several groups of lice.

Articular cartilage connective tissue covering the articular surfaces.

Articular surfaces the ends of the bones involved in a joint.

Articulation a joint.

Artificially acquired active immunity the introduction of a killed or attenuated (weakened) antigen by injection or oral solution, which causes the body to make antibodies against the antigen.

Artificially acquired passive immunity the introduction

of antibodies produced by the body of another human or an animal by means of an injection.

Ascites fluid accumulation in the abdominal cavity.

Ataractic a drug that relieves anxiety and nausea.

Atherosclerosis the formation of plaque on the lining of the arterial walls; in this disease, fatty acids in the blood, called lipids, are deposited along the artery's walls.

Augment stimulate or intensify.

Avoirdupois ounces ounces that measure weight; used to differentiate from fluid ounces.

Axon end process of a neuron; transmits impulses away from a neuron.

Bacillus rod-shaped microbe; *pl.* bacilli.

Bactericidal an agent that kills bacteria.

Bacteriostatic an agent that slows or stops the growth of bacteria.

Balanced anesthesia giving other drugs to counteract the potent side effects of anesthetics.

Barbiturates a classification of drugs that are central nervous system depressants.

Bioavailability the degree that a drug can be absorbed and transported to the site of its action.

Biotransformation the process by which a drug is detoxified or turned into harmless substances; also called metabolism.

Bladder the hollow muscular organ found in the pelvic cavity that acts as a reservoir for urine.

Blood-brain barrier a chemical barrier that prevents many drugs from affecting the central nervous system.

Booster a subsequent inoculation of a vaccine at specifically spaced intervals to produce the desired level of immunity.

Broad-spectrum antibiotics antibiotics that are active against a wide range of microbes.

Bronchodilators a classification of drugs that can relax the smooth muscle of the bronchi, resulting in more open airways, eased breathing and comfort for the patient, and improved gas exchange.

Bursa a small enclosed space found in some joints, lined with synovium and containing a small amount of synovial fluid, useful in decreasing friction; *pl.* bursae.

Bursitis an inflammation of a bursa.

Candidiasis an infection caused by the fungus *Candida;* may be called moniliasis; also called by laymen a yeast infection.

Cardiac cycle the rhythmic contractions of the atria and ventricles that move the blood throughout the body.

Cardiac output the amount of blood leaving the left ventricle with each contraction.

Catabolism breaking-down phase of metabolism.

Centi one hundredth.

Central blocks a form of regional block anesthesia in which a drug is injected into or just outside of the dura mater of the spinal cord; examples include a saddle block, epidural, or caudal block.

Centrally acting the main site of action of a drug is located in the central nervous system.

Chemotherapy drugs that attempt to kill abnormal cancer cells.

Cholesterol a lipid associated with development of atherosclerosis; normal serum levels of total cholesterol <200 mg/dL.

Cholinergic agonists a classification of drugs that mimic the parasympathetic nervous system; also called parasympathomimetics.

Cholinergic blockers a classification of drugs that are antagonistic to the actions of the parasympathetic nervous system; also called parasympathomimetic blockers, parasympatholytics, or anticholinergics.

Chvostek's sign an assessment for low calcium blood levels. To assess, tap the cheek near the ear. If the nose, mouth, and eye twitch on the side tapped, the sign is present.

Cirrhosis scarring and deterioration of the liver, often from the effects of alcohol or drugs.

Clark's rule a formula used to determine a child's dosage based on the child's weight.

Cocaine a potent drug made from the leaves of the cocoa plant of South America. It is an illegal, addicting drug.

Coccus round or spherical microbe; *pl.* cocci.

Conduction system of the heart the collection of nervous system stimuli that cause the heart muscle to contract and relax; controlled by the medulla oblongata of the brain stem.

Contacts persons spending considerable time in a shared airspace with a person who has a contagious disease.

Coryza the common cold.

Crack cocaine a form of cocaine that has been concentrated into rocks, flakes, or chips. It is then smoked in a pipe.

Cubic centimeter a unit of measurement of liquid. It is equal to the milliliter. Abbreviated cc.

Cumulation the increase of drug effects due to an imbalance between drug absorption and drug excretion.

Cycloplegia paralysis of the ciliary muscles of the eye that allow the eye to accommodate.

Decongestants a classification of drugs that decrease edema of the nasal passageways.

Delirium tremens withdrawal from alcohol; effects may include both delirium and tremors as well as gastric upset, insomnia, seizures, hallucinations, confusion, and hypoglycemia.

Demulcence one of the four major drug actions; soothing of a part of the body, normally skin or mucous membranes.

Dendrites beginning processes of a neuron that transmit impulses to the neuron.

Denial a defense mechanism used by people in light of a situation or circumstance that they cannot accept and therefore refuse to admit exists.

Depression one of the four major actions; the lowering or lessening of activity of some body part; includes respiratory, cardiac, nervous system, motor, mental, and excretory depression.

Detoxification the elimination of poisons, as in one of the functions of the liver; the elimination of alcohol from the body of an alcoholic as a portion of treatment of alcoholism.

Digestants a classification of drugs made up of digestive enzymes that are normally produced by the body, but which must be supplemented to some persons with certain diseases or disorders.

Diplo- a pair of.

Disinfectant an agent that can kill microbes. It cannot be used on skin.

Distribution the progression of a drug from the blood stream to its particular site of action.

Diuretics a classification of drugs that can be used to reduce excess fluid retention.

Drug abuse the use of any drug not prescribed by a physician or the improper or excessive use of a drug.

Drug addiction the compulsive, excessive, or continued use of habit-forming drugs that are harmful to self, society, or both.

Drug dependency the physical or psychological need to use drugs to achieve a sense of well-being or avoid withdrawal. The use may be continuous or periodic.

Drug habit often used synonymously with addiction; implies having taken the drug for a lengthy time and difficulty is experienced on attempting to stop.

Drug habituation the frequent use of a drug so that the use becomes a part of the activities of daily (or weekly) living.

Drug paraphernalia items or devices used in the use, abuse, distribution, or processing of drugs or other substances.

Drug tolerance the need to increase the dose of a drug to achieve the original effect.

Dysphagia choking and difficult swallowing.

Dysphasia hoarseness and difficulty speaking or perceiving the meaning of the spoken word.

Effects that which happens in the body as a direct or indirect result of the actions of a drug.

Efficacy ability of a drug to produce a desired chemical change in the body.

Endorphins chemicals released by the brain that may control or moderate pain; also, substances produced in the body that control emotions, especially depression and happiness.

Enkephalins chemicals released by the brain that may control or moderate pain.

Enteral the route of drug administration that refers to the gastrointestinal tract; includes the oral and nasogastric routes.

Enteric coated medications that have been treated so they will not dissolve until they reach a lower portion of the digestive tract, generally the small intestine.

Enterovirus a group of viruses that reproduce in the intestinal tract.

Enzyme inhibitors a group of drugs that decrease the production of uric acid by inhibiting the enzyme that causes uric acid to form.

Episodic alcoholic one who drinks only at specific times and is sober throughout the rest of a period.

Erythema redness of the skin.

Erythropoietin an enzyme produced by the kidneys that may act to stimulate the bone marrow to produce more red blood cells.

Esophageal varices distended blood vessels in the esophagus that are capable of hemorrhage.

Etiology cause.

ETOH abbreviation for ethyl alcohol, the type of alcohol in beverages.

Euthyroid the normal thyroid state.

Excretion the elimination of a drug from the body through respiration, perspiration, defecation, or urination.

Exophthalmos protruding eyeballs.

Expectorants a classification of drugs that reduce the viscosity of the patient's sputum by increasing the production of watery respiratory secretions. The mixing of these secretions with the thick mucus makes it easier for the patient to clear the lungs with coughing.

Extracellular outside the cell.

Extrapyramidal effects adverse effects of medication that include a shuffling gait, pill rolling, agitation, rigidity, and spasms.

Fetal alcohol syndrome effects on the infant of a woman who drank during pregnancy; may include withdrawal symptoms, growth and mental retardation, and external or internal physical abnormalities.

Fetal demise fetal death.

Free drug the portion of a drug that remains circulating in the bloodstream; also called unbound drug.

Fried's rule a formula used to determine dosage for a child whose age is measured in months.

Fungicidal a drug or substance capable of killing a fungus.

Fungistatic a drug or substance that reduces the growth of a fungus, allowing the body's own defenses to work against the fungus.

Fungus a plant with no coloring or chlorophyll.

Gastritis inflammation of the stomach lining.

General anesthesia administration of anesthesia to directly affect the brain centers and depress the nerve cells at their origin.

Germicide an agent that kills microbes and can be used on the skin and possibly on mucous membranes.

Gingival hyperplasia an overgrowth of gum tissue.

Glucocorticoids aid in the metabolism of carbohydrates, proteins, and fats; help maintain a "carbohydrate reserve" in the body for use in times of stress.

Glue sniffing a term that indicates the inhalation of a volatile substance for its mood- or mind-altering abilities.

Glycogenolysis the breakdown of glycogen into glucose.

Glycosuria presence of glucose in the urine.

Gout see gouty arthritis.

Gouty arthritis a form of arthritis characterized by the increase in the amount of circulating serum uric acid, producing symptoms of inflammation of joints and deposits of crystals in tissues called tophi; also called gout.

Gram unit of measurement used to determine the weight of a dry substance.

Gram-negative those microbes that do not retain a purple stain with use of the staining methods developed by Christian Gram. These microbes are then counterstained red for ease of viewing.

Gram-positive those microbes that retain a purple stain with use of the staining methods developed by Christian Gram.

Gynecomastia enlargement and tenderness of breasts in men or women.

Half-life the amount of time it takes for the body to inactivate half of the available drug.

Hallucinations believing one sees, hears, tastes, smells, or feels something that is not there without any physical stimulation to produce the effects.

Hallucinogens a classification of drugs that produce hallucinations.

HDL (cholesterol) high-density lipoproteins; promote mo-

bilization and metabolism of cholesterol and thereby protect against atherosclerosis; normal serum values >35 mg/dL.

Helminths worms that invade the human body; can be intestinal or extraintestinal.

Hematopoiesis the process of making blood.

Hepatotoxic capable of producing toxic effects to the liver.

Herpesvirus a group of viruses that cause some types of skin lesions; means "creeping skin disease."

Hirsutism increase in facial and body hair.

Histamine a substance released by the body any time there is a chemical or physical injury. Actions include redness, warmth, swelling, opened air passages, increased respiratory mucus, decreased gastrointestinal motility, and increased gastrointestinal mucus.

Homeostasis the uniform state of the body's internal environment.

Hormones secretions of endocrine (ductless) glands; carried by blood or lymph to other glands or tissues.

Household system an imprecise method of measurement using teaspoons, tablespoons, drops, fluid ounces, cups, pints, quarts, and gallons to measure liquid; pounds and ounces to measure weight; and inches, feet, and yards to measure length.

Hypercalcemia an increased level of calcium in the blood.

Hyperglycemia serum glucose levels above 80 to 120 mg/100 mL.

Hyperkalemia an increased level of potassium in the body.

Hypermagnesemia an increased level of magnesium in the blood.

Hypernatremia an increased level of sodium in the blood.

Hyperplasia enlargement.

Hypertension also known as high blood pressure, a diagnosis made when the mean arterial blood pressure is above 140/90 mm Hg on two or more measurements on two or more different occasions.

Hyperthyroid increased secretion of thyroid hormones.

Hypervitaminosis those symptoms experienced when the body contains an excess of a particular vitamin.

Hypervolemia an excess of fluid circulating in the body systems or deposited in a body space; a fluid imbalance.

Hypocalcemia a decreased level of calcium in the blood.

Hypoglycemia less than normal levels of blood glucose; serum glucose levels below 70 mg/100 mL.

Hypokalemia a decreased level of potassium in the blood.

Hypomagnesemia a decreased level of magnesium in the blood.

Hyponatremia a decreased level of sodium in the blood.

Hypoprothrombinemia decreased prothrombin levels in the blood.

Hypothalamic releasing factors (neurohormones) hormones from the hypothalamus gland that transmit their messages by way of the nervous and circulatory systems.

Hypothyroid insufficient secretion of thyroid hormones.

Hypovolemia a lack of fluid circulating in the body systems; a fluid imbalance.

Idiosyncratic effects effects that are not expected or desired but are highly individualized; also called paradoxical effects.

Immunity the ability of the body to fight off an antigen with the use of a specific antibody after the initial introduction of the antigen.

Immunization the introduction of a solution into the body for the purposes of producing immunity.

Impotence inability to achieve or maintain an erection of the penis.

Induration a hardened area under the skin with clearly defined edges.

Infestation an invasion of the human body by a parasite.

Inhaler a device that delivers a fine mist of medication from a special canister when it is depressed.

Inscription the second portion of a prescription, the line that contains the name of the drug, the dosage strength, and the drug form.

Intercellular between the cells.

Intracellular within the cell walls.

Iodophor an agent produced by combining iodine and a water-soluble agent.

Irritation one of four major drug actions; the production of symptoms of inflammation at the site of application.

Jaundice a yellow cast to skin and mucous membranes, often due to liver dysfunction.

Joint cavity the space between two bones.

Ketonuria presence of ketones in the urine.

Kidney a bean-shaped organ located in the back below the chest on either side of the spine and behind the peritoneum, the kidney is a major part of the urinary system.

Kilo one thousand.

Laxatives a classification of drugs that are given to produce a bowel movement.

LDL (cholesterol) low-density lipoproteins; associated with an increased risk of atherosclerosis and coronary artery disease; normal serum values <130 mg/dL.

Libido conscious or unconscious sex drive.

Lipid-soluble drug the portion of a drug that binds with fat; also called lipid-bound drug. Lipid-soluble drugs tend to have longer lasting effects.

Liter the unit of measurement used to determine the volume of a liquid.

Liver function profile a group of blood tests that show how well the liver functions.

Loading dose a larger than subsequent dose, given at the start of drug therapy to help the body reach therapeutic blood levels quickly.

Local anesthesia anesthesia administered topically, by infiltration or injection, or by regional blocks to affect only one area of the body without affecting the central nervous system.

Long-acting medications that are specially prepared to dissolve slowly, thereby providing a slower absorption, distribution, and biotransformation of the drug; also called sustained-release, timed-release.

Macronutrient those minerals of which the body needs a greater quantity, including calcium, magnesium, and phosphorus.

Maintenance dose a dose smaller than a loading dose, given throughout the rest of drug therapy to maintain therapeutic blood levels.

Margin of safety the difference between dosages that produce desirable effects and those that produce toxic effects.

Meniscus the top level of liquid as it sits in a container; because of surface tension, the edges of the meniscus are higher than the middle portion.

Metabolic acidosis a state produced by the loss of bicarbonate ions.

Metabolic alkalosis a state produced by an excess of bicarbonate ions.

Meter the unit of measurement used to determine the length of an item.

Metric system the most common system of measurement of drugs; the system is based on a factor of 10 and is widely recognized around the world, which makes communication with other caregivers more accurate.

Micro one millionth.

Micronutrients those minerals of which the body needs a lesser quantity, including iron, fluoride, iodine, and sulfur.

Milli one thousandth.

Mineralocorticoids aid in the regulation of electrolytes by controlling the reabsorption of sodium and the secretion of potassium by the kidney tubules.

Minerals essential elements to our bodies that help maintain the fluid balance in the body, regulate body systems, and regulate metabolism but have no caloric value.

Miosis decrease in pupil size caused by constriction of the circular muscles of the eye.

Mitotic inhibitors antineoplastic medications that interfere with cell division or mitosis through an unknown mode of action.

Moniliasis see candidiasis

Mucolytics a classification of drugs that are delivered by inhalation. The drug combines with viscous sputum in the lungs, adds moisture, and causes the breakup of microdroplets, thereby thinning the mucus and allowing easier expectoration.

Muscle relaxants a classification of drugs that are used to produce the relaxation of muscles necessary for treatment of such disorders as spasm, strains, and sprains.

Mycotic infection an infection of the human body by a fungus.

Mydriasis dilation of the pupil caused by constriction of the radial muscles of the eye.

Myxovirus a group of viruses that are found in or on mucus or that need mucus to survive and reproduce; also called paramyxovirus.

Narcotic antagonists drugs that act to block the activity of a previously administered narcotic by displacing the narcotic at receptor cells.

Naturally acquired active immunity the production of antibodies by the body due to the presence of an antigen introduced by nonmedical means, such as by having the disease.

Naturally acquired passive immunity the passing of antibodies from one person to another through nonmedical means, such as through the placenta or colostrum.

Nebulizer a device, attached by tubing to an air compressor, that delivers medication in the form of a fine mist to be inhaled by the patient.

Negative feedback the process by which the hypothalamus regulates the function of the anterior pituitary gland.

Neoplasm a tumor; a mass of cells that may be benign or malignant.

Nephron the microscopic filtering system of the kidney, found in both the renal cortex and the renal medulla;

made up of the Bowman's capsule, convoluted tubule, loop of Henle, and glomerulus.

Nephrotoxic capable of producing toxic effects to the kidneys.

Neurohormones (hypothalamic releasing factors) hormones from the hypothalamus gland that transmit their messages by way of the nervous and circulatory systems.

Neurotoxic capable of producing toxic effects to the nervous system.

Neurotransmitter a special chemical released into a synapse of a neuron to carry the nerve impulse across this space.

Neutropenia decrease in the number of neutrophils (a type of white blood cell).

Nits the ova of a louse, considered a diagnostic symptom of lice.

Normal flora those microbes that normally live in or on our bodies in a synergistic relationship.

Nursing process a systematic method of identifying and solving the actual and potential problems that people may experience during the course of an illness or disease.

Oligospermia low sperm count.

Ommaya reservoir device used to administer chemotherapeutic drugs into the cerebrospinal fluid, to measure the pressure of cerebrospinal fluid, or to remove a sample of the fluid for laboratory testing.

Oncology the study of cancer.

Ophthalmic preparations medications administered into the eye.

Opiates those substances derived from opium, which comes from the poppy seed. The most common of these include opium, codeine, morphine, and heroin.

Osteoblasts cells responsible for the building of new bone.

Osteoclasts cells responsible for bone breakdown.

Otic preparations medications administered into the ear.

Oxidizing agents solutions that release a free oxygen molecule on coming in contact with protein. The excess oxygen kills microorganisms present.

Palliative offers comfort or relief.

Pancreatitis inflammation of the pancreas.

Pannus the formation of overgrowth tissue in the joint space and surrounding bone in rheumatoid arthritis.

Paradoxical effects effects that are not expected or desired but are highly individualized; also called idiosyncratic effects.

Paramyxovirus a group of viruses that are found in or on mucus or that need mucus to survive and reproduce; also called myxovirus.

Parasite a creature that lives off another living thing, deriving its nourishment from the host, often from the blood of the host.

Parasympatholytics a classification of drugs that are antagonistic to the actions of the parasympathetic nervous system; also called cholinergic blockers, anticholinergics, or parasympathomimetic blockers.

Parasympathomimetic blockers a classification of drugs that are antagonistic to the actions of the parasympathetic nervous system; also called cholinergic blockers, anticholinergics, or parasympatholytics.

Parasympathomimetics a classification of drugs that mimic the actions of the parasympathetic nervous system; also called adrenergic blockers, sympatholytics, or sympathomimetic blockers.

Parenteral the route of drug administration that refers to intravenous, subcutaneous, intradermal, and intramuscular injections.

Parkinsonian crisis a sudden and severe deterioration of the symptoms of parkinsonism.

Parkinsonism a disorder caused by a lack of dopamine availability at the synapses, characterized by loss of control of movements and characteristic tremors; also called Parkinson's syndrome.

Parkinson's syndrome see parkinsonism.

Partial agonist a drug that attaches weakly to a receptor site, eliciting a weak response and preventing other reactions from occurring.

Pediculicides a group of drugs used to treat an infestation by lice.

Pediculosis an infestation of the human body by one of several types of lice; includes pediculosis capitis (head), pediculosis corporis (body), and pediculosis pubis (pubic area).

-penia decrease in the number of a particular type of cell; as in leukopenia, neutropenia, thrombocytopenia.

Percentage a certain number of parts of the whole item, where the whole item is represented by the number 100.

Percutaneous the route of drug administration that includes topical applications to the skin or mucous membranes; sublingual and buccal preparations; and instillations into the eyes, ears, nose, throat, lungs, bladder, vagina, and rectum.

Percutaneous route the application of medication to the skin or mucous membranes.

Peripheral block a form of regional block anesthesia in which a drug is injected into a nerve or group of nerves that supply feeling to the area to be incised; examples may include sciatic, femoral, ulnar, intercostal, trigeminal, and pudendal blocks.

Peripherally acting the main site of action of a drug is located outside the central nervous system.

Peritonitis inflammation of the abdominal cavity, can be fatal.

Pharmacodynamics the study of the actions and effects of drugs on the body.

Pharmacokinetics the use of a drug in the body by four steps absorption, distribution, biotransformation, and excretion.

Pharmacology a science that deals with the study of chemicals, their preparations, and their actions and effects on living tissues.

Phosphate binders a classification of drugs that work to remove phosphates by preventing their absorption from food.

Picornavirus a group of small viruses that have a strand of RNA as their core.

Placental barrier a chemical barrier that prevents many drugs from crossing over to the fetus and affecting the fetus.

Polydipsia increased thirst.

Polyhydramnios excessive amniotic fluid.

Polyphagia increased hunger.

Polyuria increased urine output.

Potency or strength of a drug a standard for drugs; determined by the concentration of the active ingredient in the preparation.

Potentiation when the effects of one drug are added to the effects of another drug, the combined effect is greater than would be expected by simple addition; also called synergism.

Prescription a form of medication order given in the medical office setting or on discharge from an institution; must contain four parts (1) superscription, (2) inscription, (3) subscription, and (4) signature.

Priapism prolonged, painful penile erections.

Primary hypertension also known as essential hypertension; most common type; familial tendency; actual cause is unknown.

Productive cough a cough that is raising mucus from the lungs.

Prohibition the period between 1919 and 1933 when alcohol was illegal as a result of the Volstead Act.

Protein-bound drug a portion of a drug that binds with protein, most commonly albumin, in the bloodstream. Protein-bound drugs are released more quickly than lipid-bound drugs are.

Protozoacides a group of drugs that work against protozoa, a class of mostly unicellular animals; also called antiprotozoals.

Protozoan a class of mostly unicellular animals.

Protrusion reflex a natural response of infants when something is placed on the tongue, causing the tongue to be "stuck out."

Pruritus itching of the skin.

Psychotherapeutic drugs a classification of drugs that are used to treat disorders of the mind; also called psychoactive drugs.

Psychotropic drugs those that affect the functioning of the mind; include sedatives, hypnotics, analgesics, anesthetics, and others.

Pulse deficit the difference between the apical pulse and the radial pulse when they are assessed simultaneously. This is an abnormal finding.

Purity a standard for drugs; a pure drug contains only one specific chemical.

Radiation therapy a mode of treatment that attempts to shrink or destroy abnormal cells.
External sources are the x-ray machines, cobalt machines, and linear accelerators.
Internal sources are isotopes or elements that are injected or ingested into the body or implanted into a body cavity; examples are gold Au 198, sodium iodide I 131 or sodium iodide I 125, sodium phosphate P 32, and radium and cesium implants.

Rationalization a defense mechanism used by people in light of a situation or circumstance that they cannot accept and for which they therefore fabricate possible logical or illogical reasons.

Rebound phenomenon after overuse of a medication, the symptoms for which the medication was prescribed return and worsen.

Receptor a chemical to which a free drug is attached.

Receptor site a place on a chemical to which a free drug is attracted and can become attached.

Refraction bending of light rays.

Regional block a form of local anesthesia injection that affects only a particular area of the body; includes peripheral blocks and central blocks.

Renal cortex the outer rim of the kidney.

Renal hilum the inner border of the kidney where the renal artery, vein, and ureter are connected.

Renal medulla the inner tissue of the kidney.

Renal pelvis a collecting space inside the kidney.

Renin an enzyme produced by the kidneys that may act to raise the blood pressure.

Rescue procedure used with administration of some chemotherapeutic drugs; involves the administration at a specific time of an antidote specific for the drug in use. The procedure is vital to counteract the potentially lethal effects of some drugs.

Reticular activating system (RAS) the part of the brain in the midbrain that functions to keep a person conscious.

Rheumatoid arthritis a form of arthritis characterized by joint inflammation, the formation of pannus, synovitis, scar tissue, and eventual ankylosis.

Rhinovirus a group of viruses that cause the common cold.

SA (sinoatrial) term used in discussion of the conduction system of the heart.

Salicylism a group of symptoms that characterize an overdose of a salicylate. Symptoms include tinnitus, tachycardia, hyperventilation, headache, fever, dehydration, sweating, drowsiness, vertigo, confusion, electrolyte imbalances, and altered blood pH.

Secondary hypertension a symptom of an underlying disease, such as heart disease or a renal tumor.

Serum a solution produced from the blood of another human or an animal that contains antibodies for the purposes of producing artificially acquired passive immunity.

Signature the fourth line of a prescription; beginning with the abbreviation Sig., a line containing directions to the patient on the proper use of the medication.

Speedballing a dangerous mixture of cocaine and heroin that is self-administered intravenously.

Spinhaler a capsule that is broken apart so that the powder may be inhaled with a special inhaler.

Spirilla spiral or curved microbes.

Splenomegaly enlargement of the spleen.

Standing orders orders prewritten and signed by the physician to be used by the nurse when needed. These generally apply to all patients universally.

Staphylo- a cluster of.

Stat orders orders from a physician for a medication to be given immediately; usually verbal and usually an emergency.

Stimulation one of the four major drug actions; the increasing of the function or activity of a part of the body; includes respiratory, cardiac, nervous, motor, mental, and excretory stimulation.

Strepto- a chain of.

Subcortical areas of the brain located below the cortex.

Subscription the third part of a prescription, beginning with either the symbol # or N, which stands for number. Following is the number of tablets, milliliters, or other appropriate directions to the pharmacist explaining the amount to be dispensed.

Summation when the effects of one drug are added to the effects of another drug, you can estimate the combined effect by simply adding them; also called addition.

Superinfections the overgrowth of normal flora, including bacteria and fungi, which then produces symptoms including glossitis, stomatitis, diarrhea, and rectal itching. These most often result from the use of antibiotics that killed other normal flora, disturbing the natural balance.

Superscription the first part of a prescription; ℞, which means "take thou."

Suppressants a group of drugs given to decrease the function of a body part or system; most often refers to those drugs given to depress the cough center of the medulla.

Sustained-release medications prepared in a special way to dissolve slowly, thereby providing slower absorption, distribution, and biotransformation of the drug; also called long-acting, timed-release.

Sympatholytics a classification of drugs that prohibit the actions of the sympathetic nervous system; also called adrenergic blockers or sympathomimetic blockers.

Sympathomimetic blockers a classification of drugs that prohibit the actions of the sympathetic nervous system; also called adrenergic blockers or sympatholytics.

Sympathomimetics a classification of drugs that mimic the sympathetic nervous system; also called adrenergic agonists.

Synapse the small space between the axon of one neuron and the dendrites of another.

Synergism 1. with regard to medications when the effects of one drug are added to the effects of another drug, the combined effect is greater than would be expected by simple addition; also called potentiation. 2. with regard to microbes those microbes that normally live in or on our bodies in a mutually beneficial relationship; also called normal flora.

Synovial fluid fluid in the joint cavity that promotes the smooth movement of the joint by decreased friction.

Synovial membrane a moist tissue in the joint cavity that produces fluid and promotes the smooth movement of the joint by decreasing friction; also called synovium.

Synovitis an inflammatory process of the synovium and the synovial fluid.

Synovium see synovial membrane.

Systemic throughout the whole body.

Tardive dyskinesia the most serious of the neurological syndromes that occur as adverse effects of some medications. Symptoms include involuntary buccofaciomandibular or buccolingual movements, such as sucking, smacking lips, and lateral movements of the jaw and tongue.

Teratogenic may cause birth defects.

Tetany a collection of symptoms resulting from irritability of the neuromuscular system; usually begins with numbness and tingling of the lips and then the extremities. Cardiac arrhythmias, tremors, spasms, and convulsions will follow if tetany is untreated.

Therapeutic expected to relieve, improve, or cure.

THIQ substance produced in the brains of alcoholics when acetaldehyde (a by-product of alcohol metabolism) reacts with dopamine. It is addictive.

Timed-release medications specially prepared to dissolve slowly, thereby providing slower absorption, distribution, and biotransformation of the drug; also called long-acting, sustained-release.

Tinea barbae a fungal infection of the bearded portion of the neck and face; also called barber's itch.

Tinea capitis a fungal infection of the scalp, most often ringworm.

Tinea corporis a fungal infection of the body, most often ringworm.

Tinea cruris a fungal infection of the genitalia; also called jock itch.

Tinea pedis a fungal infection of the feet; also called athlete's foot.

Tinea versicolor a fungal infection that causes a yellowing of the skin.

Tolerance the lessening of the effects of a drug due to the continual presence of the drug.

Tophi deposits of crystals in the skin and other tissues, found in gouty arthritis; *sing.* tophus.

Toxoid a solution that contains a weakened toxin, or poison, from a specific antigen for the purposes of producing artificially acquired active immunity.

Toxin a poison.

Transfusion reaction a reaction to blood products.

Triglycerides make up the core structure of lipoproteins (along with cholesterol); serum levels >500 mg/dL are associated with pancreatitis and possibly atherosclerosis.

Tuberculosis a primarily pulmonary disease caused by the tubercle bacillus, *Mycobacterium tuberculosis.* Symptoms include cough (possibly with production), fever, night sweats, fatigue or malaise, weight loss, and later production of bloody sputum.

Unit-dose system a method of providing medications for disbursement in individually packaged doses.

Ureter the tube that leads from the kidney to the bladder.

Urethra the tube that leads from the bladder to the outside of the body.

Uricosuric agents a group of drugs that cause the body to excrete more uric acid.

Vaccine a solution containing antigens that have been attenuated (weakened) for the purpose of producing artificially acquired active immunity.

Verbal order oral ordering of a medication; examples include emergency or stat drugs and telephone orders. This type of order must be written and signed by the physician at a later time.

Virus a parasite so small it is seen only with an electron microscope. A virus is made of a single strand of DNA or RNA covered by a protein capsule.

Virustatic a term used to denote a substance that stops the growth of viruses.

Vital signs the temperature, pulse, respirations, and blood pressure of a person.

Vitamin organic compound normally found in the daily diet that helps regulate the metabolism and promote the efficient use of other nutrients.

Withdrawal the effect experienced from stopping a drug to which the person was either physiologically or psychologically addicted.

Written order the most common way for medications to be ordered within an institution; the physician writes the name of the drug to be given, the dosage, the route, and the frequency. The order must be signed by the physician.

Young's rule a formula used to determine the dosage for a child whose age is measured in years.

Anderson, K. N., Anderson, L. E., & Glanze, W. D. (Eds.) (1994). *Mosby's medical, nursing, & allied health dictionary* (4th ed.). St. Louis: Mosby–Year Book.

Belcaster, A. (February 1994). Caring for the alcohol abuser. *Nursing94*, 56–59.

Core curriculum on tuberculosis: What the clinician should know (3rd ed.) (1994). Atlanta, Georgia: U.S. Department of Health and Human Services Public Health Services, Centers for Disease Control and Prevention, National Center for Prevention Services, Division of Tuberculosis Elimination.

Deglin, J. H., Vallerand, A, H., & Russin, M. H. (1993). *Davis's drug guide for nurses* (3rd ed.). Philadelphia: F. A. Davis.

Guralnik, D. B. (Ed.) (1972). *Webster's new world dictionary* (2nd College ed.). New York: World Publishing.

Hodgson, B. B., Kizior, R. J., & Kingdon, R. T. (1995). *Nurse's drug handbook 1995.* Philadelphia: W. B. Saunders.

Johnson, G. E., Hannah, K. J., & Zerr, S. R. (1992). *Pharmacology and the nursing process* (3rd ed.). Philadelphia: W. B. Saunders.

Lehne, R. A. (1994). *Pharmacology for nursing care* (2nd ed.). Philadelphia: W. B. Saunders.

Martin, F. L. (August 1992). When the liver breaks down. *RN,* 52–57.

Nursing95 drug handbook. (1995). Springhouse, PA: Springhouse.

NursingNow: Pain. (1985). Springhouse, PA: Nursing85 Books.

Physician's desk reference 1995 (49th ed.) (1995). Oradell, NJ: Medical Economics.

Physician's desk reference for ophthalmology 1995 (23rd ed.) (1995). Oradell, NJ: Medical Economics.

Smith, C. M., & Reynard, A. M. (1992). *Textbook of pharmacology.* Philadelphia: W. B. Saunders.

Spencer, R. T., Nichols, L. W., Lipkin, G. B., Sabo, H. M., & West, F. M. (1993). *Clinical pharmacology and nursing management* (4th ed.). Philadelphia: J. B. Lippincott.

Tasota, F. J., & Wesmiller, S. W. (May 1994). Assessing ABGs: Maintaining the delicate balance. *Nursing94,* 34–44.

Thibodeau, G. A., & Patton, K. T. (1992). *The human body in health and disease.* St Louis: Mosby–Year Book.

Thomas, C. L. (Ed.) (1993). *Taber's cyclopedic medical dictionary* (17th ed.). Philadelphia: F. A. Davis.

Zenk, K. (March 1993). Drug hot line: Beware of overdose (air bubble). *Nursing93,* 28–31.

INDEX

Note: Page numbers in *italics* indicate figures; those followed by t indicate tables.